PROFESSOR PETER J. BARNES M.A. D.M. FRCP.

AF684400

PULMONARY COMPLICATIONS OF SYSTEMIC DISEASE

LUNG BIOLOGY IN HEALTH AND DISEASE

Executive Editor

Claude Lenfant
Director, National Heart, Lung, and Blood Institute
National Institutes of Health
Bethesda, Maryland

1. Immunologic and Infectious Reactions in the Lung, *edited by Charles H. Kirkpatrick and Herbert Y. Reynolds*
2. The Biochemical Basis of Pulmonary Function, *edited by Ronald G. Crystal*
3. Bioengineering Aspects of the Lung, *edited by John B. West*
4. Metabolic Functions of the Lung, *edited by Y. S. Bakhle and John R. Vane*
5. Respiratory Defense Mechanisms (in two parts), *edited by Joseph D. Brain, Donald F. Proctor, and Lynne M. Reid*
6. Development of the Lung, *edited by W. Alan Hodson*
7. Lung Water and Solute Exchange, *edited by Norman C. Staub*
8. Extrapulmonary Manifestations of Respiratory Disease, *edited by Eugene Debs Robin*
9. Chronic Obstructive Pulmonary Disease, *edited by Thomas L. Petty*
10. Pathogenesis and Therapy of Lung Cancer, *edited by Curtis C. Harris*
11. Genetic Determinants of Pulmonary Disease, *edited by Stephen D. Litwin*
12. The Lung in the Transition Between Health and Disease, *edited by Peter T. Macklem and Solbert Permutt*
13. Evolution of Respiratory Processes: A Comparative Approach, *edited by Stephen C. Wood and Claude Lenfant*
14. Pulmonary Vascular Diseases, *edited by Kenneth M. Moser*
15. Physiology and Pharmacology of the Airways, *edited by Jay A. Nadel*
16. Diagnostic Techniques in Pulmonary Disease (in two parts), *edited by Marvin A. Sackner*
17. Regulation of Breathing (in two parts), *edited by Thomas F. Hornbein*
18. Occupational Lung Diseases: Research Approaches and Methods, *edited by Hans Weill and Margaret Turner-Warwick*
19. Immunopharmacology of the Lung, *edited by Harold H. Newball*
20. Sarcoidosis and Other Granulomatous Diseases of the Lung, *edited by Barry L. Fanburg*
21. Sleep and Breathing, *edited by Nicholas A. Saunders and Colin E. Sullivan*

22. *Pneumocystis carinii* Pneumonia: Pathogenesis, Diagnosis, and Treatment, *edited by Lowell S. Young*
23. Pulmonary Nuclear Medicine: Techniques in Diagnosis of Lung Disease, *edited by Harold L. Atkins*
24. Acute Respiratory Failure, *edited by Warren M. Zapol and Konrad J. Falke*
25. Gas Mixing and Distribution in the Lung, *edited by Ludwig A. Engel and Manuel Paiva*
26. High-Frequency Ventilation in Intensive Care and During Surgery, *edited by Graziano Carlon and William S. Howland*
27. Pulmonary Development: Transition from Intrauterine to Extrauterine Life, *edited by George H. Nelson*
28. Chronic Obstructive Pulmonary Disease: Second Edition, Revised and Expanded, *edited by Thomas L. Petty*
29. The Thorax (in two parts), *edited by Charis Roussos and Peter T. Macklem*
30. The Pleura in Health and Disease, *edited by Jacques Chrétien, Jean Bignon, and Albert Hirsch*
31. Drug Therapy for Asthma: Research and Clinical Practice, *edited by John W. Jenne and Shirley Murphy*
32. Pulmonary Endothelium in Health and Disease, *edited by Una S. Ryan*
33. The Airways: Neural Control in Health and Disease, *edited by Michael A. Kaliner and Peter J. Barnes*
34. Pathophysiology and Treatment of Inhalation Injuries, *edited by Jacob Loke*
35. Respiratory Function of the Upper Airway, *edited by Oommen P. Mathew and Giuseppe Sant'Ambrogio*
36. Chronic Obstructive Pulmonary Disease: A Behavioral Perspective, *edited by A. John McSweeny and Igor Grant*
37. Biology of Lung Cancer: Diagnosis and Treatment, *edited by Steven T. Rosen, James L. Mulshine, Frank Cuttitta, and Paul G. Abrams*
38. Pulmonary Vascular Physiology and Pathophysiology, *edited by E. Kenneth Weir and John T. Reeves*
39. Comparative Pulmonary Physiology: Current Concepts, *edited by Stephen C. Wood*
40. Respiratory Physiology: An Analytical Approach, *edited by H. K. Chang and Manuel Paiva*
41. Lung Cell Biology, *edited by Donald Massaro*
42. Heart–Lung Interactions in Health and Disease, *edited by Steven M. Scharf and Sharon S. Cassidy*
43. Clinical Epidemiology of Chronic Obstructive Pulmonary Disease, *edited by Michael J. Hensley and Nicholas A. Saunders*
44. Surgical Pathology of Lung Neoplasms, *edited by Alberto M. Marchevsky*
45. The Lung in Rheumatic Diseases, *edited by Grant W. Cannon and Guy A. Zimmerman*

46. Diagnostic Imaging of the Lung, *edited by Charles E. Putman*
47. Models of Lung Disease: Microscopy and Structural Methods, *edited by Joan Gil*
48. Electron Microscopy of the Lung, *edited by Dean E. Schraufnagel*
49. Asthma: Its Pathology and Treatment, *edited by Michael A. Kaliner, Peter J. Barnes, and Carl G. A. Persson*
50. Acute Respiratory Failure: Second Edition, *edited by Warren M. Zapol and Francois Lemaire*
51. Lung Disease in the Tropics, *edited by Om P. Sharma*
52. Exercise: Pulmonary Physiology and Pathophysiology, *edited by Brian J. Whipp and Karlman Wasserman*
53. Developmental Neurobiology of Breathing, *edited by Gabriel G. Haddad and Jay P. Farber*
54. Mediators of Pulmonary Inflammation, *edited by Michael A. Bray and Wayne H. Anderson*
55. The Airway Epithelium, *edited by Stephen G. Farmer and Douglas Hay*
56. Physiological Adaptations in Vertebrates: Respiration, Circulation, and Metabolism, *edited by Stephen C. Wood, Roy E. Weber, Alan R. Hargens, and Ronald W. Millard*
57. The Bronchial Circulation, *edited by John Butler*
58. Lung Cancer Differentiation: Implications for Diagnosis and Treatment, *edited by Samuel D. Bernal and Paul J. Hesketh*
59. Pulmonary Complications of Systemic Disease, *edited by John F. Murray*
60. Lung Vascular Injury: Molecular and Cellular Response, *edited by Arnold Johnson and Thomas J. Ferro*

ADDITIONAL VOLUMES IN PREPARATION

Cytokines of the Lung, *edited by Jason Kelley*

The Mast Cell in Health and Disease, *edited by Michael A. Kaliner and Dean Metcalfe*

Pulmonary Disease in the Elderly Patient, *edited by Donald A. Mahler*

PULMONARY COMPLICATIONS OF SYSTEMIC DISEASE

Edited by

John F. Murray

University of California, San Francisco
San Francisco, California

Marcel Dekker, Inc. New York • Basel • Hong Kong

Library of Congress Cataloging-in-Publication Data

Pulmonary complications of systemic disease / edited by John F. Murray.
p. cm. -- (Lung biology in health and disease ; v. 59)
Includes bibliographical reference and indexes.
ISBN 0-8247-8707-2 (alk. paper)
1. Pulmonary manifestation of general diseases. I. Murray, John F. (John Frederic). II. Series.
[DNLM: 1. Lung Diseases--etiology. W1 LU62 v. 59 / WF 600 P98248]
RC732.P84 1992
616.2'4--dc20
DNLM/DLC
for Library of Congress 92-18424
CIP

This book is printed on acid-free paper.

Copyright © 1992 by Marcel Dekker, Inc. All Rights Reserved.

Neither this book nor any part may be reproduced or transmitted in any form or by any means, electronic or mechanical, including photocopying, microfilming, and recording, or by any information storage and retrieval system, without permission in writing from the publisher.

Marcel Dekker, Inc.
270 Madison Avenue, New York, New York 10016

Current printing (last digit):
10 9 8 7 6 5 4 3 2 1

PRINTED IN THE UNITED STATES OF AMERICA

INTRODUCTION

Some time ago, while browsing at an antique show, I came upon a book titled *The Conclusions of Modern Sciences: Plainly Told* by Walter Grieson ("The enquiring layman"). Although the publication date had been lost in a recent rebinding, I would place it around the turn of the century.

In the chapter "The New Knowledge," which discusses "the importance of the atom, the electron, and radiation," there is a very interesting dialogue.

> Sir James Jeans: "It may be doubted whether we shall ever properly understand the realities ultimately involved; they may well be so fundamental as to be beyond the grasp of the human mind."
>
> Professor Millikan: "What does it all mean? Simply that there is an interrelatedness, a unity, a oneness about the whole of nature, and yet still an amazing mystery."
>
> [and later] Sir Oliver Lodge: "If we understand the structure of the ether, and also the structure of the electron, we should, I am sure, understand the quantum."

The series of monographs Lung Biology in Health and Disease was conceived to describe the many facets that make the lung such a complex organ, to understand its normal functions and their alterations in disease. As the series evolved, it quickly became apparent that such an endeavor could not be complete if we ignored the ''interrelatedness,'' the ''unity,'' the essential ''oneness'' of the body. Sir Oliver Lodge was indeed very correct: we must understand both the structure of the ether and the structure of the electron to understand the quantum. This is true in physics, and it is true in biology and medicine.

Thus, while this series has included many monographs focused exclusively on particular aspects of the lung, it also has taken a broader view of the lung in the context of the whole body. In 1978, the volume *Extrapulmonary Manifestations of Respiratory Disease* was published. As its editor, Eugene D. Robin, commented in his preface, that volume was ''an attempt to bridge the gap between lung function disorders and the cellular and organ alterations produced by these disorders.'' Now we come to the flip side of the question, that is, what are ''the pulmonary complications of systemic disease?'' This ''interrelatedness,'' albeit very difficult to understand—and sometimes even to recognize, as the editor notes—must be investigated if we are to be comprehensive. Because of its complexity, the lung has many effects on the rest of the body, and, conversely, nearly all organs and body functions have an impact on the lung.

This new volume, edited by John F. Murray, describes and explains the ''pulmonary manifestations of extrapulmonary disorders.'' It clearly demonstrates an aspect of ''oneness about the whole of nature,'' especially in pathological states. Undoubtedly, the series of monographs Lung Biology in Health and Disease would be incomplete without this contribution. Dr. Murray and the experts he selected to write this volume are to be commended for their insight, which helps the reader understand the realities of nature. Personally, I gratefully acknowledge this most important contribution to the series of monographs.

Claude Lenfant, M.D.
Bethesda, Maryland

PREFACE

It is impossible to generalize about the origins of the pulmonary complications of the many different systemic disorders covered in this book. The most straightforward association between disease of the lungs and the rest of the body is when the lungs are involved as one component of a multisystem disease; this occurs commonly in the rheumatological diseases, the diffuse vasculitides, some hematological diseases, and the endocrine and metabolic diseases. In other disorders, notably the primary, disease-induced, and drug-related immunodeficiency states, the lungs as well as other organs are susceptible to the infectious, neoplastic, and infiltrative complications of immune suppression; in these disorders, however, the lungs appear particularly vulnerable because of their intimate contact with inhaled and aspirated microorganisms, and probably also because they serve as a filter for the entire venous drainage and are exposed through their blood supply to noxious products produced or absorbed anywhere in the systemic circulation.

But specific pulmonary complications may also occur as part of disorders localized to a single organ system, such as the central nervous system or skeletal muscles; the connection between the lungs and neuromuscular diseases is obvious, because the configuration of the skeleton affects the size of the thorax, and the adequacy of breathing depends on the integrity of the muscles of respiration.

Another systemic cause of pulmonary disease occurs because of the intimate hemodynamic relationships between the heart and the lungs. The lungs, normally, receive the entire output of the right heart and, after oxygenating the blood, deliver it to the left heart. Thus, an acute elevation of pressure in the left heart "backs up" into the lungs and increases pressure for fluid filtration that, in turn, leads to pulmonary edema and pleural effusions. A chronic elevation of pressure in the pulmonary circulation, regardless of its cause, sets in motion an accelerating cycle of vascular reactions that culminates in irreversible pulmonary hypertension. In some instances, the lungs may show the effect of diseases in contiguous abdominal organs because of proximity (e.g., a parainflammatory pleural effusion adjacent to a subdiaphragmatic or perinephric abscess), or because of anatomical connections between the abdominal and pleural spaces (e.g., hepatic hydrothorax or Meigs's syndrome). Finally, there are many pulmonary manifestations of systemic diseases—such as the vascular abnormalities in patients with cirrhosis of the liver that lead either to right-to-left shunting of blood or to pulmonary hypertension—for which the pathogenesis is completely unknown.

Not all the pulmonary complications of systemic diseases are covered in this book. Two important conditions that were left out are pulmonary embolism, in which the lungs bear the brunt of extrapulmonary intravascular thrombosis or entry into the venous system of fat or other debris, and the mysterious disorder known as the adult respiratory distress syndrome, in which the lungs become gravely injured as part of a complex cascade of systemic responses that are often initiated by extrapulmonary events, usually sepsis. These two disorders are dealt with in detail in other volumes of the Lung Biology in Health and Disease series. Drug-induced lung disease, an important cause of a host of different pulmonary reactions, is mentioned only in the context of how various drugs may worsen or contribute to the pulmonary complications of the systemic diseases under consideration.

The pulmonary manifestations of extrapulmonary disorders are common and often misdiagnosed. The authors of the chapters in this volume hope that their efforts lead to early recognition and prompt treatment of this extremely variable, but important, group of respiratory complications.

John F. Murray

CONTRIBUTORS

Lee R. Berkowitz, M.D. Associate Professor of Medicine, Division of Hematology, University of North Carolina at Chapel Hill, Chapel Hill, North Carolina

V. Courtney Broaddus, M.D. Assistant Professor of Medicine, and Associate Staff, Cardiovascular Research Institute, University of California, San Francisco, and Chest Service, San Francisco General Hospital, San Francisco, California

Philip A. Bromberg, M.D. Director, Center for Environmental Medicine and Lung Biology, and Bonner Professor of Medicine, University of North Carolina at Chapel Hill, Chapel Hill, North Carolina

Steven R. Duncan, M.D. Associate Medical Director of Pulmonary Transplantation and Assistant Professor of Medicine, Pulmonary and Critical Care Medicine, University of Pittsburgh, Pittsburgh, Pennsylvania

Neil A. Ettinger, M.D. Assistant Professor of Medicine, Respiratory and Critical Care Division, Washington University School of Medicine, St. Louis, Missouri

Larry J. Findley, M.D. Associate Professor of Medicine, Division of Pulmonary and Critical Care Medicine, Department of Medicine, University of Virginia Health Sciences Center, Charlottesville, Virginia

Michael R. Flick, M.D., J.D. Associate Clinical Professor of Medicine, School of Medicine, University of California, San Francisco, and Chest Service, San Francisco General Hospital, San Francisco, California

Michael A. Matthay, M.D. Associate Professor of Medicine and Anesthesia, and Senior Staff, Cardiovascular Research Institute, University of California, San Francisco, San Francisco, California

John F. Murray, M.D., D.Sc. (hon.) Professor of Medicine and Senior Staff, Cardiovascular Research Institute, University of California, San Francisco, San Francisco, California

Jean-Francois Pittet, M.D. Research Fellow, Cardiovascular Research Institute, University of California, San Francisco, San Francisco, California

Udaya B. S. Prakash, M.D., F.R.C.P.(C.), F.A.C.P., F.C.C.P. Consultant in Thoracic Diseases and Internal Medicine and Director of Bronchoscopy, Mayo Clinic and Mayo Medical Center, and Professor of Medicine, Mayo Medical School, Rochester, Minnesota

Thomas A. Raffin, M.D. Chief, Division of Pulmonary and Critical Care Medicine, and Co-Director, Stanford University Center for Biomedical Ethics, Stanford University Medical Center, Stanford, California

Dudley F. Rochester, M.D. E. Cato Drash Professor of Medicine, and Head, Division of Pulmonary and Critical Care Medicine, Department of Medicine, University of Virginia Health Sciences Center, Charlottesville, Virginia

Robert M. Senior, M.D. Dorothy R. and Hubert C. Moog Professor of Pulmonary Diseases in Medicine, Washington University School of Medicine, and Director, Respiratory and Critical Care Division, Jewish Hospital at Washington University Medical Center, St. Louis, Missouri

Jeanine P. Wiener-Kronish, M.D. Associate Professor of Anesthesia and Medicine, and Associate Staff, Cardiovascular Research Institute, University of California, San Francisco, San Francisco, California

CONTENTS

1

Pulmonary Complications of Human Immunodeficiency Virus Infection

JOHN F. MURRAY

University of California, San Francisco
San Francisco, California

I. Introduction

The first dramatic cases of what was subsequently called the acquired immunodeficiency syndrome (AIDS) were reported by the Centers for Disease Control (CDC) in mid-1981 (Gottlieb et al., 1981a); more details about these and a second cluster of cases soon followed (Gottlieb et al., 1981b; Masur et al., 1981). A few years later, scientists at the Pasteur Institute (Barré-Sinoussi et al., 1983) and National Institutes of Health (Popovic et al., 1984) discovered the causative virus, the human immunodeficiency virus (HIV), and developed the first in a series of accurate tests to detect its presence in its human host (Phair and Wolinsky, 1989). Now, one decade later, much has been learned about the natural history of evolving HIV disease, including the recognition that the hallmark of progression is steadily worsening immune suppression, and that many HIV-related complications occur at reasonably predictable stages in this continuum. For diagnostic and therapeutic reasons, especially those concerning prevention and early treatment, it is much more important to consider the entire spectrum of HIV disease rather than focus, as has been true in the past, on only its last and invariably fatal stage—AIDS (Girard et al., 1991).

The lungs are one of the principal target organs of the myriad infectious and noninfectious complications of progressive HIV disease (Table 1). Some of these disorders are AIDS-defining and some are not. In this chapter, after a brief review of the general diagnostic approach to new-onset lung disease in a patient with known or suspected HIV infection, the major HIV-associated pulmonary complications will be discussed with emphasis on their clinical features and treatment. Additional details are available in several recent reviews (Leoung and Mills, 1989; White and Matthay, 1989; Volberding and Jacobson, 1990; Murray and Mills, 1990).

II. Diagnostic Approach

There is now general agreement with the concept that (1) because of the many kinds of pulmonary disorders that may occur during the course of HIV infection, and (2) because of the serious toxicity inherent in most treatment regimens, a specific diagnosis should be made each time a new complication occurs. Empirical treatment is seldom justified, except while awaiting the results of diagnostic studies. The diagnostic algorithms that have been recommended have been heavily influenced by the importance of *Pneumocystis carinii* pneumonia, which is by far the most common HIV-related pulmonary infection in North America and Europe. However, as will be pointed out, the widespread use of chemoprophylaxis against *P. carinii* pneumonia seems to be affecting the natural history of this disease and to be influencing the relative incidence of the other pulmonary complications of HIV infection; this change may, in turn, warrant new diagnostic approaches, which are also necessary in sub-Saharan Africa and other regions where different pathogens predominate (Fleming, 1990).

A. History and Physical Examination

Most patients with subacute or chronic HIV-linked pulmonary complications complain of cough, often nonproductive, and breathlessness, which are frequently associated with weight loss and fever. Patients with pyogenic bacterial pneumonias present with the typical acute onset of fever, shortness of breath, pleuritic chest pain, and productive cough. The physical examination may be completely normal in patients with early or mild HIV-related lung disease, but may also provide important information about the presence of HIV infection or one of its complications (Hollander, 1988). Oral candidiasis or hairy leukoplakia provides presumptive evidence of HIV infection and thrush often heralds imminent progression to AIDS. Persistent generalized lymphadenopathy in regions of the body other than the thorax may or may not occur and, if it does, is one of the defined stages of evolving HIV disease; lymphadenopathy with hepatosplenomegaly is relatively common and may indicate Kaposi's sarcoma, non-Hodgkin's lymphoma, or disseminated mycobacterial or fungal infection.

Table 1 Pulmonary Complications of HIV Infection

- Infections
  - Viruses
    - Cytomegalovirus
    - Herpes simplex virus
    - Varicella-zoster virus
    - Epstein-Barr virus?
    - Human immunodeficiency virus?
  - Bacteria
    - Pyogenic organisms (esp. *Streptococcus pneumoniae, Hemophilus influenzae*)
    - *Mycobacterium tuberculosis*
    - *Mycobacterium avium*-complex
    - Other nontuberculous mycobacteria
  - Fungi
    - *Histoplasma capsulatum*
    - *Coccidiodes immitis*
    - *Cryptococcus neoformans*
    - *Candida* species
    - *Aspergillus* species
  - Parasites
    - *Pneumocystis carinii*
    - *Toxoplasma gondii*
    - *Cryptosporidia*
    - *Strongyloides stercoralis*
- Malignancies
  - Kaposi's sarcoma
  - Non-Hodgkin's lymphoma
- Interstitial pneumonias
  - Lymphocytic interstitial pneumonitis
  - Nonspecific interstitial pneumonitis
  - Drug-induced reactions
- Other
  - Adult respiratory distress syndrome
  - Secondary alveolar proteinosis
  - Sarcoidosis

Source: Reprinted with permission from Murray and Mills (1990).

B. Laboratory Tests

The diagnosis of infection with HIV itself is usually made by detecting specific antibodies to the virus using a screening ELISA assay and a confirmatory test such as the Western blot. Although culture of plasma and peripheral blood monocytes for HIV is laborious and expensive, much useful information has been learned about viral titers in various stages of HIV disease (Clark et al., 1991), the response to antiviral drugs (Ho et al., 1989), and the value of surrogate markers of viremia (Coombs et al., 1989). An extremely sensitive test, the polymerase chain reaction, which is capable of detecting a single viral genome in a specimen of peripheral blood, has proved to be a powerful tool for documenting latent infection, clarifying confusing serological profiles, and predicting whether or not an infant born to a seropositive mother has been infected in utero (Phair and Wolinsky, 1989).

Of the laboratory tests that have been used to document the state of disease and the likely outcome of progressive HIV infection, the best are the determination of the absolute number or percentage of circulating CD4+ lymphocytes; levels of p24 antigenemia are often used (Spector et al., 1989), but do not correlate well with quantitative measurements of plasma viremia (Coombs et al., 1989). Either neopterin, which is produced by interferon-stimulated macrophages, or beta$_2$-microglobulin, which reflects lymphoid activity in general, in combination with the level of CD4+ T cells, were recommended as the best markers for disease-classification schemes and for evaluating responses to therapy (Fahey et al., 1990). Other tests of the severity of disease are the hematocrit, erythrocyte sedimentation rate, and CD4+/CD8+ lymphocyte ratio. Skin tests with multiple antigens are helpful in establishing the presence or absence of both anergy and latent infection from previous exposure to various microorganisms. Serological tests are also useful in documenting previous acquisition of certain infections, particularly toxoplasmosis, histoplasmosis, and coccidioidomycosis. The presence of cryptococcal antigen in serum or cerebrospinal fluid (Chuck and Sande, 1989) or of *Histoplasma capsulatum* polysaccharide antigen in urine or serum (Wheat et al., 1986) indicates active cryptococcosis or histoplasmosis, respectively.

C. Chest Radiography

All patients with known or suspected HIV infection who have symptoms or signs suggestive of pulmonary disease should have a posteroanterior and lateral chest x-ray. As listed in Table 2, the presence and type of abnormality provide important clues to the cause of the disorder and help to direct subsequent workup. It needs to be emphasized, however, that none of the radiographic abnormalities is specific for a certain disease, and that the various patterns only suggest a certain differential diagnosis.

Table 2 Differential Diagnosis of Commonly Observed Chest Radiographic Patterns in Patients with HIV Infection

Pattern	Diseases
Diffuse reticulonodular infiltration	*Pneumocystis carinii* pneumonia
	Disseminated tuberculosis
	Disseminated histoplasmosis
	Disseminated coccidioidomycosis
	Lymphocytic interstitial pneumonitis
Focal air-space consolidation	Bacterial pneumonia
	Kaposi's sarcoma
	Cryptococcosis
Normal	*Pneumocystis carinii* pneumonia
	Disseminated *Myobacterium avium*-complex
	Disseminated histoplasmosis
Adenopathy	Tuberculosis
	Kaposi's sarcoma
	Disseminated *Mycobacterium avium*-complex
	Non-Hodgkin's lymphoma
Pleural effusion	Kaposi's sarcoma
	Tuberculosis
	Non-Hodgkin's lymphoma
	Pyogenic empyema

Source: Reprinted with permission from Murray and Mills (1990).

Other radiological imaging techniques, such as computed tomography (CT) and magnetic resonance, have not been extensively used in patients with HIV infection, probably because the abnormalities on plain chest radiographs are sufficiently straightforward to direct the workup that leads to a diagnosis. The indications for CT and other special imaging methods are similar to those in non-HIV-infected patients.

D. Pulmonary Function Studies

Toward the beginning of the AIDS epidemic, much attention was paid to the use of pulmonary function tests as a means of selecting, from among the large group of patients at risk of having *P. carinii* pneumonia, those in whom fiberoptic bronchoscopy was indicated. Now, the widespread availability and diagnostic precision of sputum induction have virtually eliminated this indication. The major role of physiological testing is to help select, from among symptomatic patients with normal or nearly normal chest radiographs, those whose function is abnormal and who, therefore, require further diagnostic evaluation, often with invasive procedures (for reviews and references, see Stover and Meduri, 1988; Murray and Mills, 1990.

Four types of functional disturbance have been identified: (1) a restrictive ventilatory defect; (2) an abnormality of oxygenation, which may be present at rest and is virtually always present in patients with *P. carinii* pneumonia during exercise; (3) a low carbon monoxide diffusing capacity, which is caused, at least in *P. carinii* pneumonia, by an alveolar-capillary block (Sankary et al., 1988); decreased diffusing capacity values have also been reported in HIV-infected patients with no clinical evidence of lung disease (Shaw et al., 1988); and (4) an obstructive ventilatory defect, which has been associated with endobronchial Kaposi's sarcoma (Meduri et al., 1986), but which may occur in the absence of detectable airways abnormalities.

E. Radionuclide Imaging

Two different radionuclides have been used to study the lungs of patients with HIV infection: gallium67citrate (^{67}Ga-citrate) and technetium99mdiethylenetriamine pentaacetate (^{99m}Tc-DTPA), and a third, thallium201, is under investigation. Like pulmonary function testing, ^{67}Ga-citrate was more extensively used during the early years of the HIV epidemic than now as a guide to further diagnostic studies, particularly for *P. carinii* pneumonia. It was soon learned that many patients with HIV disease had slight (1 to 2+) ^{67}Ga-citrate uptake, but that patients with pneumocystis pneumonia had more intense (3 to 4+) uptake (Coleman et al., 1984). The utility of gallium imaging lies in directing the subsequent workup in symptomatic patients with or at risk for HIV infection whose chest radiographs are negative: (1) if the radionuclide scan is negative, attention should be directed outside the thorax; (2) if there is parenchymal uptake (diffuse or focal), sputum induction and/or bronchoalveolar lavage is warranted; and (3) if there is hilar or mediastinal node uptake, biopsy of lymph node, liver, or bone marrow is indicated. An algorithm with a recommended role for ^{67}Ga scanning has been published (Kramer et al., 1989). At our institution we find a positive (3 to 4+) gallium scan to be of particular value in providing impetus for sputum induction and/or bronchoalveolar lavage in intravenous drug abusers, who often have slightly abnormal chest radiographs and decreased diffusing capacity measurements. Imaging with ^{99m}Tc-DTPA, which is delivered to the lungs as an aerosol, has been used to study the permeability characteristics of the lung parenchyma, especially in patients with *P. carinii* pneumonia (Mason et al., 1987) and a new HIV-related disorder called lymphocytic alveolitis (Meignan et al., 1990). The value of ^{201}Tl scintigraphy is being explored in patients with Kaposi's sarcoma (Lee et al., 1988).

F. Sputum Examination

Most patients with HIV-related pyogenic pneumonia have a cough productive of purulent sputum. Examination of a gram-stained specimen of this material is useful in selecting initial antimicrobial therapy. Final diagnosis depends on the results of cultures of sputum, blood, or, when available, pleural fluid.

Patients with *P. carinii* pneumonia and other diffuse pulmonary infections nearly always complain of cough, but the cough is usually nonproductive. Induced sputum from these patients, obtained by inhaling an aerosol of hypertonic saline (3% or 5%) generated by an ultrasonic nebulizer, has a high likelihood of revealing *P. carinii* on direct examination of the stained specimen. The first reports of the results of sputum induction in patients suspected of having *P. carinii* pneumonia had a similar yield, 55% in one series (Pitchenik et al., 1986) and 56% in the other (Bigby et al., 1986). Later methodological improvements included mycolysis with dithiothreitol and centrifugation, which increased the sensitivity of the test considerably. In the largest series reported to date (404 episodes of pulmonary disease in 358 patients), the range of sensitivity for detecting *P. carinii* in induced sputum was 74–77%, and the negative predictive value was 58-64% (Ng et al., 1989). The results of initial studies with an indirect immunofluorescent stain using monoclonal antibodies directed against *P. carinii* were even better (Kovaks et al., 1988). More recently, however, a comparison of the yield in detecting *Pneumocystis* from the indirect fluorescent-antibody test, on the one hand, with that from a rapid Giemsa-like stain (Diff-Quik), toluidine blue, and Gomori methanimine silver, on the other hand, indicated that the immunofluorescence test was more sensitive than the others, but unfortunately was less specific (i.e., there were false positive results) (Ng et al., 1990).

G. Bronchoscopy

If sputum induction is not available or if the results of an induction are negative, fiberoptic bronchoscopy is indicated. Both bronchoalveolar lavage and transbronchial biopsy were usually performed during the initial bronchoscopy at the outset of the HIV epidemic, because it was shown that the yield from the two procedures was complementary in identifying respiratory tract pathogens: bronchoalveolar lavage had a sensitivity of 86% and transbronchial biopsy of 87%; when two procedures were combined, the yield was 98% for all pathogens and 100% for *P. carinii* (Broaddus et al., 1985). Transbronchial biopsy is contraindicated in patients with severe hypoxia, in all those who are being mechanically ventilated, and in patients with intractable coagulopathy. Bronchoalveolar lavage, however, can be safely performed in these patients.

During the last few years, because the techniques and experience in identifying *P. carinii* in respiratory secretions have improved, physicians in some institutions, including our own, have abandoned transbronchial biopsy and now perform only bronchoalveolar lavage during the initial bronchoscopy (Luce and Clement, 1989). This approach has several advantages: bronchoalveolar lavage is faster and easier to perform than transbronchial biopsy; the major complication, pneumothorax, is virtually eliminated; and both diagnosis and treatment for *P. carinii* can be carried out entirely on an outpatient basis.

But there is a possible disadvantage to this approach as well. Some investigators have reported that the yield of bronchoalveolar lavage for the diagnosis of *P. carinii* pneumonia was lower in patients who had been receiving aerosolized pentamidine than in those not receiving prophylaxis and, for this reason, recommended that such patients also have a transbronchial biopsy (Jules-Elysee et al., 1990). These results, however, differ from those in our institution, where investigators have shown no difference in the yield from sputum induction in patients who had and who had not received aerosolized pentamidine (Richmond et al., 1991); moreover, there is also no influence of aerosolized pentamidine on the yield from bronchoalveolar lavage if the upper lobes, instead of the middle lobe or lingula, are lavaged routinely (Golden, J. A., personal communication); as will be pointed out subsequently, this policy follows from the effect of aerosolized pentamidine on the distribution of pneumocystis when it does occur. Another consideration is the fact that as the use and effectiveness of chemoprophylaxis for *P. carinii* become more widespread, a decreasing percentage of patients who come to bronchoscopy will have *Pneumocystis* pneumonia and an increasing percentage will have some other pulmonary complication. Bronchoalveolar lavage alone is not as effective as bronchoalveolar lavage plus transbronchial biopsy in diagnosing coccidioidomycosis (Graham et al., 1988), and the same may be true for other pulmonary infections; it is clear that biopsy, not lavage, is needed to diagnose HIV-related interstitial pneumonias. However, whether or not the reinstitution of the routine use of transbronchial biopsy at the time of bronchoalveolar lavage will increase the yield of *treatable* pulmonary disorders that complicate the course of HIV infection is unknown and needs to be studied, if the causes of these events change, as seems to be happening.

H. Other Procedures

Several other procedures have been used in the diagnostic evaluation of patients with HIV-related pulmonary disease. Percutaneous needle aspiration of the lungs has a limited role in the diagnosis of diffuse infectious processes, because the high diagnostic yield is more than offset by the substantial incidence (50%) of pneumothorax (Wallace et al., 1985); needle aspiration is more useful in the diagnosis of focal mass lesions and adenopathy (Bottles et al., 1988).

An important, but still unresolved, question is what diagnostic procedure, if any, to do next in a patient who has symptomatic and radiographic evidence of progressive lung disease, but in whom the results of sputum induction (if available) and of initial bronchoscopy are negative. Because the initial bronchoscopy now often includes bronchoalveolar lavage only, unless contraindicated, a repeat bronchoscopy with both transbronchial biopsy and repeat lavage is indicated. A second bronchoscopy is probably also recommended in the patient who has already had the procedure with both biopsy and lavage, although the yield under these circumstances is low (Barrio et al., 1987). Open lung biopsy is seldom indicated in the workup of HIV-associated pulmonary complications, although only limited data are available to support this statement (Fitzgerald et al., 1987). The reason open lung biopsy is so infrequently used is, undoubtedly, that nearly all patients can be diagnosed by bronchoscopy, as just described.

III. Infectious Complications

The hallmark of advancing HIV disease is worsening immunodepression and, ultimately, the development of one or more complications, which in most cases are infectious. The lungs are the principal target of the many infections that lead to a diagnosis of AIDS and are often involved in earlier stages of evolving HIV disease as well. In this section the major pulmonary infectious complications of HIV infection will be reviewed according to the category of infectious microorganism that causes them (Table 1).

A. Viruses

Several viruses are known to cause lung disease in immunosuppressed persons, including members of the herpesvirus family (cytomegalovirus, varicella-zoster virus, herpes simplex virus, and Epstein-Barr virus), respiratory syncytial virus, influenza virus, parainfluenza virus, adenovirus, and measles virus. All these pathogens have been reported in patients with HIV infection, but only one, cytomegalovirus, is commonly found, and its role as a cause of pneumonia is debatable (for review and references, see Murray and Mills, 1990). Epstein-Barr virus and HIV itself have also been identified in the lungs of patients with HIV disease, but whether they are innocent bystanders or pathogens is unclear.

Cytomegalovirus

Infection with cytomegalovirus (CMV) is extremely common in healthy persons. The results of serological studies indicate that more than 50% of all adults and virtually 100% of homosexual men are infected with the virus (Mintz et al., 1983). CMV disease in immunocompromised patients is believed to result chiefly from reactivation of latent infection; however, because disease has been documented from de novo infection in recipients of solid organs, bone marrow, and blood, it is possible that new infection or superinfection from exogenous sources may also occur in HIV-infected persons.

Clinical Features

Retinitis is the most common form of HIV-associated CMV disease, but clinically significant involvement of the gastrointestinal tract and adrenal gland is well described (Jacobson and Mills, 1988a). The exact incidence of pneumonitis is difficult to document because there are no clear ways of distinguishing between latent infection and active disease of the lungs during life. Moreover, the majority of patients who have CMV isolated from respiratory secretions during their workup for suspected pulmonary disease have another pathogen, often *P. carinii*, identified in the same specimen. Thus, it is impossible to sort out to what extent the CMV is contributing to the patient's signs, symptoms, and chest radiographic abnormalities (Jacobson and Mills, 1988b). When dual infection is discovered, treatment directed against the coexisting disease and not against the CMV usually results in clinical resolution; this has been nicely documented in patients with first-episode *P. carinii* pneumonia: there was no difference in either short- or long-term survival or in length of hospital stay between patients who did and those who did not have CMV isolated in the same specimen in which *P. carinii* was identified (Jacobson et al., 1991).

Diagnosis

Nevertheless, CMV can cause clinically significant pneumonitis (Wallace, 1989). When this occurs as part of documented disseminated CMV disease, all that is needed for therapeutic purposes is to exclude a coexisting pulmonary pathogen by bronchoalveolar lavage, because antiviral treatment will be given for the extrapulmonary involvement regardless of the presence or absence of the virus in the lungs. The therapeutic dilemma is much greater when just the lungs appear to be afflicted. The only precise diagnostic criterion is the demonstration of *widespread* specific cytopathic changes in the lungs themselves, and this is obviously impossible to do by bronchoalveolar lavage or even with transbronchial biopsies. Neither culturing the virus from the liquid nor finding cytopathic abnormalities in the cells recovered from lavage indicates, necessarily, that the patient has important clinical involvement; it is our policy not to treat these patients for CMV pneumonia, a conclusion recently affirmed elsewhere (Millar et al., 1990). These observations mean that clinicians must make a difficult therapeutic decision based on the limited information from bronchoalveolar lavage, the exclusion of other causes of the patient's abnormalities, and good clinical judgment.

Treatment

If it were not for the serious toxicity of the drugs currently available for the treatment of CMV disease, the accuracy of diagnosis would be less important than it is. Ganciclovir, the drug of choice, must be given intravenously, usually through an indwelling delivery system, twice daily during the 2-week induction and then once daily 5 or 6 days per week for maintenance. Ganciclovir often causes neutropenia, especially when given concurrently with zidovudine (AZT). The alternative drug, foscarnat, is used either for ganciclovir failure, sometimes because of acquired resistance to the drug, or for intolerance. The principal side effects of foscarnat are renal dysfunction and hypocalcemia. Seizures and deaths have resulted from too rapid infusion.

Other Viruses

Other herpesviruses besides CMV may cause pneumonia in HIV-infected patients, but they do so infrequently. Herpes simplex virus, for example, which is commonly found in oropharyngeal secretions and which is a known lower respiratory tract contaminant, is an unusual cause of pneumonia in AIDS patients and appears to be more frequent in other immunosuppressed hosts (Ramsey et al., 1982). Varicella-zoster virus is a rare cause of pneumonia in HIV-infected patients, although 11 cases of disseminated infection were recently reported (Cohen et al., 1988). Specific viral DNA of Epstein-Barr virus has been identified in lung biopsy specimens of infants and children with lymphocytic interstitial pneumonitis (discussed subsequently), but the precise role of the virus is uncertain (Andiman et al., 1985). Almost all homosexual men are seropositive for Epstein-Barr virus, higher titers are found in AIDS patients with lymphoma (also discussed subsequently) than in other AIDS patients (Beckhardt et al., 1988), and nuclear remnants of the virus have been observed histologically in some AIDS-related lymphomas (Hamilton-Dutoit et al., 1989). There is no doubt that HIV itself is present in the lungs of patients with lymphocytic interstitial pneumonitis (Ziza et al., 1985; Chayt et al., 1986; Resnick et al., 1987), but its pathogenic role in this and other HIV-related interstitial disorders is unclear, because HIV can also be found in bronchoalveolar lavage specimens from asymptomatic patients (Linnemann et al., 1989; Rose et al., 1991).

B. Bacteria

Bacterial infections are common in HIV-infected persons, and recurrent, severe bacterial infections at various sites are a criterion for the diagnosis of AIDS in children (CDC, 1987a). Among adults, bacterial pneumonias occur with increased frequency in patients with asymptomatic HIV infection and at all stages of HIV disease, including AIDS. The exact incidence varies from one report to another and with the population studied (e.g., the incidence is higher in intravenous drug abusers than in male homosexuals), but, overall, is 5- to 100-fold greater in HIV-seropositive than in seronegative persons (for review and references, see Chaisson, 1989). The mechanisms responsible for the high rate of bacterial complications in HIV infection are complex. Undoubtedly, the most important factor is the profound deficiency of humoral immunity, which results in a markedly reduced B-cell response to novel, specific antigens, such as encapsulated bacteria; in contrast, B cells are spontaneously activated, which accounts for the commonly observed nonspecific, polyclonal hypergammaglobulinemia in HIV-infected patients (Lane et al., 1983). However, other deficiences in host defenses are also present, including impaired chemotactic and bactericidal capabilities of neutrophils (Roilides et al., 1990), abnormal macrophage function, and, at times, drug-induced neutropenia.

Community-Acquired Bacteria

Bacterial pneumonias in persons with HIV infection, as in other patient populations, can be divided into those acquired out of the hospital, so-called community-acquired pneumonias, and those resulting from nosocomial infection, or hospital-acquired pneumonias. The etiology and pathogenesis of these two types of bacterial pneumonia are quite different (Fels, 1988). The most common organisms causing community-acquired pneumonia in patients with HIV infection are *Streptococcus pneumoniae* (the pneumococcus), *Hemophilus influenzae*, other *Hemophilus* species, group B streptococci, and *Branhamella catarrhalis*. *Staphylococcus aureus* was a frequent isolate (23%) from respiratory-tract cultures of 129 HIV-seropositive patients referred for evaluation of pulmonary disease and was believed to have caused serious community-acquired pneumonia in eight of these patients (Levine et al., 1990). Other bacteria, such as *Legionella pneumophila*, Enterobacteriaceae, *Rhodococcus equi*, and *Bordatella pertussis*, have been noted sporadically (Murray and Mills, 1990).

Clinical Features

The presenting signs and symptoms of community-acquired pneumococcal and *H. influenzae* pneumonias in patients with HIV infection are similar in many respects to those seen in patients without HIV infection. Fever (96%), cough (90%), dyspnea (70%), and pleuritic chest pain (69%) are common (Gerberding et al., 1986). Chest radiographs show focal areas of consolidation that tend to involve segments or lobes; single sites of infiltration are usually seen, but multifocal involvement appears more common than in non-HIV-infected persons. The most striking feature of HIV-linked bacterial pneumonia is the extremely high rate of bacteremia: 50–80% in patients with pneumococcal pneumonia, and 5–25% in *H. influenzae* pneumonia (Chaisson, 1989). Pneumonia was the most important source of community-acquired bacteremia in HIV-infected patients admitted to San Francisco General Hospital, but several patients were also identified who had no apparent source (Krumholz et al., 1989). Patients with *P. carinii* pneumonia may have concurrent bacterial pneumonia, which complicates diagnosis and treatment, but which can usually be distinguished by careful clinical and laboratory examinations.

Diagnosis

The diagnosis of community-acquired pneumonia is the same in HIV-infected as in non-HIV-infected persons; reliance is placed on initial Gram's stain and culture of sputum. As mentioned, blood cultures are often positive when encapsulated microorganisms are involved.

Treatment

Treatment of patients with community-acquired pneumonia is the same whether they are HIV-infected or not. Pneumococcal infections are best treated with penicillin; first-generation cephalosporins, clindamycin, or erythromycin should be reserved for penicillin-allergic patients. *H. influenzae* may be treated with ampicillin unless the organism is a beta-lactamase producer, in which case a second- or third-generation cephalosporin or trimethoprim-sulfamethoxazole may be employed. Other organisms are also treated with conventional antimicrobial therapy. Despite appropriate treatment, which is nearly always successful, 25–50% of patients with HIV-related pyogenic pneumonia have recurrences, sometimes with the same strain of bacteria that caused the initial infection. The Centers for Disease Control (CDC) (1989a) has recommended that pneumococcal vaccine be given to patients with HIV infection, but the effectiveness of this policy is uncertain and failures have been reported. For patients who have had recurrent infections, continuous chemoprophylaxis with trimethoprim-sulfamethoxazole, if tolerated, is often recommended as it will also prevent episodes of *P. carinii* pneumonia. The National Institute of Child Health and Human Development Intravenous Immunoglobulin Study Group (1991) has recently shown that infusions of immune globulin every 28 days significantly prolonged the time free from serious bacterial infections in children with clinical or immunological evidence of HIV disease whose CD4+ cell counts were greater than $200/mm^3$ when they entered the study. Some physicians also use intravenous immune globulin to treat HIV-seropositive adults with recurrent community-acquired pneumonia.

Hospital-Acquired Bacteria

Hospital-acquired pneumonias in patients with HIV infection are usually due to staphylococci or to aerobic gram-negative rods; many other microorganisms have also been found in this setting (Murray and Mills, 1990). The infections almost always develop late in the course of HIV infection, generally after an AIDS index diagnosis has been made and when multiple risk factors are also present (Witt et al., 1987). The extremely high morbidity and mortality of nosocomial bacterial pneumonia, even when recognized early and treated appropriately, is explained in large part by the fact that these patients are already desperately ill when the complication supervenes.

Mycobacterium tuberculosis

During the last 5 years, a worldwide resurgence of tuberculosis has been convincingly documented. Increased numbers of cases have been reported from developed countries, including the United States, Japan, and the Netherlands, but there has been a veritable explosion of tuberculosis in sub-Saharan Africa, which has been especially well documented in Uganda, Burundi, Tanzania, and Malawi (Slutkin et al., 1988). The fact that most of this increase is attributable to coexisting HIV infection should come as no surprise, because of the role played by cell-mediated immunity in protecting against the development of tuberculosis and because of the depletion of this immunity by HIV infection. The World Health Organization estimates that there are more than 3 million persons in the world dually infected with both HIV and *Mycobacterium tuberculosis* (Chinn, J., cited in Murray, 1991), which makes, or certainly will make, tuberculosis the most important infectious complication of HIV disease. But it should be emphasized that tuberculosis differs from virtually all other HIV-related infections in ways that make it especially important: it is transmissible, curable, and preventable (CDC, 1989b).

The natural history of tuberculosis in non-HIV-infected persons and how HIV infection upsets the delicate immunological balance that ordinarily is able to contain tubercle bacilli have recently been reviewed (Murray, 1989a). There is now no doubt that HIV infection tremendously increases the likelihood that latent tuberculous infection will progress to clinically active tuberculous disease (Selwyn et al., 1989). Both reactivation of remotely acquired tuberculosis infection and rapid progression following recent exposure have been described (for review and references, see Barnes et al., 1991).

Clinical Features

There are two distinct clinical patterns of tuberculosis in HIV-infected patients, depending on whether the disease occurs early or late during the course of evolving HIV infection (Murray, 1990). The major differences in the two forms of HIV-associated tuberculosis are shown in Table 3. Of the two types, the late ''atypical'' variety has received the greater attention, in part because its features often suggest a disease other than tuberculosis, thus delaying diagnosis and the institution of specific chemotherapy and increasing the likelihood of transmission (Pitchenik and Rubinson, 1985). It should be noted that hilar and mediastinal adenopathy are not part of the HIV-related generalized lymphadenopathy syndrome (Stern et al., 1984); the differential diagnosis of intrathoracic lymph node enlargement in a patient with HIV infection is provided in Table 2.

Table 3 Manifestations of Tuberculosis in "Early" and "Late" HIV Infection

Feature	Early	Late
Skin test	Positive	Negative
Adenopathy	Unusual	Common
Distribution	Upper	Lower-middle
Cavitation	Present	Absent
Extrapulmonary	10–15%	More than 50%

Source: Reprinted with permission from Murray (1990).

Diagnosis

The diagnosis of tuberculosis, whether HIV-associated or not, depends on the isolation and identification of *M. tuberculosis* by culture. Finding acid-fast bacilli, regardless of their source, provides an indication for empirical antituberculous treatment but does not establish *M. tuberculosis* infection. Identification by culture is mandatory in view of the increasing numbers of patients with HIV disease in developed countries who are found with nontuberculous mycobacterial disease (Jacobson, 1988); this does not appear to be the case in developing countries (Colebunders et al., 1989). Virtually any specimen can be examined for acid-fast bacilli and cultured for mycobacteria, including sputum, bronchoalveolar lavage, transbronchial biopsy, bone marrow aspirate or biopsy, fine-needle aspirate of lymph node or other lesion, and biopsy of other suspicious sites. Blood cultures using special techniques are occasionally positive (Barber et al., 1990), but not nearly as often as in disseminated *M. avium* complex disease (Horsburgh, 1991). The results of drug susceptibility studies are useful in planning definitive treatment.

Treatment

Because tuberculosis is treatable and transmissible until after treatment is begun, and because nontuberculous mycobacterial disease is noncommunicable and responds relatively poorly to medications, the CDC (1987b) has recommended that antituberculous chemotherapy be started whenever acid-fast bacilli are found in a specimen from a patient with known or suspected HIV infection and clinical evidence of mycobacterial disease. While awaiting the results of cultures to distinguish *M. tuberculosis* from *M. avium* complex and other *mycobacteria*, it is important for individual and public health reasons to initiate treatment for tuberculosis with at least three drugs: isoniazid, rifampin, and pyrazinamide; occasionally, when drug resistance is suspected (because of previous antituberculosis therapy or residence in certain regions of the world) or extensive disease is present, ethambutol is also administered until the results of drug susceptibility studies are available (ATS-CDC, 1987). It may be prudent to always begin with four drugs in view of the ominous rise in prevalence of multidrug resistant strains of *M. tuberculosis* being reported from some cities in the United States (Pitchenik et al., 1990) and an increasing rate of nosocomial transmission of these organisms (CDC, 1991). Although both the CDC (1987b) and ATS-CDC (1987) recommend that treatment be administered for a minimum of 9 months and for at least 6 months after documented culture conversion, the results of a recently reported study from San Francisco indicate that standard four-drug, 6-month therapy for otherwise uncomplicated HIV-related pulmonary tuberculosis produces excellent results (Small et al., 1991). As in the treatment of all patients with tuberculosis, compliance is essential to a successful result.

It has now become clear that patients with tuberculosis and HIV infection are more likely than non-HIV-infected persons to experience toxicity from anti-tuberculous drugs. Among the conventionally used drugs, rifampin is most likely to cause adverse reactions (Small et al., 1991), whereas in Africa there is an increased incidence of side effects from thiacetazone, widely used because of its low cost (Colebunders et al., 1989; Eriki et al., 1991).

Prevention

Chemoprophylaxis with isoniazid is likely to prevent progression of latent tuberculous infection to clinical tuberculosis in patients with HIV infection. Thus, all persons with HIV infection who have more than 5 mm induration to a tuberculin skin test (note 5 mm, not 10 mm, as is customary) should have a chest radiograph, and if it is abnormal, the patient should be evaluated for tuberculosis or other lung disease. If evidence of active disease is not found, the person should receive isoniazid chemoprophylaxis. Because of the unreliability of the tuberculin skin test for detecting tuberculous infection in HIV-immunocompromised persons, chemoprophylaxis has been recommended—on the basis of decision analysis, not clinical trials—for all HIV-seropositive drug abusers, except black women, in view of the high risk of developing tuberculosis (Jordan et al., 1991). Clinical trials are under way to compare the efficacy of standard treatment with isoniazid for 6–12 months with the results of short-course therapy with rifampin and pyrazinamide for 2 months; the latter regimen was as effective as the former in an experimental model of tuberculosis (Lecoeur et al., 1989) and has the great advantage of a shorter period of administration.

Although concern has been raised about the safety and efficacy of vaccination with bacille Calmette Guérin (BCG), recent data suggest that the incidence of local complications (ulceration and lymphadenitis) did not differ among HIV-infected babies who received BCG compared with non-HIV-infected infants (Lallemant-Le Coeur et al., 1991). Moreover, the World Health Organization (WHO) and International Union Against Tuberculosis and

Lung Diseases (IUATLD) continue to recommend using BCG in developing countries where there is a high prevalence of HIV infection, but state that the vaccine should not be given to symptomatic HIV-infected children or adults (WHO/IUATLD, 1989).

Mycobacterium avium-complex

By 1980, only 24 cases of disseminated infection with *Mycobacterium avium*-complex (MAC) had been reported (Horsburgh et al., 1985), but this has changed dramatically since the beginning of the AIDS epidemic. Although the exact incidence of disseminated MAC infection is unknown and presumably underreported, clinical studies have indicated that it occurs in 15–24% of all patients with AIDS in the United States; applying these figures to the 161,073 cases of AIDS that were reported in this country from 1981 through 1990, one can calculate that 24,000–39,000 persons have probably developed disseminated MAC (Horsburgh, 1991). Not only has the number of reported cases risen steadily since 1981, but the rate as a percentage of all cases of AIDS has increased, particularly since 1987. Disseminated MAC is an infrequent index diagnosis of AIDS, because it occurs late in the course of the HIV-induced immunosuppression, a mean of 7–15 months after the diagnosis of AIDS (for review and references, see Horsburgh, 1991). Accordingly, because patients with HIV infection are living longer and longer, more and more cases of MAC can be anticipated in the future.

Disseminated MAC is believed to result from primary acquisition of the microorganism, which is ubiquitous in the environment, not reactivation of latent infection as occurs with most HIV-associated diseases (Horsburgh and Selik, 1989). These mycobacteria probably enter the body chiefly through the gastrointestinal tract, and occasionally through the lungs (MacDonnell and Glassroth, 1989). Nearly all cases of disseminated MAC are caused by *M. avium* serotypes, which suggests that there are important differences in exposure to or virulence of these particular strains (Yakrus and Good, 1990).

Clinical Features

The most common clinical presentation of disseminated MAC disease is a wasting syndrome consisting of fever, weight loss, and cachexia; other manifestations include chronic diarrhea and abdominal pain, progressive anemia, which often requires transfusion, a chronic malabsorption syndrome, which resembles Whipple's disease, and extrabiliary obstructive jaundice (Jacobson, 1988). Respiratory symptoms are usually unimportant and the chest radiographs are typically normal, even when the organism can be cultured from respiratory tract secretions (MacDonnell and Glassroth, 1989). Localized pneumonia (Tenholder et al., 1988) and endobronchial lesions without pneumonia (Packer et al., 1988) have been reported, but are rare.

Diagnosis

MAC has been cultured from numerous sites in patients with HIV disease, but the most productive sources are blood, bone marrow, liver and lymph nodes. The reliability of special techniques of culturing blood make this the preferred way of establishing the diagnosis, and two specimens are sufficient (Yagupsky and Menegus, 1990). The organisms may be cultured initially from sputum or bronchoalveolar lavage fluid, but this finding does not necessarily indicate either invasive or disseminated disease and does not lead to the diagnosis of AIDS. The pathological findings of MAC infection are characteristic but not definitive. Acid-fast bacilli are remarkably abundant and are often packed within foamy macrophages or histiocytes; granulomas are usually absent or poorly formed.

Treatment

Although the results of early studies were discouraging, more recent trials of chemotherapy for AIDS-associated disseminated MAC have been more successful (for review and references, see Horsburgh, 1991). Various combinations of drugs including rifabutin, isoniazid, ethambutol, clofazimine, rifampin, amikacin, and ciprofloxacin have been shown to decrease blood colony counts and improve systemic symptoms; an initial regimen of ethambutol, clofazimine, ciprofloxacin, and rifampin has been recommended, because of the likelihood of a good clinical response and acceptable toxicity (Horsburgh, 1991), and similar results were reported using amikacin, ethambutol, rifampin, and ciprofloxacin (Chiu et al., 1990). A new macrolide antimicrobial drug, clarithromycin, was effective against MAC in an in vivo model and should be evaluated clinically (Perronne et al., 1990).

Other Mycobacterial Infections

Analysis of the 1906 AIDS-related case of disseminated nontuberculous mycobacterial infection reported to the CDC from 1981 through 1987 showed that nearly all (96%) were caused by MAC (Horsburgh and Selik, 1989); other species of mycobacteria included *M. kansasii* (3%) and *M. gordonae*, *M. fortuitum*, and *M. chelonei* (<1% each). The reason(s) for this striking disparity, which contrasts with the frequency with which various mycobacteria cause disseminated disease in non-HIV-immunosuppressed patients, is unknown (Horsburgh et al., 1985). Increased frequency of exposure or the presence of specific defects of host defenses might account for the predominance of MAC in AIDS patients. Rare causes of disseminated or localized disease in patients with HIV infection are *M. xenopi*, *M. bovis*, *M. scrofulaceum*, *M szulgai*, *M. flavenscens*,

M. asiaticum, *M. malmoense*, and *M. xenopi* (for review and references, see Murray and Mills, 1990); to these cases must now be added a fatal infection with a novel, unidentified mycobacterium (Hirschel et al., 1990).

Recently, Levine and Chaisson (1991) described the clinical and radiographic features and the response to therapy of 19 patients with coexisting *M. kansasii* and HIV infections. Fourteen of the nineteen patients had exclusively pulmonary disease, three had both pulmonary and extrapulmonary disease, and two had only extrapulmonary involvement. The radiographic findings were interesting: eight patients had focal upper lobe infiltrates, nine had diffuse interstitial infiltrates, and nine patients also had thin-walled cavitary lesions. The 10 patients who were treated responded to antituberculous chemotherapy. The authors emphasize that *M. kansasii* can cause serious, potentially life-threatening pulmonary disease in patients with advanced HIV infection, and that, contrary to previous reports, this opportunistic infection responds to appropriate treatment.

Bacillary Angiomatosis

Bacillary angiomatosis is a newly described infectious disease that causes a neoplastic-like proliferation of small blood vessels in the skin and visceral organs of patients who are immunocompromised from HIV disease or other disorders. The unnamed microorganism is extremely fastidious, but can be grown in culture (Slater et al., 1990), seen in tissues using special stains (Perkocha et al., 1990), and characterized using the polymerase chain reaction (Relman et al., 1990); the results of recent collaborative efforts among these authors indicate that the same or closely related bacillus causes bacillary angiomatosis, bacillary peliosis hepatis, and a syndrome of fever and bacteremia in patients with HIV disease (Relman et al., 1991).

The disease presents with varying degrees of involvement of the skin, hepatomegaly, splenomegaly, and lymphadenopathy. Although pulmonary disease has not been mentioned in most reports, it was noted in a recent Letter to the Editor (Alkan and Orenstein, 1991), and we know of four cases with pleuropulmonary manifestations, two with diffuse reticulonodular infiltrates, one with mediastinal adenopathy, and one with pleural effusion, in patients with otherwise typical bacillary angiomatosis in whom no other cause for the lung disease was identified (personal observations and Gherman, C., personal communication). Bacillary angiomatosis and related disorders should be kept in mind in patients with HIV infection, because they respond to therapy with erythromycin and, apparently, with doxycycline.

C. Fungi

Fungal infections, particularly with *Candida* species and *Cryptococcus neoformans*, were recognized as important complications of HIV infection early in the unfolding AIDS epidemic. A few years later, first disseminated histoplasmosis and then disseminated coccidioidomycosis were included among the indicator diseases diagnostic of AIDS, if they occurred in a patient with laboratory evidence of HIV infection (CDC, 1985; 1987c). Fungal infections in patients with advanced HIV disease are characterized by a high incidence of dissemination and frequent relapse after initial treatment; accordingly, lifelong suppressive therapy is nearly always required. Histological examination is notable for poorly formed granulomas and a high density of organisms.

Cryptococcus neoformans

Localized pulmonary cryptococcosis is an uncommon, but well-documented disease of otherwise healthy persons, and in the pre-AIDS era disseminated infection was recognized as an occasional opportunistic disease of immunocompromised patients (Williams et al., 1976). Now, cryptococcosis is the fourth most common infectious complication of HIV disease in the United States and occurred in 7% of the first 2087 patients with AIDS seen at San Francisco General Hospital (Chuck and Sande, 1989); cryptococcosis is also common in Africa (Quinn et al., 1986). The causative fungus, *C. neoformans*, is widespread, but is most abundant in pigeon and chicken excreta. Cryptococci in the environment are unencapsulated and much smaller (3.5–7μm diameter)—and thus respirable—than when surrounded by the 1- to 30-μm-thick polysaccharide capsule that develops after deposition in the lungs.

Clinical Features

Cryptococcosis is an AIDS-indicator disease, but more than half (55%) the patients in one series had already had a diagnosis of AIDS made by some other criteria when they developed their fungal infection, which indicates that it develops late in the course of progressive HIV-induced immunosuppression (Chuck and Sande, 1989). The clinical presentation of cryptococcosis in these patients is usually dominated by the features of meningoencephalitis; the lungs are the organs next most commonly involved, and the two manifestations frequently coexist (Grant and Armstrong, 1988). Twelve of forty-eight patients reported in a recent article had pulmonary disease as their first manifestation of disseminated cryptococcosis (Cheychani and Kamholz, 1990). Several types of pulmonary involvement have been described, of which a diffuse interstitial (often nodular) pattern is most common, but which may signify coexisting infection by some other pathogen. Solitary or multiple focal infiltrates, occasionally with cavitation, lymph node enlargement, and pleural effusion, have all been observed but are less common. Respiratory signs and symptoms may be minimal, and the chest radiograph is the best way to document the presence and severity of respiratory involvement.

Diagnosis

The definitive diagnosis of intrathoracic cryptococcosis requires the isolation of *C. neoformans* from pulmonary secretions, bronchoalveolar lavage fluid, pleural fluid, or biopsy of lung tissue, endobronchial lesion, or other involved site. However, the diagnosis is frequently made by obtaining a positive cryptococcal antigen (CRAG) test result from serum, cerebrospinal fluid, or pleural fluid; in some centers, the CRAG test is also being performed on bronchoalveolar lavage fluid. In the San Francisco General Hospital series, the CRAG test using serum was more sensitive in diagnosing AIDS-related cryptococcosis, including meningitis, than the CRAG test using cerebrospinal fluid (99% versus 92%) (Chuck and Sande, 1989). In many instances, patients with radiographically detectable lung disease and a positive cryptococcal antigen in their cerebrospinal fluid or serum are treated for cryptococcosis without further diagnostic efforts. This is permissible as long as the radiographic pattern is consistent with pulmonary cryptococcosis and improves with treatment. If not, further workup for coexisting disease is indicated (Murray and Mills, 1990).

Treatment

None of the disseminated HIV-associated fungal infections can be cured. Consequently, it is now customary to subdivide the required lifelong course of treatment into an ''induction'' phase to obtain clinical remission, followed by a ''maintenance'' phase to prevent subsequent relapse. Initial treatment for HIV-associated cryptococcosis of any organ usually begins with intravenous amphotericin B. Flucytosine may be given concurrently to patients with adequate white blood cell counts, as recommended in other immunosuppressive disorders, in order to decrease the daily dosage of amphotericin B and diminish its side effects (Dismukes et al., 1987). However, the results of retrospective studies have shown that flucytosine has substantial hematological toxicity in AIDS patients and may not confer any additional advantage over amphotericin B alone. Other new drugs are also being tried, but in one small study fluconazole did not compare favorably with amphotericin B for the initial treatment of cryptococcal meningitis (Larsen et al., 1990). Although more data are needed to define the role of alternate antifungal agents, it appears that fluconazole alone is effective in patients with mild cryptococcal disease, including those with only pulmonary involvement.

As stated, after a satisfactory initial response, maintenance therapy is obligatory, and once-weekly amphotericin B has proved effective (Zuger et al., 1986). However, fluconazole, which has been released by the Food and Drug Administration for the treatment and maintenance of AIDS-related cryptococcosis, has largely supplanted amphotericin B because it is at least as effective and it is much easier and safer to administer (Bozzette et al., 1991). Itraconazole also appears useful for maintenance, but the published experience is not as large as with fluconazole (Viviani et al., 1989), and preliminary results suggest that the relapse rate after 1 year is higher with itraconazole than with fluconazole.

Histoplasma capsulatum

Histoplasmosis is a systemic disease caused by *H. capsulatum*, a dimorphic fungus found in certain endemic areas in all continents except Antarctica; in North America the organism is chiefly found in the Mississippi, Ohio, and Saint Lawrence river valleys and the Caribbean islands. Disseminated histoplasmosis was first described as a complication of AIDS in 1982, and since then, more than 150 cases have been reported; two reviews have recently appeared (Johnson et al., 1989; Wheat et al., 1990).

Pulmonary infection develops when the tuberculate spores of the mycelial phase of the fungus are inhaled; once deposited in the distal respiratory tract, the organism transforms into its yeast (or parasitic) phase and initiates an inflammatory reaction accompanied by fungemia. Primary infections, which occur each year in tens of thousands of healthy persons living in endemic areas, are usually subclinical or inconsequential and can be detected afterward by the presence of a positive skin test reaction to histoplasmin or, less commonly, by the finding of characteristic calcified lesions in the lungs or spleen. In patients with HIV infection and profoundly depressed cell-mediated immunity, histoplasmosis is nearly always disseminated and occurs both from reactivation of remotely acquired (latent) infection and from progression of newly acquired disease. High attack rates of histoplasmosis (27–75%) were reported among all patients with AIDS who lived in known endemic areas (Bartholomew et al., 1984; Bonner et al., 1984; Wheat et al., 1990). Much lower incidence rates (5%) were reported from Houston, a city on the fringe of the endemic area (Johnson et al., 1988), and the incidence is considerably lower than that in San Francisco, a city well outside the area. Coexisting infection with another HIV-related pathogen, especially *P. carinii*, is common.

Clinical Features

The presenting complaints of AIDS-associated disseminated histoplasmosis are nonspecific and include fever and weight loss. Cough or dyspnea was noted in the majority of patients who had pulmonary radiographic abnormalities, but respiratory symptoms were infrequent in those with normal chest roentgenograms. Splenomegaly, lymphadenopathy, and hepatomegaly were each found in one-third or less of the patients, and the frequency varied (Johnson et al., 1988, Wheat et al., 1990). A clinical syndrome resembling sepsis, including the adult respiratory distress syndrome, disseminated intravascular coagulation, encephalopathy, and acute renal failure, is a well-documented, but unusual, manifestation of AIDS-associated disseminated histoplasmosis.

The most common chest radiographic abnormalities are diffuse reticulonodular infiltrates, sometimes further characterized as interstitial or alveolar, which are observed in over half the patients. Normal chest radiographs are not uncommon and were reported in 44% of patients in one series (Wheat et al., 1990).

Diagnosis

The diagnosis of histoplasmosis requires isolation and identification of the causative fungus by culture or detection of *Histoplasma* polysaccharide antigen in urine or blood. Cultures of bone marrow biopsy or of blood have the highest yield. Cultures of pulmonary specimens obtained by bronchoalveolar lavage or by transbronchial biopsy are also useful. A new and promising test to detect *H. capsulatum* polysaccharide antigen in the blood, urine, or cerebrospinal fluid has been described that provides a way of rapidly establishing the diagnosis in patients with suspected disseminated histoplasmosis (Wheat et al., 1986); such tests were positive in 70 of 72 (97.3%) recently reported cases (Wheat et al., 1990). *Histoplasma* polysaccharide antigen values fall with satisfactory therapy and rise during relapses; so they may prove useful for following patients. Neither routine skin tests nor conventional *Histoplasma* serological tests are reliable for diagnosing HIV-related histoplasmosis (Johnson et al., 1988).

Treatment

Like cryptococcosis, histoplasmosis in patients with AIDS is incurable and requires both induction and maintenance therapy. Amphotericin B is much more effective than ketoconazole and is the drug of choice for induction therapy. The optimum drug and dosage for maintenance therapy is less clear cut; amphotericin B is well tolerated and effective (McKinsey et al., 1989), but is likely to be supplanted by itraconazole, which can be taken orally, is even better tolerated, and (so far) has proved highly effective (Wheat et al., 1990); fluconazole is also being tested. The role of skin testing for the identification of HIV-seropositive persons with prior exposure who would then be candidates for chemoprophylaxis is being investigated.

Coccidioides immitis

Coccidioidomycosis, like histoplasmosis, is a frequent infection in its particular endemic areas, and in immunocompetent persons is usually a benign, self-limited disease of the lungs and regional lymph nodes. Although not a particularly common pulmonary complication, it is clear that, at least in the endemic area, *Coccidioides immitis* is an important opportunistic pathogen among HIV-infected patients (Fish et al., 1990). In Tucson, Arizona, for example, a highly endemic area, 7 of 27 patients with AIDS had coccidioidomycosis, an attack rate of 27% (Bronnimann et al., 1987). Late reactivation accounts for most cases of HIV-related disseminated coccidioidomycosis that develop outside the endemic area, including those we see in San Francisco. Within the endemic region, dissemination from both progressive primary infection and reactivation of remote infection appear to occur, but it is difficult to distinguish by serological testing which mechanism is responsible in a given patient (Fish et al., 1990).

Clinical Features

The presenting symptoms of disseminated coccidioidomycosis are nonspecific and include fever, weight loss, and fatigue; cough suggests respiratory involvement. The authors of the recent report of 77 carefully analyzed patients with HIV-related coccidioidomycosis concluded that the clinical features were much more variable than previously described (Fish et al., 1990). Most patients had lung disease with either focal radiographic densities (26%) or diffuse reticulonodular infiltration (40%); far fewer patients had cutaneous involvement (5%), meningitis (12%), extrathoracic lymph node or hepatic coccidioidomycosis (9%), or only serological evidence of disease (8%).

Diagnosis

The diagnosis of HIV-associated coccidioidomycosis is made either by isolation of the fungus on culture or by cytological or histological identification of spherules. The standard tube precipitin immunodiffusion and complement fixation serological tests are often positive (about 90%) on initial testing in patients with HIV-related coccidioidomycosis, with negative results most commonly observed in patients with diffuse pulmonary infiltrates (Galgiani and Ampel, 1990). No single diagnostic technique or source of samples is uniformly successful, and all available specimens should be examined when practicable; sputum, bronchoalveolar lavage, and transbronchial biopsy have a high yield. Blood cultures are sometimes positive (Ampel et al., 1986). Coccidioidin or spherulin skin tests are of no value.

Treatment

Like cryptococcosis and histoplasmosis, disseminated coccidioidomycosis requires both induction and maintenance therapy. But the drug of choice for the disease has not been established. Amphotericin B, ketoconazole, itraconazole, and fluconazole have all been used in small numbers of patients, but it has not been possible to discern a clear therapeutic advantage of any one of them (Fish et al., 1990). At San Francisco General Hospital, we begin treatment with intravenous amphotericin B and provide maintenance with either amphotericin B or ketoconazole; however, this may change depending on the results of trials using itraconazole or fluconazole. Sporadic reports of the use of these drugs are promising (Galgiani and Ampel, 1990; Tucker et al., 1990a,b).

Aspergillus Species

Aspergillosis is an unusual systemic disease that results from the invasion of otherwise viable tissue by any of the approximately 150 species of the genus *Aspergillus*, most commonly *A. fumigatus* (Williams et al., 1976). Although invasive aspergillosis is a well-documented complication of immunodepressive disorders, particularly leukemia and organ transplantation, it is not common in patients with HIV disease, including AIDS. In the largest series reported to date, 13 patients, pulmonary aspergillosis followed the diagnosis of AIDS by a median delay of 25 months; in these patients, risk factors for the development of aspergillosis besides HIV-induced immunosuppression included use of corticosteroids, neutropenia, marijuana smoking, and use of broad-spectrum antimicrobial drugs (Denning et al., 1991).

Two distinct patterns of HIV-associated aspergillosis have been observed: invasive pulmonary aspergillosis, characterized by prolonged cough and fever, and obstructing bronchial aspergillosis, characterized by breathlessness, cough (sometimes productive of bronchial casts formed by matted hyphae), and chest pain (Denning et al., 1991). The radiographic abnormalities are variable and include unilateral or bilateral infiltrates, cavitary lesions, and nodular and pleural-based densities. The results of transbronchial biopsy are usually negative, but specimens from bronchoalveolar lavage or percutaneous aspirates are often positive on culture. This combination, a positive culture for *Aspergillus* species but negative histological findings, always leaves some doubt about the diagnosis of invasive aspergillosis; repeated isolation of the fungus in large numbers makes the diagnosis more secure.

Not enough patients with AIDS-related aspergillosis have been diagnosed and treated to allow recommendations concerning optimum therapy. Usually, amphotericin B or itraconazole has been administered with variable results. The prognosis is poor, undoubtedly in large part because aspergillosis, when it occurs, is nearly always a very late complication of progressive HIV disease.

Candida Species

Virtually all species of the genus *Candida*, but especially *C. albicans* and *C. tropicalis*, can cause candidiasis, which is defined as the invasion of viable tissue by the microorganisms. Mucocutaneous candidiasis, particularly oral thrush, is the most common opportunistic infection of progressive HIV disease and is recognized as an ominous finding that heralds the onset of AIDS (Klein et al., 1984). *Candida* esophagitis is another relatively common manifestation. However, despite the high frequency of mucocutaneous involvement in patients with HIV infection, pulmonary candidiasis is distinctly uncommon and is rarely diagnosed antemortem (Welch et al., 1984). Because of the small number of documented cases of pulmonary candidiasis, neither the clinical features nor the therapy is established. It is clear, however, that tissue invasion must be demonstrated by transbronchial biopsy for a convincing diagnosis; identification of the fungus in respiratory secretions by culture alone is insufficient.

Other Fungi

Pulmonary infections of patients with HIV-induced immune suppression by fungi, other than those already discussed, are surprisingly rare. One patient dually infected with *H. capsulatum* and with *Paracoccidioides brasiliensis* and another with disseminated penicilliosis, caused by *Penicillium marneffei*, have been reported (Johnson et al., 1988; Piehl et al., 1988). Four cases of disseminated blastomycosis are known (Sarosi, G. A., personal communication), but details have not yet been reported. Sporadic infections with these and other fungi are likely to occur in the future as patients with severe HIV disease live longer and longer.

D. Parasites

Several unicellular and multicellular parasites are known to cause disease in immunosuppressed hosts with HIV infection. Of these, *P. carinii* is by far the most common and important serious complication, infectious or malignant, of patients with AIDS in developed countries. *P. carinii* pneumonia has been the most common index diagnosis of AIDS in the United States, accounting for nearly two-thirds of all cases, and an additional 15–20% of patients with AIDS of some other origin will develop this pneumonia at some time during the course of their disease (CDC, 1989c). However, as the use of effective chemoprophylaxis against *P. carinii* is increasing, its importance as a cause of morbidity and mortality seems to be decreasing, but precise incidence figures are not yet available. *Toxoplasma gondii* and *Cryptosporidium* usually cause central nervous system and gastrointestinal disease, respectively, but can also involve the lungs. Disseminated disease from *Strongyloides stercoralis* is a rare complication of AIDS.

Pneumocystis carinii

P. carinii is usually classified as a parasite, as shown in Table 1, but there is increasing evidence that it is a fungus (for review and references, see Murray and Mills, 1990). Organisms morphologically identical to *P. carinii* are found in virtually all mammalian species examined, and the results of recent studies have confirmed that human and rat variants of *Pneumocystis* are closely related, although immunologically distinct (Kovacs et al., 1989a). The environmental reservoir for *P. carinii* and its method of transmission are unknown, but most evidence favors airborne communication. Pneumonia in humans is believed to result from reactivation of latent infection in the lungs that, according to serological studies, is acquired early in childhood and persists through adult life (Pifer et al., 1978).

The immunological defects that lead to *P. carinii* pneumonia are not well understood but, presumably, a deficiency of cell-mediated immunity is of considerable importance. Disease begins by reactivation of latent infection in the lungs, and there is an overall correlation between the number of parasites in the lungs and the severity of the pathological abnormalities, although wide variations in this relationship are found in individual patients (Greico et al., 1989). Alveolar spaces are filled with an acellular, eosinophilic, proteinaceous material that contains cysts and trophozoites of the organism and scarce inflammatory cells (Weber et al., 1977). Direct invasion of the interstitium is uncommon. Occasionally, patients will have a granulomatous reaction to pulmonary *Pneumocystis* (Blumenfeld et al., 1988), and interstitial fibrosis may develop following successful treatment of the infection (Whitcomb et al., 1970).

The most consistent functional abnormality in patients with *P. carinii* pneumonia is impairment of gas exchange, often substantial, from either a ventilation-perfusion abnormality or a right-to-left shunt, because of poor distribution of inspired air into alveoli that are partly or completely filled with parasites and inflammatory debris (Stover and Meduri, 1988). Diffusing capacity for carbon monoxide is nearly always decreased. Reductions in lung volumes (vital capacity and total lung capacity) reflect the degree of alveolar filling. Pulmonary compliance is also reduced, perhaps because of interstitial inflammation, which is usually present to some extent, or because of abnormalities in surface forces, which have been described in an experimental model (Sheehan et al., 1986).

Clinical Features

P. carinii pneumonia is a late manifestation of HIV infection and seldom occurs in adults until their CD4+ lymphocyte counts are below $200/mm^3$; in most series the median CD4 counts have been less than $100/mm^3$ (CDC, 1989c; Masur et al., 1989a). In contrast, for reasons that are poorly understood but that probably relate to their incompletely developed immune systems, infants with HIV infection who develop *P. carinii* pneumonia are apt to have much higher CD4+ cell counts than adults (Leibovitz et al., 1990). Patients with *P. carinii* pneumonia commonly present with fever, a nonproductive cough, and dyspnea on exertion. Patients with HIV infection complicated by *P. carinii* pneumonia usually have a slowly progressive illness with a median duration of symptoms of nearly 1 month, in comparison with only 5 days in other immunosuppressed patients (Kovacs et al., 1984). However, the tempo of the illness varies greatly from patient to patient. On physical examination, the lungs of patients with *P. carinii* pneumonia are usually normal, but associated abnormalities, such as thrush, hairy leukoplakia, or Kaposi's sarcoma, may be detected that are useful in patients without a prior AIDS diagnosis and in those not known to have risk factors for HIV infection. Numerous studies have shown that serum lactate dehydrogenase levels are elevated in approximately 80% of patients with *P. carinii* pneumonia, in comparison with only about 20% in patients with other types of pulmonary infection, and that increases or decreases in serum concentrations reflect worsening or improvement in the severity of infection (Medina et al., 1987).

Although there were certainly variations on the central theme, from 1981 until a few years ago, most cases of *P. carinii* pneumonia had fairly stereotypical clinical, radiographic, and laboratory characteristics (Levine and White, 1988). Now, two unusual features of *P. carinii* infection are being encountered with apparently increasing frequency: atypical chest radiographic patterns and extrapulmonary involvement. Both these manifestations have been attributed to the recent widespread use of chemoprophylaxis with aerosolized pentamidine, although admittedly these features were observed before this form of preventive therapy was in vogue.

Typical chest radiographic findings include a diffuse alveolointerstitial infiltrate, often described as a "ground-glass" pattern, with a predominance in the lung bases. Normal chest radiographs have occurred in about 10% of our patients at San Francisco General Hospital (Goodman and Gamsu, 1987). Less frequent abnormalities are focal infiltrates, nodules, and cavities or pneumatoceles; mediastinal adenopathy and pleural effusion are rare and, when present, suggest another diagnosis (for review and references, see Murray and Mills, 1990). However, since the advent of chemoprophylaxis with aerosolized pentamidine, clinicians and radiologists have been impressed by a striking increase in the number of patients who present with upper rather than lower lobe predominance of the infiltrates (Chaffey et al., 1990) and pneumothorax (Sepkowitz et al., 1991) with or without obvious pneumatoceles (Jules-Elysee et al., 1990). The atypical distribution is probably best explained by the poorer deposition of pentamidine particles in the upper lung zones compared to the lower lung zones when the aerosol is inhaled while sitting or standing; more uniform distribution is attained when the aerosol is inhaled while supine (Baskin et al., 1990). The mechanisms underlying the apparent incidence in frequency of pneumothorax and formation of pneumatoceles are not known, but speculations concerning their pathogenesis include the effects of zidovudine (AZT) and other anti-HIV drugs; because these agents enhance immune capabilities, they also promote the development of necrosis in the lungs in response to the parasites; necrosis, in turn, could underlie the occurrence of both rupture and pneumatocele.

Virtually all cases of *P. carinii* infection involve only the lungs, although its rare ability to disseminate has been recognized for many years. The authors of a new review of the subject have related an apparent recent increase in disseminated *P. carinii* infection to topical chemoprophylaxis with aerosolized pentamidine; extrapulmonary disease has not been reported in patients receiving systemic chemoprophylaxis with trimethoprim-sulfamethoxazole or dapsone (Northfelt et al., 1990). Reported sites of dissemination include the reticuloendothelial system, the skin, pararespiratory structures, the central nervous system, and rarely elsewhere (for review and references, see Murray and Mills, 1990). Although the link between aerosolized pentamidine and extrapulmonary pneumocystosis has not been confirmed, clinicians should be aware of this possible relationship.

Diagnosis

The diagnosis of *Pneumocystis* infection in the lungs and other organs depends entirely on finding morphologically compatible stained organisms by microscopic examination of tissues or body fluids, because the parasite cannot be cultured reliably in vitro. *P. carinii* can be detected in expectorated or induced sputum, pulmonary secretions obtained by nasotracheal suction, bronchoalveolar lavage, or percutaneous aspiration of the lung parenchyma, and in pulmonary tissue obtained by either transbronchial or open lung biopsy (for review and references, see Murray and Mills, 1990). The role of induced sputum, bronchoalveolar lavage, and transbronchial biopsy for diagnosis and the yield of various staining methods for detecting *P. carinii* organisms in respiratory specimens were described earlier in this chapter in Section II "Diagnostic Approach."

Treatment

Several drugs are available to treat *P. carinii* pneumonia in patients with AIDS (Table 4), and the history of their development and usage has recently been reviewed (Murray and Mills, 1990). Two of these agents, trimethoprim-sulfamethoxazole and pentamidine, are approved in the United States for the treatment of the infection, but both are associated with a high frequency of adverse reactions (Masur et al., 1989b). The alternative drugs are used in cases of treatment failure or toxicity to the two principal agents.

Trimethoprim-sulfamethoxazole is considered the drug of choice, largely because when initially tested in non-HIV-immunocompromised hosts with *Pneumocystis* pneumonia, it was better tolerated than pentamidine. Although a therapeutic advantage to trimethoprim-sulfamethoxazole has not been found in some studies comparing the two drugs in patients with HIV disease (Wharton et al., 1986), in the largest controlled trial to date a 21-day course of trimethoprim-sulfamethoxazole was significantly more effective than pentamidine; however, toxicity occurred with equal frequency (about 90%) with both drugs (Sattler et al., 1988). Trimethoprim-sulfamethoxazole has the added advantage that its antimicrobial spectrum provides coverage against many bacteria that may cause

Table 4 Drugs Used for Treatment and Prevention of *P. carinii* Pneumonia in Patients with HIV Infection

Treatment	Prevention
Trimethoprim-sulfamethoxazole	Trimethoprim-sulfamethoxazole
Pentamidine (intravenous)	Pentamidine (aerosolization)
Dapsone-trimethoprim	Dapsone
Primaquine-clindamycin	Pyrimethamine-sulfadoxine
Trimetrexate	
Under Investigation	
BW566	
WR2096	
Not recommended	
Eflornithine	

pneumonia (sometimes coexisting) in the same patients. The drug is usually administered intravenously during the first few days of treatment, and the accepted duration of therapy in AIDS patients is 3 weeks, rather than 2 weeks as in other patients, because the response is often slow and because of the high incidence of detectable organisms at the completion of 3 weeks of therapy (Wharton et al., 1986). Mild toxic effects such as headache, nausea, and vomiting are common; more severe adverse reactions include rash, fever, neutropenia, thrombocytopenia, leukopenia, and hepatitis. All these occur much more often in patients with HIV disease than in those with other immunosuppressive disorders (Gordin et al., 1984).

Like trimethoprim-sulfamethoxazole, pentamidine treatment of *P. carinii* pneumonia results in a 60–80% rate of clinical response and approximately the same rate of adverse reactions (Glatt et al., 1988). Common toxic manifestations include tachycardia, hypotension, azotemia, elevated serum potassium, hepatitis, neutropenia, thrombocytopenia, and hypocalcemia. Pentamidine also has a cytolytic effect on the islet cells of the pancreas that may lead to overt pancreatitis and to either hypoglycemia or hyperglycemia. Patients should be switched from trimethoprim-sulfamethoxazole to pentamidine when they develop unacceptable toxicity or fail to respond to the initial drug. The first indication is usually easier to discern than the second; in general, we are reluctant to switch for "failure" until well into the second week of treatment with the drug that was started initially, because response is often slow. Pentamidine has also been administered as an aerosol to treat patients with mild to moderate first episodes of *P. carinii* pneumonia and in nonrandomized trials was reasonably effective (Montgomery et al., 1987); however, two subsequent randomized studies showed an unacceptable failure rate compared with intravenous pentamidine in patients with mild to moderately severe *Pneumocystis* pneumonia, and use of the aerosol in these patients is not recommended (Soo Hoo et al., 1990; Conte et al., 1990).

Although dapsone had an unacceptably high rate of treatment failure when used alone (Mills et al., 1988), the combination of dapsone-trimethoprim appears to be as effective as trimethoprim-sulfamethoxazole or pentamidine for the treatment of mild-moderate *P. carinii* pneumonia and may be less toxic (Medina et al., 1990). Dapsone should be used cautiously or not at all in patients with glucose-6-phosphate dehydrogenase deficiency, and it also causes methemoglobinemia, although usually clinically silent.

Trimetrexate, a congener of methotrexate, is a potent inhibitor of a key enzyme of *P. carinii*, dihydrofolate reductase, and showed good efficacy when used for both initial treatment and salvage (Allegra et al., 1987). The drug must be given intravenously and at the doses currently recommended, combined with leucovorin, which is extremely expensive. Trimetrexate is recommended only for seriously ill patients with documented *P. carinii* pneumonia who fail on or are intolerant of standard chemotherapy.

The combination of primaquine and clindamycin is active in the rat model of *Pneumocystis* pneumonia, and the results of formal clinical trials are beginning to appear. The combination was effective for the initial treatment of patients with mild to moderately severe *P. carinii* pneumonia (Black et al., 1991) and also for those who had failed on or were intolerant of other drugs (Noskin et al., 1991). Additional studies are under way.

Eflornithine (often known as difluromethylornithine, or DFMO) has been used as an investigational drug for the treatment of *P. carinii* pneumonia with variable effectiveness (Golden et al., 1984; Sahai and Berry, 1989). At present, there is no justification for using this drug to treat *Pneumocystis* pneumonia except as a last resort. New, much more promising drugs, BW566 and WR2096, are being tested in ongoing clinical trials.

Adjuvant Therapy

Despite the availability of effective anti-*Pneumocystis* drugs, the mortality rate of *P. carinii* pneumonia remains appreciable: overall, 228 of the 876 patients reported by several authors died, a mortality rate of 26% (for review and references, see Allegra et al., 1987). The majority of these deaths are caused by progressive lung disease that culminates in intractable hypoxemic respiratory failure. A frequent clinical observation is that worsening often takes place suddenly 3–5 days after initiation of anti-*Pneumocystis* therapy, even in patients whose disease had been slowly progressive (Montaner et al., 1990). Two major developments that have occurred during the last 2 years, the early use of corticosteroids and a redefinition of the role of intensive care, have served to mitigate to some extent the incidence, severity, and mortality of acute respiratory failure associated with *Pneumocystis* pneumonia.

Corticosteroids. Until recently, there was no shortage of anecdotal and retrospective reports on the benefits of corticosteroids in the management of severe *P. carinii* pneumonia, but the lack of controlled trials precluded their wide acceptance as adjuvant therapy (for review and references, see Murray and Mills 1990). Now the debate is over. The National Institutes of Health (NIH)–University of California (UC) Expert Panel for Corticosteroids as Adjunctive Therapy for *Pneumocystis* Pneumonia (1990) concluded that such therapy "can clearly reduce the likelihood of death, respiratory failure, or deterioration of oxygenation in patients with moderate-to-severe pneumocystis pneumonia." The panel further recommended that corticosteroids be used as adjunctive therapy in adults or adolescents (children >13 years old) with documented or suspected *Pneumocystis* pneumonia if they are hypoxic, as defined by an arterial P_{O_2} of <70 mmHg or an alveolar-arterial P_{O_2} difference of 35 mmHg. Adjunctive corticosteroids, either oral prednisone or intravenous methylprednisolone, should be started when specific anti-*Pneumocystis* treatment is begun; a delay in the administration of corticosteroids nullifies their effectiveness. (For a description and analysis of the five studies on which these recommendations are based, see the NIH-UC Expert Panel, 1990.) Physicians need to be careful about using corticosteroids in patients with suspected—not proved—*Pneumocystis* pneumonia. There is no reason why these drugs cannot be used along with anti-*Pneumocystis* treatment in patients who meet the indications while diagnostic efforts are under way. But if no diagnosis or some other diagnosis is made, the need for corticosteroids must be carefully reevaluated.

Intensive Care. One of the results of the first National Institutes of Health workshop on the pulmonary complications of HIV infection, at which physicians met to pool their collective experience, was the realization that respiratory failure during a first episode of *P. carinii* pneumonia, if severe enough to warrant endotracheal intubation and mechanical ventilation, had a mortality rate of 86% (Murray et al., 1984). Subsequent reports from individual hospitals confirmed this unfavorable prognosis; 39 of 45 patients died who were intubated and ventilated for *Pneumocystis* pneumonia at San Francisco General Hospital, a mortality rate of 87% (Wachter et al., 1986). Accordingly, in many institutions, including our own, aggressive treatment of *Pneumocystis*-induced acute respiratory failure in intensive care units was actively discouraged. Recently, however, this has changed because the outcome is no longer as bad as it used to be: for example, mortality at our hospital was 86% during the years 1981–1985, but decreased to 60% during the years 1986–1988 (Wachter et al., 1991). The reasons for the reduced mortality are not entirely clear, but early treatment with corticosteroids undoubtedly contributes. We believe that improved patient selection and careful restriction of fluids in these patients—whose lungs are leaky—are also helpful. As expected, the improved outcome has created increased utilization of intensive care units for the management of *P. carinii* pneumonia and its complications.

Prevention

Given the high rate of recurrence of *P. carinii* pneumonia after successful initial therapy (at least 50% within 1 year), secondary chemoprophylaxis to prevent these episodes is mandatory. Of equal importance is the CDC (1989c) recommendation that primary chemoprophylaxis to prevent the onset of infection be initiated in all HIV-seropositive patients at high risk of developing *P. carinii* infection, including persons with 200 or fewer peripheral blood CD4+ lymphocytes/mm^3, those whose CD4+ cell counts are less than 20% of total lymphocytes, and those with prolonged fever, weight loss, or oral thrush. Although the CDC (1989c) recommends the use of either oral trimethoprim-sulfamethoxazole or aerosolized pentamidine, oral dapsone also appears to be beneficial for both primary and secondary prophylaxis and has the advantage of low cost and minimal toxicity (Klein, 1989).

The results of a controlled trial in patients with advanced Kaposi's sarcoma showed that no episodes of *Pneumocystis* pneumonia occurred in 30 patients who received trimethoprim-sulfamethoxazole, whereas 16 episodes occurred in 30 patients who took placebo; however, the active drug had to be stopped in 17% of the recipients because of rash, leukopenia, hepatitis, or other serious toxicity (Fischl et al., 1988). Aerosolized pentamidine appears to be better tolerated than trimethoprim-sulfamethoxazole, but does not completely prevent new-onset *P. carinii* pneumonia (Hirschel et al., 1991) or relapses in those who have already had the disease (Leoung et al., 1990; Montaner et al., 1991). The benefits of aerosolized pentamidine must depend in large part on how much drug reaches the alveoli in which the parasites are living. Alveolar deposition depends chiefly on particle size and the delivered dose, which vary considerably from one nebulizer to another; breathing pattern is also important (Smaldone et al., 1991). It is clear that neither the optimal drug nor the optimal dose for the prevention of *Pneumocystis* pneumonia has yet been found. Trials are presently under way to compare the relative prophylactic effectiveness of oral trimethoprim-sulfamethoxazole, aerosolized pentamidine, and oral dapsone; other studies are evaluating the usefulness of dapsone-pyrimethamine and pyrimethamine-sulfadoxine (Fansidar). The results of these investigations should have considerable effect on future practice. Drugs such as trimethoprim-sulfamethoxazole, dapsone, and pyrimethamine-sulfadoxine, if safe and effective in the prevention of *P. carinii* pneumonia, would be desirable because they would also prevent toxoplasmosis (Girard et al., 1991).

Toxoplasma gondii

Infection of the brain by *T. gondii* is a well-recognized complication of late HIV disease and is the most common cause of focal brain abscesses in patients with AIDS. However, in contrast to the frequency with which this organism causes central nervous system disease, pulmonary involvement has been recognized only sporadically, and seldom during life. The incidence of HIV-related toxoplasmosis is higher in Western Europe and Africa than in North America, presumably because of differences in diet and eating habits. Patients who develop toxoplasmosis have advanced immunosuppression, as shown by the fact that many of them have already had an AIDS-defining diagnosis, and that their mean CD4+ lymphocyte counts are low; mean values were $32/mm^3$ in one series (Oksenhendler et al., 1990) and $87/mm^3$ in another (S. Matheron, cited by Girard et al., 1991).

In the largest reported series of pulmonary toxoplasmosis, 13 cases, all patients had fever and diffuse bilateral pulmonary infiltrations, extrapulmonary involvement was present in seven, and serological evidence of past infection was observed in 11 of the 12 patients in whom it was looked for (Oksenhendler et al., 1990). Similar features were noted in the seven patients with pulmonary toxoplasmosis diagnosed at San Francisco General Hospital, except that two had pleural effusions, and none had clinically significant central nervous system involvement (Schnapp et al., 1991). The diagnosis in the patients reported in both series was frequently made by finding the tachyzoites of *T. gondii* in bronchoalveolar lavage fluid; transbronchial biopsy was helpful but induced sputum was of no value. Pulmonary toxoplasmosis usually responds to treatment with pyrimethamine and sulfadiazine, and chemoprophylaxis has been recommended for HIV-infected patients with serological evidence of past *Toxoplasma* infection and CD4+ lymphocyte counts $< 200/mm^3$ (Girard et al., 1991). It now seems clear that *T. gondii* pneumonia must be considered in the differential diagnosis of diffuse pulmonary disease and, rarely, pleural effusion in patients with advanced HIV-related immune depression.

Other Parasites

Several cases of pulmonary cryptosporidiosis in patients with intestinal cryptosporidial infection have been reported (for review and references, see Murray and Mills, 1990). The hyperinfection syndrome with *Strongyloides stercoralis* has been documented in one patient with AIDS, but was unusual in that it was associated with meningitis and not with pulmonary disease (Maayan et al., 1987). We have seen two cases of pulmonary strongyloidiasis as part of widely disseminated disease, but both patients were receiving large doses of corticosteroids as treatment of AIDS-associated cerebral lymphoma. *Strongyloides* hyperinfection does not seem to be an important HIV-related complication, even in developing countries where the parasite is endemic.

IV. Noninfectious Disorders

In the evaluation of patients with known or suspected HIV-related lung disease, attention has rightly been directed toward prompt identification of the various pulmonary infections, because these are extremely common, usually treatable, and, in the case of tuberculosis, transmissible to other persons, whether HIV-infected or not. However, HIV-infected patients are also susceptible to a wide variety of noninfectious pulmonary complications of evolving immunosuppression. Some of these are AIDS-defining, some are not, but all need to be diagnosed because the indications for and types of treatment vary considerably.

A. Malignancies

Two quite different AIDS-related malignancies, Kaposi's sarcoma and non-Hodgkin's lymphoma, may involve the lung parenchyma, airways, pleura, or hilar or mediastinal lymph nodes. Intrathoracic disease from both neoplasms is usually a late manifestation of involvement already recognized elsewhere, but occasionally these malignancies begin in the thorax, and they are frequently complicated by coexisting pulmonary infections; thus, as outlined in this section, specific diagnosis is required for each instance of new respiratory manifestations.

Kaposi's Sarcoma

The most common HIV-associated malignancy is Kaposi's sarcoma, although the incidence of this neoplasm has decreased dramatically since the beginning of the AIDS epidemic. Kaposi's sarcoma was the indicator disease in one-third of the first 1000 patients diagnosed with AIDS who were reported by the CDC; the fraction decreased to one-quarter of the 16,500 cases reported up to the end of January 1986; and then decreased even further to one-tenth of the 11,000 cases reported to the CDC between January and August 1987 (Des Jarlais et al., 1987). Similar trends were noted in San Francisco, where the percentage of patients with AIDS who presented with or who developed Kaposi's sarcoma at some time during their illness declined from 60 to 20% between 1981 and 1987 (Rutherford et al., 1989). The incidence of Kaposi's sarcoma has always been higher in male homosexuals than in intravenous drug abusers. Although Kaposi's sarcoma is known to complicate other immunosuppressive disorders, the link, albeit changing, with HIV infection is by far the most impressive and may provide important clues to the pathogenesis of this curious malignancy. The two main theories of origin are either that HIV infection itself triggers cellular mechanisms that promote the development of Kaposi's sarcomatous lesions, or that HIV infection plus a cofactor, perhaps a virus such as cytomegalovirus, interact to cause malignant transformation of vulnerable cells.

Clinical Features

Three recurrent features of most reports about the intrathoracic manifestations of HIV-related Kaposi's sarcoma are (1) that respiratory involvement nearly always (in 90–95% of patients) follows rather than precedes the development of mucocutaneous lesions; (2) that the frequency of pulmonary involvement that can be documented at autopsy (50%) is higher than that detected clinically (33%); and most important, (3) that approximately two-thirds of patients with known Kaposi's sarcoma who present with new pulmonary findings actually have a coexisting, usually treatable, opportunistic infection (for review and references see White and Matthay, 1989). These observations emphasize the need to evaluate each patient with Kaposi's sarcoma who is found to have pulmonary manifestations not only for intrathoracic spread of the malignancy, but for respiratory tract infections as well.

The most common respiratory manifestations of Kaposi's sarcoma are dyspnea, nonproductive cough, and fever; chest pain and hemoptysis are less frequently noted. Physical examination of the chest is often normal, but crackles, generalized or localized wheezes, and signs of pleural effusion have been observed. Findings on chest radiographs are more helpful than those on history or physical examination in documenting the location and severity of intrathoracic involvement.

Four predominant patterns of radiographic abnormalities have been described: (1) parenchymal involvement that consists of nonuniform linear densities that follow septal lines; (2) parenchymal involvement that consists of nodular lesions of various sizes and in varying locations; (3) pleural effusions on one or both sides of the chest that may vary considerably in size; and (4) hilar and/or mediastinal adenopathy (Heitzman, 1990). Segmental or lobar infiltrations have also been reported, although less commonly. None of these patterns is specific for Kaposi's sarcoma, and all may be found in patients with various respiratory infections. Moreover, in patients with known pulmonary Kaposi's sarcoma, the onset of a complicating lung infection may produce only very subtle changes in the already abnormal chest radiograph.

Diagnosis

Patients with Kaposi's sarcoma who develop new pulmonary infiltrations should be worked up using the methods already described (i.e., induced sputum followed by bronchoalveolar lavage); at bronchoscopy the finding of characteristic red or violacious flat or slightly raised lesions is sufficient to diagnose bronchopulmonary Kaposi's sarcoma, but the presence of these lesions, obviously, does not rule out the coexistence of an infection, nor does their absence rule out either parenchymal involvement by the neoplasm or a coexisting infection. Direct or transbronchial biopsy of the airway or parenchymal abnormalities, respectively, is seldom diagnostic and is not recommended; even open lung biopsy has failed to diagnose Kaposi's sarcoma when it was present (Garay et al., 1987). Patients with pleural effusion should have a thoracentesis, primarily to exclude the presence of an infection, such as pyogenic empyema or tuberculous or fungal pleurisy. Isolated intrathoracic adenopathy should be evaluated by transbronchial (Wang) or percutaneous computed tomographic-directed biopsy, in an effort to diagnose an infection such as tuberculosis, not Kaposi's sarcoma.

Treatment

When pulmonary involvement occurs as a late complication of widespread Kaposi's sarcoma, the response to further therapy is usually unsatisfactory. The use of interferon-alpha, a biological response modifier, in conjunction with zidovudine may cause remission in patients with CD4+ T-cell counts greater than 200/mm^3 who have not had prior opportunistic infections (Kovacs et al., 1989b). For early or moderately advanced involvement, chemotherapy, usually with multiple agents, may control the rate of growth and spread. Large bulky lesions, especially those causing airway obstruction, often respond transiently to radiation treatment. Rapidly recurring pleural effusions may present a difficult therapeutic problem; sclerotherapy is recommended but is not always successful.

Non-Hodgkin's Lymphoma

There are some interesting similarities and differences between non-Hodgkin's lymphoma and Kaposi's sarcoma, the two most common AIDS-associated malignancies. The similarities are that both have been documented as complications of other immunosuppressive disorders, both may have a predilection for homosexual men, and when they occur in HIV-infected patients, both are extremely aggressive in their clinical behavior. The chief differences are that the incidence of AIDS-related Kaposi's sarcoma is decreasing, whereas that of non-Hodgkin's lymphoma appears to be increasing, and that intrathoracic involvement is more common in AIDS-associated Kaposi's sarcoma than in non-Hodgkin's lymphoma. The increasing incidence of non-Hodgkin's lymphoma is probably an important prelude to the future and is almost certainly attributable to the changing natural history of advanced HIV disease with increased survival of patients because of effective antiretroviral therapy (Plauda et al., 1990) and effective chemoprophylaxis against *P. carinii* pneumonia. Although the pathogenesis of lymphoma in patients with HIV infection is unknown, diffuse B-cell stimulation is believed to play a role, and 17 cases have been reported in which Epstein-Barr virus was implicated (for review and references, see Cohen, 1991).

Clinical Features

At the time of diagnosis, patients with AIDS-related lymphoma usually have widely disseminated disease with frequent extranodal involvement. Despite this presentation, intrathoracic involvement is not especially common; the reported incidence of respiratory tract disease varies from 0 to 25% of patients at the time of clinical diagnosis and is usually higher at the time of autopsy (for review and references, see White and Matthay, 1989). The radiographic abnormalities that were compiled from a review of 14 articles that described 23 cases included pleural effusion (47%), reticulonodular disease or alveolar consolidation (22%), hilar and/or mediastinal adenopathy (22%), and nodular or mass densities (17%); although most other investigators have observed similar manifestations, their reported frequency varies considerably (for review and references, see Haskal et al., 1990).

Diagnosis

The diagnosis of non-Hodgkin's lymphoma, with or without intrathoracic involvement, is nearly always made by histological examination of biopsy specimens obtained from nonthoracic sites. A few cases have been diagnosed by pleural biopsy (Knowles et al., 1988; Sider and Horton, 1989). Bronchoscopy does not appear to be helpful, although reported experience is limited (White and Matthay, 1989).

Treatment

Most patients with AIDS-associated non-Hodgkin's lymphoma respond poorly to treatment with multiple cytotoxic drugs. The low survival is linked to the preponderance of high-grade histological abnormalities and poor bone marrow reserve in these patients. Radiation therapy may provide some palliation from local complications, including those in the thorax, related to bulky, compressive infiltrations. New studies are testing whether marrow-stimulating cytokines can mitigate neutropenia and allow higher doses of chemotherapy to be administered.

Other Malignancies

All physicians who deal with large numbers of patients with HIV disease find occasional cases of other solid tumors, especially Hodgkin's disease and bronchogenic carcinoma. There is, however, no convincing (or "official") partnership between these malignancies and the HIV infection, and their association is explained as the coexistence of two common disorders. Nevertheless, the neoplasms are likely to be highly malignant and to be clinically very aggressive, features that are attributable to the enhanced biological behavior conferred by underlying HIV-induced immunosuppression.

B. Interstitial Pneumonitis

The term "interstitial pneumonitis" (or pneumonia) means different things to different people. In this section the heading is used in its generic sense to refer to certain pneumonias that are characterized by an inflammatory process, which may vary from an acute cellular infiltration to chronic fibrosis, that is mainly situated in the interstitial space of the interalveolar septum; there may be some "spillover" of the commonly associated alveolitis into the alveolar space, but frank alveolar consolidation is not a prominent feature (Murray, 1989b). The infectious pneumonias, which tend to be consolidative, are discussed elsewhere. This section will consider the noninfectious pneumonitides listed in Table 1.

Lymphocytic Interstitial Pneumonitis

Practically from the time it was first described by Carrington and Liebow (1966), there has been uncertainty whether lymphocytic interstitial pneumonitis (LIP) is a pathogenetically distinct entity or a disorder of multiple etiologies that all cause a similar pathological reaction. The fact that LIP occurs with increased frequency in persons with HIV infection and is diagnostic of AIDS when found in a seropositive child less than 13 years of age favors the diverse-origin theory. Histological abnormalities of LIP consist of diffuse infiltration of the lung parenchyma by mature lymphocytes, plasma cells, plasmacytoid lymphocytes, and immunoblasts; an apparently related disorder, pulmonary lymphoid hyperplasia (PLH), has similar features, but the aggregates of lymphoid cells, with or without germinal centers, are more conspicuous and are located in peribronchovascular regions (Joshi, et al., 1984). Now it is generally accepted that there is a continuum of benign lymphoid infiltrative disorders of the lung in HIV disease that includes LIP at one end and PLH at the other, with considerable overlap in between (Joshi and Oleske, 1986).

The cause of HIV-related LIP is unknown. As stated earlier (see ''Other Viruses''), Epstein-Barr virus and HIV itself have each been implicated in the cause of lymphoproliferative disorders. It is also possible that the two viruses act in concert, in view of the in vitro observation that Epstein-Barr–infected cells are unusually susceptible to infection by HIV (Montagnier et al., 1984).

Clinical Features

The truly striking feature of LIP in HIV-infected persons is its incidence in different age groups. In early reports of AIDS in infants and children, LIP accounted for nearly half of all reported cases; now, the frequency is somewhat less, perhaps one-third, but this is still remarkably higher than its incidence in adults, in whom it is rare (Pitt, 1991). Noteworthy manifestations in children include slowly progressive dyspnea and failure to thrive; clubbing is often observed. Lymphadenopathy and hepatosplenomegaly have been reported in both children and adults. In non-HIV-infected adults LIP has been associated with Sjögren's syndrome, including parotid gland enlargement and xerostomia; accordingly, it is of interest that 10 of 17 patients with an HIV-related diffuse lymphocytic disorder resembling Sjögren's syndrome also had LIP (Itescu et al., 1990).

The chest radiograph of LIP at all ages shows bilateral reticulonodular ''interstitial'' infiltrations with a lower zone predominance. Hilar and/or mediastinal adenopathy sometimes coexists. Most reports of the results of gallium scintigraphy have noted diffuse uptake. Hypergammaglobulinemia is seen in both children and adults with HIV-associated LIP, but it also occurs in patients with non-HIV-linked LIP (for review and references, see White and Matthay, 1989) and is common in otherwise uncomplicated HIV infection.

Diagnosis

Classically, the diagnosis of LIP requires histological confirmation, but this, in turn, requires open lung biopsy, which no one likes to do (or to have). There are two ways of avoiding open lung biopsy and of making a reasonably secure diagnosis of LIP: (1) by performing a bronchoalveolar lavage and finding large numbers of lymphocytes with an increased ratio of T8 to T4 cell, as shown in Table 5; (2) by documenting the radiographic presence of chronic bilateral reticulonodular infiltrations that are unresponsive to appropriate antimicrobial treatment for likely pathogens during a period of 2 or more months.

Treatment

The natural history of HIV-associated LIP is not well understood, and it is unclear whether treatment is warranted. In infants and children whose clinical course is deteriorating, corticosteroids are often administered, at times with apparently beneficial results. But because spontaneous remissions have been well documented, the effects of therapy are difficult to evaluate. It is clear, however, that the prognosis of LIP is much better in childhood AIDS than when the indicator diagnosis is either recurrent bacterial infections or *P. carinii* pneumonia (Pitt, 1991). There are so few cases among adults and the course is so variable that it is impossible to recommend a specific treatment.

Nonspecific Interstitial Pneumonitis

The pulmonary disorder nonspecific interstitial pneumonitis (NIP) has been reported with varying frequencies in patients with HIV infection (Stover et al., 1985; Suffredini et al., 1987). NIP refers to the pathological finding of an

Table 5 Cellular Composition of Bronchoalveolar Lavage Liquid

Variable	Normals	HIV asympt.	HIV-LIP
Total cells, per mm^3	150	150	500
Lymphocytes, %	<15	10–20	35
CD4+ T cells, %	50	25	3
CD8+ T cells, %	30	64	85
CD4+/CD8+	1.7	0.4	0.04

interstitial inflammatory infiltration of mononuclear cells, predominantly lymphocytes and plasma cells, with edema and fibrin deposition; known causes of inflammation, such as previous *P. carinii* pneumonia, drugs, oxygen, radiation, or occult viral infection, must be excluded, which is often difficult or impossible. Because NIP is a histological diagnosis, its incidence in HIV-infected patients depends on how often biopsy is performed during the workup for suspected lung disease and how much emphasis is put on the findings. In most instances the abnormalities are mild, and some consider them ''nondiagnostic'' (Barrio et al., 1987).

Clinical Features

The clinical findings that may accompany NIP include respiratory symptoms, usually exertional dyspnea or cough, fever, and the presence of chest radiographic abnormalities, mainly bilateral interstitial or fine reticulonodular infiltrations. These features, however, occurred in patients who were sick enough to warrant biopsy for evaluation. Now we know that identical histological abnormalities may occur in persons without symptoms and with normal chest radiographs; the only fairly consistent finding in these subjects, who were evaluated as part of a research study, was a mild reduction of carbon monoxide diffusing capacity (Ognibene et al., 1988).

Diagnosis

It seems definite that NIP is part of the spectrum of HIV-related interstitial pneumonitides, and that it must be diagnosed by histological examination. That being said, one is always uncomfortable with the diagnosis of NIP, because there are so many other important, treatable diseases that look exactly the same clinically and radiographically, and because of the possibility of sampling error at the time of biopsy.

Treatment

The natural history of HIV-associated NIP is not well understood, but it usually resolves or stabilizes without therapy. Observation is all that is required, with the proviso that, if the patient is severely sick or deteriorating, which should not occur in uncomplicated NIP, repeat bronchoscopy and biopsy is indicated to look for another disorder.

Lymphocytic Alveolitis

Another product of the widespread use of bronchoalveolar lavage in patients at various stages of evolving HIV disease has been the identification of a group of subjects who have a striking increase in both the absolute number and percentage of T lymphocytes recoverable from their lungs (Table 5), a condition now called lymphocytic alveolitis (Guillon et al., 1988). It was recognized at the outset that the excess lymphocytes were of the suppressor-cytotoxic phenotype, and the results of recent studies have further characterized the cells functionally as cytotoxic and phenotypically as bearing CD8+D44+ surface markers. Because these cells killed HIV-infected macrophages, it was postulated that lymphocytic alveolitis was caused by an HIV-specific host defense reaction in the lungs of infected persons (Autran et al., 1988). The latest development in this emerging story is the observation that those patients with the highest number of CD8+D44+ cells had increased clearance from their lungs of aerosolized ^{99m}Tc-DTPA, a test that estimates alveolar epithelial permeability; these findings supported the author's contention that lymphocytic alveolitis is the result of "immunological conflict" in the alveolar epithelium of HIV-infected patients (Meignan et al., 1990).

Excess T lymphocytes were found by bronchoalveolar lavage in 70% of HIV-infected patients without detectable pulmonary infections or malignancies (Guillon et al., 1988); the cells appear early and then gradually disappear as HIV disease evolves. Most patients had minimal symptoms, radiographic findings, and functional abnormalities, but when present, these correlated, roughly, with the number and percentage of T lymphocytes in the lavage liquid (Plata et al., 1987). Lymphocytic alveolitis has been described in primary HIV (seroconversion) disease (Longworth et al., 1990), an illness now known to be associated with high levels of viremia (Daar et al., 1991). There is no doubt that HIV infects the lungs (Rose et al., 1991; Linnemann et al., 1989), but its role in the pathogenesis of HIV-related lymphocytic alveolitis, LIP, and NIP, on the one hand, and the interrelationships among these three interstitial pneumonitides, on the other, are unknown and await further investigations.

Drug-Induced Reactions

Interstitial pneumonia may develop in HIV-infected patients who are receiving trimethoprim-sulfamethoxazole for the treatment of *P. carinii* pneumonia or cytotoxic drugs for the treatment of AIDS-associated malignancies. Fever, rash, and neutropenia are common adverse reactions to trimethoprim-sulfamethoxazole and occur more frequently than in non-HIV-infected patients (Gordin et al., 1984); in addition, the trimethoprim-sulfamethoxazole was associated with the onset of new pulmonary infiltrations and hypoxemia that recurred when the drug was reintroduced (Silvestri et al., 1987). Whether HIV-infected patients are unusually likely to develop interstitial pneumonitis when treated with cytotoxic drugs is unknown, but possible toxicity from bleomycin has been reported (for review and references, see White and Matthay, 1989). The frequent occurrence of coexisting infections and the short duration of survival complicate analysis.

C. Other Disorders

A few other disorders deserve brief comment for the sake of completeness, although all are extremely unusual pulmonary complications of HIV infection.

Adult Respiratory Distress Syndrome

The nebulous disorder adult respiratory distress syndrome (ARDS) has been associated with a wide variety of systemic and pulmonary disorders in the absence of HIV infection. (Murray et al., 1988). ARDS has also been diagnosed in patients with HIV-associated disorders, usually sepsis (Stover et al., 1985). Patients with *P. carinii* pneumonia may present with all the radiographic and physiological features of ARDS of unknown etiology, but, obviously, the implications for diagnosis and treatment differ between the two varieties. Patients with AIDS-related tuberculosis may also have a sepsis-like presentation, complete with ARDS, presumably caused by septicemia from *M. tuberculosis* alone (Gachot, 1990); similar features have been observed in disseminated histoplasmosis (Wheat et al., 1990).

Secondary Alveolar Proteinosis

Two cases of what were called ''secondary alveolar proteinosis'' have been reported by Rubin and Talamo (1986). Both patients had had AIDS-related opportunistic infections; later, when they did not improve, histological examination revealed extensive intra-alveolar deposits of a lipoproteinaceous material that stained strongly with periodic acid–Schiff. The authors speculate that the alveolar proteinosis was secondary to infection, as has been reported in non-HIV-infected persons. Recently, both light and ultrastructural examination of bronchoalveolar liquid from 9 of 26 patients with *P. carinii* pneumonia showed lipoproteinaceous material highly suggestive of that described in pulmonary alveolar proteinosis (Van Nhieu et al., 1990).

Sarcoidosis

Sarcoidosis is one of the last disorders one might expect to find among the pulmonary complications of HIV infection, because in many respects the coexistence of the two diseases is incompatible: sarcoidosis is characterized by granuloma formation, which HIV infection inhibits; moreover, sarcoid-induced alveolitis consists predominantly of CD4+ lymphocytes, whereas HIV-alveolitis consists chiefly of CD8+ lymphocytes. Nevertheless, several cases of sarcoidosis associated with HIV infection have been reported (for review and references, see Lowery et al., 1990). There is overlap between the two diseases in symptoms, radiographic findings, physiological abnormalities, and lymphocyte function. The results of bronchoalveolar lavage can distinguish the cause of any associated alveolitis (see above) and help determine whether corticosteroid treatment is indicated.

V. Summary

In this review the major pulmonary complications of HIV infection have been discussed. The workup of a patient with known or suspected HIV infection and new-onset pulmonary disease has become fairly straightforward. If community-acquired pneumonia is not a consideration, diagnostic efforts begin with sputum induction, if available, and if not, with fiberoptic bronchoscopy for bronchoalveolar lavage, and in selected patients, transbronchial biopsy. If a second bronchoscopy is required, transbronchial biopsy is certainly indicated. Cultures of blood and bone marrow are useful for diagnosing disseminated mycobacterial and fungal diseases, as is biopsy of accessible lesions for diagnosing malignancies. These relatively simple methods will provide the diagnosis of virtually all the treatable pulmonary complications of HIV infection. More invasive procedures such as open lung biopsy are rarely necessary.

In contrast to the uniformity of the diagnostic approach, the concepts and methods of treatment are changing rapidly with new and rightful emphasis being placed on prevention. Increasingly wide use of zidovudine and other anti-HIV drugs and primary prevention of *Pneumocystis* pneumonia with aerosolized trimethoprim-sulfamethoxazole, pentamidine, or dapsone seem to be altering the natural history of HIV disease, largely by postponing the onset of the usual complications and, apparently, by modifying the type and/or clinical manifestations of those that finally supervene. It is important to realize that these changes are occurring, because diagnostic and therapeutic efforts need to change with them.

Acknowledgment

This work was supported by a grant from the National Heart, Lung and Blood Institute (Pulmonary Vascular SCOR, HL19155).

References

Alkan, S., and Orenstein, J. M. (1991). Bacillary peliosis hepatis (letter). *N. Engl. J. Med.* **324**:1513–1514.

Allegra, C. J., Chabner, B. A., Tuazon, C. V., Ogata-Arakaki, D., Baird, B., Drake, J. C., Simmons, J. T., Lack, E. E., Shelhamer, J. H., Balis, J., Walker, R., Kovacs, J. A., Lane, H. C., and Masur, H. (1987).

Trimetrexate for the treatment of *Pneumocystis carinii* pneumonia in patients with the acquired immunodeficiency syndrome. *N. Engl. J. Med.* **317**:978–985.

Ampel, N. W., Ryan, K. J., Carry, P. J., Wieden, M. A., and Schifman, R. B. (1986). Fungemia due to *Coccidioides immitis*. An analysis of 16 episodes in 15 patients and a review of the literature. *Medicine* **65**:312–321.

Andiman, W. A., Martin, K., Rubinstein, A., Pahwa, S., Eastman, R., Katz, B. Z., Pitt, J., and Miller, G. (1985). Opportunistic lymphoproliferations associated with the Epstein-Barr viral DNA in infants and children with AIDS. *Lancet* **2**:1390–1393.

ATS-CDC. (1987). Mycobacterioses and the acquired immunodeficiency syndrome. *Am. Rev. Respir. Dis.* **136**:492–496.

Autran, B., Mayaud, C. M., Parhael, M., Plata, F., Denis, M., Bourguin, A., Guillon, J. M., Debre, P., and Akoun, G. (1988). Evidence for a cytotoxic T lymphocyte alveolitis in HIV-infected patients. *AIDS* **2**:179–183.

Barber, T. W., Craven, D. E., and McCabe, W. R. (1990). Bacteremia due to *Mycobacterium tuberculosis* in patients with human immunodeficiency virus infection. A report of 9 cases and a review of the literature. *Medicine* **69**:375–383.

Barnes, P. F., Bloch, A. B., Davidson, P. T., and Snider, D. E., Jr. (1991) Tuberculosis in patients with human immunodeficiency virus infection. *N. Engl. J. Med.* **324**:1644–1650.

Barré-Sinoussi, F., Chermann, J. C., Rey, F., Nugeyre, M. T., Chamaret, S., Gruest, J., Dauget C., Axler-Blin, C., Vézinet-Brun, F., Rouzioux, F., Rozenbaum, W., and Montagnier, L. (1983). Isolation of a T-lymphotropic retrovirus from a patient at risk for acquired immune deficiency syndrome (AIDS) *Science* **220**:868–871.

Barrio, J. I., Harcup, C., Baier, H. J., and Pitchenik, A. E. (1987). Value of repeat fiberoptic bronchoscopies and significance of nondiagnostic bronchoscopic results in patients with the acquired immunodeficiency syndrome. *Am. Rev. Respir. Dis.* **135**:422–425.

Bartholomew, C., Raju, C., Patrick, A., Penco, F., and Jankey, N. (1984). AIDS on Trinidad (letter). *Lancet* **1**:103.

Baskin, M. I., Abd, A. G., and Ilowite, J. S. (1990). Regional deposition of aerosolized pentamidine. Effects of body position and breathing pattern. *Ann. Intern. Med.* **113**:677–683.

Beckhardt, R. N., Farady, N., May, M., Torres, R. A., and Strauchen, J. A. (1988). Increased incidence of malignant lymphoma in AIDS: a comparison of risk groups and possible etiologic factors. *Mt. Sinai J. Med.* **55**:383–389.

Bigby, T. D., Margolskee, D., Curtis, J. L., Michael, P. F., Sheppard, D., Hadley, W. K., and Hopewell, P. C. (1986). The usefulness of induced sputum in the diagnosis of *Pneumocystis carinii* pneumonia in patients with the acquired immunodeficiency syndrome. *Am. Rev. Respir. Dis.* **133**:515–518.

Black, J. R., Akil, B. J., Murphy, R., Fass, R., Feinberg, J., Mills, J., and Sattler, F. (1991). Oral clindamycin plus primaquine therapy for *Pneumocystis carinii* pneumonia (PCP) in AIDS patients (abstract). Presented at the VII International Conference on AIDS, Florence, Italy, p. 66.

Blumenfeld, W., Basgoz, N., Owen, W. F., Jr., and Schmidt, D. M. (1988). Granulomatous pulmonary lesions in patients with AIDS and *Pneumocystis carinii* infection. *Ann. Intern. Med.* **109**:505–507.

Bonner, J. R., Alexander, J., Dismukes, W. E., App, W., Griffin, F. M., Little, R., and Shin, M. S. (1984). Disseminated histoplasmosis in patients with the acquired immune deficiency syndrome. *Arch. Intern. Med.* **144**: 2178–2181.

Bottles, K., McPhaul, L. W., and Volberding, P. (1988). Fine-needle aspiration in patients with the acquired immunodeficiency syndrome (AIDS): experience in an outpatient clinic. *Ann. Intern. Med.* **108**:42–45.

Bozzette, S. A., Larsen, R. A., Chiu, J., Leal, M. A. E., Jacobsen, J., Rothman, P., Robinson, P., Gilbert, G., McCutchan, J. A., Tilles, J., Leedom, J. M., Richman, D. D., and the California Collaborative Treatment Group. (1991). Placebo-controlled trial of maintenance therapy with fluconazole after treatment of cryptococcal meningitis in the acquired immunodeficiency syndrome. *N. Engl. J. Med.* **324**:580–584.

Broaddus, V. C., Dake, M. D., Stulbarg, M. S., Blumenfeld, W., Hadley, W. K., Golden, J. A., and Hopewell, P. C. (1985). Bronchoalveolar lavage and transbronchial biopsy for the diagnosis of pulmonary infections in the acquired immunodeficiency syndrome. *Ann. Intern. Med.* **102**: 747–752.

Bronnimann, D. A., Adam, R. D., Galgiani, J. N., Habib, M., Petersen, E. A., Porter, B., and Bloom, J. W. (1987). Coccidioidomycosis in the acquired immunodeficiency syndrome. *Ann. Intern. Med.* **106**:372–379.

Carrington, C. B., and Liebow, A. A. (1966). Lymphocytic interstitial pneumonia (abstract). *Am. J. Pathol.* **48**:36a.

CDC (1985). Revision of the case definition of acquired immune deficiency syndrome for national reporting—United States. *MMWR* **34**:373–375.

CDC (1987a). Classification system for human immunodeficiency virus (HIV) infection in children under 13 years of age. *MMWR* **36**:225–236.

CDC (1987b). Diagnosis and management of mycobacterial infection and disease in persons with human immunodeficiency virus infection. *Ann. Intern. Med.* **106**:254–256.

CDC (1987c). Revision of the CDC surveillance case definition for acquired immunodeficiency syndrome. *MMWR* **36**:3s–15s.

CDC (1989a). General recommendations on immunization. *MMWR* **38**: 205–228.

CDC (1989b). Tuberculosis and human immunodeficiency virus infection: recommendations of the Advisory Committee for the Elimination of Tuberculosis (ACET). *MMWR* **39**:236–250.

CDC (1989c). Guidelines for prophylaxis against *Pneumocystis carinii* pneumonia for persons with human immunodeficiency virus infection. *MMWR* **38**:1–8.

CDC (1991). Nosocomial transmission of multidrug-resistant tuberculosis among HIV-infected persons—Florida and New York, 1988–1991. *MMWR* **40**:585–591.

Chaffey, M. H., Klein, J. S., Gamsu, G., Blanc, P., and Golden, J. A. (1990). Radiographic distribution of *Pneumocystis carinii* pneumonia in patients with AIDS treated with prophylactic inhaled pentamidine. *Radiology* **175**:715–719.

Chaisson, R. E. (1989). Bacterial pneumonia in patients with human immunodeficiency virus infection. *Semin. Resp. Infect.* **4**:133–138.

Chayt, K. J., Harper, M. E., Marselle, L. M., Lewin, E. B., Rose, R. M., Oleske, J. M., Epstein, L. G., and Wong-Staal, F. (1986). Detection of HTLV-III RNA in lungs of patients with AIDS and pulmonary involvement. *JAMA* **256**:2356–2359.

Cheychani, V., and Kamholz, S. L. (1990). Pulmonary manifestations of disseminated cryptococcosis in patients with AIDS. *Chest* **98**:1060–1066.

Chiu, J., Nussbaum, J., Bozette, S., Tilles, J. G., Young, L. S., Leedom, J., Heseltine, P. N. R., McCutchan, J. A., and the California Collaborative Treatment Group. (1990). Treatment of disseminated *Mycobacterium avium* complex infection in AIDS with amikacin, ethambutol, rifampin, and ciprofloxin. *Ann. Intern. Med.* **113**:358–361.

Chuck, S. L., and Sande, M. A. (1989). Infections with *Cryptococcus neoformans* in the acquired immunodeficiency syndrome. *N. Engl. J. Med.* **321**:794–799.

Clark, S. J., Saag, M. S., Decker, W. D., Campbell-Hill, S., Roberson, J. L., Veldkamp, P. J., Kappes, J. C., Hahn, B. H., and Shaw, G. M. (1991). High titers of cytopathic virus in plasma of patients with symptomatic primary HIV-1 infection. *N. Engl. J. Med.* **324**:954–960.

Cohen, J. I. (1991). Epstein-Barr virus lymphoproliferative disease associated with acquired immunodeficiency. *Medicine* **70**:137–160.

Cohen, P. R., Beltrani, V. P., and Grossman, M. E. (1988). Disseminated herpes zoster in patients with human immunodeficiency virus infection. *Am. J. Med.* **84**:1076–1080.

Colebunders, R. L., Ryder, R. W., Nzilambi, N., Dikilu, K., Willame, J.-C., Kaboto, M., Bagala, N., Jeugmans, J., Muepo, K., Francis, H. L.,

Mann, J. M., Quinn, T. C., and Piot, P. (1989). HIV infection in patients with tuberculosis in Kinshasa, Zaire. *Am. Rev. Respir. Dis.* **139**: 1082–1085.

Coleman, D. L., Hattner, R. S., Luce, J. M., Dodek, P. M., Golden, J. A., and Murray, J. F. (1984). Correlation between gallium lung scans and fiberoptic bronchoscopy inpatients with suspected *Pneumocystis carinii* pneumonia and the acquired immunodeficiency syndrome. *Am. Rev. Respir. Dis.* **130**:1166–1169.

Conte, J., Chernoff, D., Feigal, D. W., Jr., Joseph, P., McDonald, C., and Golden, J. A. (1990). Intravenous or inhaled pentamidine for treating *Pneumocystis carinii* pneumonia in AIDS (1990). *Ann. Intern. Med.* **113**:203–209.

Coombs, R. W., Collier, A. C., Allain, J-P., Nikora, B., Leuther, M., Gjerset, G. F., and Corey, L. (1989). Plasma viremia in human immunodeficiency virus infection. *N. Engl. J. Med.* **321**:1626–1631.

Daar, E. S., Moudgil, T., Meyer, R. D., and Ho, D. (1991). Transient high levels of viremia in patients with primary human immunodeficiency virus type 1 infection. *N. Engl. J. Med.* **324**:961–964.

Denning, D. W., Follansbee, S. E., Scolaro, M., Norris, S., Edelstein, H., and Stevens, D. A. (1991). Pulmonary aspergillosis in the acquired immunodeficiency syndrome. *N. Engl. J. Med.* **324**:654–662.

Des Jarlais, D. C., Stoneburner, R., Thomas, P., and Friedman, S. R. (1987). Declines in proportion of Kaposi's sarcoma among cases of AIDS in multiple risk groups in New York City (letter). *Lancet* **2**:1024–1025.

Dismukes, W. E., Cloud, G., Gallis, H. A., Kerkering, J. M., Medoff, G., Craven, P. C., Kaplowitz, L. G., Fisher, J. F., Gregg, C. R., Bowles, C. A., Shadomy, S., Stamm, A. M., Diasio, R. B., Kaufman, L., Soong, S-J., Blackwelder, W. C., and (1987) NIAID Mycoses Study Group. Treatment of cryptococcal meningitis with combination amphotericin B and flucytosine for four as compared with six weeks. *N. Engl. J. Med.* **317**:334–341.

Eriki, P. P., Okwera, A., Aisu, T., Morrissey, A. B., Ellner, J. J., and Daniel, T. M. (1991). The influence of human immunodeficiency virus infection on tuberculosis in Kampala, Uganda. *Am. Rev. Respir. Dis.* **143**:185–187.

Fahey, J. L., Taylor, J. M. G., Detels, R., Hofman, B., Melmed, R., Nishanian, P., and Giorgi, J. V. (1990). The prognostic value of cellular and serologic markers in infection with human immunodeficiency virus type I. *N. Engl. J. Med.* **322**:166–172.

Fels, A. O. S. (1988). Bacterial and fungal pneumonias. In White, D. A., and Stover, D. E. (eds.). Pulmonary effects of AIDS. *Clin. Chest Med.* **9**:449–457.

Fischl, M. A., Dickinson, G. M., and LaVoie, L. (1988). Safety and efficacy of sulfamethoxazole and trimethoprim chemoprophylaxis for *Pneumocystis carinii* pneumonia in AIDS. *JAMA* **259**:1185–1189.

Fish, D. G., Ampel, N. M., Galgiani, J. N., Dols, C. L., Kelly, P. C., Johnson, C. H., Pappagianis, D., Edwards, J. E., Wasserman, R. B., Clark, R. J., Antoniskis, D., Larsen, R. A., Englender, S. J., and Petersen, E. A. (1990). Coccidioidomycosis during human immunodeficiency virus infection. A review of 77 patients. *Medicine* **69**:384–391.

Fitzgerald, W., Bevelaqua, F. A., Garay, S. M., and Aranda, C. P. (1987). The role of open lung biopsy in patients with the acquired immunodeficiency syndrome. *Chest* **91**:659–661.

Fleming, A. F. (1990). Opportunistic infections in AIDS in developed and developing countries. *Trans. Roy. Soc. Trop. Med.* **84**:1–6.

Gachot, B., Wolff, B., Clair, B., and Régnier, B. (1991). Severe tuberculosis in patients with human immunodeficiency virus infection. *Intensive Care Med.* **16**:491–493.

Galgiani, J. N., and Ampel, N. M. (1990). Coccidioidomycosis in human immunodeficiency virus-infected patients. *J. Infect. Dis.* **162**:1165–1169.

Garay, S. M., Belenko, M., Fazzini, E., and Schinella, R. (1987). Pulmonary manifestations of Kaposi's sarcome. *Chest* **91**:39–43.

Gerberding, J. L., Krieger, J., and Sande, M. A. (1986). Recurrent bacteremic infection with *S. pneumoniae* in patients with AIDS virus (AV) infection (abstract 443). Program and abstracts of the 26th Interscience Conference on Antimicrobial Agents and Chemotherapy. Washington, D.C., American Society for Microbiology, p. 177.

Girard, P-M., Pocidalo, J-J., and Murray, J. F. (1991). Primary prophylaxis against common infectious diseases in persons with human immunodeficiency virus infection. *Am. Rev. Respir. Dis.* **143**:447–450.

Glatt, A. E., Chirgwin, K., and Landesman, S. H. (1988). Current concepts: treatment of infections associated with human immunodeficiency virus. *N. Engl. J. Med.* **318**:1439–1448.

Golden, J. A., Sjoerdsma, A., and Santi, D. V. (1984). *Pneumocystis carinii* pneumonia treated with alpha-difluoromethylornithine. *West J. Med.* **141**:613–623.

Goodman, P. C., and Gamsu, G. (1987). Pulmonary radiographic findings in the acquired immunodeficiency syndrome. *Postgrad. Radiol.* **7**:3–15.

Gordin, F. M., Simon, G. L., Wofsy, C. B., and Mills, J. (1984). Adverse reactions to trimethoprim-sulfamethoxazole in patients with the acquired immunodeficiency syndrome. *Ann. Intern. Med.* **100**:495–499.

Gottlieb, M. S., Schanker, H., Fan, P., Saxon, A., and Weisman, J. D. (1981a). Pneumocystis pneumonia—Los Angeles. *MMWR* **30**:250–252.

Gottlieb, M. A., Schroff, R., Schanker, H. M., Weisman, J. D., Fan, P. T., Wolf, R. A., and Saxon, A. (1981b). *Pneumocystis carinii* pneumonia and mucosal candidiasis in previously healthy homosexual men. Evidence of a new acquired cellular immunodeficiency. *N. Engl. J. Med.* **305**: 1425–1431.

Graham, A. R., Sobonya, R. E., Bronnimann, D. A., and Galgiani, J. N. (1988). Quantitative pathology of coccidioidomycosis in acquired immunodeficiency syndrome. *Hum. Pathol.* **19**:800–806.

Grant, I. H., and Armstrong, D. (1988). Fungal infections in AIDS. Cryptococcosis. *Infect. Dis. Clin. North Am.* **2**:457–464.

Greico, M. J., Helmann, A., Steigbigel, R. T., and Smaldone, G. C. (1989). Severity of *Pneumocystis carinii* pneumonia correlates with number of organisms recovered from lavage (abstract). *Am. Rev. Respir. Dis.* **139**(suppl):A149.

Guillon, J-M., Autran, B., Dennis, M., Fouret, P., Plata, F., Mayaud, C. M., and Akoud, G. M. (1988). HIV-related lymphocytic alveolitis. *Chest* **94**:1264–1270.

Hamilton-Dutoit, S. J., Pallesen, G., Karkow, J., Skinhoj, P., Franzmann, M. B., and Pedersen, C. (1989). Identification of EBV-DNA in tumour cells of AIDS-related lymphomas by in situ-hybridisation. *Lancet* **1**:554–555.

Haskal, Z. J., Lindan, C. E., and Goodman, P. C. (1990). Lymphoma in the immunocompromised patient. *Radiol. Clin. North Am.* **28**:885–899.

Heitzman, E. R. (1990). Pulmonary neoplastic and lymphoproliferative disease in AIDS: a review. *Radiology* **177**:347–351.

Hirschel, B., Chang, H. R., Mach, N., Piguet, P-F., Cox, J., Piguet, J-D., Silva, M. T., Larsson, L., Klatser, P. R., Thole, J. E. R., Rigouts, L., Portaels, F. (1990). Fatal infection with a novel unidentified *Mycobacterium* in a man with the acquired immunodeficiency syndrome. *N. Engl. J. Med.* **323**:109–113.

Hirschel, B., Lazzarin, A., Chopard, P., Oparavil, M., Furrer, H-J., Ruttimann, S., Vernazza, P., Chave, J-P., Anagarani, F., Gabriel, V., Heald, A., King, R., Malinverni, R., Martin, J-L., Mermillod, B., Nicod, L., Simoni, L., Vivirito, M. C., Zerboni, R., and the Swiss Group for Clinical Studies on AIDS (1991). A controlled study of inhaled pentamidine for primary prevention of *Pneumocystis carinii* pneumonia. *N. Engl. J. Med.* **324**:1079–1083.

Ho, D. D., Moudgil, T., and Alam, J-P. (1989). Quantitation of human immunodeficiency virus type 1 in the blood of infected persons. *N. Engl. J. Med.* **321**:1621–1625.

Hollander, H. (1988). Work-up of the HIV-infected patient. Practical approach. *Infect. Dis. Clin. North Am.* **2**:353–358.

Horsburgh, C. R., Jr. (1991). *Mycobacterium avium* complex infection in the acquired immunodeficiency syndrome. *N. Engl. J. Med.* **324**:1332–1338.

Horsburgh, C. R., Jr., and Selik, R. M. (1989). The epidemiology of disseminated nontuberculous mycobacterial infection in the acquired immunodeficiency syndrome (AIDS). *Am. Rev. Respir. Dis.* **139**:4–7.

Horsburgh, C. R., Jr., Mason, U. G., Farhi, D. C., and Iseman, M. D. (1985). Disseminated infection with *Mycobacterium avium-intracellulare*. *Medicine* **64**:36–48.

Itescu, S., Brancato, L. J., Buxbaum, J., Gregersen, P. K., Rizk, C. C., Croxson, T. S., Solomon, G. E., and Winchester, R. (1990). A diffuse infiltrative CD8 lymphocytosis syndrome in human immunodeficiency virus (HIV) infection: a host immune response associated with HLA-DR5. *Ann. Intern. Med.* **112**:3–10.

Jacobson, M. A. (1988). Mycobacterial diseases: tuberculosis and *Mycobacterium avium* complex. *Infect. Dis. Clin. North Am.* **2**:465–474.

Jacobson, M. A., and Mills, J. (1988a). Serious cytomegalovirus disease in the acquired immunodeficiency syndrome (AIDS). Clinical findings, diagnosis and treatment. *Ann. Intern. Med.* **108**:585–594.

Jacobson, M. A., and Mills, J. (1988b). Cytomegalovirus infection. In White, D. A., and Stover, D. E. (eds.). Pulmonary effects of AIDS. *Clin. Chest Med.* **9**:443–448.

Jacobson, M. A., Mills, J., Rush, J., Peiperl, L., Seru, V., Mohanty, P. K., Hopewell, P. C., Hadley, W. K., Broaddus, V. C., Leoung, G. L., and Feigal, D. W. (1991). Morbidity and mortality of patients with AIDS and first-episode *Pneumocystis carinii* pneumonia unaffected by concomitant pulmonary cytomegalovirus infection. *Am. Rev. Respir. Dis.* **144**:6–9.

Johnson, P. C., Khardori, N., Najjar, A. F., Butt, F., Mansell, P. W. A., and Sarosi, G. A. (1988). Progressive disseminated histoplasmosis in patients with acquired immunodeficiency syndrome. *Am. J. Med.* **85**:152–158.

Johnson, P. C., Hamil, R. J., and Sarosi, G. A. (1989). Clinical review: progressive disseminated histoplasmosis in the AIDS patient. *Semin. Respir. Infect.* **4**:139–146.

Jordan, T. J., Lewit, E. M., Montgomery, R. L., and Reichman, L. B. (1991). Isoniazid as preventive therapy in HIV-infected intravenous drug abusers. A decision analysis. *JAMA* **265**:2987–2991.

Joshi, V. V., and Oleske, J. M. (1986). Pulmonary lesions in children with the acquired immunodeficiency syndrome: a reappraisal based on data in additional cases and follow-up study of previously reported cases. *Hum. Pathol.* **17**:641–642.

Joshi, V., Oleske, J. M., Minnefor, A. B., Singh, R., Bokhari, T., and Rapkin, R. H. (1984). Pathologic pulmonary findings in children with the acquired immune deficiency syndrome. *Pediatr. Pathol.* **2**:71–87.

Jules-Elysee, K. M., Stover, D. E., Zamen, M. B., Bernard, E. M., and White, D. A. (1990). Aerosolized pentamidine: effect on diagnosis and presentation of *Pneumocystis carinii* pneumonia. *Ann. Intern. Med.* **112**:750–757.

Klein, R. S. (1989). Prophylaxis of opportunistic infections in individuals infected with HIV. *AIDS* **3**(suppl):161–173.

Klein, R. S., Harris, C. A., Small, C. B., Moll, B., Lesser, M., and Friedland, G. H. (1984). Oral candidiasis in high-risk patients as the initial manifestation of the acquired immuno-deficiency syndrome. *N. Engl. J. Med.* **311**:354–358.

Knowles, D. M., Chamulak, G. A., Subar, M., Burke, J. S., Dugan, M., Wernz, J., Slywotzky, C., Pelicci, P-G., Dalla-Favera, R., and Raphael, B. (1988). Lymphoid neoplasia associated with the acquired immunodeficiency syndrome (AIDS). *Ann. Intern. Med.* **108**:744–753.

Kovacs, J. A., Heimenz, J. W., Macher, A. M., Stover, D., Murray, H. W., Shelhamer, J., Lane, H. C., Urmacher, C., Honig, C., Longo, D. L., Parker, M. M., Natanson, C., Parrillo, J. E., Fauci, A. S., Pizzo, P. A., and Masur, H. (1984). *Pneumocystis carinii* pneumonia: a comparison between patients with the acquired immunodeficiency syndrome and patients with other immunodeficiencies. *Ann. Intern. Med.* **100**:663–671.

Kovacs, J. A., Ng, V. L., Masur, H., Leoung, G., Hadley, W. K., Evans, G., Lane, H. C., Ognibene, F. P., Shelhamer, J., Parrillo, J. E., and Gill, V. J. (1988). Diagnosis of *Pneumocystis carinii* pneumonia: improved detection in sputum with use of monoclonal antibodies. *N. Engl. J. Med.* **318**:589–593.

Kovacs, J. A., Halpern, J. L., Lundgren, B., Swan, J. C., Parillo, J. E., and Masur, H. (1989a). Monoclonal antibodies to *Pneumocystis carinii*: identification of specific antigens and characterization of antigenic differences between rat and human isolates. *J. Infect. Dis.* **159**:60–70.

Kovacs, J. A., Deyton, L., Davey, R., Falloon, J., Zunich, K., Lee, D., Metcalf, J. A., Bigley, J. W., Sawyer, L. A., Zoon, K. C., Masur, H., Fauci, A. S., and Lane, H. C. (1989b). Combined zidovudine and interferon-alpha therapy in patients with Kaposi sarcoma and the acquired immunodeficiency syndrome (AIDS). *Ann. Intern. Med.* **111**:280–287.

Kramer, E. L., Sanger, J. H., Garay, S. M., Grossman, R. J., Tin, S., and Banner, H. (1989). Diagnostic implications of Ga-67 chest-scan patterns in human immunodeficiency virus-seropositive patients. *Radiology* **170**: 671–676.

Krumholz, H., Sande, M. A., and Lo, B. (1989). Community-acquired bacteremia in patients with acquired immunodeficiency: clinical presentation, bacteriology and outcome. *Am. J. Med.* **86**:776–779.

Lallemant-Le Coeur, S., Lallemant, M., Cheynier, D., Nzingoula, S., Drucker, J., and Larouze, B. (1991). Bacillus Calmette-Guérin immunization in infants born to HIV-1-seropositive mothers. *AIDS* **5**:195–199.

Lane, H. C., Masur, H., Edgar, L. C., Whalen, G., Rook, A. H., and Fauci, A. S. (1983). Abnormalities of B-cell activation and immunoregulation in patients with the acquired immunodeficiency syndrome. *N. Engl. J. Med.* **309**:453–458.

Larsen, R. A., Leal, M. A. E., and Chan, L. S. (1990). Fluconazole compared with amphotericin B plus flucytosine for cryptococcal menigitis in AIDS. A randomized trial. *Ann. Intern. Med.* **113**:183–187.

Lecoeur, H. F., Truffot-Pernot, C., and Grosset, J. H. (1989). Experimental short-course preventive therapy of tuberculosis with rifampin and pyrazinamide. *Am. Rev. Respir. Dis.* **140**:1189–1193.

Lee, V. W., Rosen, M. P., Baum, A., Cohen, S. E., Cooley, T. P., and Liebman, H. A. (1988). AIDS-related Kaposi sarcoma: findings on thallium-201 scintigraphy. *AJR* **151**:1233–1235.

Leibovitz, E., Rigaud, M., Pollack, H., Lawrence, R., Chandwani, S., Krasinski, K., and Borkowsky, W. (1990). *Pneumocystis carinii* pneumonia in infants infected with the human immunodeficiency virus with more than 450 CD4 T lymphocytes per cubic millimeter. *N. Engl. J. Med.* **323**:531–533.

Leoung, G. S., and Mills, J. (eds.). (1989). *Opportunistic Infections in Patients with the Acquired Immunodeficiency Syndrome*. Marcel Dekker, New York, pp. 1–480.

Leoung, G. S., Feigal, D. W., Montgomery, A. B., Corkery, K., Wardlaw, L., Adams, M., Busch, D., Gordon, S., Jacobson, M. A., Volberding, P. A., Abrams, D., and the San Francisco County Community Consortium. (1990). Aerosolized pentamidine for prophylaxis against *Pneumocystis carinii* pneumonia. The San Francisco community prophylaxis trial. *N. Engl. J. Med.* **323**:769–775.

Levine, B., and Chaisson, R. E. (1991). *Mycobacterium kansasii*: a cause of treatable pulmonary disease associated with advanced human immunodeficiency virus (HIV) infection. *Ann. Intern. Med.* **114**:861–868.

Levine, S. J., and White, D. A. (1988). *Pneumocystis carinii* (infections in patients with AIDS). *Clin. Chest Med.* **9**:395–423.

Levine, S. J., White, D. A., and Fels, A. O. S. (1990). The incidence and significance of *Staphylococcus aureus* in respiratory cultures from patients infected with the human immunodeficiency virus. *Am. Rev. Respir. Dis.* **141**:89–93.

Linnemann, C. C., Jr., Baughman, R. P., Frame, P. T., and Floyd, R. (1989). Recovery of human immunodeficiency virus and detection of p24 antigen in bronchoalveolar lavage fluid from adult patients with the acquired immunodeficiency syndrome. *Chest* **96**:64–67.

Longworth, D. L., Spech, T. J., Ahmad, M., Sharp, D. E., Fishleder, A. J., Yen-Lieberman B., and Profitt, M. R. (1990). Lymphocytic alveolitis in primary HIV infection. *Cleve. Clin. J. Med.* **57**:379–382.

Lowery, W. S., Whitlock, W. L., Dietrich, R. A., and Fine, J. M. (1990). Sarcoidosis complicated by HIV infection: three case reports and a review of the literature. *Am. Rev. Respir. Dis.* **142**:887–889.

Luce, J. M., and Clement, M. J. (1989). Pulmonary diagnostic evaluation in patients suspected of having an HIV-related disease. *Semin. Respir. Infect.* **4**:93–101.

Maayan, S., Wormser, G., Widerhorn, J., Sy, E. R., Kim, Y. H., and Ernst, J. A. (1987). *Strongyloides stercoralis* hyperinfection in a patient with the acquired immunodeficiency syndrome. *Am. J. Med.* **83**:945–948.

MacDonnell, K. B., and Glassroth, J. (1989). *Mycobacterium avium* complex and other nontuberculous mycobacteria in patients with HIV infection. *Semin. Respir. Infect.* **4**:123–132.

Mason, G. R., Duane, G. B., Mena, I., and Effros, R. M. (1987). Accelerated solute clearance in *Pneumocystis carinii* pneumonia. *Am. Rev. Respir. Dis.* **135**:864–868.

Masur, H., Michelis, M. A., Green, J. B., Onorato, I., Vande Stouwe, R. A., Holzman, R. S., Wormser, G., Brettman, L., Lange, M., Murray, H. W., and Cunningham-Rundles, S. (1981). An outbreak of community-acquired *Pneumocystis carinii* pneumonia. *N. Engl. J. Med.* **305**:1431–1438.

Masur, H., Frederick, P., Ognibene, F. P., Yarchoan, R., Shelhamer, J. R., Baird, B. F., Travis, W., Suffredini, A. F., Deyton, L., Kovacs, J. A., Metcalf, J., Falloon, J., Davey, R., Polis, M., Metcalf, J., Baseler, M., Wesley, R., Gill, V. J., Fauci, A. S., and Lane, H. C. (1989a). CD4 counts as predictors of opportunistic pneumonias in human immunodeficiency virus (HIV) infection. *Ann. Intern. Med.* **111**:223–231.

Masur, H., Lane, C., Kovacs, J. A., Allegra, C. J., and Edman, J. C. (1989b). *Pneumocystis* pneumonia: from bench to bedside. *Ann. Intern. Med.* **111**:8813–826.

McKinsey, D. S., Gupta, M. R., Riddler, S. A., Driks, M. R., Smith, D. L., and Kurtin, P. J. (1989). Long-term amphotericin B therapy for disseminated histoplasmosis in patients with the acquired immunodeficiency syndrome (AIDS). *Ann. Intern. Med.* **111**:655–659.

Medina, I., Mills, J., and Wofsy, C. (1987). Serum lactate dehydrogenase levels in *Pneumocystis carinii* pneumonia in AIDS: possible indicator and predictor of disease activity (abstract). III International Conference on AIDS, Washington, D.C., p. 109.

Medina, I., Mills, J., Leoung, G., Hopewell, P. C., Lee, B., Modin, G., Benowitz, N., and Wofsy, C. (1990). Oral therapy for *Pneumocystis carinii* pneumonia in the acquired immunodeficiency syndrome. A controlled trial of trimethoprim-sulfamethoxazole versus trimethoprim-dapsone. *N. Engl. J. Med.* **323**:776–782.

Meduri, G. U., Stover, D. E., Lee, M., Myskowski, P. L., Caravelli, J. F., and Zaman, M. B. (1986). Pulmonary Kaposi's sarcoma in the acquired immune deficiency syndrome. Clinical, radiographic and pathologic manifestations. *Am. J. Med.* **81**:11–18.

Meignan, M., Guillon, J-M., Denis, M., Joly P., Rosso, J., Carette, M-F., Baud, L., Parquin, F., Plata, F., Debre, P., Akoun, G., Autran, B., and Mayaud, C. (1990). Increased lung epithelial permeability in HIV-infected patients with isolated cytotoxic t-lymphocytic alveolitis. *Am. Rev. Respir. Dis.* **141**:1241–1248.

Millar, A. B., Patou, G., Miller, R. F., Grundy, J. E., Katz, D. R., Weller, I. V., and Semple, S. J. (1990). Cytomegalovirus in the lungs of patients with AIDS. Respiratory pathogen or passenger? *Am. Rev. Respir. Dis.* **141**:1474–1477.

Mills, J., Leoung, G., Medina, I., Hopewell, P. C., Hughes, W. T., and Wofsy, C. (1988). Dapsone treatment of *Pneumocystis carinii* pneumonia in the acquired immunodeficiency syndrome. *Antimicrob. Agents Chemother.* **32**:1057–1060.

Mintz, L., Drew, W. L., Miner, R. C., and Braf, E. H. (1983). Cytomegalovirus infections in homosexual men: an epidemiologic study. *Ann Intern. Med.* **98**:326–329.

Montagnier, L., Gruest, J., Charmaret, S., Dauguet, C., Axler, C., and Guetard, D. (1984). Adaptation of lymphadenopathy associated virus (LAV) to replication in EBV-transformed B lymphoblastoid cell lines. *Science* **225**:63–66.

Montaner, J. S. G., Lawson, L. M., Levitt, N., Belzberg, A., Schechter, M. T., and Ruedy, J. (1990). Corticosteroids prevent early deterioration in patients with moderately severe *Pneumocystis carinii* pneumonia and the acquired immunodeficiency syndrome (AIDS). *Ann. Intern. Med.* **113**:14–20.

Montaner, J. S. G., Lawson, L. L., Gervais, A., Hyland, R. H., Chan, C. K., Falutz, J. M., Renzi, P. M., MacFadden, D., Rachlis, A. R., Fong, I. W., Garbner, G. E., Simor, A., Gilmore, N., Fanning, M., Taylor, G. D., Martel, A. H., Schlech, W. F., and Schechter, M. T. (1991). Aerosol pentamidine for secondary prophylaxis of AIDS-related *Pneumocystis carinii* pneumonia. A randomized, placebo-controlled study. *Ann. Intern. Med.* **114**:948–953.

Montgomery, A. B., Debs, R. J., Luce, J. M., Corkery, K. J., Turner, J., Brunette, E. N., Lin, E. T., and Hopewell, P. C. (1987). Aerosolized pentamidine as sole therapy for *Pneumocystis carinii* pneumonia in patients with acquired immunodeficiency syndrome. *Lancet* **2**:480–483.

Murray, J. F. (1989a). The J. Burns Amberson Lecture. The white plague: down and out or up and coming? *Am. Rev. Respir. Dis.* **140**:1788–1796.

Murray, J. F. (1989b). Interstitial pneumonias associated with human immunodeficiency virus infection. In *Interstitial Pneumonia of Unknown Etiology.* Edited by M. Harasawa, Y. Fukuchi, and H. Morinari. University of Tokyo Press, Tokyo, pp. 71–81.

Murray, J. F. (1990). Cursed duet: HIV infection and tuberculosis. *Respiration* **57**:210–220.

Murray, J. F. (1991). Tuberculosis and human immunodeficiency virus infection during the 1990's. *Bull. Int. Union Tuberc. Lung Dis.* **66**:21–25.

Murray, J. F., and Mills, J. (1990). Pulmonary infectious complications of human immunodeficiency virus infection. *Am. Rev. Respir. Dis.* **141**:1356–1372, 1582–1598.

Murray, J. F., Felton, C. P., Garay, S., Gottlieb, M. S., Hopewell, P. C., Stover, D. E., and Teirstein, A. S. (1984). Pulmonary complications of the acquired immunodeficiency syndrome. Report of a National Heart, Lung, and Blood Institute Workshop. *N. Engl. J. Med.* **310**:1682–1688.

Murray, J. F., Matthay, M. A., Luce, J. M., and Flick, M. R. (1988). An expanded definition of the adult respiratory distress syndrome. *Am. Rev. Respir. Dis.* **138**:720–723.

National Institute of Child Health and Human Development Intravenous Immunoglobulin Study Group (1991). Intravenous immune globulin for the prevention of bacterial infections in children with symptomatic human immunodeficiency virus infection. *N. Engl. J. Med.* **324**:73–80.

National Institutes of Health-University of California Expert Panel (1990). Consensus statement on the use of corticosteroids as adjunctive therapy for *Pneumocystis* pneumonia in the acquired immunodeficiency syndrome. *N. Engl. J. Med.* **323**:1500–1504.

Ng, V. L., Gartner, I., Weymouth, L. A., Goodman, C. D., Hopewell, P. C., and Hadley, W. K. (1989). The use of mucolysed induced sputum for the identification of pulmonary pathogens associated with human immunodeficiency virus infection. *Arch. Pathol. Lab. Med.* **113**:488–493.

Ng, V. L., Yajko, D. M., McPhaul, L. W., Gartner, I., Byford, B., Goodman, C. D., Nassos, P. S., Sanders, C. A., Howes, E. L., Leoung, G., Hopewell, P. C., and Hadley, W. K. (1990). Evaluation of an indirect fluorescent-antibody stain for detection of *Pneumocystis carinii* in respiratory specimens. *J. Clin. Microbiol.* **28**:975–979.

Northfelt, D. W., Clement, M. J., and Safrin, S. (1990). Extrapulmonary pneumocytosis: clinical features in human immunodeficiency virus infection. *Medicine* **69**:392–398.

Noskin, G., Murphy, R. L., Black, J. R., and Phair, J. P. (1991). Clindamycin/primaquine as salvage therapy for *Pneumocystis carinii* pneumonia (abstract). Presented at the VII International Conference on AIDS. Florence, Italy, p. 239.

Ognibene, F. P., Masur, H., Rogers, P., Travis, W. D., Suffredini, A. F., Fenerstein, I., Gill, V. J., Baird, B. F., Carrasquillo, J. A., Parillo, J. E., Lane, H. C., and Shelhamer, J. H. (1988). Nonspecific interstitial pneumonitis without evidence of *Pneumocystis carinii* in asymptomatic patients infected with human immunodeficiency virus (HIV). *Ann. Intern. Med.* **109**:874–879.

Oksenhendler, E., Cadranel, J., Sarfati, C., Katlama, C., Datry, A., Marche, C., Wolf, M., Roux, P., Derovin, F., and Clauvel, J-P. (1990). *Toxoplasma gondii* pneumonia in patients with the acquired immunodeficiency syndrome. *Am. J. Med.* **88**:18–21.

Packer, S. J., Ceesario, T., and Williams, J. H., Jr. (1988). *Mycobacterium avium* complex infection presenting as endobronchial lesions in immunosuppressed patients. *Ann. Intern. Med.* **109**:389–393.

Perkocha, L. A., Geaghan, S. M., Yen, T. S. B., Nishimura, S. L., Chan, S. P., Garcia-Kennedy, R., Honda, G., Stoloff, A. C., Klein, H. Z, Goldman, R. L., Van Meter, S., Ferrell, L. D., and LeBoit, P. E. (1990). Clinical and pathological features of bacillary peliosis hepatis in association with human immunodeficiency virus infection. *N. Engl. J. Med.* **323**: 1581–1586.

Perronne, C., Gikas, A., Truffot-Pernot, C., Grosset, J., Pocidalo, J-J., and Vilde, J-L. (1990). Activities of clarithromycin, sulfisoxazole, and rifabutin against *Mycobacterium avium* complex multiplication within human macrophages. *Antimicrob. Agents Chemother.* **34**:1508–1511.

Phair, J. P., and Wolinsky, S. (1989). Diagnosis of infection with the human immunodeficiency virus. *J. Infect. Dis.* **159**:320–323.

Piehl, M. R., Kaplan, R. L., and Haber, M. H. (1988). Disseminated penicilliosis in a patient with acquired immunodeficiency syndrome. *Arch. Pathol. Lab. Med.* **112**:1262–1264.

Pifer, L. L., Hughes, W. T., Stagno, S. S., and Woods, D. (1978). *Pneumocystis carinii* infection: evidence for a high prevalence in normal and immunosuppressed children. *Pediatrics* **61**:35–41.

Pitchenik, A. E., and Rubinson, H. A. (1985). The radiographic appearance of tuberculosis in patients with the acquired immune deficiency syndrome (AIDS) and pre-AIDS. *Am. Rev. Respir. Dis.* **131**:393–396.

Pitchenik, A. E., Ganjei, P., Torres, A., Evans, D. A., Rubin, E., and Baier, H. (1986). Sputum examination for the diagnosis of *Pneumocystis carinii* pneumonia in the acquired immunodeficiency syndrome. *Am. Rev. Respir. Dis.* **133**:226–229.

Pitchenik, A. E., Burr, J., Lauffer, M., Miller, G., Cacciatore, R., Bigler, W. J., Witte, J. J., and Cleary, T. (1990). Outbreaks of drug-resistant tuberculosis at AIDs Centre. *Lancet* **2**:440–441.

Pitt, J. (1991). Lymphocytic interstitial pneumonia. *Pediatr. Clin. North Am.* **38**:89–95.

Plata, F., Autran, B., Martins, L. P., Wain-Hobson, S., Raphael, M., Mayaud, C., Denis, M., Guillon, J-M., and Debre, P. (1987). AIDS-virus specific cytotoxic T lymphocytes in lung disorders. *Nature* **328**:348–351.

Plauda, J. M., Yarchoan, R., Jaffe, E. S., Feuerstein, I. M., Solomon, D., Steinberg, S. M., Wyvill, K. M., Raubitschek, A., Katz, D., and Broder, S. (1990). Development of non-Hodgkin lymphoma in a cohort of patients with severe human immunodeficiency virus (HIV) infection on long-term antiretroviral therapy. *Ann. Intern. Med.* **113**:276–282.

Popovic, M., Sarngadharan, M. D., Read, E., and Gallo, R. C. (1984). Detection, isolation, and continuous production of cytopathic retroviruses (HTLV-III) from patients with AIDS and pre-AIDS. *Science* **224**: 497–500.

Quinn, T. C., Mann, J. M., Curran, J. W., and Piot, P. (1986). AIDS in Africa: an epidemiologic paradigm. *Science* **234**:955–963.

Ramsey, P. G., Fife, K. H., Hackman, R. C., Meyers, J. D., and Corey, L. (1982). Herpes simplex virus pneumonia. Clinical, virologic, and pathologic features in 20 patients. *Ann. Intern. Med.* **97**:813–820.

Relman, D. A., Loutit, J. S., Schmidt, T. M., Falkow, S., and Tompkins, L. S. (1990). The agent of bacillary angiomatosis—an approach to the identification of uncultured pathogens. *N. Engl. J. Med.* **323**:1573–1580.

Relman, D. A., Falkow, S., LeBoit, P. E., Perkocha, L. A., Min, K-W., Welch, D. F., Slater, L. N. (1991). The organism causing bacillary angiomatosis, peliosis hepatis, and fever and bacteremia in immunocompromised patients (letter). *N. Engl. J. Med.* **324**:1514.

Resnick, L., Pitchenik, A. E., Fisher, E., and Croney, R. (1987). Detection of HTLV-III/LAV-specific IgG and antigen in bronchoalveolar lavage fluid from two patients with lymphocytic interstitial pneumonitis associated with AIDS-related complex. *Am. J. Med.* **82**:553–556.

Richmond, G. J., Imoto, E. M., Doherty, J. J., Beck, J. M., and Brown, J. K. (1991). Prophylaxis with inhaled pentamidine does not diminish the yield of sputum induction for diagnosis of *Pneumocystis carinii* pneumonia (abstract). *Am. Rev. Respir. Dis.* **143**:A716.

Roilides, E., Mertins, S., Eddy, J., Walsh, T. J., Pizzo, P. A., and Rubin, M. (1990). Impairment of neutrophil chemotactic and bactericidal function in children infected with human immunodeficiency virus type 1 and partial reversal after in vitro exposure to granulocyte-macrophage colony-stimulating factor. *J. Pediatr.* **117**:531–540.

Rose, R. M., Krivine, A., Pinkston, P., Gillis, J. M., Huang, A., and Hammer, S. M. (1991). Frequent identification of HIV-1 DNA in bronchoalveolar lavage cells obtained from individuals with the acquired immunodeficiency syndrome. *Am. Rev. Respir. Dis.* **143**:850–854.

Rubin, F. L., and Talamo, T. S. (1986). Secondary alveolar proteinosis in two patients with acquired immune deficiency syndrome. *Am. J. Med.* **80**:1187–1190.

Rutherford, G. W., Schwarcz, S. K., Lemp, G. F., Barnhart, J. L., Rauch, K. J., Warner, W. L., Piland, T. H., and Werdegar, D. (1989). The epidemiology of AIDS-related Kaposi's sarcoma in San Francisco. *J. Infect. Dis.* **159**: 569–572.

Sahai, J., and Berry, A. J. (1989). Eflornithine for the treatment of *Pneumocystis carinii* pneumonia in patients with the acquired immunodeficiency syndrome: a preliminary review. *Pharmacotherapy* **9**:29–33.

Sankary, R. M., Turner, J., Lipavsky, A., Howes, E. L., Jr., and Murray, J. F. (1988). Alveolar-capillary block in patients with AIDS and *Pneumocystis carinii* pneumonia. *Am. Rev. Respir. Dis.* **137**:443–449.

Sattler, F. R., Cowan, R., Nielsen, D. M., and Ruskin, J. (1988). Trimethoprim--sulfamethoxazole compared with pentamidine for treatment of *Pneumocystis carinii* pneumonia in the acquired immunodeficiency syndrome. A prospective, noncrossover study. *Ann. Intern. Med.* **109**:280–287.

Schnapp, L. M., Geaghan, S., Campagna, A., Fahy, J. V., Steiger, D., Ng., V., Hadley, W. K., Hopewell, P. C., and Stansell, J. D. (1991). *Toxoplasma gondii* pneumonitis in patients infected with the human immunodeficiency virus. *Arch. Int. Med.* (in press).

Selwyn, P. A., Hartel, D., Lewis, V. A., Schoenbaum, E. E., Vermund, S. H., Klein, R. S., Walker, A. T., and Friedland, G. H. (1989). A prospective study of the risk of tuberculosis among intravenous drug users with human immunodeficiency virus infection. *N. Engl. J. Med.* **320**:545–550.

Sepkowitz, K. A., Telzak, E. E., Gold, J. W. M., Bernard, E. M., Blum, S., Carrow, M., Dickmeyer, M., and Armstrong, D. (1991). Pneumothorax in AIDS. *Ann. Intern. Med.* **114**:455–459.

Shaw, R. J., Roussak, C., Forster, S. M., Harris, J. R. W., and Pinching, A. J. (1988). Lung function abnormalities in patients infected by the human immunodeficiency virus with and without overt pneumonitis. *Thorax* **43**:436–440.

Sheehan, P. M., Stokes, D. C., Yeh, Y-Y., and Hughes, W. T. (1986). Surfactant phospholipids and lavage phospholipase A2 in experimental *Pneumocystis carinii* pneumonia. *Am. Rev. Respir. Dis.* **134**:526–531.

Sider, L., and Horton, E. S. (1989). Pleural effusion as a presentation of AIDS-related lymphoma. *Invest. Radiol.* **24**:150–153.

Silvestri, R. C., Jensen, W. A., Zibrak, J. D.., Alexander, R. C., and Rose, R. M. (1987). Pulmonary infiltrates and hypoxemia in patients with the acquired immunodeficiency syndrome re-exposed to trimethoprim-sulfamethoxazole. *Am. Rev. Respir. Dis.* **136**:1003–1004.

Slater, L. N., Welch, D. F., Hensel, D., and Coody, D. W. (1990). A newly recognized fastidious gram-negative pathogen as a cause of fever and bacteremia. *N. Engl. J. Med.* **323**:1587–1593.

Slutkin, G., Leowski, J., and Mann, J. (1988). The effects of the AIDS epidemic on the tuberculosis problem and tuberculosis programmes. *Bull. Int. Union Tuberc. Lung Dis.* **63**:21–24.

Smaldone, G. C., Fuhrer, J., Steigbigel, R. T., and McPeck, M. (1991). Factors determining pulmonary deposition of aerosolized pentamidine in patients with human immunodeficiency virus infection. *Am. Rev. Respir. Dis.* **143**:727–737.

Small, P. M., Schecter, G. F., Goodman, P. C., Sande, M. A., Chaisson, R. E., and Hopewell, P. C. (1991). Treatment of tuberculosis in patients with advanced human immunodeficiency virus infection. *N. Engl. J. Med.* **324**:289–294.

Soo Hoo, G. W., Mohsenifar, Z., and Meyer, R. (1990). Inhaled or intravenous pentamidine therapy for *Pneumocystis carinii* pneumonia in AIDS. *Ann. Intern. Med.* **113**:195–202.

Spector, S. A., Kennedy, C., McCutchan, J. A., Bozzette, S. A., Straube, R. G., Connor, J. D., and Richman, D. D. (1989). The antiviral effect of zidovudine and ribavirin in clinical trials and the use of p24 antigen levels as a virologic marker. *J. Infect. Dis.* **159**:822–828.

Stern, R. G., Gamsu, G., Golden, J. A., Hirji, M., Webb, W. R., and Abrams, D. I. (1984). Intrathoracic adenopathy: differential feature of AIDS and diffuse lymphadenopathy syndrome. *AJR* **142**:689–692.

Stover, D. E., and Meduri, G. U. (1988). Pulmonary function tests. In White, D. A., and Stover, D. E. (eds.). Pulmonary effects of AIDS. *Clin. Chest Med.* **9**:473–479.

Stover, D. E., White, D. A., Romano, P. A., Gellene, R. A., and Robeson, W. A. (1985). Spectrum of pulmonary diseases associated with the acquired immune deficiency syndrome. *Am. J. Med.* **78**:429–437.

Suffredini, A. F., Ognibene, F. P., Lack, E. E., Simmons, J. T., Brenner, M., Gill, V. J., Lane, H. C., and Fauci, A. S. (1987). Nonspecific interstitial pneumonitis: a common cause of pulmonary disease in the acquired immunodeficiency syndrome. *Ann. Intern. Med.* **107**:7–13.

Tenholder, M. F., Moser, R. J., and Tellis, C. J. (1988). Mycobacteria other than tuberculosis: pulmonary involvement in patients with acquired immunodeficiency syndrome. *Arch. Intern. Med.* **148**:953–955.

Tucker, R. M., Denning, D. W., Dupont, B., and Stevens, D. A. (1990a). Itraconazole therapy for chronic coccidioidal meningitis. *Ann. Intern. Med.* **112**:108–112.

Tucker, R. M., Galgiani, J. N., Denning, D. W., Hanson, L. H., Graybill, J. R., Sharkey, K., Eckman, M. R., Salemi, C., Libke, R., Klein, R. A., and Stevens, D. A. (1990b). Treatment of coccidioidal meningitis with fluconazole. *Rev. Infect. Dis.* (suppl 3):S380–S389.

Van Nhieu, J. T., Vojek, A-M., Bernaudin, J-F., Escudier, E., and Fleury-Feith, J. (1990). Pulmonary alveolar proteinosis associated with *Pneumocystis carinii*. Ultrastructural identification in bronchoalveolar lavage in AIDS and immunocompromised non-AIDS patients. *Chest* **98**:801–805.

Viviani, M. A., Tortorano, A. M., Langer, M., Almaviva, M., Negri, C., Cristina, S., and Scocia, S., DeMaria, R., Fiocchi, R., and Ferrazzi, P. (1989). Experience with itraconazole in cryptococcosis and aspergillosis. *J. Infect.* **18**:151–165.

Volberding, P., and Jacobson, M. A. (eds.) (1990). *AIDS Clinical Review 1990*. Marcel Dekker, New York, pp. 1–288.

Wachter, R. M., Luce, J. M., Turner, J., Volberding, P., and Hopewell, P. C. (1986). Intensive care of patients with the acquired immunodeficiency syndrome. *Am. Rev. Respir. Dis.* **134**:891–896.

Wachter, R. M., Russi, M. B., Bloch, D. A., Hopewell, P. C., and Luce, J. M. (1991). *Pneumocystis carinii* pneumonia and respiratory failure in AIDS. Improved outcomes and increased use of intensive care units. *Am. Rev. Respir. Dis.* **143**:251–256.

Wallace, J. M. (1989). Pulmonary infection in human immunodeficiency disease: viral pulmonary infections. *Semin. Respir. Infect.* **2**:147–154.

Wallace, J. M., Batra, P., Gong, H., Jr., and Ovenfors, C-O (1985). Percutaneous needle lung aspiration for diagnosing pneumonitis in the patient with acquired immunodeficiency syndrome (AIDS). *Am. Rev. Respir. Dis.* **131**:389–392.

Weber, W. R., Askin, F. B., and Dehner, L. P. (1977). Lung biopsy in *Pneumocystis carinii* pneumonia: a histopathologic study of typical and atypical features. *Am. J. Clin. Pathol.* **67**: 11–19.

Welch, K., Finkbeiner, W., Alpers, C. E., Blumenfeld, W., Davis, R. L., Smuckler, E. A., and Beckstead, J. H. (1984). Autopsy findings in the acquired immune deficiency syndrome. *JAMA* **252**:1152–1159.

Wharton, J. M., Coleman, D. L., Wofsy, C. B., Luce, J. M., Blumenfeld, W., Hadley, W. K., Volberding, P. A., and Hopewell, P. C. (1986). Trimethoprim-sulfamethoxasole or pentamidine for *Pneumocystis carinii* pneumonia in the acquired immunodeficiency syndrome. *Ann. Intern. Med.* **105**:37–44.

Wheat, L. J., Kohler, R. B., and Tewari, R. P. (1986). Diagnosis of disseminated histoplasmosis by detection of *Histoplasma capsulatum* antigen in serum and urine specimens. *N. Engl. J. Med.* **314**:83–88.

Wheat, L. J., Connolly-Stringfield, P. A., Baker, R. L., Curfman, M. F., Eads, M. E., Israel, K. S., Norris, S. A., Webb, D. H., and Zeckel, M. L. (1990). Disseminated histoplasmosis in the acquired immune deficiency syndrome: clinical findings, diagnosis and treatment, and review of the literature. *Medicine* **69**:361–374.

Whitcomb, M. E., Schwarz, M. I., Charles, M. A., and Larson, P. H. (1970). Interstitial fibrosis after *Pneumocystis carinii* pneumonia. *Ann. Intern. Med.* **73**:761–765.

White, D. A., and Matthay, R. A. (1989). Noninfectious pulmonary complications of infection with the human immunodeficiency virus. *Am. Rev. Respir. Dis.* **140**:1783–1787.

WHO/IUATLD. Tuberculosis and AIDS. (1989). Statement on AIDS and tuberculosis, Geneva, March 1989. *Bull. Int. Union Tuberc. Lung Dis* **64**:8–11.

Williams, D. M., Krick, J. A., and Remington, J. S. (1976). State of the art. Pulmonary infections in the compromised host. *Am. Rev. Respir. Dis.* **114**:359–394, 593–627.

Witt, D. J., Craven, D. E., and McCabe, W. R. (1987). Bacterial infections in adult patients with the acquired immunodeficiency syndrome (AIDS) and AIDS-related complex. *Am. J. Med.* **82**:900–906.

Yagupsky, P., and Menegus, M. A. (1990). Cumulative positivity rates of multiple blood cultures for *Mycobacterium avium-intracellulare* and *Cryptococcus neoformans* in patients with the acquired immunodeficiency syndrome. *Arch. Pathol. Lab. Med.* **114**:923–925.

Yakrus, M. A., and Good, R. C. (1990). Geographic distribution, frequency, and specimen source of *Mycobacterium avium* complex serotypes isolated from patients with and without acquired immunodeficiency syndrome. *J. Clin. Microbiol.* **28**:926–929.

Ziza, J-M., Brun-Vezinet, F., Venet, A., Rouzioux, C. H., Traversat, J., Israel-Biet, B., Barré-Sinoussi, F., and Cherman, J-C. (1985). Lymphadenopathy-associated virus isolated from bronchoalveolar lavage fluid in AIDS-related complex with lymphoid interstitial pneumonitis (letter). *N. Engl. J. Med.* **313**:183.

Zuger, A., Louie, E., Holzman, R. S., Simberkoff, M. S., and Rahal, J. J. (1986). Cryptococcal disease in patients with the acquired immunodeficiency syndrome. *Ann. Intern. Med.* **104**:234–240.

2

Pulmonary Complications of Immunosuppressive Diseases Other Than Human Immunodeficiency Virus Infection

STEVEN R. DUNCAN

University of Pittsburgh
Pittsburgh, Pennsylvania

THOMAS A. RAFFIN

Stanford University Medical Center
Stanford, California

I. Introduction

The numerous and diverse pulmonary complications of immunosuppression seen in contemporary practice are, to a very large extent, a phenomenon of medical progress. Recent gains in the understanding of basic pathogenetic mechanisms have resulted in a proliferation of the indications for immunosuppressive treatment of autoimmune and neoplastic diseases. Striking advances in therapeutics and surgical techniques during the last decade, moreover, have turned organ transplantation into a practical reality for large numbers of patients with otherwise incurable diseases. Considerable experience has accumulated in the last few years with respect to diagnosis, management, and prevention of complications in these compromised patients. Despite some notable successes, however, serious pulmonary sequlae of immunosuppression remain distressingly all to frequent (Rosenow et al., 1985; Ettinger and Trulock, 1991).

Evaluation and management of immunosuppressed patients with pulmonary complications are particularly challenging because of the wide range of possible diagnoses in these populations. Immunosuppression places patients at great risk for rapidly progressive infections with a variety of unusual organisms. Many of these patients are also prone to develop noninfectious pulmonary sequelae of their underlying diseases or side effects of treatments. Furthermore, the diagnosis of acute pulmonary processes in the immunocompromised cannot often be ascertained reliably by noninvasive clinical or radiographic evaluations (Rubin and Greene, 1981). In most cases, the ultimate assessment of these complex problems requires specimen acquisition by invasive procedures, i.e., fine-needle aspiration, open thoracotomy, or, most frequently, fiberoptic bronchoscopy (Stover et al., 1984). Despite the limitations of routine, noninvasive assessments, astute clinical insights into the likely etiologies of the pulmonary disease are an invaluable aid to delivery of optimal care.

This chapter will highlight some of the most common pulmonary problems of patients with immunosuppressive diseases other than the acquired immunodeficiency syndrome (AIDS). The discussion will begin with an overview of the primary deficiencies of immunity and their associated pulmonary manifestations. For the most part, these entities are seldom encountered outside of selected referral centers. Investigations into the nature of the primary immunodeficiencies, however, have furnished important insights into the function of normal immune mechanisms. Most of this chapter is devoted to discussion of the pulmonary complications associated with secondary, and often iatrogenic, immune system abnormalities. These disorders occur far more frequently than the primary deficiencies and often comprise a significant proportion of pulmonary medicine practices.

II. Primary Immunodeficiencies

The primary immunodeficiencies are, by convention, classified into defects of humoral immunity, abnormalities or inadequate numbers of phagocytes, and impairments of cellular immunity (Table 1). Although these simplified schema are conceptually and practically useful, in reality the various components of the immune system do not function in isolation, but instead comprise elements of an intricate and interwoven system. Many of the primary immunodeficiencies defy ready categorization as a simple limited defect because significant abnormalities are present in two or even all three limbs of the immune system.

Detailed descriptions of immune mechanisms and their integrated responses, as applied to the respiratory tract, can be found elsewhere in comprehensive reviews (Kaltreider, 1976; Reynolds, 1987). The following discussion of the primary immunodeficiency diseases will be limited to those entities most often encountered in clinical practice and/or selected representative prototypes of the various classifications.

A. Disorders of Humoral Immunity

Primary abnormalities of humoral immunity can be further subdivided into deficiencies of immunoglobulins or complement components. Defects of either system result in impairment of microbial agglutination, opsonization, and neutralization, as well as antibody-complement-mediated cytolysis and granulocyte recruitment to sites of inflammation. In general, patients afflicted with primary humoral deficiencies are prone to recurrent or refractory infections of the sinopulmonary tract and skin with extracellular encapsulated bacteria (e.g., *Streptococcus pneumoniae, Hemophilus influenza, Neisseria* spp.) and *Staphylococcus aureus* (Johnston, 1984).

Immunoglobulin Deficiencies

X-Linked Agammaglobulinemia

Also commonly known as Bruton's agammaglobulinemia, this disorder of B-lymphocyte maturation was the first inborn error of immunity described in detail (Bruton, 1952). The disease is characterized by an inability to make antibodies, hypoplastic lymph node germinal centers, and very low levels of circulating immunoglobulins (Conley, 1985). Afflicted patients have marked reductions in numbers of fully differentiated B cells and plasma cells, whereas normal numbers of B-cell precursors are found in bone marrow (Pearl et al., 1978). Intrinsic T-cell functions appear to be unaffected by this disorder.

Classic descriptions of sex-linked recessive inheritance are based on very few pedigree analyses. Variable phenotypic expression of the disorder is suggested by findings that relatives of index cases may manifest with other, less global, deficiencies of immunoglobulin production (Kirkpatrick and Schimke, 1967) or onset of disease late in life (Buckley and Sidbury, 1968). An otherwise indistinguishable syndrome with apparent autosomal recessive heredity has been described in a small number of female patients (Hoffman et al., 1977).

Typical onset of refractory or recurrent sinopulmonary infections, meningitis, otitis media, and eczema occur in infants between 4 and 6 months of age, as levels of passively transferred maternal immunoglobulins decrease. The importance of immunoglobulin opsonization for microbial clearance is illustrated by the predilection of these patients for persistent viral and parasitic infections of the central nervous system and gastrointestinal (GI) tract (Rosen et al., 1984a). Attenuated live virus vaccination has been associated with the development of serious viral infection (Wright et al., 1977). Occasional patients present with pneumonias due to *Pneumocystis carinii* (Saulsbury et al., 1979). Adult hypogammaglobulinemic patients appear uniquely predisposed to *Mycoplasma* respiratory tract infections (Roifman et al., 1986).

In addition to specific antimicrobial treatment of active infections, patients may benefit from intermittent prophylactic antibiotics. The cornerstone of maintenance therapy, however, is regular replacement of γ-globulin by intravenous infusions (Cunningham-Rundles et al., 1984; Rosen et al., 1984a; Roifman and Gelfand, 1988). Current recommendations, based largely on inference,

Table 1 Pulmonary Infections of Selected Primary Immunodeficiencies

	Defect	Pulmonary pathogens
Humoral deficiencies		
X-linked agammaglobulinemia	B-lymphocyte maturation	Encapsulated bacteria–e.g., *H. influenzae*, *S. pneumoniae* or *pyogenes S. aureus*
Hypogammaglobulinemia hyper-IgM		*Mycoplasma*
Common variable immunodeficiency		Less common: *P. carinii*, viruses
IgA and IgG subclass deficiency		Pyogenic bacteria
Phagocyte abnormalities		
Chronic and cyclic neutropenias	Neutrophil maturation	Occasional: *S. aureus*, streptococci, and Enterobacteriaceae
Chronic granulomatous disease	Various defects of superoxide and H_2O_2 generation, i.e., ''respiratory burst''	*S. aureus*, Enterobacteriaceae *Aspergillus, Candida* Occasional: mycobacteria, viruses, *Nocardia, P. carinii*

Job's syndrome	Neutrophil chemotaxis (and others—see text)	*S. aureus* Encapsulated bacteria *Candida, Aspergillus* Enterobacteriaceae
Cellular immune deficiencies		
Severe combined immunodeficiency disease	Lymphoid stem cell maturation (B and T cells affected) 50% idiopathic 25% adenosine deaminase deficiency	*P. carinii* Herpes viruses *Influenza* Measles *Legionella* Other bacteria, occasional *Candida*
Ataxia-telangeictasia	T-cell proliferation Immunoglobulin synthesis	*S. aureus* Encapsulated bacteria
DiGeorge syndrome	Thymic hypoplasia	Herpes viruses Measles *P. carinii* Enterobacteriaceae

call for monthly intravenous immunoglobulin administration of doses adequate to maintain γ-globulin trough levels at approximately 400 mg/dl (Buckley and Schiff, 1991). γ-Globulin replacement has been shown to decrease frequencies of upper and lower airway infections and successfully reverse persistent viral infections (Rosen et al., 1984a; Roifman and Gelfand, 1988). Replacement therapy has not yet been proven, however, to also result in a decreased prevalence of the bronchiectasis and fibrosis that ultimately develop in many patients with hypogammaglobulin syndromes (Hermans et al., 1976; Cunningham-Rundles, 1989).

Hypogammaglobulinemia with Hyperimmunoglobulin M

This abnormality of B lymphocytes has also been reported with both X-linked and autosomal recessive heredity, as well as occasional onset in later life. The primary functional defect of this syndrome appears to be a block in the normal ontogeny of IgM+ B cells to more differentiated IgG- and IgA-secreting B cells (Rosen et al., 1984a). Although measures of cellular immunity are normal in these patients, the underlying abnormality of B-cell differentiation may be due to dysregulation by intrinsically defective T cells (Fiorilli et al., 1986). Like Bruton's syndrome, hypogammaglobulinemia with increased IgM is associated with an inability to synthesize IgG and IgA antibodies (Geha et al., 1979). In contrast, however, patients with the hyperimmunoglobulin M syndrome have circulating B lymphocytes and plasma cells (though limited to IgM and IgD phenotypes) and hypertrophied lymphoid tissue (Schwaber et al., 1981). Furthermore, serum levels of IgM (and IgD) are usually elevated in patients with this disorder.

Under normal circumstances, IgA isotype antibodies predominate in upper airway secretions, whereas lower airway protection is primarily afforded by IgG antibodies. IgM is not usually present in respiratory or GI secretions, however, as the molecules are too large for ready diffusion. Accordingly, patients with the hypogammaglobulinemia-hyperimmunoglobulin M syndrome are especially prone to pyogenic infections of the respiratory and gastrointestinal tracts, despite increased serum IgM. Affected patients are also predisposed to develop lymphoproliferative disorders, autoimmune thrombocytopenia, hemolytic anemia, and profound neutropenia. Treatment of the antibody deficiency with regular γ-globulin replacement is similar to that described above for Bruton's agammaglobulinemia. One patient with hyperimmunoglobulin M syndrome reportedly showed improvements of several indices of humoral immunity while treated with cimetidine, a putative result of blockade of histamine-mediated suppressor T-cell inhibition (Ciboddo et al., 1987).

Common Variable Immunodeficiency

Common variable immunodeficiency (CVI) is a relatively frequently encountered syndrome characterized by failure of B-lymphocyte differentiation.

Whereas the total number of circulating B cells is often normal, serum levels of IgG are low or absent and IgA and IgM are variably depressed in afflicted patients. CVI occurs with approximately equal frequency in both genders, and patients generally present in the second or third decade of life (Hermans et al., 1976). Most often the disorder appears to occur spontaneously, although an association with Epstein-Barr virus infections has also been described (Provisor et al., 1975). A genetic basis seems to account for at least some cases (Rosen et al., 1984b).

CVI is the common manifestation of myriad heterogeneous B-cell defects. Pathogenetic mechanisms identified in various CVI patients include intrinsic failures of antibody synthesis or secretion, abnormal production of T-cell immunoregulatory factors, or, rarely, autoantibodies directed against B or T lymphocytes (Geha et al., 1974; Waldman et al., 1974; Siegal, 1978; Saiki et al., 1982; Rosen et al., 1984b). A significant proportion of CVI patients have demonstrable impairments of T-cell cytokine production or other regulatory functions, and as many as 50% have some defect of T-lymphocyte-mediated immunity (Ichkikawa et al., 1982; Pastorelli et al., 1989).

CVI patients are prone to frequent sinopulmonary infections and recurrent otitis media with encapsulated bacteria. Sprue-like malabsorption also occurs in a majority of these patients. An association between CVI, or an essentially identical syndrome, and thymomas has also been identified in approximately 10% of patients with the neoplasm (Hermans et al., 1976; Rosenow and Hurley, 1984). CVI is also an established risk for eventual development of GI carcinomas and non-Hodgkin's lymphomas. As many as 40% of hypogammaglobulinemic patients ultimately present with clinically significant bronchiectasis or other debilitating airway diseases (Hermans et al., 1976; Dukes et al., 1978; Cunningham-Rundles, 1989).

Maintenance treatment consists of γ-globulin replacement therapy, as previously described. IgE antibodies directed against IgA have been detected in serum of some CVI patients without detectible levels of IgA (Burks et al., 1986). Consequently, these patients are at considerable risk for anaphylactoid reactions to immune globulin preparations that contain IgA. Commercially available preparations with low levels of IgA (Gammagard, Baxter Healthcare, Glendale, CA) can be safely administered, however, in carefully controlled settings (Buckley and Schiff, 1991).

A number of recent studies have employed novel treatment approaches in attempts to modify the immunological defect associated with this syndrome. Cimetidine has been shown to increase production of immunoglobulins and ameliorate deficiencies of T-cell functions in small numbers of CVI patients (White and Ballow, 1985; Segal et al., 1989). Preliminary data show administration of 13-*cis* retinoic acid promotes the in vivo differentiation of B lymphocytes among afflicted persons (Adelman et al., 1991). Interleukin-2 (IL-2) treatment of CVI patients with defective T-cell production of the cytokine has been reported to result in increased serum levels of immunoglobulins (Welte and Mertelsmann, 1985). Administration of thymic factors has also been described as increasing immunoglobulin levels and antibody responses, as well as decreasing numbers of infections in a small number of patients (Bordiogoni et al., 1982).

Selective Immunoglobulin Deficiencies

Isolated deficiency of IgA is the most commonly encountered humoral immune deficit, occurring in as many as 1 in 700 individuals (Rosen et al., 1984a). Most patients with this defect are probably asymptomatic, although there are numerous reports of an association between IgA deficiency and diarrhea (which may be the result of *Giardia lamblia* infections) as well as a propensity for autoimmune and collagen vascular diseases. A distinct minority of patients with isolated IgA deficiency have serious recurrent respiratory tract infections.

Individuals with combined deficiencies of IgA and IgG subclasses (IgG2 and IgG4), however, appear to have a much greater than normal incidence of pneumonias and middle ear infections (Umetsu et al., 1985; Shackelford et al., 1986). The IgA deficiency may be a relatively innocent bystander, since patients with selective deficits of both IgG2 and IgG4, or IgG4 alone, are similarly likely to develop recurrent bacterial infections and bronchietasis (Umetsu et al., 1985; Shackelford et al., 1986). Isolated IgG4 deficits have been particularly implicated as a significant risk factor for progression to chronic airway disease (Heiner, 1984). Patients with low levels of IgG3 deficiencies have also been reported to develop recurrent pneumonias, although this association is somewhat less conclusive. The presence of isolated subclass deficiencies is by no means an invariable predilection for disease, however, since many patients with very low levels of IgG2 appear to be asymptomatic (Shackelford et al., 1990).

Total serum IgG levels are often normal in patients with selective subclass deficiencies. Accordingly, diagnosis of these abnormalities requires quantitative IgG subclass assays (Reynolds, 1988). Because IgG1 comprises two-thirds of serum IgG concentrations, patients with selective deficiencies of this subclass are overtly hypogammaglobulinemic and readily detected by measurement of total IgG. Immunoglobulin replacement, at least with preparations containing normal concentrations of the deficit IgG subclass(es), is beneficial among symptomatic patients with recurrent infections.

Forty percent of patients with isolated IgA deficiency have demonstrable anti-IgA antibodies. These individuals are obviously at great risk for adverse reactions to immunoglobulin infusions, and, in any event, there is no clinical indication for replacement of deficient IgA (Buckley and Schiff, 1991). Among patients with concomitant IgA and IgG subclass deficiencies who have recurrent infections, immunoglobulin can usually be administered safely following guidelines discussed elsewhere (Buckley and Schiff, 1991).

Complement Component Deficiencies

Clinically evident immune suppression from congenital deficiencies of complement components are rare (Ross and Densen, 1984). Deficiencies of either C3 or C5 result in impairment of the full range of complement-mediated functions, including microbial opsonification and cytolysis, as well as neutrophil recruitment. Manifestations of C3 deficiency resemble those described for agammaglobulinemia syndromes, but tend to be even more severe (Alper et al., 1976; Ross and Densen, 1984). Patients with congenital C5 deficiency are particularly prone to recurrent infections with enteric gram-negative and encapsulated bacteria, as well as candidiasis (Miller and Nisson, 1970). Primary deficiencies of C3 or C5 can be replaced with infusions of fresh frozen plasma. Due to the lability of C5, however, plasma stored for ≥24 h has little remaining factor activity. Secondary deficiencies of C3 and C5 have been described in association with a variety of systemic diseases, particularly systemic lupus erythematosus (Ginzler et al., 1978; Nived et al., 1985a), nephrotic syndrome, and hepatic failure, and occur much more frequently than the congenital defects.

Small numbers of patients have been found to have various other deficiencies of complement components (Hill, 1981). Absence of C6, C7, or C8 is associated with high rates of serious infections with *Neisseria* spp. and *S. pneumoniae* (Leddy et al., 1974).

B. Phagocyte Abnormalities

Impairments of phagocyte-mediated immunity may be attributable to either absolute reductions in number or functional defects of granulocytes, macrophages, or fixed-tissue histiocytes. The spectrum of pathogens among patients with phagocyte abnormalities overlaps considerably with those of the humoral defects. Skin infections are especially problematic among individuals with defects of phagocyte function. Pyogenic bacterial and fungal infections of the respiratory tract are among the most acutely life-threatening manifestations of these disorders.

Inadequate Numbers of Granulocytes

Granulocytopenia is almost always an acquired abnormality of various disorders, including hematological malignancies, splenomegaly, idiosyncratic drug reactions, or cytotoxic chemotherapies (Price and Dale, 1978). Pulmonary complications of profound secondary granulocytopenia are discussed in the section "Acute Nonlymphocytic Leukemia."

Chronic neutropenia with counts as low as 50–200/mm^3 occurs in a small number of sporadic or inherited cases (Dale et al., 1979). Infections are infrequent among all but the most profoundly neutropenic of these patients. The distinct entity of cyclical neutropenia is characterized by reductions of granulocyte counts with a 21-day periodicity (Price and Dale, 1978). These patients are prone to develop fever and oral ulcers during the neutropenic phase, but deep visceral infections are unusual. The low incidence of serious infectious complications in these disorders of neutrophil number may be attributable to the frequent presence of concomitant monocytosis. The neutropenia associated with both these disorders can be ameliorated by administration of corticosteroids, although therapy should probably be reserved for judicious use in severely affected patients (Wright et al., 1978).

Defects of Phagocyte Function

Chronic Granulomatous Disease

Chronic granulomatous disease (CGD) is a syndrome of heterogeneous disorders characterized by defective "respiratory burst" mechanisms and impaired intracellular killing of specific microbes by phagocytes (Babior and Woodman, 1990). Granulocytes, alveolar macrophages, and tissue histiocytes of patients with CGD are able to ingest microbes normally, but cannot produce superoxide anion (O_2^-), hydrogen peroxide (H_2O_2), or other reduction products of O_2. These highly reactive oxidants are not only direct-acting microbicides, but are also used as substrates for myeloperoxidase-catalyzed halogenation reactions of microbial proteins and nucleic acids. In the last few years, a number of discrete defects of the phagocyte electron transport mechanism have been identified, any one of which may result in a failure of respiratory burst activities and clinical presentation with CGD (Babior and Woodman, 1990; Smith and Curnutte, 1991).

The onset of CGD can be as late as 16 years of age, although most often manifestations of the disease are evident during infancy (Mouy et al., 1989). The majority of cases are X-linked, but autosomal recessive heredity has also been described (Weening et al., 1985). Afflicted patients present with repeated, refractory lymphadenitis, infections of the oropharynx, skin, and GI tract, as well as rapidly progressive pneumonias. Pathogens tend to be catalase positive, thus neutralizing the minute amount of hydrogen peroxide produced as a byproduct of microbial metabolism or, alternatively, organisms inherently incapable of synthesizing hydrogen peroxide. *Aspergillus* pneumonia is an especially common manifestation of CGD and is lethal in approximately 50% of cases. Other frequently identified pathogens include *S. aureus*, *Candida*, enteric gram-negative bacteria, and *Salmonella*. Much less commonly, disease is due to *S. epidermidis*, *M. tuberculosis* or atypical mycobacteria (Mouy et al., 1989). Pneumonia among patients with CGD has also, on relatively rare occasions, been caused by cytomegalovirus, *Nocardia*, or *P. carinii*.

Reconstitution with normally functioning phagocytes by bone marrow transplantation is the definitive treatment of CGD (Lenarsky and Parkman,

1990). CGD patients have normal cellular immunity, however, and immunosuppressive prophylaxis for graft-versus-host disease is necessary. Thus, successfully treated patients avoid the infectious complications of CGD at the cost of potential complications of bone marrow transplantation (see "Bone Marrow Transplantation"). The administration of recombinant human interferon-gamma (rHuIFN-γ) was recently shown to decrease the number and severity of infections in patients with CGD (Ezekokwitz et al., 1988; ICGDCS, 1991). Efficacy of rHuIFN-γ has been attributed to increased granulocyte superoxide production (Jeppson et al., 1991). Other investigators note little change of oxidative capacity among rHuIFN-γ-treated neutrophils, however, and suggest alternative mechanisms of macrophage activation may be responsible for the effectiveness of this therapy (Bernhisel-Broadbent et al., 1991; ICGDCS, 1991). Regular prophylaxis with trimethoprim-sulfamethoxazole (TMP-SMX) is well tolerated and decreases the incidence of bacterial infections among CGD patients by two- to threefold (Mouy et al., 1989; Margolis et al., 1990). Trials of antifungal prophylaxis, however, have not shown yet been shown to be effective for the prevention of *Aspergillus* infections (Mouy et al., 1989).

Chediak-Higashi Syndrome (CHS)

CHS is a rare autosomal recessive defect of neutrophil and monocyte microbicidal activity (Root et al., 1972). Although phagocytosis and respiratory burst functions of these cells appear to be normal, chemotaxis and microbial killing functions are impaired due to an abnormality of intracellular lysozomal granules (Root et al., 1972; Gallin et al., 1980). Afflicted patients are prone to develop skin and lethal respiratory tract infections with *S. aureus* and encapsulated bacteria.

Job's Syndrome (JS)

Also known as the hyperimmunoglobulin E syndrome, this unusual disorder of phagocyte function has autosomal dominant heredity with variable penetrance (Van Scoy et al., 1975). Numerous diverse defects of immune system components have been described in patients with JS, and the predominant deficiency accounting for clinical manifestations of the syndrome remains arguable. Phagocytes of affected patients have normal capacities for microbial ingestion and killing. Neutrophils of these patients, however, show variably impaired chemotaxis. The motility defect appears to be due to an underlying abnormality of mononuclear cells, which inappropriately either produce inhibitory cytokines or fail to elaborate chemotactic facilitators (Donabedian and Gallin, 1982). Derangements of lymphocyte immunoregulatory functions could also account for the concomitant findings of markedly increased levels of IgE, deficient production of some other immunoglobulins (notably a defect of secretory IgA directed against *S. aureus*), decreased suppressor T cells, abnormal cytokine production, and depressed lymphocyte proliferation (Donabedian and Gallin, 1983; Leung et al., 1988; Del Prete et al., 1989).

The most common clinical features of this syndrome are frequent respiratory and skin infections, whereas deep visceral infections and sepsis are rare. Cold abscesses due to *S. aureus* infection are prominent, as well as mucocutaneous candidias (Donabedian and Gallin, 1983). Recurrent *S. aureus* pneumonias and empyemas are especially common respiratory tract manifestations. A lesser incidence of pneumonias are attributable to *H. influenzae* and other bacterial pathogens (Buckley et al., 1972; Donabedian and Gallin, 1983). Patients with JS often live well into adulthood, although pulmonary sequlae of repeated necrotizing lung infections become increasingly problematic (Merten et al., 1979).

Treatment approaches with afflicted patients include the use of intermittent antistaphlococcal prophylaxis, which appears to reduce the frequency of infections with this organism. Anecdotal reports that administration of levamisole restored some immune defects associated with JS were not corroborated by a randomized double-blind trial (Donabedian et al., 1982). A recent preliminary trial in seven patients with the disorder showed that treatment with H_2-receptor blockers resulted in a decreased frequency of infections, presumably by augmentation of neutrophil chemotaxis (Thompson and Kummararatne, 1989). Findings that mononuclear lymphocytes of patients with JS have deficient production of interferon-γ may ultimately provide important new treatment approaches (Jeppson et al., 1991). Incubation of neutrophils from afflicted patients with rHuIFN-γ has been demonstrated to increase chemotactic responsiveness of these cells by threefold (Jeppson et al., 1991). Moreover, a recent in vivo study showed that treatment of JS patients with rHuIFN-γ resulted in marked, dose-dependent decreases of abnormally high IgE levels (King et al., 1989).

C. Disorders of Cellular Immunity

The disorders that comprise the cellular immunodeficiencies are characterized by absent or functionally impaired T lymphocytes. Accordingly, afflicted patient have depressed T-cell proliferative responses to mitogens, skin test anergy, and a predisposition for a wide variety of infections with opportunistic pathogens, including herpes viruses, *P. carinii*, *Legionella* spp., mycobacteria, *Nocardia*, and *Listeria*. For the most part, these opportunists are intracellular pathogens that are readily phagocytized by alveolar macrophages or fixed-tissue histiocytes. The relatively unimpeded intracellular proliferation of these pathogens in patients with impaired cell-mediated immunity, however, is a reflection of the importance of T cells for macrophage activation and cytotoxicity. Furthermore, T lymphocytes have a central role in regulation of other immune system components, notably including proliferation and differentiation of B lymphocytes.

Accordingly, in addition to primary defects of cell-mediated immunity, many of the disorders described in this section also present with concomitant deficits of humoral and/or phagocyte defense mechanisms.

Severe Combined Immunodeficiency Disease

The myriad immune defects associated with severe combined immunodeficiency disease (SCID) result from any of several diverse abnormality(ies) of lymphoid stem cell maturation. Common manifestations of these entities include hypoplastic lymphoid tissue, absence of delayed hypersensitivity, defects of antibody production, and hypogammaglobulinemia (Buckley, 1983; Rosen et al., 1984b). Profound lymphopenia of both B and T cells is usual, although some individuals have normal absolute counts due to increased numbers of circulating immature lymphocytes.

Affected neonates often develop a morbilliform rash within a few days after birth, which has been ascribed to graft-versus-host disease from passively transferred maternal lymphocytes (Rosen et al., 1984b). In addition, SCID infants classically present with a triad of mucocutaneous candidias, intractable diarrhea, and *P. carinii* pneumonia (Leggiadro et al., 1981). Viral pathogens, particularly herpes viruses (herpes simplex, cytomegalovirus, varicella), measles, and influenza are other common causes of severe early pneumonia. A few cases of disseminated *Legionella* have also been reported (Cutz et al., 1982). Administration of attenuated live-virus vaccines results in fatal infections (Rosen et al., 1984b).

Several variants of this syndrome have been described. An X-linked recessive variant, in which the basis for the underlying defect has not yet been discovered, accounts for nearly one-half of SCID cases. The preponderance of remaining patients appear to have autosomal recessive heredity. About one-half of the autosomal recessive cases are attributable to a deficiency of adenosine deaminase (ADA) (Hirschhorn, 1990). ADA catalyzes an early step in the purine salvage pathway and is ubiquitous in mammalian cells. Toxic effects of the enzyme deficiency are due to accumulation of adenosine metabolites. ADA deficiency, however, has not been identified as a cause of significant disease of cells other than lymphocytes (Rosen et al., 1984b).

The lifespan of infants with SCID is usually limited to a very few years. Enzyme replacement by infusion of red blood cells has been attempted in ADA-deficient patients, with variable success. Frequent administration of polyethylene-glycol–bonded ADA has recently been demonstrated to ameliorate B- and T-cell defects of enzyme-deficient patients (Levi et al., 1988). A possible future role for cytokine therapy has been suggested by observations that T-cell mitogen responses of ADA-deficient patients are enhanced by exposure to interleukin-2 (IL-2) (Cowan et al., 1989). Insertion of the cloned human gene for ADA is a promising potential treatment of enzyme-deficient patients (Kantoff et al., 1986). Allogeneic bone marrow transplantation remains the definitive therapy for patients with SCID, although resistance to engraftment and posttransplant abnormalities of B-lymphocyte function have been serious problems (O'Reilly et al., 1989).

A clinically similar entity ascribed to purine-nucleoside phosphorylase deficiency has been described in a small number of patients (Rosen et al., 1984b). The metabolic toxicity of purine-nucleoside phosphorylase deficiency preferentially affects T lymphocytes. Patients with this disorder usually have normal numbers of circulating B lymphocytes, and antibody production is unimpaired. Approximately one-half of affected patients also have profound neurological disorders (Hirschhorn, 1986). In the not too distant future, this rare disease may also be amenable to treatment by gene transfer (McIvor et al., 1987).

DiGeorge's Syndrome

DiGeorge's syndrome is a congenital defect that appears to represent a dysfunction of neural crest cell migration or other failure of these cells to normally interact with the third and fourth pharyngeal pouches during embryogenesis (Rosen et al., 1984b). In addition to thymic and parathyroid aplasia, the constellation of overt findings associated with this disorder includes various craniofacial deformities, as well as great-vessel anomalies and congenital cardiac defects. The cardiovascular abnormalities and neonatal hypocalcemic tetany account for most deaths among affected infants (Lischner, 1972; Freedom et al., 1972; Rosen et al., 1984b).

Unlike most of the other cell-mediated immunodeficiencies, the defect of DiGeorge's syndrome is entirely limited to cellular immune functions. T-cell numbers are markedly reduced and cell-mediated immunity is depressed to variable degrees, whereas circulating B lymphocytes are normal in number and function, and humoral immunity is intact. Neonates who survive hypocalcemic events and effects of cardiovascular anomalies are at risk for viral pneumonias, especially herpes viruses and measles. A number of cases of *P. carinii* pneumonia have also been reported. Spontaneous recovery of cellular immunity has been reported, although the immunodeficiencies may alternatively worsen with age. Implants of fetal thymus, epithelium, or extracts have successfully ameliorated the deficiency (Rosen et al., 1984b).

Wiskott-Aldrich Syndrome

Wiskott-Aldrich syndrome is an X-linked recessive disorder with an estimated occurrence in four infants per one million male births. The manifestations of this rare disorder include a predilection for opportunistic infection, thrombocytopenia, eczema, and an increased relative risk for hematological malignancies. Infection accounts for 60% of deaths among affected individuals (Perry et al., 1980).

Both cellular and humoral immunity are impaired in this syndrome. Afflicted patients typically have a progressive decline in numbers and functions of T cells, low levels of IgM, elevated concentrations of IgA and IgE, and impaired antibody responses to challenges with polysaccharide antigens (Rosen et al., 1984b). The underlying defect may be related to the absence of a T-lymphocyte membrane glycoprotein, although the exact function of this cell surface marker is uncertain (Remold-O'Donnell et al., 1984). Successful bone marrow transplantation results in a reversal of the myriad hematological and immune defects associated with the syndrome (Rimm 1990).

Ataxia-Telangiectasia

This autosomal recessive syndrome is characterized by the constellation of progressive cerebellar ataxia, telangiectasias, a variable predilection for infections, and a very high incidence of malignancies. Ataxia is usually detected during the second year of life. Telangiectasias have a later onset, usually at about 5 years of age. Lesions are most prominent in conjunctivae and on skin exposed to sunlight. The majority of toddlers with the syndrome have an increased prevalence of bacterial and viral sinopulmonary infections (McFarlin et al., 1972). Chronic bronchiectasis ultimately develops in approximately one-third of cases. Patients with ataxia-telangiectasia syndrome also have a relative risk of 100 for the development of neoplasms, especially non-Hodgkin's lymphoma (Kersey et al., 1988). Otherwise unaffected heterozygous family members have a reported fivefold greater incidence of malignancies (Swift et al., 1976).

The pathogenesis of the syndrome is complex and not completely elucidated. Fibroblasts of patients with ataxia-telangiectasia are exquisitely sensitive to ionizing radiation (Taylor et al., 1975) and chromosomal aberrations are frequent (McCaw et al., 1975; Kamatsu et al., 1990), which suggests a basic defect of DNA repair mechanisms. A yet to be identified enzymatic deficiency has also been postulated (Waldmann et al., 1983).

The spectrum of immunodeficiencies associated with ataxia-telangiectasia is heterogeneous and complex. The majority of patients exhibit varying degrees of reductions in levels of IgA, IgE, and IgG subclasses. T-helper cells of these patients are dysfunctional and may account for the underlying abnormalities of B-cell activity and humoral immunity. Deficient interleukin-2 (IL-2) production by mononuclear leukocytes of patients with ataxia-telangiectasia has recently been demonstrated, and administration of recombinant IL-2 restored at least some measures of B- and T-cell functions in an afflicted individual (Doi et al.,

1989). Treatment with synthetic thymic factors has been reported to increase immunoglobulin levels and decrease the incidence of infections in a small number of patients (Bordiogoni et al., 1982).

The propensity for development of serious respiratory tract infections among ataxia-telangiectasia patients is significantly correlated with the presence of IgG-subclass deficiencies (Oxelius et al., 1982). Despite the well-documented impairment of T-helper activity, *P. carinii* pneumonias have not been reported to occur in patients with this syndrome.

III. Secondary Immunodeficiencies

A. Renal Insufficiency

Rates of pneumonia among chronic renal failure patients may be as great as 50%, and up to half these infections are fatal (Montgomerie et al., 1968; Keane et al., 1977; Kjellstrand, 1978). The epidemiology of pulmonary infections in uremic patients reflects the prevalence of upper airway colonization; as expected, gram-negative pathogens predominate in hospitalized populations (Montgomerie et al., 1968; Keane et al., 1977). Pulmonary infections with *Legionella* spp. also occur at higher rates in these patients than among the general population (England et al., 1981). Renal failure is also a predisposing risk for skin and upper airway colonization with *S. aureus* (Goldblum and Reed, 1980), and several cases of pneumonia due to this virulent pathogen have been noted in large series (Montgomerie et al., 1968; Keane et al., 1977). The incidence of mycobacterial disease is increased severalfold by chronic renal failure (Andrew et al., 1980), prompting liberal recommendations for isoniazid prophylaxis in tuberculin-positive uremic patients (American Thoracic Society–Center for Disease Control Consensus Statement, 1986).

Despite the apparent predilection for infection in renal failure patients, the clinical significance of the various immune deficits described in this population has not been clearly defined. Absolute numbers of circulating B and T lymphocytes tend to be reduced in the presence of uremia, and specific impairments of lymphocyte responsiveness are noted (Anagnoston and Kurtzman, 1986). Uremia also has deleterious effects on neutrophil maturation, metabolism, and chemotaxis (Briggs and Silliz, 1983; Anagnoston et al., 1986). Although chronic renal failure patients are capable of febrile responses to infection, these responses tend to be attenuated (Wolk and Apicell, 1978). Despite these myriad in vitro functional immunological abnormalities, however, assessments of bacterial clearance in experimental animals have generally shown only relatively minor defects due to uremia per se (Clarke et al., 1983).

The high rate of pulmonary infections among dialysis patients may be, at least in part, a result of underlying uremic lung injuries. Significant histological abnormalities of pulmonary parenchyma and airways, putative effects of uremic toxicity, have been well documented in renal failure patients. These structural changes could interfere with local defense mechanisms, including mucociliary clearance, and predispose renal failure patients to bacterial infections (Goldblum and Reed, 1980). Furthermore, these patients are generally more likely to develop infections because of repeated vascular cannulation, indwelling vascular catheters, malnutrition, and widespread antibiotic use.

B. Collagen-Vascular Disease

A wide range of pulmonary complications associated with the collagen-vascular diseases have been described (Hunninghake and Fauci, 1979), and are discussed in Chapter 8, "Rheumatological Diseases." Of particular relevance here, certain collagen-vascular disorders appear to predispose patients to significant infectious pulmonary complications as a result of inherent and/or iatrogenic defects of immune defenses.

Systemic Lupus Erythematosus

Of the various collagen-vascular diseases, the evidence linking underlying immune deficits with a predilection for pulmonary infections is strongest in systemic lupus erythematosus (SLE). Overall, infectious disease accounts for approximately one-third of deaths in SLE patients (Rosner et al., 1982), and pneumonias are the most frequently lethal of these infections (Hellmann et al., 1987).

SLE is associated with defects of both humoral and cell-mediated immune function. Complement level is depressed and serum opsonizing activity is impaired in patients with SLE, particularly during disease flares (Ginzler et al., 1978; Nived et al., 1985a). Various T-cell functional abnormalities have also been identified in SLE patients, and the severity of these aberrations is, similarly, much more pronounced during disease exacerbations (Rosenthal and Franklin, 1975; Landry, 1977).

Not surprisingly, the propensity for development of pulmonary and other infections is strongly correlated with SLE activity (Staples et al., 1974; Ginzler et al., 1978; Nived et al., 1985b). Further, fulminant SLE flares are often treated with augmentation of immunosuppressant medications, which further depress intrinsic defense mechanisms (Staples et al., 1974; Ginzler et al., 1978; Nived et al., 1985b; Hellmann et al., 1987).

Respiratory tract infections in SLE patients are most often attributable to bacterial pathogens, including enteric gram-negative organisms, *S. aureus*, and *S. pneumoniae*. Opportunistic pathogens, however, account for significant proportions of the pneumonias in SLE patients, especially those undergoing corticosteroid or cytotoxic therapy. As in other patients with defects of cellular immunity, a wide range of opportunistic organisms have been identified as agents of pneumonitis, including *P. carinii*, *Aspergillus*, *Candida*, locally endemic fungi, cytomegalovirus, *Nocardia*, and mycobacteria (Staples et al., 1974; Ginzler et al., 1978; Gorevic et al., 1980; Hellmann et al., 1987).

Opportunistic pathogens are difficult to diagnose in this population because numerous, and more common, noninfectious complications have similar presentations (Hunninghake and Fauci, 1979). The diagnostic difficulty is perhaps best highlighted by the report of Hellmann et al. (1987), who noted that 80% of opportunistic pathogens in their series of SLE patients were not recognized prior to death. Early use of invasive diagnostic procedures is, therefore, especially likely to be warranted in high-risk SLE patients with acute pulmonary disease (e.g., ongoing disease flare or antecedent immunosuppressive therapy).

Rheumatoid Arthritis (RA)

RA is a remarkable systemic disease with especially protean pulmonary manifestations (see Chapter 8, ''Rheumatological Diseases''). There is currently no clear consensus on the intrinsic propensity for pulmonary infections among RA patients, aside from a recognized risk among those treated with immunosuppressants. Early reports implied that stable patients not receiving immunosuppressive medications have increased risk for death from pneumonia and other infections (Cobb et al., 1953; Mitchell et al., 1986), but these findings are disputed by more recent investigations (Vandenbroucke et al., 1987; Albada-Kuipers et al., 1988).

There is little question, however, that patients with Felty's syndrome have a much greater than normal incidence of recurrent respiratory tract infections (Breedveld et al., 1987). The predilection for infection associated with this disorder is inversely correlated with absolute granulocyte counts $< 100\ mm^3$ (Breedveld et al., 1987). In contrast, infection risks are markedly augmented in acute leukemia patients as counts fall below $1000\ mm^3$ (Bodey et al., 1966), suggesting that the neutrophils of Felty's syndrome patients are more fully functional and lack the intrinsic defect(s) associated with leukemia. The predominant manifestation of lower respiratory tract infections in patients with the syndrome are lobar or bronchopneumonias with gram-positive cocci (e.g., *S. aureus*, *S. pneumonia*), enteric gram-negative rods, and occasionally *Candida* (Barnes et al., 1971; Goldberg and Pinals, 1980; Breedveld et al., 1987).

Treatment of RA with immunosuppressive medications unequivocally increases risk of infectious diseases. As in other populations, corticosteroids in doses greater than 15–20 mg/day of prednisone (or equivalent) are associated with a propensity for bacterial and opportunistic infections (Hoffman and Fauci, 1991). Low-dose methotrexate (MTX) is being increasingly utilized in treatment of severe or refractory RA. These MTX regimens have not generally been demonstrated to suppress cellular immune function and are, accordingly, much less immunosuppressive than the large doses of corticosteroids or cyclophosphamide used in SLE patients during exacerbations. Nonetheless, widespread use of low-dose MTX has resulted in a small number of infections with opportunistic organisms, including *P. carinii* (Wollner et al., 1991), *Nocardia* (Keegan and Byrd, 1988), and *Cryptococcus* (Altz-Smith et al., 1987).

Polymyositis-Dermatomyositis

Upper airway motor abnormalities, as well as weakness of respiratory muscles, is a common complication of these disorders. The resultant frequent aspirations of oropharyngeal secretions, in conjunction with impaired cough, predisposes these patients to recurrent pneumonias. Opportunistic infections are unusual among afflicted patients unless they are being treated with immunosuppressive therapy. Many polymyositis/dermatomyositis patients are maintained on high-dose corticosteroids or other immunosuppressants, however, and as many as 5% of all acute episodes of pulmonary abnormalities among those so treated have been shown to be due to infections with opportunistic organisms (Dickey and Myers, 1984).

Other Collagen-Vascular Diseases

Systemic sclerosis is not known to predispose afflicted patients to opportunistic infections, aside from risks that accrue from immunosuppressant therapies. Owing to esophageal dysmotility, many of these patients are also at considerable risk for recurrent aspiration and its pulmonary consequences. Sjögren's syndrome is associated with at least some predilection for suppurative airway disease and bacterial pneumonias (Hunninghake and Fauci, 1979).

C. Malignancies

Leukemias

Lung diseases are extremely common sequlae of the various leukemias and occur at some time in from 60 to 90% of afflicted patients (Tenholder and Hooper, 1980; Maile et al., 1983). These same series describe a nearly equal distribution of infectious and noninfectious complications.

Noninfectious pulmonary complications of the leukemias are often difficult to diagnose and are readily mistaken for infections. Pulmonary infiltration with leukemic cells may occur in one-third of patients and is especially common in those with peripheral leukocyte counts showing > 40% blasts. The diagnosis of leukemic infiltration requires lung biopsy, which is often infeasible in seriously ill or thrombocytopenic patients, and, thus, the disorder often goes unappreciated (Prakash et al., 1979; Maile et al., 1983). Pleural effusions may also be the result of leukemic pleural infiltration and can easily be misdiagnosed as signs of congestive heart failure or infection. Pulmonary vascular leukostasis is not infrequent in patients with leukocyte counts greater than 200,000/mm^3 and large proportions of blasts (McKee and Collins, 1974; Vernant et al., 1979). Occasional leukoagglutination reactions to infused blood products present as increased permeability pulmonary edema. A particularly fulminant interaction between transfused granulocytes and amphotericin B is a reported cause of severe lung injury and death (Wright et al., 1981). Spontaneous alveolar hemorrhage occurs in a significant proportion of patients with platelet counts $< 15,000/mm^3$ or with other bleeding dyscrasias and are particularly difficult to discriminate from infections solely by the clinical presentation (Goodall and Vosti, 1975; Tenholder and Hooper, 1980). Hydrostatic pulmonary edema is a common sequla of volume overload in these patients, especially among those with cardiac dysfunction due to anthracycline chemotoxicity, but should be apparent by assessments of fluid balance and responses to diuretics.

Acute Nonlymphocytic Leukemia

Acute nonlymphocytic leukemia (ANLL) provides a model for the pulmonary complications of neutropenia, because the spectrum of infections associated with this disease and their diagnosis and management are, in general, similar to those found in other granulocytopenic disorders.

Before receiving induction chemotherapy, nonneutropenic ANLL patients have an otherwise nearly intact immune system and are at relatively small risk for developing pulmonary infections with opportunistic organisms. The overwhelming majority of the infections that occur prior to treatment are due to common community-acquired organisms, and most of these present with typical clinical features, including focal radiographic abnormalities. Diffuse infiltrates that appear prior to induction chemotherapy are most frequently noninfectious complications of leukemia (Tenholder and Hooper, 1980).

The neutropenia that develops during induction therapy predisposes these patients to overwhelming infections from bacterial and fungal pathogens. The risk for these nosocomial infections increases with the duration of neutropenia and number of chemotherapy cycles (Tenholder and Hooper, 1080). Concomitant reduction of both leukocytes and lymphocytes to $<1000/mm^3$ doubles the rate of infection, compared to patients with only granulocytopenia (Bodey et al., 1966).

Functional defects of granulocytes that could further predispose to infection have also been identified in morphologically normal-appearing peripheral cells of patients with acute leukemias (Gregory et al., 1972; Cline 1973). Treatment with antileukemic cytotoxic agents results in additional impairments of neutrophil bactericidal activity (Nedelkova et al., 1981), as well as depressions of humoral and cell-mediated immune functions (Heppner and Calabresi, 1976; Bolivar et al., 1980). Despite in vitro abnormalities of granulocytes, however, the propensity for infections in ANLL patients correlates most closely with absolute reductions of neutrophil numbers (Bodey et al., 1966). Furthermore, despite chemotherapy-associated defects of cell-mediated immune mechanisms, opportunistic infections other than fungi (e.g., *P. carinii* and viruses) account for only 5% or less of all pneumonias among ANLL patients (Tenholder and Hooper, 1980; Pizzo et al., 1982a; O'Hanley et al., 1989).

In general, gram-negative bacteria have been the most commonly isolated pathogens from granulocytopenic patients (Armstrong et al., 1971; Pizzo et al., 1982a). Infections due to *Legionella* spp. may also occur, but vary from one location to another. More recently, increasing proportions of the infections among granulocytopenic patients appear to be caused by gram-positive organisms; a possible result of microbial selection with broad-spectrum antibiotics and use of indwelling intravenous lines (Bodey et al., 1982). *S. aureus* and *Enterococcus* as well as otherwise avirulent *S. epidermidis*, *Corneybacterium* spp., and saphrophytes of the oral cavity, including *Streptococcus mitis*, are being increasingly recognized as respiratory tract pathogens of granulocytopenic patients (Bodeyet al., 1982; Wade et al., 1982; O'Hanley et al., 1989).

As in most other populations, aspiration of secretions laden with upper airway and/or alimentary tract organisms is the usual precursor of pulmonary infection among ANLL patients. Disruption of epithelial integrity due to chemotherapy-induced mucositis is also a likely risk factor (Walsh et al., 1991). Because inflammatory responses are often markedly depressed in the absence of granulocytes, the clinical manifestations of pneumonias among neutropenic ANLL patients can be quite subtle (Sickles et al., 1975).

Persistence of neutropenia predisposes these patients to primary and superinfections with fungi. *Aspergillus* spp. are the most frequent of these pathogens, although recent reports describe a seemingly increasing prevalence of pneumonias due to *Candida*, Mucoraceae, and unusual dermatophytic species (Walsh and Pizzo, 1988). The mortality associated with fungal pneumonias among granulocytopenic patients has, in most series, been in excess of 80%. Recent uncontrolled, but encouraging, trials with high-dose amphotericin B (1.0–1.5 mg/kg/day) plus flucytosine have reported greatly improved survival rates of patients with pulmonary or disseminated fungal disease (Burch et al., 1987). This regimen also appears effective for the prevention of recurrent fungal disease among patients who survive the initial *Aspergillus* infection (Karp et al., 1988).

The management of neutropenic patients with pulmonary infiltrates is an extremely controversial subject that suffers from lack of rigorously controlled studies (Wardman and Cooke, 1984). Given the predominance of bacteria as the etiology of early infections, there is general agreement that empirical antimicrobial drugs are appropriate initial therapy in most cases of pulmonary infiltrates, and that immediate utilization of invasive diagnostic procedures is not usually indicated (Tenholder and Hooper, 1980; O'Hanley et al., 1989; Walsh et al., 1991).

There is much less consensus about the indications for empirical amphotericin B therapy and the optimal sequence and timing of invasive diagnostic studies in granulocytopenic patients with possible pulmonary infections. Clearly, suspicion for fungal disease should be heightened in patients not responding to broad-spectrum antibiotics or in whom new pulmonary infiltrates appear during the course of antibiotic therapy (Commers et al., 1984). Owing to the predilection of *Aspergillus* for angiocentric invasion and thrombosis, the presence of signs or symptoms of pulmonary thromboemboli in granulocytopenic patients (Fig. 1) can be viewed as evidence of fungal pneumonitis (Young et al., 1970). The manifestations of fungal pneumonias are indistinguishable from those of bacterial infections or other processes, however, in the vast majority of patients (Jochelson et al., 1986; Tenholder and Hooper, 1980). Given the seriousness of fungal disease, institution of appropriate therapy appears especially important in those relatively few patients with characteristic clinical features. Moreover, two randomized trials have shown substantially increased survival in granulocytopenic patients who received empirical amphotericin B therapy for persistent or recurrent fever after a few days of antibiotic treatment (EORTC Antimicrobial Therapy Cooperative Group 1989; Pizzo et al., 1982b).

In practice, many clinicians are understandably reluctant to commit patients to protracted courses of amphotericin B in the absence of definite evidence of fungal disease (Walsh et al., 1991), especially given the substantial toxicities of aggressive contemporary treatment protocols (Burch et al., 1987; Karp et al., 1988). Unfortunately, the diagnosis of fungal pneumonitis is fraught with

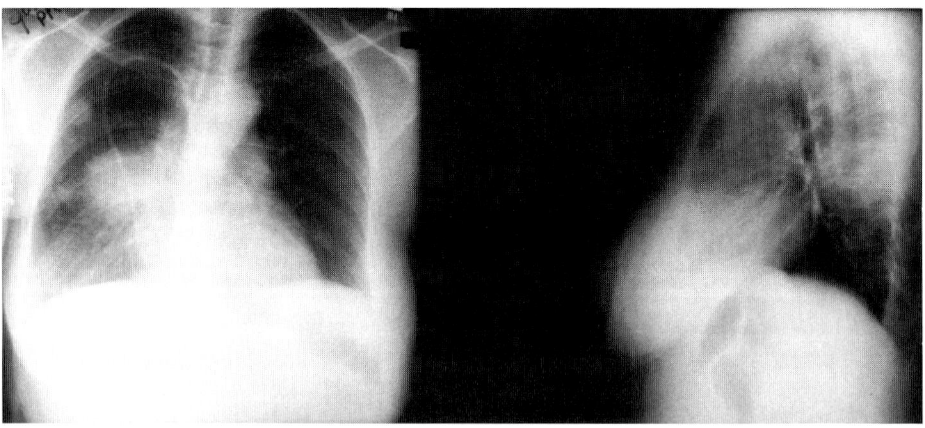

Figure 1 Chest radiograph of a neutrophilic patient with acute nonlymphocytic leukemia demonstrates characteristic peripheral nodular lesions of *Aspergillus* pulmonary infection.

considerable technical difficulties, and the disease often goes unrecognized until autopsy. The isolation of *Aspergillus* in nasal swabs or expectorated sputa has high predictive value for the presence of invasive lower respiratory tract disease in granulocytopenic patients, but false negative results are common (Yu et al., 1986).

Transtracheal aspiration, fine-needle transthoracic aspiration, fiberoptic bronchoscopy with the use of either protected brush or bronchoalveolar lavage (BAL), and open thoracotomy have all been employed with variable degrees of success and have been briefly reviewed elsewhere (Saito et al., 1988). In general, fine-needle aspiration is the initial diagnostic procedure of choice for small peripheral focal lesions, although there are many contraindications to the procedure (e.g., profound thrombocytopenia) and the diagnostic yield is far from perfect (Castellino and Blank, 1979; Chan et al., 1989). During the last few years, bronchoalveolar lavage (BAL) has become the favored invasive procedure at most centers for the evaluation of pulmonary infiltrates in immunocompromised hosts (Stover et al., 1984). The sensitivity of BAL for bacterial infections (Thorpe et al., 1987) and most opportunistic pathogens (Stover et al., 1984) is generally excellent, but the procedure has a yield of little better than 50% for invasive fungal pneumonitis in most credible reports (Kahn et al., 1986; Saito et al., 1988). The tendency of *Aspergillus* to invade the interstitial compartment with relative sparing of airspaces probably accounts for the numerous false negative BAL studies. Transbronchial biopsies are positive for *Aspergillus* in slightly more than 10% of cases and add specificity for the diagnosis of invasive disease, but do not appreciably increase the detection rate of BAL alone (Kahn et al., 1986). Even the most definitive test, open lung biopsy by thoracotomy, has less than 100% sensitivity for *Aspergillus*, according to McCabe et al. (1985). These investigators further maintained that diagnostic confirmation of fungal infections by open lung biopsy probably did not appreciably alter the ultimate outcomes of patients in their series.

Given the imperfect sensitivity of most (if not all) currently available diagnostic procedures, and the high mortality of untreated fungal disease, there are several unresolved dilemmas in the management of granulocytopenic patients with refractory fever and pulmonary infiltrates. Whereas the presence of fungi in lung specimens obtained by invasive or other procedures is usually considered sufficient indication for treatment, negative results do not reliably exclude the diagnosis of fungal pneumonitis. Accordingly, the soundness of denying potentially lifesaving therapy to high-risk patients on the basis of often falsely negative tests is arguable. On the other hand, the toxicities of potentially curative antifungal therapy (Burch et al., 1987; Karp et al., 1988) may be too great to justify empirical administration to all patients, relatively few of whom actually have invasive fungal disease (O'Hanley et al., 1989). Similarly, the morbidity and small, but finite, mortality associated with open thoracotomy of seriously ill patients (Potter et al., 1985) may not warrant use of this procedure in all granulocytopenic patients with persistent undiagnosed pneumonias. Ultimate resolution of these and related questions awaits determination by prospective randomized trials (Wardman and Cooke, 1984). Alternatively, the development of new sensitive diagnostic tests, such as assays for fungal antigens (Andrews and Weiner, 1982), or the introduction of efficacious but less toxic prophylactic or therapeutic agents (Walsh et al., 1991) could render these issues moot.

Acute Lymphocytic Leukemia

Many of the pulmonary complications of acute lymphocytic leukemia (ALL) are similar to those described previously for ANLL. Noninfectious lung problems, in particular, are practically indistinguishable between the two diseases, except for a somewhat lesser propensity for patients with ALL to present with leukemic pulmonary infiltration (Maile et al., 1983). Functional neutropenia associated with high proportions of circulating lymphoblasts or an absolute neutropenia resulting from induction chemotherapy also predisposes ALL patients to the same spectrum of bacterial or fungal pathogens seen in those with ANLL (Bodey et al., 1982; Maile et al., 1983).

Patients will ALL are much more likely than those with ANLL, however, to develop opportunistic pulmonary infections with viruses and *P. carinii* (Hughes et al., 1975). The predilection for *P. carinii* pneumonia is sufficiently great that prophylaxis with trimethoprim-sulfamethoxazole (SMX-TMP) is of proven benefit in high-risk ANLL patients undergoing intense chemotherapy (Hughes et al., 1977). Given the high likelihood of infection due to opportunistic pathogens, especially in cases with diffuse radiographic infiltrates, early definitive diagnosis by invasive diagnostic procedures is generally recommended.

The frequent occurrence of opportunistic pneumonias in this population reflects a significant leukemia-associated impairment of humoral and cell-mediated immune functions. In large part, these deficiencies result from a relative paucity of fully mature and functional lymphocytes. In addition, aggressive therapeutic regimens for ALL unavoidably lead to further defects of lymphocyte function. Corticosteroids and vincristine are widely used in current induction protocols, and both agents have significant deleterious effects on antibody-dependent and natural killer cytotoxicities against viral-infected cells (Bolivar et al., 1980). Corticosteroids also have an often-described lympholytic effect, but, at least in humans, the lymphopenia following steroid administration is primarily due to sequestration rather than true cytolysis (Hoffman and Fauci, 1991). Prophylactic central nervous system irradiation also has an adverse effect on phagocyte and cellular immune functions that results in a demonstrably greater incidence of infection in treated ALL patients (Aur et al., 1972). In contrast to transplant populations, however, cytomegalovirus pneumonitis among

ALL patients is not necessarily associated with a severe or progressive disease course.

Chronic Myelogenous Leukemia

During blast crises or cycles of intense chemotherapy, patients with chronic myelogenous leukemia (CML) may have reductions of functional granulocytes and, accordingly, face many of the same risks for infection seen in patients with ANLL (Bodey et al., 1982). While patients are in the chronic phase of their illness, however, they do not appear to have greater than normal risks for infection, despite their abnormally high granulocyte counts.

Chronic Lymphocytic Leukemia

Although the peripheral lymphocytes of patients with chronic lymphocytic leukemia (CLL) appear morphologically normal, these cells are often functionally inert. Consequently, CLL patients are frequently hypogammaglobulinemic and have impaired antigen-specific antibody production. Cellular immune functions may be also be significantly impaired. Overall, the relative risk for infection is increased fivefold by CLL, and infectious processes are a contributing or causal factor in the death of at least 30% of afflicted patients. The most frequently identified pathogens are encapsulated bacteria and, a to a lesser extent, herpes-zoster. Opportunistic infections with *Nocardia* and locally endemic fungi have also been reported (Kauffman et al., 1978). Prophylactic therapy with intravenous immune globulin (IVIG) has recently been shown in a large prospective trial to decrease the incidence of bacterial disease in patients with recurrent infections (Cooperative Group for the Study of Immunoglobulin in Chronic Lymphocytic Leukemia, 1988).

Pulmonary parenchymal and endobronchial infiltration with CLL is also frequent in this population and may present with recurrent localized pneumonias (Palosaari and Colby, 1986).

Myelodysplastic Syndromes

The myelodysplastic syndromes (MDS), often referred to as "preleukemias," are a diverse group of disorders characterized by refractory cytopenias and morphological aberrations of myeloid or erythroid cell lines. Progression to overt leukemia is common. Patients with MDS have a generally increased risk of infections with a spectrum of bacterial and fungal organisms similar to that of overtly neutropenic patients. A recent report attributed two-thirds of the mortality in a large group of these patients to infectious disease, with pneumonias being the most frequent serious infection (Pomeroy et al., 1991). The risk of infection among these patients could be stratified on the basis of the underlying morphological abnormality and was inversely correlated with absolute neutrophil counts.

Plasma Cell Dyscrasias

Multiple myeloma (MM) is an indolent disease of B-cell hyperproliferation that results in profound impairments of humoral immunity and a high prevalence of pulmonary infections. Afflicted patients typically have gross deficiencies of antigen-specific antibody responses and overall reductions of normal immunoglobulin levels. Gram-positive bacteria, particularly *S. aureus* and *S. pneumoniae*, account for 50% of all infections, with most of the remainder attributable to enteric gram-negative rods (Savage et al., 1982). Opportunistic infections in MM patients are extremely unusual.

Infections occur at an overall rate of 1.5/MM patients/year, account for 70% of all deaths in this population, and most frequently involve the lungs (Perri et al., 1981). The greatest risk for infections among MM patients occurs during the immediate few weeks after initial chemotherapy (Perri et al., 1981); the relative risk then decreases among patients responding to these treatments, but it substantially increases again if the disease relapses. Recent trials have shown that prophylactic therapy with IVIG significantly decreases the incidence of infections in these patients (Schedel, 1986).

Waldenström's macroglobulinemia results in similar defects of humoral immunity and a predilection for bacterial infections. Hyperviscosity syndrome is a major noninfectious pulmonary manifestation of the disease (Rausch and Herion, 1980).

Hairy Cell Leukemia

Hairy cell leukemia is an uncommon B-cell neoplasm with a smoldering course reminiscent of the chronic leukemias. Afflicted patients are extremely susceptible to respiratory tract and other infections with bacteria, mycobacteria, fungi, cytomegalovirus, and parasites (Stewart and Bodey, 1981). The predilection for these infections appears to be attributable to a reduction of circulating monocytes as well as abnormal monocyte chemotaxis (Yam et al., 1977).

Lymphomas

Pulmonary infections are a leading cause of death in lymphoma patients (Feld and Bodey, 1977; Ostrow et al., 1981; Bishop et al., 1981). The underlying neoplasm is associated with specific defects of cellular immune function, and these impairments are augmented as a consequence of chemotherapy. Thus, lymphoma patients, especially those undergoing chemotherapy, are at considerable risk for a spectrum of opportunistic infections similar to those of transplant populations (Ostrow et al., 1981; Bishop et al., 1981). Further, the intense cytotoxicity associated with therapeutic protocols for lymphoma may cause transient neutropenia, thus increasing risk for bacterial and fungal infections, at least during the period of granulocytopenia.

P. carinii is the most frequent opportunistic pulmonary pathogen of lymphoma patients and accounts for approximately 4–15% of acute pulmonary infiltrates (Chuang et al., 1981; McCabe et al., 1989; Catterall et al., 1989; Campbell et al., 1989). Other opportunistic pathogens of this population include *Aspergillus* and *Candida* spp., herpes viruses (cytomegalovirus, herpes simplex, and varicella-zoster), zygomycetes, *Cryptococcus*, *Nocardia*, *Listeria monocytogenes*, and *Mycobacterium* spp.

Bronchoscopic techniques have excellent sensitivity for the detection of most of these infections, with the exception of invasive fungi (see ANLL) (Chuang et al., 1981; Stover et al., 1984; Campbell et al., 1989). There appear to be fewer organisms in the lung parenchyma of *P. carinii*–infected lymphoma and other non-AIDS patients than in those associated with AIDS (Limper et al., 1989). Furthermore, the pathogen is often localized primarily in pulmonary interstitium of affected non-AIDS patients, whereas massive airspace involvement is usual in those with underlying HIV infection. Accordingly, the diagnostic sensitivity of BAL for *P. carinii* among lymphoma and other non-AIDS populations is likely to be reduced (Dunn et al., 1988; Limper et al., 1989) in comparison to the 90% yield reported in patients with AIDS (Broaddus et al., 1985). Silver stains of transbronchial biopsies can detect many, if not most, of these BAL-negative cases.

Noninfectious complications account for a large proportion of acute pulmonary diseases among lymphoma patients (Chuang et al., 1981; McCabe et al., 1989; Catterall et al., 1989; Campbell et al., 1989). Over one-half of the noninfectious episodes are due to recurrences of the malignancy. Altogether, direct pulmonary involvement with the underlying malignancy eventually occurs in up to 60% of all patients with Hodgkin's disease, and to a somewhat lesser extent in non-Hodgkin's lymphomas (Castellino et al., 1973; Costello and Mauch, 1979; Rosenow et al., 1985). Recurrences can present as focal or (more often) multifocal nodules, localized consolidations, diffuse infiltrates, or pleural effusions. Hilar and/or mediastinal adenopathy is prominent in most cases of initial presentation with lymphoma, although pulmonary parenchymal involvement without apparent adenopathy frequently occurs in cases with antecedent mediastinal irradiation. Further, relapses in or adjacent to the treatment field are not unusual (Castellino et al., 1973).

Transbronchial biopsies (TBB) often yield specimens adequate for the diagnosis of pulmonary parenchymal infiltration by non-Hodgkin's lymphomas, at least in those cases of diffuse disease or large lesions that can be fluoroscopically localized (Chuang et al., 1981; Campbell et al., 1989). The yield of TBB for pulmonary Hodgkin's disease, however, may be somewhat lower. Isolated cases have been diagnosed by recovery of Reed-Sternberg cells in BAL or brushing specimens. The availability of histological markers for abnormal lymphocytes should increase the yield of transbronchial biopsy and transthoracic aspiration.

Two recent series have examined the role of open lung biopsy in this population (Potter et al., 1985; Hall et al., 1987). Both studies found that there were no outcome differences between groups randomized to open lung biopsy versus empirical therapy with trimethoprim-sulfamethoxazole and erythromycin. Infections, primarily *P. carinii*, were the only treatable causes of diffuse pulmonary infiltrates in these reports. Despite these nihilistic implications, however, other investigators maintain that the diagnosis of recurrent pulmonary lymphoma by biopsy can result in improved patient outcome by reimplementation of chemotherapy (McCabe et al., 1989; Catterall et al., 1989).

Radiation pneumonitis (RP) occurs in up to one-third of treated lymphoma patients (Kaplan and Stewart, 1973) and, in conjunction with cases of drug-induced lung injury, probably accounts for many of the nonspecific biopsies reported in various series (Chuang et al., 1981; McCabe et al., 1989; Catterall et al., 1989; Campbell et al., 1989). Clinical manifestations of RP are often indistinguishable from those of pulmonary lymphoma or opportunistic infections. Radiation injury classically presents 2–4 months after treatment with a nonproductive cough, low-grade fever, and, in progressive cases, eventual fibrosis with worsening dyspnea and hypoxemia. The usual radiographic appearance consists of nondescript fibrotic infiltrate(s) in the field of irradiation, but diffuse disease that extends well outside the treated area is not infrequent. A recent investigation of patients undergoing localized thoracic irradiation reported that pulmonary segments distant from the treatment fields had abnormally increased gallium uptake and BAL lymphocytosis (Gibson et al., 1988). This evidence of global pulmonary inflammation was interpreted by the observers as the result of a generalized hypersensitivity reaction, an injury mechanism that could well explain the occurrences of diffuse RP.

Cytotoxic drug-induced pneumonitis mimics disease due to diffuse RP and has, likewise, nonspecific clinical features and nondiagnostic histopathological findings (Cooper et al., 1986). The lung injuries of most cytotoxic agents are dose-dependent, although there are wide variations of toxic thresholds. Moreover, modest doses of individual agents that would otherwise be well tolerated may, in fact, cause significant cytotoxic lung injuries when given in combination, or in conjunction with radiation therapy. Idiosyncratic hypersensitivity reactions, independent of cumulative doses, have also been described for bleomycin, procarbazine, and methotrexate.

Solid Tumors

Pulmonary infections occur with high frequencies in cancer patients and are among the most common proximate causes of death in this population (Singer et al., 1977). In some cases, the increased risk of pneumonia is due to mechanical effects of the tumor that alter local defense mechanisms, e.g., abnormalities of deglutition with head and neck tumors or obstructing endobronchial tumors. Other neoplastic complications may have secondary effects on immune function, e.g., renal failure and malnutrition.

With very few exceptions (e.g., Cushing's syndrome associated with malignancy) untreated carcinomas are not known to have substantive direct effects on immune system function. Accordingly, HIV testing is indicated among untreated cancer patients who develop *P. carinii* pneumonia (Walsh et al., 1991). Neutropenia, with resultant markedly increased risk for bacterial and fungal infections (Bodey et al., 1966), may be a complication of chemotherapies and/or radiation therapy. Further, the immunosuppressive effects of cytotoxic chemotherapy and irradiation can result in significant impairments of humoral and cellular immune functions. Intensely treated carcinoma patients have an increased relative risk for the development of a spectrum of opportunistic infections frequently observed in organ transplantation recipients, including *P. carinii*, fungi, herpes viruses, and intracellular bacterial pathogens (e.g., *Legionella, Listeria*, mycobacteria, and *Nocardia*).

IV. Bone Marrow Transplantation

Bone marrow transplantation (BMT) is associated with an unparalleled range of pulmonary complications. On the one hand, the intense immunosuppression of BMT predisposes these patients to the full spectrum of infectious complications seen in solid-organ transplant recipients. The unique lung injuries that ensue from cytotoxic therapies and graft-versus-host disease, moreover, result in a high frequency of devastating pulmonary diseases with nondescript clinical features and poorly understood pathogenesis.

Serious lung disease occurs in approximately 50% of allogeneic bone marrow transplant recipients (Krowka et al., 1985; Cordonnier et al., 1986). Autologous BMT recipients have a lower, but still considerable, incidence of pulmonary sequlae (Pecego et al., 1986). For purposes of discussion, these processes can be grouped into early (< 100 days after transplantation) and later complications. These two groups can be further illuminated by stratification into infectious, idiopathic, graft-versus-host, and vascular etiologies. In practice, however, these general classifications are not necessarily mutually exclusive, but often overlap considerably and/or coexist.

A. Early complications

Infectious Complications

During the first 2–4 weeks after transplantation, prior to engraftment of the marrow, profound neutropenia is the major predisposing risk factor for pulmonary infections. Mechanical impairments of respiratory tract defenses during this early period are also substantial, including severe mucositis and narcotic analgesia resulting in aspiration of pooled secretions, and immobility and inanition that lead to atelectasis (Krowka et al., 1985).

In early reports, bacterial pneumonias occurred in as many as 20–30% of BMT recipients during the preengraftment period (Sloane et al., 1983; Cordononnier et al., 1986). Enteric gram-negative rods are the most frequently isolated etiological agents, with a few cases of gram-positive cocci (Krowka et al., 1985; Cordonnier et al., 1986). *Legionella pneumophila* has been sporadically reported and is associated with an especially high mortality (Kugler et al., 1983). The etiology of a large proportion of presumed bacterial pneumonias eludes diagnosis (Cordonnier et al., 1986). Anaerobic organisms may be important causal agents, but are probably underreported owing to shortcomings of isolation and culture techniques. With the exception of infections due to singularly unusual or virulent organisms, however, bacterial pneumonias are not a major cause of mortality in BMT recipients. Empirically selected antimicrobial therapy, followed by eventual return of the white blood cell count, usually results in a favorable response. The prevalence of bacterial infections also appears to be decreased somewhat by prophylactic antibiotics and intravenous immune globulin (IVIG) during the neutropenic phase (Krowka et al., 1985; Peterson et al., 1987; Sullivan et al., 1990).

Fungal Pneumonias

Neutropenia during the preengraftment period also predisposes these patients to fungal pneumonias. *Aspergillus* and *Candida* are the most frequent fungal pathogens, but Mucoraceae and another unusual organisms have been sporadically reported. The overall incidence of fungal pneumonias among BMT recipients is approximately 10–20% (Winston et al., 1979; Meyers, 1990). As in other granulocytopenic patients, the prediliction for fungal disease among BMT recipients is a direct function of the duration and severity of neutropenia. Even in cases of successful early diagnosis and appropriate therapy, nearly 80% of fungal pneumonias among BMT recipients are fatal and these infections may account for up to 30% of all deaths in this population (Winston et al., 1979; Krowka et al., 1985; Meyers, 1990).

Aggressive measures to prevent fungal pneumonias are warranted by the diagnostic difficulties and seriousness of these infections (also, see section on ANLL). Reverse isolation in high-efficiency particulate air filters reduces the prevalence of *Aspergillus* colonization and probably, though less certainly, decreases the incidence of fungal infections in BMT recipients (Sherertz et al., 1987). Administration of low-dose amphotericin (~0.3 mg/kg/day) during the neutropenic phase is widely used and generally believed to have prophylactic efficacy, but data in support of this policy are scant. High-dose amphotericin B, in conjunction with flucytosine, has been reported to be much more effective in neutropenic acute leukemic patients with fungal infections than traditional regimens (Burch et al., 1987), but experience with this therapy in BMT recipients is limited. There is also as yet insufficient experience to assess the role and utility of newly formulated imidazoles that appear to have substantial antifungal activity, but less toxicity than amphotericin B. Itraconazole, which remains an experimental agent at the time of this writing, has been especially promising in preliminary investigations of other patient populations (Denning et al., 1989).

P. carinii Pneumonia

Prophylaxis with trimethoprim-sulfamethoxazole has nearly eradicated *P. carinii* pneumonia among BMT recipients, a former scourge of these patients with a high mortality rate (Krowka et al., 1985). The median onset of *P. carinii* was approximately 2 months following transplantation, with the risk period for this infection persisting for up to 4 months in uncomplicated patients. BMT recipients with chronic GVHD are predisposed to *P. carinii* infections for even more prolonged periods, thus justifying indefinite prophylaxis in these patients. Trimethoprim-sulfamethoxazole prophylaxis has also been credited with an incidental decrease in frequency of infections due to susceptible bacteria (Sullivan et al., 1984). Aerosolized pentamidine is widely used and appears effective for the prevention of *P. carinii* infection in patients unable to tolerate trimethoprim-sulfamethoxazole.

Cytomegalovirus Pneumonia

The single most serious pulmonary infection of BMT recipients is cytomegalovirus (CMV) pneumonia. Overall, CMV pneumonias occur in ~20% of allogeneic recipients (Meyers et al., 1982), and in a lesser 7% of autologous transplant recipients (Reusser et al., 1990). Risk factors for CMV infections in this population (Table 2) are cumulative: the probability of pneumonia in a seropositive patient older than 35 years with moderate to severe GVHD may approach 50% (Meyers et al., 1982, 1986). For practical purposes, CMV disease is limited to patients with preexistent infection or, among patients with negative anti-CMV

Table 2 Risk Factors for Cytomegalovirus Infections in Bone Marrow Transplant Recipients

CMV-seropositive recipient (pretransplant)
CMV-seropositive donor(s) (of either marrow or blood products)
Treatment with total-body irradiation
Increasing age
Occurrence of acute graft-versus-host disease (GVHD)
Severity (grade) of acute GVHD
Use of antithymocyte globulin

Source: Meyers et al., 1982, 1986; Cordonnier et al., 1986; Reusser, et al., 1990.

serologies, recipients of bone marrow from CMV-seropositive donors. CMV infections in this population most often occur from 40 to 120 days after transplantation, a period that overlaps the time when the cellular immunity of these patients is severely impaired.

CMV pneumonitis typically presents with nonspecific dyspnea, hypoxemia, and interstitial infiltrates that may progress in severity over a few hours or days. The diagnosis can be rapidly established by demonstration of characteristic viral cytopathic changes in pulmonary specimens. The sensitivity of BAL cytology is < 30%, however, and yields of transbronchial biopsies are highly variable (Springmeyer et al., 1982; Crawford et al., 1988; Paradis et al., 1988; Heurlin et al., 1989). Assays using fluroscent-linked monoclonal antibodies directed against intermediate-early CMV antigens (shell vial cultures) are positive in at least 60% of cases, and results can be available in 24–48 hours (Crawford et al., 1988; Erice et al., 1988; Schmidt et al., 1991). Conventional viral cultures in fibroblast tissue cultures remain the diagnostic "gold standard," but results may take 2 to 3 weeks. The natural history of CMV pulmonary infections has been particularly well described in BMT recipients. Positive shell vial or conventional cultures of BAL specimens, in the absence of histological or cytopathic findings, do not unequivocally establish the diagnosis of concurrent CMV disease or exclude the possibility of other ongoing processes. At least two longitudinal studies have established that this viral shedding (infection), however, is the eventual precursor to overt CMV pneumonitis in at least 70% of cases (Ruutu et al., 1990; Schmidt et al., 1991).

Until quite recently, CMV pneumonitis among BMT recipients was nearly always fatal (Meyers et al., 1982). Various trials of antiviral agents, including acyclovir, vidarabine, and interferon, showed no therapeutic benefit in patients with established CMV disease. Administration of intravenous immune globulin (IVIG) as a single agent may have some therapeutic effect, although results of trials have been inconsistent (Blacklock et al., 1985; Reed et al., 1987). Treatment with ganciclovir, a recently developed nucleoside analog, was demonstrated to quickly eradicate CMV in BMT recipients with pneumonitis, but did not alter the natural history of the disease (Shepp et al., 1985). A trial of ganciclovir plus corticosteroids was also unsuccessful (Reed et al., 1986). Recent regimens that combine ganciclovir and IVIG have shown a 50–75% reduction of mortality due to CMV pneumonitis, especially when therapy is instituted promptly after presentation with infection (Emmanuel et al., 1988; Reed et al., 1988).

The immunopathogenesis of CMV disease in bone marrow and other transplant recipients is an intricate process of considerable ongoing interest. Infection with CMV results in further impairment of host defense responses and a predisposition to superinfections with *P. carinii*, fungal, and bacterial pathogens (Rand et al., 1978; Rubin, 1989). A strong positive association exists between

CMV infections and GVHD in that the occurrence of either disease is an important risk factor for the development of the other (Miller et al., 1986; Meyers et al., 1986). An analogous correlation between CMV and allograft rejection has often been described in recipients of solid-organ transplantations (Rubin, 1989; Grattan et al., 1989; Duncan and Cook, 1991; Keenan et al., 1991).

Several investigators postulate that the mechanism of injury with CMV infections in transplant recipients is predominantly the result of cytotoxic or delayed-type hypersensitivity T-cell responses against new, or up-regulated, cell-surface antigens (Grundy et al., 1987). The target of these responses could be either products of the viral genome or up-regulated host MHC antigens. Deleterious immunopathogenic effects of CMV can occur in the absence of virion replication per se (Shepp et al., 1985; Grundy et al., 1987), a possible explanation for the failure of therapies limited to agents that prevent viral DNA synthesis (e.g., single-agent ganciclovir, a competitive inhibitor of viral thymidine kinase). The efficacy of the immunoglobulin preparations in combination regimens (with ganciclovir) appears to be independent of neutralizing antibody titers and is unlikely to be attributable to direct IVIG antiviral activity (McKeating et al., 1987). The mechanism of the synergistic effect of IVIG with ganciclovir has not been explained, but is presumably related to modification of host responses to the infection (Grundy et al., 1987).

Efforts have increasingly focused on prevention of CMV infection by use of antiviral prophylaxis. The use of CMV-seronegative blood products in recipients without past infection or exposure from the donor is of proven benefit (Bowden et al., 1986). Both IVIG and acyclovir appear to have partial efficacy as CMV prophylactic agents (Winston et al., 1987; Meyers et al., 1988; Sullivan et al., 1990). Recently Schmidt and colleagues (1991) demonstrated virtually complete prevention of CMV pneumonitis in high-risk allogeneic BMT recipients who completed a course of ganciclovir from 35 to 120 days after transplantation. The renal and bone marrow toxicities of ganciclovir were acceptable, but the regimen is somewhat cumbersome in requiring long-term administration of the intravenous medication. Prophylactic trials are currently underway with antivirals suitable for oral administration, including foscarnet, and an orally active formulation of ganciclovir, as well as monoclonal anti-CMV antibodies that require only infrequent parenteral dosing (Drobyski et al., 1991).

Other Viral Infections

Compared to CMV, other viral pathogens are much less troublesome in the early period following BMT. Herpes simplex viruses (HSV) have been isolated in 9% of lung tissue specimens from BMT recipients obtained at autopsy, although the actual prevalence of attributable pulmonary disease in these cases is uncertain (Ramsey et al., 1982). HSV is an unequivocal cause of pneumonitis in a small number of patients (Meyers et al., 1982), although the virus is more frequently associated with infections of the upper airways. Asymptomatic HSV respiratory tract infection occurs in the majority of untreated BMT recipients and, owing to rapid growth of the virus in culture, often results in overgrowth of BAL specimens obtained for isolation of CMV. Acyclovir and ganciclovir are both effective prophylactic and therapeutic agents for HSV infections.

An epidemic of infections due to respiratory syncytial virus (RSV), an otherwise uncommon pathogen of adults, was recently described in a small series of BMT recipients (Hertz et al., 1989). The etiology of these cases was convincingly demonstrated by either viral culture or ELISA of BAL specimens. Cough and upper airway symptoms appeared to be particularly prominent clinical feature of this disease. Chest radiographs usually showed nonspecific findings, but in some cases remained entirely normal. Mortality of these infections was 50%, despite treatment with aerosolized ribavirin.

Idiopathic Complications

A large number of the pulmonary problems following BMT have uncertain etiologies. Mild pulmonary restriction is common following BMT, but these mechanical defects tend to resolve by approximately 1 year after transplantation (Springmeyer et al., 1984; Depledge et al., 1983). Diffusing capacity abnormalities are also noted in the majority of these patients and may persist indefinitely (Depledge et al., 1983). The pulmonary function test abnormalities of BMT recipients are likely due, at least in part, to cumulative toxicities of pre- or post-transplant chemotherapies or irradiation. Krowka and colleagues (1990) recently showed BMT candidates often demonstrated hyperreactive bronchial responses to methacholine challenge prior to transplantation, another putative (but unproven) sequla of pretransplant chemotherapies. Unpublished observations during the course of a large study of BMT recipients (Schmidt et al., 1991) suggested that there was a high incidence of airway hyperreactivity among these patients, and that bronchoscopy may be facilitated by pretreatment with aerosolized β_2-agonists.

Diffuse Alveolar Hemorrhage

Several recent reports describe a clinical syndrome of diffuse alveolar hemorrhage (DAH) in BMT recipients (Sloane et al., 1983; Robbins et al., 1989; Jules-Elysee et al., 1990; Chao et al., 1991). As detailed by observers, DAH is a distinct idiopathic entity and not to be confused with alveolar hemorrhage due to *Aspergillus* or other necrotizing infections. DAH occurs in 5–35% of autologous BMT recipients (Robbins et al., 1989; Jules-Elysee et al., 1990; Chao et al., 1991) and in a much smaller percentage of allogeneic transplantation patients (Cordonnier et al., 1986). This disorder is an early complication of BMT, with a median onset the 12th day after transplantation. Clinical features of DAH are (again) nonspecific, with very rapidly progressive dyspnea, hypoxemia, and cough (Robbins et al., 1989). In rare cases, onset may be heralded by scant hemoptysis. More typically, hemoptysis is not present because extravasated blood in the distal lung parenchyma does not often freely communicate with proximal airways. The earliest radiographic abnormality may be innumerable 1 to 4-mm densities that represent individual hemorrhage-filled acinii. This finding is easily missed, however, since densities quickly evolve into confluent, nonsegmental consolidations. Risk features for DAH in autologous BMT recipients include age $>$ 40 years, severe mucositis, high fevers, underlying solid malignancy, renal insufficiency, and return of the white blood cell count (WBC) (Robbins et al., 1989). Neither the platelet count nor measures of coagulation appear to be strongly associated with a propensity for DAH.

The profound thrombocytopenia usually present at the time of DAH onset does, however, preclude safe biopsy of the lung. Histopathological specimens obtained in patients with DAH have, in any event, failed to show definite diagnostic findings or provide insight into possible pathogenetic mechanisms (Sloane et al., 1983; Robbins et al., 1989). Successive BAL aliquot returns are characteristically productive of increasingly hemorrhagic returns that, in the absence of pathogenic organisms, are diagnostic of the syndrome. DAH has an especially fulminant course and, in most series, has been associated with a mortality of 80–100% (Robbins et al., 1989; Jules-Elysee et al., 1990). The correlation of disease onset with WBC recovery is suggestive of an immunopathogenic etiology, a speculation further supported by a recent trial of high-dose steroids in a small number of patients which, quite promisingly, resulted in complete resolution and survival of all patients (Chao et al., 1991).

Interstitial Pneumonitis

Interstitial pneumonitis (IP) is an especially dreaded complication of BMT, which occurs in as many as one-half of allogeneic recipients, usually within 90 days after transplantation (Meyers et al., 1982; Weiner et al., 1986; Wingard et al., 1988). The prevalence of IP is somewhat lower (~8–20%) in syngeneic and autologous BMT recipients (Pecego et al., 1986; Weiner et al., 1989). IP is typified by diffuse, interstitial infiltrates and nonspecific clinical findings of cough, dyspnea, and hypoxemia. In many instances, the underlying lung injury can be attributed to infectious organisms, especially CMV. The etiology of 40–60% of episodes remains unknown, however, despite thorough diagnostic evaluations. The seriousness of idiopathic IP is underscored by the nearly identical mortality rate of 80% in two large series (Weiner, 1986; Wingard et al., 1988). These reports, and others (Cordonnier et al., 1986), also describe a better prognosis in cases with an identifiable etiology.

The clinical and radiographic abnormalities of idiopathic IP tend to have a more insidious onset and slower progression than most infections. Nonetheless, there are wide interindividual variations in manifestations of both idiopathic IP and the various opportunistic pathogens, and a diagnosis cannot be reliably assumed on the basis of presentation. Furthermore, a fulminant variant of idiopathic IP with a rapidly progressive course to respiratory failure has also been described in a small number of patients. Diagnostic procedures are useful primarily for the exclusion of infection. Lung biopsy specimens of these cases are nondescript; most show mononuclear parenchymal infiltration with varying degrees of fibrosis and hyperplasia of type II pneumocytes (Sloane et al., 1983). Histopathological examination of the more explosive cases often reveals diffuse alveolar damage, a nonspecific manifestation of diverse lung injuries also seen in patients with adult respiratory distress syndrome.

A number of risk factors for IP have been identified, including age, performance rating prior to transplantation, dose rate of total-body irradiation, elapsed time between diagnosis and BMT, severity of GVHD, and the type of GVHD prophylaxis (being greatest among patients receiving regimens other than cyclosporine A) (Weiner et al., 1986; Wingard et al., 1988; Sullivan et al., 1990). The variety of predisposing factors suggests IP is likely a heterogeneous entity with numerous causes. The strong association between IP and chemotherapy and/or irradiation implicates cytotoxicities of these treatments in the etiology of IP. The relative risk attributable to GVHD is also consistent with an immunological pathogenesis accounting for a least some cases of IP. The possibility of an immune-mediated mechanism is further supported by the demonstration of large numbers of activated CD8 lymphocytes (suppressor/cytotoxic–type T cells) in the BAL of patients with IP (Milburn et al., 1990). Moreover, a promising recent study showed that prophylactic therapy with IVIG resulted in a decreased incidence of IP in association with a reduction of acute GVHD (Sullivan et al., 1990). The much lower rate of IP in syngeneic and autologous BMT patients is consistent with either possible etiology (i.e., side effects of treatment versus immunological mechanisms) because patients with perfect donor-recipient HLA matches do not develop GVHD or require cytotoxic GVHD prophylaxis.

Acute Graft-Versus-Host Disease

Acute GVHD typically presents with a constellation of skin, GI tract, and liver involvement; manifestations of this disease in the lower respiratory tract remain largely inferential. As discussed above, acute GVHD has been implicated in the pathogenesis of IP. Acute GVHD has also been causally associated with early post-BMT adult respiratory distress syndrome and the syndrome of lymphocytic bronchitis (Beschorner et al., 1978). The very existence of this latter entity, however, is controversial. Adherents maintain the disorder is a discrete entity characterized by complaints of nonproductive cough and dyspnea, the presence of normal chest radiographs, and a predisposition to lower respiratory tract infections (Chan et al., 1990). Airway inflammation is attributed to bronchial mucosal infiltration with small lymphocytes demonstrable by bronchial biopsy or BAL. Disease manifestations are said to reflect the activity of acute GVHD in other sites and are likewise ameliorated, without residual airflow obstruction, by increased immunosuppression for the GVHD. Observations that lymphocytic bronchitis is found with equal frequencies in autopsies of BMT recipients and nontransplanted patients (Hackman and Sale, 1981), however, raise questions regarding this etiology of this entity.

Pulmonary Vascular Complications

In comparison to other general categories of complications following BMT, pulmonary vascular sequelae are relatively straightforward and seldom associated with long-term morbidity. Pulmonary edema is common in the early period after transplantation, a possible result of any combination of intravenous volume loading, total parenteral nutrition, hypoalbuminemia, acute GVHD, hepatic veno-occlusive disease, or renal tubular dysfunction from cyclosporine toxicity (Dickout et al., 1987). Underlying myocardial dysfunction secondary to pretransplant cardiotoxic chemotherapy is likely to also play a role in some cases (Appelbaum et al., 1976). Early trials with high doses of hematopoietic stem-cell growth factors, particularly granulocyte-monocyte colony-stimulating factor (GM-CSF), resulted in several cases of severe increased permeability pulmonary edema and pleural effusions, but the incidence of these side effects has been ameliorated by use of more modest doses (Brandt et al., 1988). Increased permeability pulmonary edema also occasionally occurs due to leukoagglutination reactions with transfused blood products (Krowka et al., 1985). While drug- or transfusion-related edema is an especially acute and severe cause of pulmonary dysfunction, these cases tend to resolve promptly over a few days with supportive care. Pulmonary emboli due to thrombi or infused bone fragments have been documented in a surprisingly large number of BMT recipients (Krowka et al., 1990), but are generally occult and not usually associated with clinical or physiological manifestations (Abrahams and Catchatourian, 1983).

B. Late Complications

Bacterial Infections

In the absence of GVHD, most functions of the immune system are reconstituted by 1 year following BMT (Sullivan, 1989). As expected, therefore, the frequency and seriousness of infections in BMT recipients with uncomplicated courses generally diminish with elapsed time after transplantation. BMT recipients with antecedent GVHD, however, are predisposed to recurrent bacterial infections of the respiratory tract. Sinopulmonary bacterial infections with gram-positive organisms, including *S. aureus*, are especially common among patients with chronic GVHD. High rates of respiratory tract colonization with pathogenic bacteria are also prevalent in this population, as well as frequent recurrences of bronchitis (Atkinson et al., 1979; Sullivan et al., 1984).

Risk factors for respiratory tract infections among BMT recipients with chronic GVHD include local abnormalities of airways and systemic defects of immune responses. Bronchiectasis and granulation plugs in small airways, a putative result of GVHD-mediated injuries, impair ciliary function and clearance of secretions. BMT recipients with chronic GVHD also have much more protracted deficiencies of humoral immunity than transplant recipients with uncomplicated courses. Whereas serum IgG and IgM levels normalize within 4 months in unaffected allogeneic BMT recipients, persistent hypogammaglobulinemia occurs in 15% of patients with chronic GVHD (Sullivan et al., 1988). The latter population also appears to have a much greater prevalence of IgG subclass deficiencies (Aucouturier et al., 1987) and depressed levels of secretory IgA (Izutsu et al., 1983). Chronic use of prophylactic trimethoprim-sulfamethoxazole decreases the incidence of late sinopulmonary infections in patients at risk (Peterson et al., 1987). Immunoglobulin replacement may also be beneficial for prevention of recurrent infections (Sullivan, 1989).

Varicella-Zoster Infection

Cutaneous varicella-zoster virus (VZV) occur in 40% of BMT recipients and eventually disseminate in from 20 to 40% of untreated patients (Sullivan et al., 1984; Krowka et al., 1985). Prophylaxis with acyclovir has markedly decreased the incidence of the disease and effectively prevents progression to lung infection. Ganciclovir prophylaxis for CMV could likely have even further impact on VZV prevention, given the severalfold greater activity of this agent against herpes viruses, including VZV, compared to acyclovir.

Relapses of Underlying Malignancy

Pulmonary recurrences of the underlying leukemia occur in a small number of BMT recipients. In most cases, pulmonary infiltration is a relatively incidental and late finding of leukemic recurrences (see previous leukemia sections). Recurrent disease is most often diagnosed by examinations of blood or bone marrow specimens.

Obliterative Bronchiolitis

Expiratory airflow obstruction due to obliterative bronchiolitis (OB) occurs in about 10% of long-term BMT survivors (Springmeyer et al., 1983; Clark et al.,

1987; Chan et al., 1987). Affected patients present with symptoms of chronic cough and progressively worsening dyspnea. The usual onset of the disease is from 6 to 12 months after BMT, although cases have been reported as early as 41 days after transplantation (Clark et al., 1987; Chan et al., 1987). Chest radiographs are typically normal or show some degree of hyperinflation or, less frequently, low-grade nondescript infiltrates. Pulmonary function tests usually demonstrate fixed expiratory airflow obstruction, with hyperinflation and impaired diffusing capacities. In particularly severe cases with massive small-airway obliteration, pulmonary restriction may be the predominant abnormality of spirometrical or helium equilibration studies. Plethysmography may be useful in these patients to demonstrate the large volumes of trapped intrathoracic gas.

Obliterative bronchiolitis in BMT recipients is almost certainly an immunologically mediated injury of GVHD. The disease rarely, if ever, occurs in BMT recipients without a history of preexisting GVHD (Clark et al., 1987; Chan et al., 1987). Identified predisposing factors for OB among these patients include methotrexate therapy (Clark et al., 1987), as well as two independent

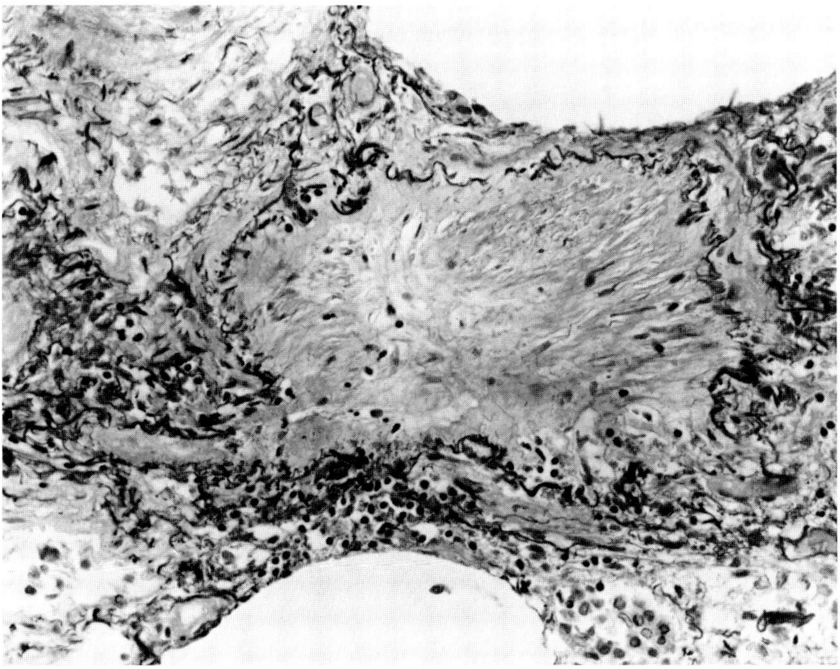

Figure 2 Obliterative bronchiolitis. Elastic stain of a lung biopsy specimen highlights the basal elastica of a terminal bronchiole that is completely occluded by dense fibrous connective tissue (magnified 350×).

risks for GVHD: a history of CMV infections (Chan et al., 1987) and low serum immunoglobulin levels prior to transplantation (Holland et al., 1988). BAL differential cell counts among patients with OB show increased numbers of active inflammatory cells (St. John et al., 1990). Biopsy specimens (Fig. 2), although seldom needed for diagnosis, reveal desquamation and metaplasia of bronchiolar and aveolar duct epithelium, peribronchial inflammation, and varying degrees of luminal obstruction with tufts of dense connective tissue (Chan et al., 1987). Pathological findings of BMT-associated OB are indistinguishable from those seen in cases of chronic rejection of pulmonary allografts (Yousem et al., 1985). Like lung transplant recipients with OB, BMT patients with small airway injury are predisposed to chronic respiratory tract colonization and recurrent infection with a variety of pathogens, including *Pseudomonas* spp.

In most cases, OB can usually be diagnosed on the basis of clinical and physiological findings and is, thus, relatively unique among the pulmonary complications of BMT. For prognostic and therapeutic purposes, OB should be distinguished from reversible airway disorders of BMT recipients, including recurrent bronchitis, asthma, and/or possible lymphocytic bronchitis. The severity of clinical abnormalities appears to be highly variable (Springmeyer et al., 1983; Clark et al., 1987). Management of BMT patients with rapidly progressive OB, however, is generally frustrating. Symptoms are usually unremitting to therapy with bronchodilators. Augmentation of immunosuppression is frequently tried and, by anecdotal report, occasionally results in stabilization or amelioration of disease manifestations (Chan et al., 1990). All too frequently, however, afflicted patients inexorably progress despite immunosuppressive therapy. The overall mortality associated with progressive OB may be as great as 80% (Chan et al., 1987; Clark et al., 1987).

V. Renal Transplantation

Pulmonary abnormalities complicate the course of up to one in four renal allograft recipients and have an associated mortality rate as great as 50% (Simmons et al., 1972; Munda et al., 1978; Ramsey et al., 1980). Approximately two-thirds of the pulmonary problems following renal transplantation in these early series are the result of infection. Several recent reviews, however, emphasize an evolving spectrum of infectious pathogens among these patients and, most important, reductions in the incidence of respiratory tract infections (Peterson et al., 1982; Masur et al., 1982; Hesse et al., 1986).

A. Infectious Complications

As in other transplant populations, bacteria are the predominant cause of respiratory tract infection among renal allograft recipients during the first month following their procedure. Similarly, the majority of these infections are attributable to typical nosocomial pathogens, notably enteric gram-negative organisms, with a lesser incidence of gram-positive cocci (Ramsey et al., 1980; Masur et al., 1982; Peterson and Anderson, 1986). The clinical presentation of early bacterial pneumonias in renal allograft recipients is characteristically acute and often rapidly progressive. A number of risk factors for these infections have been identified by various investigators (Table 3). Altogether, however, early bacterial pneumonias occur in < 10% of renal transplant patients, a rate much lower than in other allograft recipients (Heino et al., 1986). The comparative infrequency of pneumonia after renal transplantation is probably due to the reduced incidence of postoperative pulmonary complications associated with the low abdominal surgical procedure. Community-acquired pneumonias that occur after hospital discharge are similar to those of immunologically competent patients, at least in terms of clinical manifestations, spectrum of pathogens, and response to therapy (Ramsey et al., 1980).

Opportunistic pathogens assume greater significance in these patients after a few weeks of cumulative immunosuppression. *Nocardia*, *Legionella*, and other unusual opportunists are the cause of a small number of infections (Gump et al., 1979). Fungal infections are especially prevalent in the first few months after transplantation and are, moreover, associated with a poor response to therapy and very high mortality (Simmons et al., 1972; Munda et al., 1978; Ramsey et al., 1980). Although the majority of fungal infections are due to *Aspergillus*, a variety of other species have been reported, including *Candida*, *Cryptococcus*, and, in respective endemic locales, *Coccidioides* and *Histoplasma* (Peterson et al., 1982; Cohen et al., 1982; Wheat et al., 1983). The risk for development of fungal infections (and *Nocardia* infections) is significantly correlated with the intensity of immunosuppression, particularly the number of treatments with antirejection regimens (Bach et al., 1973). Fungal disease in renal transplant

Table 3 Risk Factors for Bacterial Pneumonia After Renal Transplantation

High-dose prednisone
Hyperglycemia
Age > 40 years
Leukopenia
Renal failure
Malnutrition
Previous pulmonary complication (including pulmonary emboli, CMV infection)
Retransplantation

Source: Simmons et al., 1972; Anderson et al., 1973; Ramsey et al., 1980.

patients, as well as in other solid-organ transplant recipients, tends to have a more insidious onset than bacterial infections. In most cases, pulmonary involvement is radiographically characterized by focal or multifocal infiltrates that often cavitate; necrotizing upper lobe nodules are classically, if far from invariably, described with *Aspergillus* lesions. Especially unusual infiltrates and clinical features have been reported with infections due to *Coccidioides* and *Histoplasma* (Wheat et al., 1983).

Because of the apparent efficacy of trimethoprim-sulfamethoxazole prophylaxis, *P. carinii* pneumonias are primarily of historical interest in renal transplant recipients. Cases still occur in patients unable to tolerate sulfa medications, but these few instances could likely be reduced further by prophylaxis with aerosolized pentamidine.

Cytomegalovirus Infection

CMV infections are the single most frequent, and probably most morbid, infectious pathogen of renal allograft recipients (Simmons et al., 1972; Ramsey et al., 1980). The epidemiology of the disease in these patients is remarkably similar to that in other solid-organ transplant populations: infections occur in approximately 75% of all recipients; pulmonary involvement occurs in about one-third of cases; and onset is usually between 1 and 4 months following transplantation. Furthermore, CMV infections in renal and other solid-organ transplant recipients are often temporally associated with episodes of allograft rejection and/or antecedent treatment with high-dose corticosteroids or anti-T-cell immunoglobulin therapy (Rubin et al., 1977, 1981; Peterson et al., 1980). In addition to direct and attributable CMV disease, significant unaccountable morbidity accrues due to indirect (and often delayed) secondary effects of CMV infections, including induction of allograft rejection and a heightened propensity for superinfections with other organisms (Schooley et al., 1983; Rubin, 1989).

Treatment of CMV disease in renal allograft and other solid-organ transplant populations has been frustratingly disappointing. CMV infections were associated with an overall mortality rate of 48% in untreated renal transplant recipients (Peterson et al., 1980). High-dose acyclovir has no apparent therapeutic efficacy. A recent compilation of ganciclovir trials in CMV-infected renal transplant recipients, all of which were uncontrolled, describes a wide range of response rates, with survival varying from 33 to 100% (Ettinger and Trulock, 1991).

Methodological differences between these studies are notable, however, especially in terms of inclusion of variable proportions of subjects with mere viral shedding. Unlike BMT recipients, the isolation of CMV in solid-organ transplant populations does not necessarily presage the eventual development of viral disease. Furthermore, the natural history of limited CMV shedding in solid-organ transplant recipients appears to be much more benign than in patients with demonstrable visceral disease (Simmons et al., 1977; Rubin et al., 1977). Accordingly, the true effectiveness of ganciclovir therapy in cases of invasive CMV disease is not readily apparent. Overall results with antiviral therapy may be much less impressive in serious cases with visceral organ involvement than among patients with mere viral shedding (Duncan and Cook, 1991).

Studies of CMV prophylaxis using IVIG have shown disparate results, with greatest efficacy ascribed to high-titer anti-CMV globulin (Snydman et al., 1987). Somewhat similarly, high-dose acyclovir has been variously reported as showing significant prophylactic usefulness (Balfour et al., 1989) or no apparent protective effect (Wong et al., 1991). Ganciclovir prophylaxis trials are presently ongoing, but results are not yet unavailable.

Tuberculosis

Renal allograft recipients are unique among transplant populations for their apparent predilection for mycobacterial infections. These infections may occur at any time, but peak prevalence appears to be at least several months after transplantation (Coutts et al., 1979; Riska et al., 1987). Incidences as great as 10% have been reported (Malhotra et al., 1986), although rates in most centers are substantially less. The majority of infections are attributable to *M. tuberculosis*; however, up to one-third of mycobacterial infections are due to atypical species (Lichtenstein and MacGregor, 1983). Many reports highlight the varied and unusual presentations of mycobacterial infections in this population: pulmonary infections are often cryptic, lower lobe infiltrates are not uncommon, and extrapulmonary disease is unusually frequent (Coutts et al., 1979; Dautzenberg et al., 1984). Treatment with conventional antituberculosis chemotherapy is usually effective, but may require longer courses (Dautzenberg et al., 1984; Malhotra et al., 1986) and has the propensity for greater than usual toxicity in these patients (Coutts et al., 1979). The role of isoniazid (INH) prophylaxis in these patients is controversial. Standard recommendations suggest use of prophylactic INH in tuberculin-positive transplant recipients (ATS-CDC Statement, 1986). The universal validity of this recommendation can be questioned, however, except for those with documented recent tuberculin conversion, given the low rate of reactivation observed in renal transplant patients with distant conversion (Rubin, 1988).

B. Noninfectious Complications

In addition to their importance as direct causes of pulmonary dysfunction, the noninfectious pulmonary complications of renal transplantation are notable for the ease with which they are misdiagnosed as disease due to opportunistic pathogens. Hydrostatic pulmonary edema due to renal dysfunction is exceptionally common among these patients in the early postoperative period and during episodes of allograft rejection (Simmons et al., 1972; Ramsey et al., 1980). The fever that accompanies rejection, in conjunction with the dyspnea and diffuse radiographic infiltrates of pulmonary edema, is a constellation of findings readily misdiagnosed as due to opportunistic infection.

Renal transplant recipients are also unusually prone to development of deep venous thrombosis (Brunkwall et al., 1987) and pulmonary thromboemboli within the first month after transplantation (Simmons et al., 1972; Ramsey et al., 1980). These early series describe pulmonary thromboemboli as the cause of 16% of lung complications in these patients, but there is a somewhat lower incidence in more recent reports (Brunkwall et al., 1987). Pulmonary thromboemboli present with especially nondescript symptoms in renal allograft recipients. The most frequently observed radiographic findings are peripheral focal infiltrates, but less specific lesions are common (Simmons et al., 1972; Ramsey et al., 1980). Infarcts due to these emboli often cavitate, thus mimicking fungal or other necrotizing infections. Pulmonary emboli in this population, moreover, act as the nidus for bacterial superinfections in a surprisingly high proportion of cases (Ramsey et al., 1980).

Transplant-associated malignancies occur in a small number of renal allograft recipients and should be considered in the differential diagnosis of stable or slowly growing pulmonary infiltrates among long-term survivors. Pulmonary presentations of posttransplant lymphoproliferative disease (PTLD) have been sporadically reported (Penn, 1989), although most often PTLD in these patients is a subdiaphragmatic disease. Extrapulmonary Kaposi's sarcoma (KS) occurs in a markedly disproportionate number of renal transplant recipients, and a few patients present with significant lung involvement (Chanez et al., 1988).

VI. Liver Transplantation

A. Infectious Complications

The incidence of bacterial respiratory tract infectious following liver transplantation ranges from ~5 to 20% in various recent series and may be associated with a roughly 50% mortality (Kusne et al., 1988; Thompson et al., 1988; Colonna et al., 1988; Paya et al., 1989). The high rate and seriousness of bacterial pneumonias in these patients, relative to recipients of renal allografts, is likely a reflection of the more extensive surgery and overall higher incidence of postoperative pulmonary complications following liver transplantation (Ekberg et al., 1986). Furthermore, liver transplant recipients are much more predisposed to develop postoperative abdominal infections and bacteremias than are renal transplant patients (Kusne et al., 1988; Colonna et al., 1988; Paya et al.,

1989). Selective bowel decontamination appears to significantly decrease the prevalence of bacterial pneumonias after liver transplantation, although the relative proportion of infections due to gram-positive organisms appears to be somewhat increased (Colonna et al., 1988; Paya et al., 1989).

Opportunistic pulmonary infections in liver transplant recipients are similar to those previously described following renal transplantation. This topic has also been extensively described in large series of patients (Schroter et al., 1976; Kusne et al., 1988; Paya et al., 1989).

B. Noninfectious Complications

Liver transplantation is a relatively complex and prolonged procedure, with extensive upper abdominal dissection and massive fluid shifts (Krowka and Cortese, 1989; Ekberg et al., 1986). Protracted intubation, diaphragmatic dysfunction, pleural effusions, and pulmonary atelectasis are ubiquitous among early postoperative liver transplant patients (Ekberg et al., 1986; Jensen et al., 1986). The adult respiratory distress syndrome occurs in approximately 5% of liver allograft recipients and is nearly always fatal (Jensen et al., 1986; Takaoka et al., 1989). The myriad medical and surgical postoperative complications following liver transplantation result in an often indecipherable array of signs and symptoms and render the diagnosis of supervening pulmonary infections extremely complex.

VII. Heart Transplantation

A. Infectious Complications

Infectious pneumonias remain a major cause of morbidity and mortality in heart transplant recipients. Early reports described incidences of serious lung infections in these patients that approached 50% (Remington et al., 1972; Pennock et al., 1982; Cooper et al., 1983). The introduction of cyclosporine in the early 1980s has, by most accounts (Hofflin et al., 1987; Dummer, 1990), resulted in a reduction of infectious complications. Widespread use of anti-T-cell immunoglobulins (e.g., ATG, OKT3), however, seems to have resulted in greater rates of CMV infections and posttransplant lymphoproliferative disease (Dummer, 1990; Swinnen et al., 1990).

The pathogens that cause pulmonary infections in heart transplant patients are quite similar to those seen in other solid-organ transplant recipients. With the exception of occasional infections with fungi (notable *Aspergillus* spp.), pneumonias during the first month after heart transplantation are primarily due to bacteria, with a predominance of gram-negative enteric organisms (Cooper et al., 1983; Brooks and Remington, 1986; Schulman et al., 1988; Austin et al.,

1989). Heart transplant recipients are extraordinarily predisposed to postoperative nosocomial pneumonias because of risks associated with the thoracic surgical procedure, e.g., retained secretions and atelectasis due to painful or ineffectual cough, shallow respirations, and impaired respiratory muscle function (Tisi, 1979). A small, but finite, number of these patients also develop postoperative mediastinitis, with an associated high mortality (Trento et al., 1984).

Opportunistic pathogens assume much greater importance in the second and later months following transplantation. In general, opportunistic infections after cardiac transplantation often present with singularly unusual clinical and radiographic features, a probable function of these patients' characteristically intense immunosuppression (Schulman 1987, Austin 1989, Cook 1990). Nodular or focal Legionella and P. carinii infiltrates are not rare in these series, and CMV infections have been the occasional cause of nodular lesions, focal consolidations, or pleural effusions (Schulman, 1987; Austin et al., 1989; Cook et al., 1990; Duncan and Cook, 1991). Cardiac transplant patients have been described as having a particularly high incidence of infections with *Nocardia* and *Legionella* spp. (Redd et al., 1988), although these diseases appear to be abating in more contemporary reports (Hofflin et al., 1987). The cardiac allograft is an excellent vehicle for transmission of *Toxoplasma gondii*, but these infections rarely involve the lungs (Luft et al., 1983). Mycobacterial infections are distinctly unusual (Cook et al., 1990; Dummer, 1990). In most other respects, the spectrum of pulmonary infections in these patients is remarkablly similar to that of other organ transplant recipients. Accordingly, the following discussion will focus on features of these diseases that are unique to heart transplant recipients.

Many reports have emphasized that the relative risk of pulmonary infection in recipients of cardiac allografts is markedly reduced after approximately 2 years have elapsed (Cooper et al., 1983; Schulman et al., 1988). Nonetheless, a substantial number of late infections have been documented in transplant centers with a large population of survivors followed for long periods, thus delineating the need for prolonged vigilance in these patients (Cook et al., 1990; Dummer, 1990). The epidemiology of infections in these longitudinal studies also highlights the reemergence of bacteria as relatively frequent pathogens of long-term survivors (Fig. 3).

As in other transplant populations, CMV is a major pathogen in heart transplant recipients and is found in nearly 80% of these patients. Pulmonary CMV infections ultimately develop in approximately one of eight cardiac transplant recipients (Dummer et al., 1985). Aside from disease attributable to direct cytopathic effects, CMV infections in cardiac allograft recipients are also compellingly (albeit circumstantially) associated with pulmonary superinfections (Rand et al., 1978) and allograft rejection, including accelerated coronary atherosclerosis (Grattan et al., 1989). Initial anecdotal trials suggested 2-week

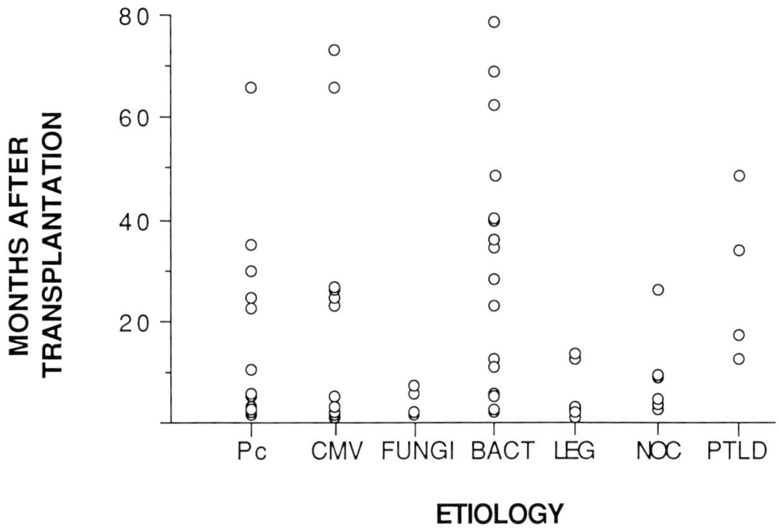

Figure 3 Spectrum and timing of pneumonias among heart transplantation recipients at Stanford University Medical Center. A subset of these patients has been more fully described elsewhere (Dunn et al., 1988). Pc. *Pneumocystic carinii*; CMV, cytomegalovirus; BACT, bacteria; LEG, *Legionella* spp.; NOC, *Nocardia*; PTLD, posttransplant lymphoproliferative disease.

courses of single-agent ganciclovir was effective treatment of CMV infections in these patients (Keay et al., 1988; Watson et al., 1988). Many of the patients in these series, however, appeared to have mere (and relatively benign) viral shedding, rather than proven invasive disease. Furthermore, the posttreatment observation periods of these series tended to be short. A recent, longitudinal study of heart transplant recipients with cytologically or histologically proven CMV pneumonitis treated with ganciclovir, however, found that 75% of these patients ultimately succumbed within 6 months of their infection, despite frequent early clinical improvement with therapy (Duncan and Cook, 1991). In nearly all cases, deaths in this series were attributable to allograft rejection, thus reemphasizing the considerable, and often delayed, indirect effects of CMV infections (Rubin, 1989; Grattan et al., 1989). Such findings are obviously distressing and evoke a need for development of improved therapies, perhaps using combinations of antiviral agents with intravenous immunoglobulin, as per current regimens in bone marrow transplant recipients (Emanuel et al., 1988; Reed et al., 1988), and/or efficacious prophylaxis (Schmidt et al., 1991).

Historically, *P. carinii* has also been a significant cause of pulmonary disease in these patients. Sensitivity of BAL for *P. carinii* pneumonia among heart transplant recipients may be as low as 70% (Dunn et al., 1988). The relative insensitivity of BAL is likely attributable to a small burden of pathogens and a predominantly interstitial distribution (Limper et al., 1989). Bronchoscopic yield may be considerably improved by performing concurrent transbronchial biopsies. Currently, most transplant centers routinely employ trimethoprim-sulfamethoxazole or aerosolized pentamidine for *P. carinii* prophylaxis. Although there is yet no conclusive data in these population, *P. carinii* prophylaxis regimens will almost certainly result in a substantial reduction of pneumonia due to this pathogen and likely decrease the incidence of infections from *Nocardia* and susceptible bacteria.

B. Noninfectious Complications

Postoperative pulmonary complications in the immediate postsurgical period are nearly ubiquitous following cardiac surgery (Carter et al., 1983). Left lower lobe atelectasis is especially frequent and persistent, in large part due to left phrenic nerve injury from cardioplegia and mechanical torsion (Wheeler et al., 1985). Pleural effusions and pulmonary edema are also extremely common (Henry et al., 1989). Pulmonary edema has been attributed to a number of factors related to the nature of cardiac surgery and cardiopulmonary bypass, but may also be a manifestation of hyperacute or acute allograft rejection (Stinson et al., 1971; Henry et al., 1989). Right ventricular failure resulting from postoperative pulmonary artery hypertension is an often fatal complication that cannot be entirely foreseen by preoperative hemodynamic assessments (Armitage et al., 1987). In addition to predisposing patients to postoperative bacterial pneumonias, the noninfectious complications of cardiac surgery may also be problematic because of occasional confusion with infectious processes.

A number of noninfectious pulmonary complications also occur among long-term survivors of heart transplantation. Residual radiographic changes as a result of the throacotomy are common, but are rarely the cause of clinical problems (Shirazi et al., 1983). Hydrostatic pulmonary edema resulting from cardiac dysfunction, a common manifestation of allograft rejection, is an obvious serious noninfectious etiology of acute radiographic infiltrates in these patients. With a few notable exceptions, pulmonary edema is fairly readily distinguished from infectious etiologies on the basis of clinical features or results of invasive hemodynamic assessment. Posttransplant lymphoproliferative disorder (PTLD) is an extremely serious complication of cardiac transplantation, with a mortality that may be as great as 90% (Cleary et al., 1984). Isolated pulmonary parenchymal involvement with the lymphoma, however, is unusual in these patients (Nalesnik et al., 1988). A large proportion of heart transplant recipients have residual mild to moderate restrictive pulmonary function defects that persist indefinitely following the transplantation (Duncan et al., 1991a).

The mechanism(s) of the abnormality is unknown, but is likely a sequela of interstitial fibrosis from chronic pulmonary vascular congestion and edema prior to the transplantation (Heard et al., 1968).

VIII. Lung Transplantation

Advances are readily apparent in the field of lung transplantation, which has evolved in very few years from an experimental procedure to an acceptable treatment of end-stage cardiopulmonary diseases (Theodore and Lewiston, 1990). Recent trends in lung transplantation are notable for gratifying improvements of survival, now approximating success rates in other solid-organ transplant procedures (McCarthy et al., 1990), and progressively selective utilization of single-lung and double-lung allografts, in lieu of earlier heart-lung en bloc preparations (Grossman et al., 1990). Complications following pulmonary transplantation include infections that, with few exceptions, are epidemiologically similar to those of other transplant populations, as well as a unique set of problems referable to the distinct nature of the allograft.

A. Infectious Complications

Bacterial pneumonias are an especially severe problem during the first month after lung transplantation (Dauber et al., 1990). Risk factors for postoperative infections in lung allograft recipients are, in certain respects, similar to those common to other patients recovering from major thoracic surgical procedures, including endotracheal intubation, retained secretions, and atelectasis (Tisi, 1979). Additional risks for development of pulmonary infections accrue from denervation of the allograft, with resultant loss of cough reflexes, and impaired mucociliary clearance due to mucosal ischemia, as well as granulation tissue (or dehiscence) at the airway anastomosis (Mancini and Tauxe, 1986). Local host defense mechanisms following transplantation are further hindered by postoperative edema due to reimplantation injury (Herman, 1990) and disruption of bronchial and lymphatic circulations that slows ingress of immune effector cells (Muggenburg et al., 1986).

Lung transplant recipients are unique, moreover, in that the transplanted allograft is in direct communication with the environment and is constantly exposed to inhaled or aspirated organisms. During implantation, the transplanted lung is sutured directly into often nonsterile tissue, i.e., the native trachea or mainstem bronchus. Airways are especially heavily colonized in recipients with underlying suppurative pulmonary disease, including chronic bronchitis, bronchiectasis, and cystic fibrosis. The course of lung allograft recipients with cystic fibrosis is likely to be marked by recurrent tracheobronchitis and pneumonias that appear due to aspiration of purulent drainage from residual sinus infections.

Further, preterminal events that occurred in the donor prior to organ harvest (e.g., intubation and mechanical ventilation, small-volume aspirations) may result in colonization of the allograft and possibly, in some cases, subclinical infection (Zenati et al., 1990).

The prevention of pneumonias and other infections is one of major emphasis in the postoperative care of these patients. Most centers routinely employ aggressive chest physiotherapy and postural drainage, at least until recipients are ambulatory. Aerosolized β_2 agonists are important in the care of single-lung transplant patients, who have airflow obstruction in the remaining native lung, to minimize hyperinflation with resultant compression of the allograft. Repeated aspiration and drainage of paranasal sinuses in cystic fibrosis patients may decrease the incidence of lower respiratory tract infections following lung transplantation.

Although most data are preliminary, prophylactic therapy with antimicrobial agents appears to have an important role in the management of lung transplant recipients. A dramatic reduction of early bacterial infections (from an incidence of 45% to 13%) was reported by the University of Pittsburgh group after implementation of directed posttransplant antimicrobial prophylaxis (Dauber et al., 1990; Zenati et al., 1990). The recent incidence of mediastinitis in these patients is also much decreased from a historical rate of 14% (Trento et al., 1984). The lesser occurrence of mediastinits in recent compilations may primarily be the result of fewer airway anastomosis complications and other improvements in surgical techniques. Low-dose amphotericin B prophylaxis appears to have resulted in a marked decrease in early fungal pneumonias and infections of the aortic anastomosis, with minimal and acceptable clinical toxicity (Dauber et al., 1990). Routine use of low-dose trimethoprim-sulfamethoxazole has virtually eliminated *P. carinii* infections, in a manner similar to the efficacy observed in other transplant populations.

CMV infections remain a major affliction of these patients despite the use of seronegative blood products and high-dose acyclovir (Dummer et al., 1985; Burke et al., 1986). As in other transplant recipients, CMV in this population is a relatively early infection, with a mean onset of about 50 days following the procedure. Nearly all cases occur between 14 and 90 days after transplantation (Fig. 4). The proportion of CMV infections involving the lungs appears to be greater than in other solid-organ transplant recipients (Dauber et al., 1990). Mortality can be directly attributed to CMV disease in at least 40% of primary lung infections (Dummer et al., 1985; Dauber et al., 1990). A lesser, but still significant, number of deaths occur with reactivation (secondary infections) pneumonitis. Substantial, if unquantifiable, morbidity due to pulmonary allograft rejection also results from infection with CMV in these patients (Keenan et al., 1991). Preliminary data from the University of Pittsburgh suggest that the incidence of CMV infection in high-risk lung transplant recipients has been

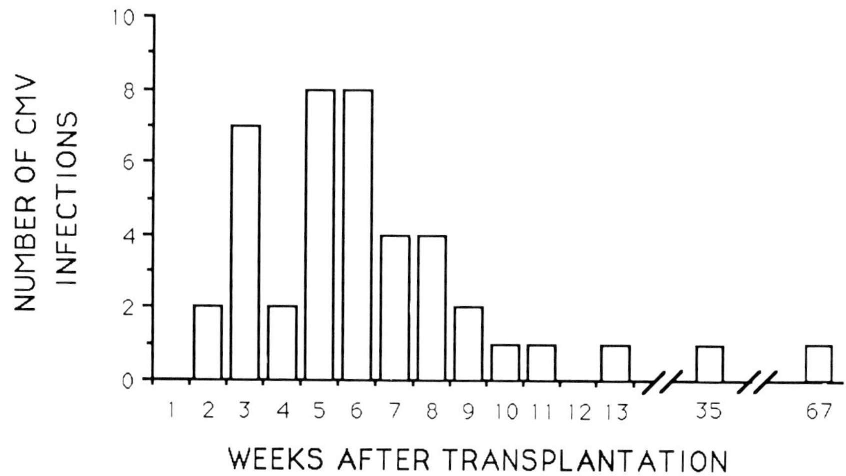

Figure 4 Cytomegalovirus infections among the first 90 pulmonary allograft recipients at the University of Pittsburgh Medical Center. Mean onset was 53 days following transplantation. Cases clustered between the second and twelfth weeks after transplantation.

substantially reduced from approximately 80% to less than 15% by a protracted course of intravenous ganciclovir starting 1 week after transplantation (Duncan et al., 1992).

B. Noninfectious Complications

Early noninfectious, and generally transient, surgically related causes of pulmonary edema in these patients include volume overload, fluid shifts, transient myocardial depression, or increased vascular permeability resulting from cardiopulmonary bypass (Royston et al., 1985). More serious and refractory pulmonary dysfunction with the radiographic appearance of edema may be due to either reperfusion injury or acute rejection. Reperfusion injury, also referred to as reimplantation response or preservation injury, is a poorly characterized syndrome of early allograft dysfunction that appears to be associated with lung ischemia during organ harvesting and/or transport. Typically, afflicted patients develop diffuse parenchymal radiographic infiltrates that may occur immediately after transplantation or become progressively more apparent during the first 2–4 days (Herman, 1990). To a certain extent, this injury may be expressed, albeit subclinically, in the majority of pulmonary allografts; severe cases requiring prolonged mechanical ventilation have been noted in as many as 20–30% of lung transplant recipients (Chiles et al., 1985; Montefusco and Veith, 1986; Griffith et al., 1987; Holland et al., 1989). Although incomplete preservation undoubtedly plays a central role, simple measures of organ ischemic time correlate poorly with subsequent development of the syndrome. Other factors that may be involved in this injury include allograft trauma, lung denervation, and disruption of the lymphatic circulation. Recent experiences with single-lung transplantations of patients with pulmonary artery hypertension suggest that reperfusion injury is, at least to some extent, exacerbated by elevated postransplant pulmonary arterial pressures and/or flow.

In most cases, the pulmonary infiltrates and gas exchange abnormalities associated with this syndrome resolve after a few days of supportive care, including aggressive diuresis (Herman, 1990). Clinical manifestations of the more unremitting cases, however, are indistinguishable from typical adult respiratory distress syndrome. Lung biopsies of patients, prior to development of nosocomial infections, show nonspecific diffuse alveolar damage characteristic of myriad severe lung injuries. Overall mortality of clinically evident cases may be in excess of 30% (Griffith et al., 1987; Herman, 1990); most deaths are attributable to complications of prolonged life support rather than intractable respiratory failure. Patients who survive have residual restrictive pulmonary mechanics that ultimately resolve (Chen et al., 1991).

Clinical features of acute allograft rejection are remarkably similar to reperfusion injuries and other causes of increased permeability pulmonary edema. Hyperacute (within hours) rejection sometimes seen in other organ transplant recipients has rarely been documented in lung allografts. Depending on the intensity of the perioperative rejection prophylaxis regimen used, however, acute rejection may occur as early as 7 days after transplantation (Starnes et al., 1989). Thus, acute rejection may overlap considerably with other causes of early pulmonary dysfunction and can be reliably diagnosed only by lung biopsy demonstration of lymphocytic perivascular and interstitial infiltrates (Higenbottam et al., 1988; Tazelaar and Yousem, 1988; Starnes et al., 1989). Asynchronous rejection is typical among heart-lung recipients, in that the pulmonary allograft is much more likely to show rejection than is the transplanted heart (Griffith et al., 1985). More typical cases of acute rejection appearing 2 or more weeks after transplantation may mimic pulmonary infections (Burke et al., 1986).

Nearly all pulmonary allograft recipients show restrictive pulmonary function following transplantation that tends to resolve (although not invariably) over a period of a few weeks or months (Theodore et al., 1984). In at least some cases, these mechanical defects can be attributed to alterations of chest wall compliance rather than intrinsic abnormalities of pulmonary parenchyma (Glanville et al., 1988). Despite early concerns that pulmonary denervation would result in profound disturbances of control of breathing, as seen in subprimate mammals (Nakae et al., 1967), human lung transplantation recipients appear to have normal perception of flow-resistive loads (Tapper et al., in press), and to maintain appropriate ventilatory regulation during sleep (Shea et al., 1988) and exercise (Sciurba et al., 1988). Hypercarbic ventilatory responses of heart-lung transplant patients with normal pulmonary mechanics are also well maintained (Kagawa et al., 1991; Duncan et al., 1991a), although recipients with moderate pulmonary restriction have severely blunted responses (Duncan et al., 1991b). The inability of heart-lung allograft recipients to hyperventilate appropriately in response to inhaled CO_2 in the presence of mild restrictive impedances is suggestive of an inherent defect of elastic load compensation that could predispose these patients to respiratory failure during otherwise well-tolerated acute illnesses.

Chronic Rejection

Chronic rejection of the transplanted lung is histologically characterized by mononuclear inflammation of small airways with intraluminal plugs of granulation tissue, a lesion that is virtually identical to obliterative bronchiolitis among bone marrow transplant recipients (Fig. 2) (Burke et al., 1984; Yousem et al., 1985; Tazelaar and Yousem, 1988). Published series report a prevalence of greater than 50% among long-term pulmonary allograft survivors (Theodore et al., 1990). Early observations suggested a greater incidence of obliterative bronchiolitis in recipients of heart-lung transplant patients, compared to single- or double-lung allograft patients, but recent experiences suggests this difference is more apparent than real. The clinical presentation of obliterative bronchiolitis is also strikingly similar to that seen with the airway injuries of chronic GVHD in BMT recipients. Both entities are typified by progressive expiratory airflow obstruction, an onset several weeks after transplantation, and an increased relative risk in patients with antecedent acute rejection or pulmonary infections (Paradis et al., 1989; Keenan et al., 1991). Moreover, both patient populations are predisposed by the presence of obliterative bronchiolitis to develop lower airway colonization and recurrent infections with virulent bacteria, especially *S. aureus* and *Pseudomonas*.

Most centers now rely heavily on transbronchial biopsy for diagnosis of both acute and chronic rejection (Higenbottam et al., 1988; Starnes et al., 1989). Clinical and radiographic features, as well as pulmonary function tests, may provide useful clues, but are generally too insensitive and nonspecific to permit empirical therapy with increased immunosuppression (Theodore et al., 1990). Unlike obliterative bronchiolitis associated with BMT, potential reversibility of the obstructive abnormality in lung transplant recipients is much better documented. Several reports show that early detection and treatment with high-dose steroids or antilymphocyte globulins can arrest and/or reverse the obliterative bronchiolitis of chronic allograft rejection (Allen et al., 1986; Glanville et al., 1987). Nonetheless, obliterative bronchiolitis is the single greatest cause of functional disability in long-term survivors of lung transplantation and accounts for very substantial, if poorly delineated, excess mortality owing to the predilection of these patients to develop infections (Theodore et al., 1990).

Posttransplant Lymphoproliferative Disorder

In contrast to other solid-organ transplant populations, posttransplant lymphoproliferative disease (PTLD) among pulmonary allograft recipients has a unique porpensity to present with primary involvement of the lung parenchyma and mediastinum and, moreover, tends to occur earlier after transplantation (Randhawa et al., 1989). To date, PTLD has developed in 8 of the 77 lung allograft recipients at the University of Pittsburgh who have survived more than 2 months. Cases tended to cluster at 2–4 months following transplantation, but occurrences range from as early as 43 days to as late as 6 years. These lymphomas may be focal or multifocal and often rapidly progress to surprisingly large size prior to detection (Fig. 5) Although intrathoracic PTLD eventually causes symptoms due to mass effects, patients are equally or more likely to present with vague and nonspecific constitutional complaints, such as nightsweats, fever, weight loss, and malaise.

With very few exceptions, PTLD is a high-grade lymphoma of B-cell lineage, which may be either monoclonal or polyclonal (Cleary et al., 1984; Nalesnik et al., 1988). The introduction of cyclosporine A has led to an increased incidence of PTLD in transplant recipients, compared to previous immunosuppressive regimens (Penn, 1983). Occurrences of PTLD are strongly associated with serological evidence of primary or reactivation infections of Epstein-Barr virus (EBV), and EBV genomes can be identified in the majority of tumors (Ho et al., 1985). Peripheral blood smears usually reveal variable numbers of lymphocytes with a high proportion of atypical cells.

Cumulative numbers of lung allograft recipients with PTLD are too small to provide definitive data regarding therapy, and in any event, most experiences are anecdotal. Many lung transplant recipients with PTLD have at least partial responses to reductions of immunosuppression. Uncontrolled observations in other transplant populations describe beneficial results with antiviral therapy using acyclovir (Hanto et al., 1985) or ganciclovir (Pirsch et al., 1989). Surgical excision, chemotherapy, irradiation, and α-interferon have been used with variable success in other small series (Shapiro et al., 1988). A recent promising report described a number of favorable responses with use of anti-B-cell monoclonal antibodies (Fischer et al., 1991). Conservative management by decreases of immunosuppression may more likely result in remissions of polymorphic polyclonal tumors. At least one group advocates early use of irradiation and/or chemotherapy for the more refractory monoclonal tumors (Cleary et al., 1984). Despite various sequential therapies, however, the majority of the lymphomas eventually recur and/or disseminate and ultimately cause the death of at least 60% of afflicted patients (Randhawa et al., 1989).

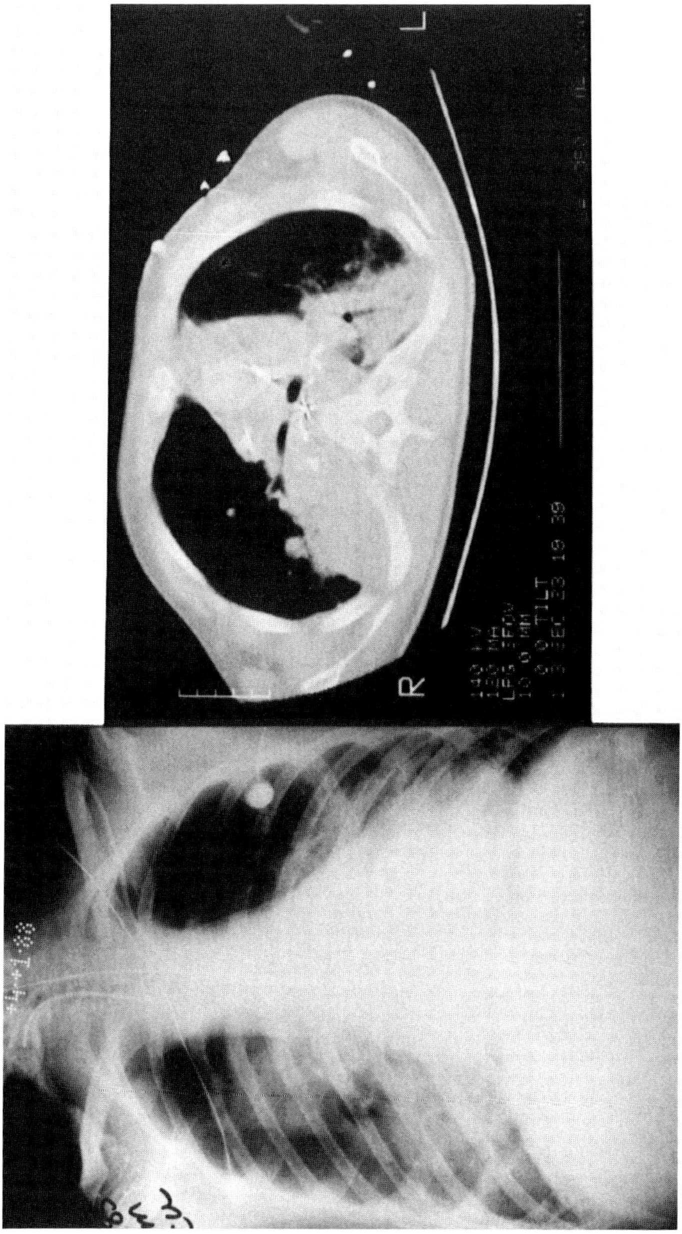

Figure 5 Posttransplantation lymphoproliferative disease in an 18-year-old pulmonary allograft recipient. Chest radiograph and CT scan demonstrate extensive intrathoracic lymphoma 43 days after transplantation.

IX. Summary

This chapter has focused on the pulmonary complications associated with primary and secondary immunodeficiency diseases and with bone marrow and solid-organ transplantation. The discussion has not dealt with the consequences of specific and common drugs, such as corticosteriods, cyclosporine, and the numerous cytotoxic and antineoplastic agents, except insofar as these worsen or contribute to the immunosuppressive effects of the various disorders under consideration. Moreover, we have scarcely mentioned many ordinary, but less dramatic, influences, including protein depletion, other forms of malnutrition, alcoholism, and drug addiction; these prosaic, but powerful, immunosuppressive factors undoubtedly contribute to the development of more lung disease than all the various conditions we have highlighted.

A decade ago, however, the great majority of the patients with the disorders we chose to address would have died of their underlying disease. Thus, the facts that so many of these patients are alive today and that their pulmonary complications warrant a chapter in this book represent a triumph of modern medical science. But these remarkable advances have, in turn, left in their wake a host of new, unforeseen clinical problems. As pointed out, there are certain patterns to the infectious and noninfectious pulmonary complications that arise in the various disease-related and induced immunodepressive disorders, and to the time sequences during which they occur. Nevertheless, there remain formidable obstacles to prompt and accurate diagnosis of most of these disorders; consequently, we are often left with imprecise, or empirical therapy for life-threatening conditions. Although the ''state of the art'' today leaves much to be desired, we are confident that great progress is imminent in this rapidly moving, extremely complex field.

References

Abrahams, C., and Catchatourian, R. (1983). Bone fragment emboli in the lungs of patients undergoing bone marrow transplantation. *Am. J. Clin. Pathol.* **79**:360–363.

Adelman, D. C., Yen T. Y., Cumberland, W. G., Sidell, N., and Saxon, A. (1991). 13-*cis* retinoic acid enhances in vivo B-lymphocyte differentiation in patients with common variable immunology. *J. Allergy Clin. Immunol.* (in press).

Albada-Kuipers, G. A., Linthorst, J., Peeters, E. A. J., Breedreld, F. C., Kijkmans, B. A. C., Hermans, J., Vandenbroucke, J. P., and Cats, A. (1988). Frequency of infection among patients with rheumatoid arthritis versus patients with osteoarthritis or soft tissue rheumatism. *Arthritis Rheum.* **31**:667–671.

Allen, M., Burke, C., McGregor, C., Baldwin, J. C., Jamieson, S. W., and Theodore, J. (1986). Steroid-responsive bronchiolitis after human heart-lung transplantation. *J. Thorac. Cardiovasc. Surg.* **92**:449–451.

Alper, C. A., Colten, H. R., Gear, J. S. S., Rabson, A. R., and Rosen, F. S. (1976). Homozygous human C3 deficiency. *J. Clin. Invest.* **57**:222–229.

Altz-Smith, M., Kendall, L. G., and Stamm, A. M. (1987). Cryptococcosis associated with low-dose methotrexate for arthritis. *Am. J. Med.* **83**:179–181.

American Thoracic Society–Center for Disease Control Joint Statement (1986). Treatment of tuberculosis and tuberculosis infection in adults and children. *Am. Rev. Respir. Dis.* **134**:355–363.

Anagnoston, A., and Kurtzman, N. A. (1986). Hematological consequences of renal failure. In *The Kidney*, 3rd ed. Edited by B. M. Brenner and F. C. Rector. Saunders, Philadelphia, pp. 1640–1643.

Anderson, R. J., Schafer, L. A., Olin, D. B., and Eickhoff, T. X. (1973). Infectious risk factors in the immunosuppressed host. *Am. J. Med.* **54**:453–460.

Andrew, O. T., Schoenfeld, P. Y., Hopewell, P. C., and Humphreys, M. H. (1980). Tuberculosis in patients with end-stage renal disease. *Am. J. Med.* **68**:59–65.

Andrews, C. P., and Weiner, M. H. (1982). *Aspergillus* antigen detection in bronchoalveolar lavage fluid from patients with invasive aspergillosis and aspergillomas. *Am. J. Med.* **73**:372–380.

Appelbaum, F. R., Strauchen, J. A., Graw, R. G., Savage, D. D., Kent, K. M., Ferrans, V. J., and Herzig, G. P. (1976). Lethal carditis caused by high dose combination chemotherapy: a unique clinical and pathological entity. *Lancet* **1**:58–67.

Armitage, J. M., Hardesty, R. L., and Griffith, B. P. (1987). Prostaglandin E1: an effective treatment of right heart failure after orthotopic heart transplantation. *J. Heart Transplant.* **6**:348–351.

Armstrong, D., Young, L. S., Meyer, R. D., and Blevins, A. H. (1971). Infectious complications of neoplastic disease. *Med. Clin. North Am.* **55**: 729–745.

Atkinson, K., Storb, R., Prentice, R. L., Weiden, P. L., Witherspoon, R. P., Sullivan, K., Noel, D., and Thomas, E. D. (1979). Analysis of late infections in 89 long-term survivors of bone marrow transplantation. *Blood* **53**:720–731.

Aucouturier, P., Barra, A., Intrator, L., Cordonnier, C., Schulz, D., Duarte, F., Vernant, J. P., and Preud'homme, J. L. (1987). Long lasting IgG subclass and antibacterial polysaccharide antibody deficiency after allogeneic marrow transplantation. *Blood* **70**:779–785.

Aur, R. J. A., Simone, J. V., Hustu, H. O., and Verzosa, M. S. (1972). A comparative study of central nervous system irradiation and intensive chemotherapy early in remission of childhood acute lymphoctic leukemia. *Cancer* **29**:381–391.

Austin, J. H. M., Schulman, L. L., and Mstrobattista, J. D. (1989). Pulmonary infection after cardiac transplantation: clinical and radiologic correlations. *Radiology* **172**:259–265.

Babior, B. M., and Woodman, R. C. (1990). Chronic granulomatous disease. *Semin. Hematol.* **27**:247–259.

Bach, M. C., Adler, J. L., Breman, J., Fank-Ku, P., Sahyoun, A., Schlesinger, R. M., Madras, P., and Monaco, A. P. (1973). Influence of rejection therapy on fungal and nocardial infections in renal transplant recipients. *Lancet* **1**:180–184.

Balfour, H. H., Chace, B. A., Stapleton, J. T., Simmons, R. L., and Fryd, D. S. (1989). Randomized, placebo controlled trial of oral acyclovir for the prevention of cytomegalovirus disease in recipients of renal allografts. *N. Engl. J. Med.* **320**:1381–1387.

Barnes, C. G., Turnball, A. L., and Vernon-Roberts, B. (1971). Felty's syndrome. A clinical and pthological survey of 21 patients and their response to treatment. *Ann. Rheum. Dis.* **30**:359–374.

Bernhisel-Broadbent, J., Camargo, E. E., Jaffe, H. S., and Lederman, H. M. (1991). Recombinant human interferon-gamma as adjunct therapy for *Aspergillus* infection in a patient with chronic granulomatous disease. *J. Infect. Dis.* **163**:901–911.

Beschorner, W. E., Saral, R., Hutchins, G. W., Tutschka, P. J., and Santos, G. W. (1978). Lymphocytic bronchitis associated with graft-vs-host disease in recipients of bone marrow transplants. *N. Engl. J. Med.* **299**:1030–1036.

Bishop, J. F., Schimpff, S. C., Diggs, C. H., and Wirnik, P. H. (1981). Infections during intensive chemotherapy for non-Hodgkin's lymphoma. *Ann. Intern. Med.* **95**:549–555.

Blacklock, H. A., Griffiths, P., Stirk, P., and Prentice, P. G. (1985). Specific hyperimmune globulin for cytomegalovirus pneumonitis. *Lancet* **1**:152–153.

Bodey, G. P., Bolivar, R., and Fainstein, V. (1982). Infectious complications in leukemic patients. *Semin. Hematol.* **19**:193–226.

Bodey, G. P., Buckley, M., Sath, Y. S., and Freireich, E. J. (1966). Quantitative relationships between circulating leukocytes and infection in patients with acute leukemia. *Ann. Intern. Med.* **64**:328–340.

Bolivar, R., Kohl, S., and Pickering, L. K. (1980). Effect of anti-neoplastic drugs on antibody dependent cellular cytotoxicity mediated by human leukocytes against herpes simplex virus infected target cells. *Cancer* **46**:1555–1561.

Bordiogoni, P., Faure, G., Bene, M. C., Dardenne, M., Bach, J. F., Duheille, J., and Olive, D. (1982). Improvement of cellular immunity and IgA production in immunodeficient children after treatment with synthetic serum thymic factor (FTS). *Lancet* **2**:293–297.

Bowden, R. A., Sayers, M. Flournoy, N., Newton, B., Banaji, M., Thomas, E. D., and Meyers, J. D. (1986). Cytomegalovirus immune globulin and seronegative blood products to prevent primary cytomegalovirus infection after marrow transplantation. *N. Engl. J. Med.* **314**:1006–1010.

Brandt, S. J., Peters, W. P., Atwater, S. K., Kurtzberg, J., Borowitz, M. J., Jones, R. B., Shpall, E. J., Bast, R. C., Gilbert, C. J., and Oette, D. H. (1988). Effect of recombinant human granulocyte-macrophage colony stimulating factor on hematopoietic reconstitution after high dose chemotherapy and autologous bone marrow transplantation. *N. Engl. J. Med.* **318**:869–876.

Breedveld, F. C., Fibbe, W. E., Hermans, J., Van der Meer, J. W. M., and Cats, A. (1987). Factors influencing the incidence of infections in Felty's syndrome. *Arch. Intern. Med.* **147**:915–920.

Briggs, W. A., and Silliz, D. H. (1983). Leukocyte metabolism and function in uremia. *Kidney Int.* **24**(suppl): 593–596.

Broaddus, C., Dake, M. D., Stulbarg, M. S., Blumenfeld, W., Hadley, W. K., Golden, J. A., and Hopewell, P. C. (1985). Bronchoalveolar lavage and transbronchial biopsy for the diagnosis of pulmonary infec tions in the acquired immune deficiency syndrome. *Ann. Intern. Med.* **102**:747–752.

Brooks, R. G., and Remington, J. S. (1986). Transplant-related infections. In *Hospital Infections*, 2nd ed. Edited by J. V. Bennett and P. S. Brachman. Little, Brown & Little, Boston, pp. 581–618.

Brunkwall, J., Bergqvist, D., Bergentz, S. E., Bornmyr, S., and Husberg, B. (1987). Postoperative deep venous thrombosis after renal transplantation. *Transplantation* **43**:647–649.

Bruton, O. C. (1952). Agammaglobulinemia. *Pediatrics* **9**:722–728.

Buckley, R. H. (1983). Immunodeficiency. *J. Allergy Clin. Immunol.* **72**:627–641.

Buckley, R. H., and Schiff, R. I. (1991). The use of intravenous immune globulin in immunodeficiency diseases. *N. Engl. J. Med.* **325**:110–117.

Buckley, R. H., and Sidbury, J. B. (1968). Hereditary alterations in the immune response: coexistence of "agammaglobulinemia," acquired hypogammaglobulinemia and selective immunoglobulin deficiency in a sibship. *Pediatr. Res.* **2**:72–84.

Buckley, R. H., Wray, B. B., and Belmaker, E. Z. (1972). Extreme hyperimmunoglobulinemia E and undue susceptibility to infection. *Pediatrics* **49**:59–70.

Burch, P. A., Karp, J. E., Mers, W. G., Kuhlman, J. E., and Fishman, E. K. (1987). Favorable outcome of invasive aspergillosis in patients with acute leukemia. *J. Clin. Oncol.* **5**:1985–1993.

Burke, C. M., Theodore, J., Dawkins, K. D., Yousem, S. A., Blank, N., Billingham, M. E., VanKessel, A., Jamieson, S. W., Oyer, P., Baldwin, J. C.,

Stinson, E. B., Shumway, N. E., and Robin, E. D. (1984). Post transplant obliterative bronchiolitis and other later lung sequelae in human heart-lung transplantation. *Chest* **86**:824–829.

Burke, C. M., Glanville, A. R., Macoviak, J. A., O'Connell, B. M., Tazelaar, H. D., Baldwin, J. C., Jamieson, S. W., and Theodore, J. (1986). The spectrum of cytomegalovirus infection following human heart-lung transplantation. *J. Heart Transplant.* **5**:267–272.

Burks, A. W., Sampson, H. A., and Buckley, R. H. (1986). Anaphylactic reactions after gamma globulin administration in patients with hypogammaglobulinemia: detection of IgE antibodies to IgA. *N. Engl. J. Med.* **314**:560–564.

Campbell, J. H., Raina, V., Banham, S. W., Cunningham, D., and Soukop, M. (1989). Pulmonary infiltrates—diagnostic problems in lymphoma. *Postgrad. Med. J.* **65**:881–884.

Carter, A. R., Sostman, H. D., Curtis, A. M., and Swett, H. A. (1983). Thoracic alterations after cardiac surgery. *AJR* **140**:475–481.

Castellino, R. A., and Blank, N. (1979). Etiologic diagnosis of focal pulmonary infection in immunocompromised patients by fluroscopically guided percutaneous needle aspiration. *Radiology* **132**:563–567.

Castellino, R. A., Blank, N., Cassady, J. R., and Kaplan, H. S. (1973). Roentgenologic aspects of Hodgkin's disease. II. Role of routine radiographs in detecting initial relapse. *Cancer* **31**:316–323.

Catterall, J. R., McCabe, R. E., Brooks, R. G., and Remington, J. S. (1989). Open lung biopsy in patients with Hodgkin's disease and pulmonary infiltrates. *Am. Rev. Respir. Dis.* **139**:1274–1279.

Chan, C. K., Hyland, R. H., Hutcheon, M. A., Minden, M. D., Alexander, M. A., Kossakowska, A. E, Urbanski, S. J., Fyles, G. M., Fraser, I. M., Curtis, J. E., and Messner, H. A. (1987). Small-airways disease in recipients of allogeneic bone marrow transplants. *Medicine* **66**:327–340.

Chan, C. K., Hyland, R. H., and Hutcheon, M. A. (1990). Pulmonary complications following bone marrow transplantation. *Clin. Chest Med.* **11**:323–332.

Chan, J. C., Dunn, C. J., Bergin, C. J., and Duncan, S. R. (1989). Diagnosis of pneumonia in heart transplant recipients using percutaneous fine needle aspiration (abstract). *Am. Rev. Respir. Dis.* **139**:A428.

Chanez, P., Mourad, G., Aubas, P., Guillot, B., Godard, P., Mion, C., and Michel, F. B. (1988). Kaposi's sarcoma of the bronchial tree in a renal transplant recipient. *Respiration* **53**:259–261.

Chao, N. J., Duncan, S. R., Long, G. D., Horning, S. J., and Blume K. G. (1991). Corticosteroid therapy for diffuse alveolar hemorrhage in autologous bone marrow transplant recipients. *Ann. Intern. Med.* **114**:145–146.

Chen, B., Couch, L., Burdine, J., Bolman, R., and Hertz, M. (1991). Severe acute lung injury following heart-lung transplantation: impact on long-term pulmonary function (abstract). *Am. Rev. Respir. Dis.* **143**:A462.

Chiles, C., Guthaner, D. F., Jamieson, S. W., Stinson, E. B., Oyer, P. E., and Silverman, J. F. (1985). Heart-lung transplantation: the postoperative chest radiograph. *Radiology* **154**:299–304.

Chuang, M. T., Teirstein, A. S., Gribetz, A. R., Berman, L. B., and Nieburgs, H. E. (1981). Flexible fiberoptic bronchoscopy in the diagnosis of pulmonary complication of lymphoma. *Cancer Detect. Prev.* **4**:347–350.

Ciboddo, G., Crosti, F., Di Lucca, G. D., and Bellone, M. (1987). Cimetidine treatment in hyper-IgM hypogammaglobulinemia *JAMA* **258**:1892.

Clark, J. G., Schwartz, D. A., Flournoy, N., Sullivan, K. M. Crawford, S. W., and Thomas, E. D. (1987). Risk factors for airflow obstruction in recipients of bone marrow transplants. *Ann. Intern. Med.* **107**:648–656.

Clarke, I. A., Ormrod, D. J., and Miller, T. E. (1983). Host immune status in uremia. Effect of uremia on resistance to bacterial infection. *Kidney Int.* **24**:66–73.

Cleary, M. L., Warnke, R., and Sklar, J. (1984). Monoclonality of lymphoproliferative lesions in cardiac-transplant recipients. *N. Engl. J. Med.* **310**:477–482.

Cline, M. J. (1973). A test of individual phagocyte function in a mixed population of leukocytes. Identifications of a neutrophil abnormality in acute myelocytic leukemia. *J. Lab. Clin. Med.* **81**:311–315.

Cobb, S., Anderson, F., and Bauer, W. (1953). Length of life and cause of death in rheumatoid arthritis. *N. Engl. J. Med.* **249**:553–556.

Cohen, I. M., Galgiani, J. N., Potter, D., and Ogden, D. A. (1982). Coccidiodomycosis in renal replacement therapy. *Arch. Intern. Med.* **142**:489–494.

Colonna, J. D., Winston, D. J., Brill, J. E., Goldstein, L. I., Hoff, M. P., Hiatt, J. R., Quiones-Baldrich, W., Ramming, K. P., and Busuttil, R. W. (1988). Infectious complications in liver transplantation. *Arch. Surg.* **123**:360–364.

Commers, J., Robichaud, K. J., and Pizzo, P. A. (1984). New pulmonary infiltrates in granulocytopenic patients being treated with antibiotics. *Pediatr. Infect. Dis.* **3**:423–428.

Conley, M. (1985). B cells in patients with X-linked agammaglobulinemia. *J. Immunol.* **134**:3070–3074.

Cook, D. J., Chan, J., Dunn, C. J., Bergen, C. J., and Duncan, S. R. (1990). Late occurring pneumonia in heart transplant recipient (abstract). *Am. Rev. Respir. Dis.* **141**:A604.

Cooper, D. K. C., Lanza, R. P., Oliver, S., Forder, A. A., Rose, A. G., Uys, C. J., Novitsky, D., and Barnard, C. N. (1983). Infectious complications after heart transplantation. *Thorax* **38**:822–828.

Cooper, J. A. D., White, D. A., and Matthay, R. A. (1986). Drug induced pulmonary disease. Part 1: Cytotoxic drugs. *Am. Rev. Respir. Dis.* **133**:321–340.

Cooperative Group for the Study of Immunoglobulin in Chronic Lymphocytic Leukemia (1988). Intravenous immunoglobulin for the prevention of infection in chronic lymphocytic leukemia. *N. Engl. J. Med.* **319**:902–907.

Cordonnier, C., Bernaudin, J. F., Bierling, P., Huet, Y., and Vernant, J. P. (1986). Pulmonary complications occurring after allogeneic bone marrow transplantation. *Cancer* **58**:1047–1054.

Costello, P., and Mauch, P. (1979). Radiographic features of recurrent intrathoracic Hodgkin's disease following radiation therapy. *Am. J. Roentgenol.* **133**:201–206.

Coutts, I. I., Jegarajah, S., and Stark, J. E. (1979). Tuberculosis in renal transplant recipients. *Br. J. Dis. Chest* **73**:141–148.

Cowan, M. J., Smith W., and Amman, A. J. (1989). Interleukin-2 responsive lymphocytes in patients with adenosine deaminase deficiency. *Clin. Immunol. Immunopathol.* **53**:59–67.

Crawford, S. W., Bowden, R. A., Hackman, R. C., Gleaves, C. A., Meyers, J. D., and Clark, J. G. (1988). Rapid detection of cytomegalovirus pulmonary infection by bronchoalveolar lavage and centrifugation culture. *Ann. Intern. Med.* **108**:180–185.

Cunningham-Rundles, C. (1989). Clinical and immunological analysis of 103 patients with common variable immunodeficiency. *J. Clin. Immunol.* **9**:22–23.

Cunningham-Rundles, C., Siegal, F., Smithwick, E., Siegal, F. P., Smithwich, E. M., Lion-Boulé, A., Cunningham-Rundles, S., O'Malley, J., Barandun, S., and Good, R. A. (1984). Efficacy of intravenous immunoglobulin in primary humoral immunodeficiency disease. *Ann. Intern. Med.* **101**:435–439.

Cutz, E., Throner, P. S., Rao, C. P., Toma, S., Gold, R., and Gelfand, E. W. (1982). Disseminated *Legionella* pneumophila infection in an infant with severe combined immunodeficiency. *J. Pediatr.* **100**:760–762.

Dale, D. C., DuPont, G., IV, Wewerka, J. R., Bull, J. M., and Chusid, M. J. (1979). Chronic neutropenia. *Medicine* **58**:128–144.

Dauber, J. H., Paradis, I. L., and Dummer, J. S. (1990). Infectious complications in pulmonary allograft recipients. *Clin. Chest Med.* **11**:291–308.

Dautzenberg, B., Grosset, J., Fechner, J., Lucciani, J., Debre, P., Herson, S., Truffot, C., and Sors, C. (1984). The management of thirty immunocompromised patients with tuberculosis. *Am. Rev. Respir. Dis.* **129**:494–495.

Del Prete, G., Tiri, A., Maggi, E., De Carli, M., Macchia, D., Parronchi, P., Rossi, M. E., Pietrogrande, M. C., Ricci, M., and Romagnani, S. (1989). Defective in vitro production of gamma-interferon and tumor necrosis factor-alpha by circulating T cells from patients with the hyper-immunoglobulin E syndrome. *J. Clin. Invest.* **84**:1830–1835.

Denning, D. W., Tucker, R. M., Hanson, L. H., and Stevens, D. A. (1989). Treatment of invasive aspergillosis with intraconazole. *Am. J. Med.* **86**:791–800.

Depledge, M. H., Barrett, A., and Powles, R. L. (1983). Lung function after bone marrow grafting. *Int. J. Radiation Oncol. Biol. Phys.* **9**:145–151.

Dickey, B. F. and Myers, A. R. (1984). Pulmonary disease in polymyositis/dermatomyositis. *Semin. Arthritis Rheum.* **14**:60–76.

Dickout, W. J., Chan, C. K., Hyland, R. H., Hutcheon, M. A., Fraser, I. M., Morgan, C. D., Curtis, J. E., and Messner, H. A. (1987). Prevention of acute pulmonary edema after bone marrow transplantation. *Chest* **92**:303–309.

Doi, S., Saiki, O., Hara, T., Sugita, T., Ha-Kawa, K., Tanaka, T., Hara, H., Negoro, S., Yabuuchi, H., and Kishimoto, S. (1989). Administration of recombinant IL-2 augments the level of serum IgM in an IL-2 deficient patient. *Eur. J. Pediatr.* **148**:630–633.

Donabedian, H., and Gallin, J. I. (1982). Mononuclear cells from patients with hyperimmunoglobulin E-recurrent infection syndrome produce an inhibitor of leukocyte chemotaxis. *J. Clin. Invest.* **69**:1155–1163.

Donabedian, H., and Gallin, J. I. (1983). The hyperimmunoglobulin E recurrent-infection (Job's) syndrome. *Medicine* **62**:195–208.

Donabedian, H., Alling, D. W., and Gallin, J. I. (1982). Levamisole is inferior to placebo in the hyperimmunoglobulin E recurrent-infection (Job's) syndrome. *N. Engl. J. Med.* **307**:290–292.

Drobyski, W. R., Gottlieb, M., Carrigan, D., Ostberg, L., Grebenau, M., Schran, H., Magid, D., Ehrlich, P., Nadler, P. I., and Ash, R. C. (1991). Phase I study of safety and pharmacokinetics of a human anticytomegalovirus monoclonal antibody in allogeneic bone marrow transplant recipients. *Transplantation* **51**:1190–1196.

Dukes, R. J., Rosenow, E. C., and Hermans, P. E. (1978). Pulmonary manifestations of hypogammaglobulinaemia. *Thorax* **33**:603–607.

Dummer, J. S. (1990). Infectious complications of transplantation. In *Cardiac Transplantation*. Edited by M. E. Thompson. F. A. Davis, Philadelphia, pp. 163–178.

Dummer, J. S., White, L. T., Ho, M., Griffith, B. P., Hardesty, R. L., and Bahnson, H. T. (1985). Morbidity of cytomegalovirus infection in recipients of heart or heart-lung transplants who received cyclosporine. *J. Infect. Dis.* **152**:1182–1191.

Duncan, S. R., and Cook, D. J. (1991). Survival of ganciclovir-treated heart transplant recipients with cytomegalovirus pneumonitis. *Transplantation* **52**:910–913.

Duncan, S. R., Kagawa, F. T., Starnes, V. A., and Theodore, J. (1991a). Hypercarbic ventilatory responses of human heart-lung transplant recipients to progressive hypercarbia. *Am. Rev. Respir. Dis.* **144**:126–130.

Duncan, S. R., Kagawa, F. T., Kramer, M. R., Starnes, V. A., and Theodore, J. (1991b). Effects of pulmonary restrictions on hypercapnic responses of heart-lung transplant recipients. *J. Appl. Physiol.* **71**:322–327.

Duncan, S. R., Paradis, I. L., Williams, P., Dauber, J. H., Yousem, S., Johnson, B., and Griffith, B. P. (1992). Prevention of cytomegalovirus infections in lung transplant recipients. (abstract). *Am Rev. Respir. Dis.* (in press).

Dunn, C., Chan, J., Rizk, N., and Duncan, S. R. (1988). Diagnosis of pneumonia in heart transplant recipients using fiberoptic bronchoscopy (abstract). *Chest* **94**:S395.

Ekberg, H., Tranberg, K. G., Anderson, R., Jeppsson, B., and Bengmark, S. (1986). Major liver resection: perioperative course and management. *Surgery* **100**:1–7.

Emanuel, D., Cummingham, I., Jules-Elyses, K., Brochstein, J. A., Kernan, N. A., Laver, J., Stover, D., White, D. A., Fels, A., Polsky, B., Castro-Malaspina, H., Peppard, J. R., Bartus, P., Hammerling, U., and O'Reilly, R. J. (1988). Cytomegalovirus pneumonia after bone marrow transplantation successfully treated with the combination of ganciclovir and high-dose intravenous immune globulin. *Ann. Intern. Med.* **109**:777–782.

England, A. C., Fraser, D. W., Plikaytis, B. D., Tsai, T. F., Storch, G., and Broome, C. V. (1981). Sporadic legionellosis in the United States: the first thousand cases. *Ann. Intern. Med.* **94**:164–170.

EORTC Antimicrobial Therapy Cooperative Group (1989). Empiric antifungal therapy infebrile granulocytopenic patients. *Am. J. Med.* **86**:668–672.

Erice, A., Hertz, M. I., Snyder, L. S., Englund, J., Edelman, C. K., and Balfour, H. H. (1988). Evaluation of centrifugation cultures of bronchoalveolar lavage fluid for the diagnosis of cytomegalovirus pneumonitis. *Diagn. Microbiol. Infect. Dis.* **10**:205–212.

Ettinger, N. A., and Trulock, E. P. (1991). Pulmonary considerations of organ transplantation. Parts 1–3. *Am. Rev. Respir. Dis.* **143**:1386–1405; **144**:213–223, 433–451.

Ezekokwitz, A., Phil, D., Dinauer, M., Jaffe, H. S., Orkin, S. H., and Newburger, P. E. (1988). Partial correction of the phagocyte defect in patients with X-linked chronic granulomatosus disease by subcutaneous interferron gamma. *N. Engl. J. Med.* **319**:146–150.

Feld, R., and Bodey, G. P. (1977). Infections in patients with malignant lymphoma treated with combination chemotherapy. *Cancer* **48**:779–782.

Fiorilli, M., Russo, G., Paanelli, R., Papetti, C., Carbonari, M., Crescenzi, M., Calvani, M., Quinti, I., and Aiuti, F. (1986). Hypogammaglobulinemia with hyper-IgM, severe T-cell defect, and abnormal recirculation of OKT4 lymphocytes in a girl with chronic lymphadenopathy. *Clin. Immunol. Immunopathol.* **38**:256–264.

Fischer, A., Blanche, S., Le Bidois, J., Bordigoni, P., Garnier, J. L., Niavdet, P., Morinet, F., LeDeist, F., Fischer, A. M., Griscelli, C., and Hirn, M. (1991). Anti-B-cell monoclonal antibodies in the treatment of severe B-cell lymphoproliferative syndrome following bone marrow and organ transplantation. *N. Engl. J. Med.* **324**:1451–1456.

Freedom, R. M., Rosen, F. S., and Nadas, A. S. (1972). Congenital cardiovascular disease and anomalies of the third and fourth pharyngeal pouch. *Circulation* **46**:165–172.

Gallin, J. I., Wright, D. G., Malech, H. L., Davis, J. M., Klempner, M. S., and Kirkpatrick, C. H. (1980). Disorders of phagocyte chemotaxis. *Ann. Intern. Med.* **92**:520–538.

Geha, R. S., Schereebeyer, E., Merler, E., and Rosen, F. S. (1974). Heterogeneity of "acquired" or common variable agammaglobulinemia. *N. Engl. J. Med.* **291**:1–6.

Geha, R. S., Hyslop, N., Alami, S., Farah, F., Schneeberger, E. E., and Rosen, F. S. (1979). Hyperimmunoglobulin M immunodeficiency (dysgammaglobulinemia): presence of immunoglobulin M-secreting plamacytoid cells in peripheral blood and failure of immunoglobulin M-immunoglobulin-G switch in B-cell differentiation. *J. Clin. Invest.* **64**:385–391.

Gibson, P. G., Bryant, D. H., Morgan, G. W., Yeates, M., Fernandez, V., Penny, R., and Breit, S. N. (1988). Radiation-induced lung injury: a hypersensitivity pneumonitis? *Ann. Intern. Med.* **109**:288–291.

Ginzler, E., Diamond, H., Kaplan, D., Weiner, M., Schlesinger, M., and Seleznick, M. (1978). Computer analysis of factors influencing frequency of infection in systemic lupus erythermatosus. *Arthritis Rheum.* **21**:37–44.

Glanville, A., Baldwin, J., Burke, C., Theodore, J., and Robin, E. D. (1987). Obliterative bronchiolitis after heart-lung transplantation: apparent arrest by augmented immunosuppression. *Ann. Intern. Med.* **107**:300–304.

Glanville, A., Theodore, J., Harvey, J., and Robin, E. D. (1988). Elastic behavior of the transplanted lung. Exponential analysis of static pressure-volume relationships. *Am. Rev. Respir. Dis.* **137**:308–312.

Goldberg, J. G., and Pinals, R. S. (1980). Felty syndrome. *Semin. Arthritis Rheum.* **10**:52–65.

Goldblum, S. E., and Reed, W. P. (1980). Host defenses and immunologic alterations associated with chronic hemodialysis. *Ann. Intern. Med.* **93**:597–613.

Goodall, P. T., and Vosti, K. L. (1975). Fever in acute myelogenous leukemia. *Arch. Intern. Med.* **135**:1197–1203.

Gorevic, P. D., Katler, E. I., and Agus, B. (1980). Pulmonary nocardiosis in men with SLE. *Arch. Intern. Med.* **140**:361–363.

Grattan, M. T., Moreno-Cabral, C. E., Starnes, V. A., Oyer, P. E., Stinson, E. B., and Shumway, N. E. (1989). Cytomegalovirus infections is associated with cardiac allograft rejection and atherosclerosis. *JAMA* **261**:3561–3566.

Gregory, L., Williams, R., and Thompson, E. (1972). Leukocyte function in Down's syndrome and acute leukemia. *Lancet* **1**:1359–1368.

Griffith, B. P., Hardest, R. L., Trento, A., and Bahnson, H. T. (1985). Asynchronous rejection of heart and lungs following cardiopulmonary transplantation. *Ann. Thorac. Surg.* **40**:488–493.

Griffith, B. P., Hardesty, R. L., Trento, A., Paradis, I. L., Duquesnoy, R. J., Zeevi, A., Dauber, J. H., Dummer, J. S., Thompson, M. E., Gryzan, S., and Bahnson, H. T. (1987). Heart-lung transplantations: lessons learned and future directions. *Ann. Thorac. Surg.* **43**:6–16.

Grossman, R. F., Frost, A., Zamel, N., Patterson, G. A., Cooper, J. D., Myron, P. R., Dear, C. L., Maurer, J., and Toronto Lung Transplant Group (1990). Results of single-lung transplantation for bilateral pulmonary fibrosis. *N. Engl. J. Med.* **322**:727–733.

Grundy, J. E., Shanley, J. D., and Griffiths, P. D. (1987). Is cytomegalovirus interstitial pneumonitis in transplant recipients an immunopathological condition? *Lancet* **2**:996–999.

Gump, D. W., Frank, R. O., Winn, W. C., Foster, R. S., Broome, C. V., and Cherry, W. B. (1979). Legionnaires' disease in patients with associated serious disease. *Ann. Intern. Med.* **90**:538–542.

Hackman, R. C., and Sale, G. E. (1981). Large airway inflammation as a possible manifestation of a pulmonary graft-vs-host disease in recipients of bone marrow transplants (abstract). *Lab. Invest.* **44**:26A.

Hall, T. S. Hutchins, G. M., and Baker, R. R. (1987). A critical review of the use of open lung biopsy in the management of the oncologic patient with acute pulmonary infiltrates. *Am. J. Clin. Oncol.* **10**:249–252.

Hanto, D. W., Frizzera, G., Gajl-Peczalska, K. J., Balfour, H. H., Simmons, R. L., and Najarian, J. S. (1985). Acyclovir therapy of Epstein-Barr virus-induced posttransplant lymphoproliferative diseases. *Transplant. Proc.* **17**:89–92.

Heard, B. E., Path, F. C., Steiner, R. E., Herdan, A., and Gleason, D. (1968). Oedema and fibrosis of the lungs in left ventricular failure. *Br. J. Radiol.* **41**:161–171.

Heiner, D. C. (1984). Significance of immunoglobulin G subclasses. *Am. J. Med.* **76**(suppl 3A): 1–6.

Heino, A., Orko, R., and Rosenberg, P. H. (1986). Anaesthesiological complications in renal transplantation: a retrospective study of 500 transplantations. *Acta Anesthesiol. Scand.* **30**:574–580.

Hellmann, D. B., Petri, M., and Whiting-O'Keefe, Q. (1987). Fatal infections in systemic lupus erythematosus: the role of opportunistic organisms. *Medicine* **66**:341–348.

Henry, D. A., Jolles, H., Berberich, J. J., and Schmetzer, V. (1989). The post-cardiac surgery radiograph: a clinically integrated approach. *J. Thorac. Imaging* **4**:20–41.

Heppner, G. H., and Calabresi, P. (1976). Selective suppression of humoral immunity by antineoplatic drugs. *Annu. Rev. Pharmacol. Toxicol.* **16**:367–379.

Herman, S. J. (1990). Radiologic assessment after lung transplantation. *Clin. Chest Med.* **11**:333–346.

Hermans, P. E., Diaz-Buxo, J. A., and Stobo, J. O. (1976). Idiopathic late-onset immunoglobulin deficiency. Clinical observations in 50 patients. *Am. J. Med.* **61**:221–237.

Hertz, M. I., Englund, J. A., Snover, D., Bitterman, P. B., and McGlave, P. B. (1989). Respiratory syncytial virus-induced acute lung injury in adult patients with bone marrow transplants: a clinical approach and review of the literature. *Medicine* **68**:269–281.

Hesse, U. J., Fryd, D. S., Chatterjee, S. N., Simmons, R. L., Sutherland, D. E. R., and Najarian, J. S. (1986). Pulmonary infections: the Minnesota randomized prospective trial of cyclosporine vs azathioprine-antilymphocyte globulin for immunosuppression in renal allograft recipients. *Arch. Surg.* **121**:1056–1060.

Heurlin, J., Lonnqvist, B., Tollemar, J., and Ehrnst, A. (1989). Fiberoptic bronchoscopy for diagnosis of opportunistic pulmonary infections after bone marrow transplantation. *Scand. J. Infect. Dis.* **21**:358–366.

Higenbottam, T., Stewart, S., and Penketh, A. (1988). Transbronchial lung biopsy for the diagnosis of rejection in heart-lung transplant patients. *Transplantation* **46**:532–539.

Hill, H. R. (1981). Infections complicating congenital immunodeficiency syndromes. In: *Clinical Approach to Infection in the Compromised Host*. Edited by R. H. Rubin and L. S. Young. Plenum Press, New York, pp. 417–460.

Hirschhorn, R. (1986). Inherited enzyme deficiencies and immunodeficiency: adensosine deaminase (ADA) and purine nuclesoside phosphorylase (PNP) deficiencies. *Clin. Immunol. Immunopathol.* **40**:157–165.

Hirschhorn, R. (1990). Adenosine deaminase deficiency. *Immunodefic. Rev.* **2**:175–198.

Ho, M., Miller, G. R., Atchison, R. W., Breinig, M. K., Dummer, J. S., Andiman, W., Starzl, T. E., Eastman, R., Griffith, B. P., Hardesty, R. L., Bahnson, H. T., Hakala, T. R., and Rosenthal, J. T. (1985). Epstein-Barr virus infections and DNA hybridization studies in post-transplantation lymphoma and lymphoproliferative lesions: the role of primary infection. *J. Infect. Dis.* **152**:876–886.

Hofflin, J. M., Potasman, I., Baldwin, J. C., Oyer, P. E., Stinson, E. B., and Remington, J. S. (1987). Infectious complications in heart transplant recipients receiving cyclosporine and corticosteroids. *Ann. Intern. Med.* **106**:209–216.

Hoffman, G. S., and Fauci, A. S. (1991). Respiratory disease in patients treated with glucocorticoids. In *Respiratory Disease in the Immunocompromised Host*. Edited by J. Shelhamer, P. A. Pizzo, J. E. Parrillo, and H. Masur. Lippincott, Philadelphia, pp. 682–689.

Hoffman, T., Winchester, R., Schulkind, M., Frias, J. L. Ayoub, E. M., and Good, R. A. (1977). Hypogammaglobulinemia with normal T cell function in female siblings. *Clin. Immunol. Immunopathol.* **7**:364–371.

Holland, H. K., Wingard, J. R., Beschorner, W. E., Saral, R., and Santos, G. W. (1988). Bronchiolitis obliterans in bone marrow transplantation and its relationship to chronic graft-vs-host disease and low serum immunoglobulin. *Blood* **72**:621–627.

Holland, S. A., Hutton, L. C., and McKenzie, F. N. (1989). Radiologic findings in heart-lung transplantation: a preliminary experience. *J. Can. Assoc. Radiol.* **40**:94–97.

Hughes, W. T., Feldman, S., Aur, R. J. A., Verzosa, M. S., Husta, H. O., and Simone, J. V. (1975). Intensity of immunosuppressive therapy and the incidence of *Pneumocystis carinii* pneumonitis. *Cancer* **36**:2004–2009.

Hughes, W. T., Kuhn, S., Chaudhury, S., Feldman, S., Versoza, M., Aur, R. J. A., Pratt, C., and George, S. L. (1977). Successful chemoprophylaxis for *Pneumocystis carinii* pneumonitis. *N. Engl. J. Med.* **297**:1419–1426.

Hunninghake, G. W., and Fauci, A. S. (1979). Pulmonary involvement in the collagen vascular diseases. *Am. Rev. Respir. Dis.* **119**:471–503.

Ichikawa, Y., Ganzales, E. B., and Daniels, J. C. (1982). Suppressor cells of mitogen-induced lymphocyte proliferation in the peripheral blood of patients with common variable hypogammaglobulinemia. *Clin. Immunol. Immunopathol.* **25**:252–263.

International Chronic Granulomatous Disease Cooperative Study Group (1991). A controlled trial of interferon gamma to prevent infection in chronic granulomatous disease. *N. Engl. J. Med.* **324**:509–516.

Izutsu, K. T., Sullivan, K. M., Schubert, M. M., Truelove, E. L., Shulman, H. M., Sale, G. E., Morton, T. H., Rice, J. C., Witherspoon, R. P.,

Storb, R., and Thomas, E. D. (1983). Disordered salivary immunoglobulin secretion and sodium transport in human chronic graft-versus-host disease. *Transplantation* **35**:441–446.

Jensen, W. A., Rose, R. M., Hammer, S. M., Jenkins, R. L., Bothe, A., Benotti, P. N., Dzik, W. H., Costello, P., Khettry, U., Trey, C., Eliopoulos, G. M., and Karchmer, A. W. (1986). Pulmonary complications of orthotopic liver transplantation. *Transplantation* **42**:484–490.

Jeppson, J. D., Jaffe, H. S., and Hill, H. R. (1991). Use of recombinant human interferon gamma to enhance neutrophil chemotactic responses in Job's syndrome of hyperimmunoglobulinemia E and recurrent infections. *J. Pediatr.* **118**:383–387.

Jochelson, M., Altschuler, J., and Stomper, P. (1986). The yield of chest radiography in febrile and neutropenic patients. *Ann. Intern. Med.* **105**:708–709.

Johnston, R. B. (1984). Recurrent bacterial infections in children. *N. Engl. J. Med.* **310**:1237–1243.

Jules-Elysee, K., Gulati, S., Stover, D. E., and White, D. A. (1990). Pulmonary complications in autologous bone marrow transplantation. (abstract). *Am. Rev. Respir. Dis.* **141**:A604.

Kagawa, F. T., Duncan, S. R., and Theodore, J. (1991). Inspiratory timing of heart-lung transplant recipients during progressive hypercapnia. *J. Appl. Physiol.* **71**:945–950.

Kahn, R. W., Jones, J. M., and England, D. M. (1986). The role of bronchoalveolar lavage in the diagnosis of invasive pulmonary aspergillosis. *Am. J. Clin. Pathol.* **86**:518–523.

Kaltreider, H. B. (1976). State of the art: expression of immune mechanisms in the lung. *Am. Rev. Respir. Dis.* **113**:347–379.

Kantoff, P. W., Kohn, D. B., Mitsuya, H., Armentano, D., Sieberg, M., Zweibel, J. A., Eglitis, M. A., McLachlin, J. R., Wiginton, P. A., Hutton, J. J., Herowitx, S. D., Gilboa, E., Blaese, R. M., and Anderson, W. F. (1986). Correction of adenosine deaminase deficiency in cultured human T and B cells by retrovirus-mediated gene transfer. *Proc. Natl. Acad. Sci. USA* **83**:6563–6567.

Kaplan, H. S., and Stewart, J. R. (1973). Complications of intensive megavoltage radiotherapy for Hodgkin's disease. *Natl. Cancer Inst. Monogr.* **36**:439–444.

Karp, J. E., Burch, P. A., and Merx, W. G. (1988). An approach to intensive antileukemia therapy in patients with previous invasive aspergillosis. *Am. J. Med.* **85**:203–206.

Kauffman, C. A., Israel, K. S., Smith, J. W., White, A. C., Schwarz, J., and Brooks, G. F. (1978). Histoplasmosis in immunosuppressed patients. *Am. J. Med.* **64**:923–932.

Keane, W. F., Shapiro, F. L., and Raij, L. (1977). Incidence and type of infections occurring in 445 chronic hemodialysis patients. *Trans. Am. Soc. Artif. Intern. Organs* **23**:41–46.

Keay, S., Petersen, E., Icenogle, T., Zeluff, B. J., Samo, T., Busch, D., Newman, C. L., Buhles, W. C., and Merigan T. C. (1988). Ganciclovir treatment of serious cytomegalovirus infection in heart and heart-lung transplant recipients. *Rev. Infect. Dis.* **10**:S563–S572.

Keegan, J. M., and Byrd, J. W. (1988). Nocardiosis associated with low dose methotrexate for rheumatoid arthritis. *J. Rheumatol.* **15**:1585–1586.

Keenan, R. J., Lega, M. E., Dummer, J. S., Paradis, I. L., Dauber, J. H., Rabinowich, H., Yousem, S. A., Hardesty, R. L., Griffith, B. P., Duquesnoy, R. J., and Zeevi, A. (1991). Cytomegalovirus serologic status and postoperative infection correlated with risk of developing chronic rejection after pulmonary transplantation. *Transplantation* **51**:433–438.

Kersey, J. H., Shapiro, R. S., and Filipovich, A. H. (1988). Relationship of immunodeficiency to lymphoid malignancy. *Pediatr. Infect. Dis. J.*(suppl 7): S10–S12.

King, C. L., Gallin, J. I., Malech, H. L., Abramsom, S. L., and Nutman, T. B. (1989). Regulation of immunoglobulin production in hyperimmunoglobulin E recurrent-infection syndrome by interferon gamma. *Proc. Natl. Acad. Sci. USA* **86**:1085–1089.

Kirkpatrick, G. H., and Schimke, R. N. (1967). Paternal immunoglobulin abnormalities in congenital hypogammaglobulinemia. *JAMA* **200**:105–113.

Kjellstrand, C. M. (1978). The Achilles heel of the hemodialysis patient. *Arch. Intern. Med.* **138**:1063–1064.

Komatsu, K., Kodama, S., Okumura, Y., Koi, M., and Oshimura, M. (1990). Restoration of radiation resistance in atazia telangiectasia cells by the introduction of normal human chromosom 11. *Mutat. Res.* **235**:59–63.

Krowka, M. J., and Cortese, D. A. (1989). Pulmonary aspects of liver disease and liver transplantation. *Clin. Chest Med.* **10**:593–616.

Krowka, M. J., Rosenow, E. C. III, and Hoagland, H. C. (1985). Pulmonary complications of bone marrow transplantation. *Chest* **87**:237–246.

Krowka, M. J., Staats, B. A., and Hoagland, H. C. (1990). A prospective study of airway reactivity before bone marrow transplantation. *Mayo Clin. Proc.* **65**:5–12.

Kugler, J. W., Armitage, J. W., and Helms, C. M. (1983). Nosocomial Legionnaires' disease: occurrence in recipients of bone marrow transplants. *Am. J. Med.* **74**:281–288.

Kusne, S., Dummer, J. S., Singh, N., Iwatsuki, S., Makowka, L., Esquivel, C., Tzakis, A. G., Starzl, T. E., and Ho, M. (1988). Infections after liver transplantation: an analysis of 101 consecutive cases. *Medicine* **67**:132–143.

Landry, M. (1977). Phagocyte function and cell-mediated immunity in systemic lupus erythematosus. *Arch. Dermatol.* **113**:147–154.

Leddy, J. P., Frank, M. M., Gainer, I., Baum, J., and Klemperer, M. R. (1974). Hereditary deficiency of the sixthe component of complement in man. *J. Clin. Invest.* **53**:544–553.

Leggiadro, R. J., Winkelstein, J. A., and Hughes, W. T. (1981). Prevalence of *Pneumocystis carinii* pneumonitis in severe combined immunodeficiency. *J. Pediatr.* **99**:96–98.

Lenarsky, C., and Parkman, R. (1990). Bone marrow transplantation for the treatment of immune deficiency states. *Bone Marrow Transplant.* **6**:361–369.

Leung, D. Y., Ambrosino, D. M., Arbeit, R. D., Newton, J. L., and Geha, R. S. (1988). Impaired antibody responses in the hyperimmunoglobulin E syndrome. *J. Allergy Clin. Immunol.* **81**:1082–1087.

Levi, Y., Hershfield, M. S., Fernandez-Mejia, C., Polmar, S. H., Scudiery, D., Berger, M., and Sorensen, R. U. (1988). Adenosine deaminase deficiency with late onset recurrent infections: response to treatment with polyethylene glycol-modified adenosine deaminase. *J. Pediatr.* **113**:312–317.

Lichtenstein, I. H., and MacGregor, R. R. (1983). Mycobacterial infections in renal transplant recipients: report of five cases and review of the literature. *Rev. Infect. Dis.* **5**:216–226.

Limper, A. H., Offord, K. P., Smith, T. F., and Martin, W. J. (1989). *Pneumocystis carinii* pneumonia. Differences in lung parasite number and inflammation in patients with and without AIDS. *Am. Rev. Respir. Dis.* **140**:1204–1209.

Lischner, H. W. (1972). DiGeorge syndrome(s). *J. Pediatr.* **81**:183–192.

Luft, B. J., Naot, Y., Araujo, F. G., Stinson, E. B., and Remington, J. S. (1983). Primary and reactivated *Toxoplasma* infection in patients with cardiac transplants. *Ann. Intern. Med.* **99**:27–31.

Maile, C. W., Moore, A. V., Ulreich, S., and Putman, C. E. (1983). Chest radiographic-pathologic correlation in adult leukemia patients. *Invest. Radiol.* **18**:495–499.

Malhotra, K. K., Dash, S. C., Dhawan, I. K., Bhuyan, U. N., and Gupta, A. (1986). Tuberculosis and renal transplantation-observations from an endemic area of tuberculosis. *Postgrad. Med. J.* **62**:359–362.

Mancini, M. C., and Tauxe, W. N. (1986). Assessment of pulmonary clearance in heart lung transplant recipients using technetium 99-m minimicronized albumin colloid (abstract). *Am. Rev. Respir. Dis.* **133**:A11.

Margolis, D. M., Melnick, D. A., Alling, D. W., and Gallin, J. I. (1990). Trimethoprim-sulfamethoxazole prophylaxis in the management of chronic granulomatous disease. *J. Infect. Dis.* **162**:723–726.

Masur, H., Cheigh, J. S., and Stubenbord, W. T. (1982). Infection following renal transplantation: a changing pattern. *Rev. Infect. Dis.* **4**:1208–1219.

McCabe, R. E., Brooks, R. G., Mark, J. B. D., and Remington, J. S. (1985). Open lung biopsy in patients with acute leukemia. *Am. J. Med.* **78**:609–616.

McCabe, R. E., Brooks, R. G., Catteral, J. R., and Remington, J. S. (1989). Open lung biopsy in patients with non-Hodgkin's lymphoma and pulmonary infiltrates. *Chest* **96**:319–324.

McCarthy, P., Starnes, V., Theodore, J., Stinson, E. B., Oyer, P. E., and Shumway, N. E. (1990). Improved survival following heart-lung transplant. *J. Thorac. Cardiovasc. Surg.* **99**:54–60.

McCaw, B. K., Hecht, F., Harnden, D. G., and Teplitz, R. L. (1975). Somatic rearrangement of chromosome 14 in human lymphocytes. *Proc. Natl. Acad. Sci. USA* **72**:2071–2075.

McFarlin, D. D., Strober, W., and Waldmann, T. A. (1972). Ataxia-telangiectasia. *Medicine* **51**:281–314.

McIvor, R. S., Johnson, M. J., Miller, A. D., Pitts, S., Williams, S. R., and Valerio, D. (1987). Human purine nucleoside phosphorylase and adenosine deaminase: gene transfer into cultured cells and murine hematopoietic stem cells by using recombinant amphotropic retroviruses. *Mol. Cell. Biol.* **7**:838–846.

McKeating, J. A., Griffiths, P. D., and Grundy, J. E. (1987). Cytomegalovirus in urine specimens has host β_2-microglobulin bound to the virus envelope: a mechanism of evading the host immune response? *J. Gen. Virol.* **68**:785–792.

McKee, L. C., and Collins, R. D. (1974). Intravascular leukocyte thrombi and aggregates as a cause of morbidity and mortality in leukemia. *Medicine* **53**:463–478.

Merten, D. F., Buckley, Pratt, P. C., Effmann, E. L., and Grossman, H. (1979). Hyperimmunoglobulinemia E syndrome: radiographic observations. *Radiology* **132**:71–78.

Meyers, J. D. (1990). Fungal infections in bone marrow transplant patients. *Semin. Oncol.* **17**:10–13.

Meyers, J. D., Flounoy, N., and Thomas E. D. (1982). Nonbacterial pneumonia after allogeneic marrow transplantation: a review of ten years' experience. *Rev. Infect. Dis.* **4**:1119–1132.

Meyers, J. D., Flournoy, N., and Thomas, E. D. (1986). Risk factors for cytomegalovirus infection after human marrow transplantation. *J. Infect. Dis.* **153**:478–488.

Meyers, J. D., Reed, E. C., Shepp, D. H., Thornquist, M., Dandliker, P. S., Vicary, C. A., Flournoy, N., Kirk, L. E., Kersey, J. H., Thomas, E. D., and Balfour, H. H. (1988). Acyclovir for prevention of cytomegalovirus infection and disease after allogeneic marrow transplantation. *N. Engl. J. Med.* **318**:70–75.

Milburn, H. J., Du Bois, R. M., Prentice, H. G., and Poulter, L. W. (1990). Pneumonitis in bone marrow transplant recipients results from a local immune response. *Clin. Exp. Immunol.* **81**:232–237.

Miller, M. E., and Nilsson, U. R. (1970). A familial deficiency of the phagocytosis-enhancing activity of serum related to a dysfunction of the fifth component of complement (C5). *N. Engl. J. Med.* **282**:354–358.

Miller, W., Flynn, P., McCullough, J., Balfour, H. H., Goldman, A., Haake, R., McGlave, P., Ramsay, N., and Kersey, J. (1986). Cytomegalovirus infection after bone marrow transplantation: an association with acute graft-v-host disease. *Blood* **67**:1162–1167.

Mitchell, D. M., Spitz, P. W., Young, D. Y., Bloch, D. A., McShane, D. J., and Fries, J. F. (1986). Survival, prognosis and causes of death in rhematoid arthritis. *Arthritis Rheum.* **29**:706–714.

Montefusco, C. M., and Veith, F. J. (1986). Lung transplantation. *Surg. Clin. North Am.* **66**:503–515.

Montgomerie, J. Z., Kalmanson, G. M., and Guze, L. B. (1968). Renal failure and infection. *Medicine* **47**:1–32.

Mouy, R., Fischer, A., Vilmer, E., Seger, R., and Griscelli, C. (1989). Incidence, severity, and prevention of infections in chronic granulomatous disease. *J. Pediatr.* **114**:550–560.

Muggenburg, B. A., Bice, D. E., Haley, P. J., Mauderly, J. L., Dauber, J. J., Herlan, K., and Griffith, B. P. (1986). Immune response in the transplanted canine lung (abstract). *Am. Rev. Respir. Dis.* **134**:A103.

Munda, R., Alexander, J. W., First, M. R., Gartside, P. S., and Fidler, J. P. (1978). Pulmonary infections in renal transplant recipients. *Ann. Surg.* **187**:126–133.

Nakae, S., Webb, W., Heodorides, T., and Sugg, W. L. (1967). Respiratory function following cardiopulmonary denervation in the dog, cat, and monkey. *Surg. Gynecol. Obstet.* **125**:1285–1291.

Nalesnik, M. A., Jaffe, R., Starzl, T. E., Demetris, J. A., Porter, K., Burnham, J. A., Makowka, L., Ho, M., and Locker, J. (1988). The pathology of postransplant lymphoproliferative disorders occurring in the setting of cyclosporin A–prednisone immunosuppression. *Am. J. Pathol.* **133**:173–192.

Nedelkova, M., Bacolova, S., and Georgieva, B. (1981). Infectious complications and host immune defense in acute leukemia. *Eur. J. Cancer* **17**:617–622.

Nived, O., Linder, C., Odeberg, H., and Svensson, B. (1985a). Reduced opsonization of protein A containing *Staphylococcus aureus* in sera with cryoglobulins from patients with active systemic lupus erythematosus. *Ann. Rheum. Dis.* **44**:252–259.

Nived, O., Stufelt, G., and Wolheim, F. (1985b). Systemic lupus erythematosus and infection: a controlled and prospective study including an epidemiological group. *Q. J. Med.* **55**:271–287.

O'Hanley, R., Easaw, J., Rugo, H., and Easaw, S. (1989). Infectious disease management of adult leukemic patients undergoing chemotherapy: 1982 to 1986 experience at Stanford University Hospital. *Am. J. Med.* **87**:605–613.

O'Reilly, R. J., Keever, C. A., Small, T. N., and Brochstein, J. (1989). The use of HLA-non-identical T-cell-depleted marrow transplants for correction of severe combined immunodeficiency disease. *Immunodefic. Rev.* **1**:273–309.

Ostrow, S., Diggs, C. H., Sutherland, J., and Wiernik, P. H. (1981). Causes of death in patients with non-Hodgkin's lymphoma. *Cancer* **48**:779–782.

Oxelius, V. A., Berkel, A. I., and Hanson, L. A. (1982). IgG2 deficiency in ataxia-telangiectasia. *N. Engl. J. Med.* **306**:515–517.

Palosaari, D. E., and Colby, T. V. (1986). Bronchiolocentric chronic lymphocytic leukemia. *Cancer* **58**:1695–1698.

Paradis, I. L., Grgurich, W. F., Drummer, J. S., Dekker, A., and Dauber, J. H. (1988). Rapid detection of cytomegalovirus pneumonia by evaluation of bronchoalveolar cells. *Am. Rev. Respir. Dis.* **138**:697–702.

Paradis, I. L., Dummer, J. S., and Dauber, J. H. (1989). Risk factors for the development of chronic rejection of the human lung allograft (abstract). *Am. Rev. Respir. Dis.* **139**:A529.

Pastorelli, G., Roncarolo, M. G., Touraine, J. L., Peronne, G., Tovo, P. A., and de Vries, J. E. (1989). Peripheral blood lymphocytes of patients with common variable immunodeficiency (CVI) produce reduced levels of interleukin-4, interleukin-2 and interferon-gamma, but proliferate normally upon activation by mitogens. *Clin. Exp. Immunol.* **78**:334–340.

Paya, C. V., Hermans, P. E., Washington, J. A., Smith, T. F., Anhalt, J. P., Wiesner, R. H., and Krom, R. A. F. (1989). Incidence, distribution, and outcome of episodes of infection in 100 orthotopic liver transplantations. *Mayo Clin. Proc.* **64**:555–564.

Pearl, E. R., Vogler, L. B., Okos, A. J., Crist, W. M., Lawton, A. R., and Cooper, M. D. (1978). B lymphocyte precursors in human bone marrow: an analysis of normal individuals and patients with antibody-deficient states. *J. Immunol.* **120**:1169–1175.

Pecego, R., Hill, R., Appelbaum, F. R., Amos, D., Buckner, C. D., Fefer, A., and Thomas, E. D. (1986). Interstitial pneumonitis following autologous bone marrow transplantation. *Transplantation* **42**:515–517.

Penn, I. (1983). Lymphomas complicating organ transplantation. *Transplant. Proc.* **15**:2790–2797.

Penn, I. (1989). Risk of cancer in the transplant patient. In *Principles of Organ Transplantation*. Edited by M. Flye. Saunders, Philadelphia, pp. 634–643.

Pennock, J. L., Oyer, P. E., Reitz, B. A., Jamieson, S. W., Bieber, C. P., Wallwork, J., Stinson, E. B., and Shumway, N. E. (1982). Cardiac transplantation in perspective for the future. *J. Thorac. Cardiovasc. Surg.* **83**:168–177.

Perri, R. T., Hebbel, R. P., and Oken, M. M. (1981). Influence of treatment and response status on infection risk in multiple myeloma. *Am. J. Med.* **71**:935–940.

Perry, G. S. III, Spector, B. D., Schuman, L. M., Mandel, J. S., Anderson, E., McHugh, R. B., Hanson, M. R., Falhstrom, S. M., Krivit, W., and Kersey, J. H. (1980). The Wiskott-Aldrich syndrome in the United States and Canada (1892–1979). *J. Pediatr.* **97**:72–80.

Peterson, F. B., Bowden, R. A., Thornquist, M., Meyers, J. D., Buckner, C. D., Counts, G. W., Nelson, N., Newton, B. A., Sullivan, K. M., McIver, J., and Thomas, E. D. (1987). The effect of prophylactic intravenous immune globulin on the incidence of septicemia in marrow transplant recipients. *Bone Marrow Transplant.* **2**:141–148.

Peterson, P. K., and Anderson, R. C. (1986). Infection in renal transplant recipients. *Am. J. Med.* **81**:2–10.

Peterson, P. K., Balfour, H. H., Marker, S. C., Fryd, D. S., Howard, R. J., and Simmons, R. L. (1980). Cytomegalovirus disease in renal allograft recipients: a prospective study of the clinical features, risk factors, and impact on renal transplantation. *Medicine* **59**:283–300.

Peterson, P. K., Ferguson, R., Fryd, D. S., Balfour, H. H., Rynasiewicz, J., and Simmons, R. L. (1982). Infectious diseases in hospitalized renal transplant recipients: a prospective study of a complex and evolving problem. *Medicine* **61**:360–372.

Pirsch, J. D., Stratta, R. J., Sollinger, H. W., Havez, G. R., D'Alessandro, A. M., Kalayoglu, M., and Belzer, F. O. (1989). Treatment of severe Epstein-Barr after solid organ transplantation. *Am. J. Med.* **86**:241–244.

Pizzo, P. A., Robichaud, K. J., Wesley, R., and Commers, J. R. (1982a). Fever in the pediatric and young adult patient with cancer: a prospective study of 1001 episodes. *Medicine* **61**:153–165.

Pizzo, P. A., Robichaud, K. J., and Gill, F. A. (1982b). Empiric antibiotic and antifungal therapy for cancer patients with prolonged fever and granulocytopenia. *Am. J. Med.* **72**:101–110.

Pomeroy, C., Oken, M. M., Rydel, R. E., and Filice, G. A. (1991). Infection in the myelodysplastic syndromes. *Am. J. Med.* **90**:338–344.

Potter, D., Pass, H. I., Brower, S., Macher, A., Browne, M., Thaler, M., Cotton, D., Hathorn, J., Wesley, R., Longo, D., Pizzo, P., and Roth, J. A. (1985). Prospective randomized trial of open lung biopsy versus empirical antibiotic therapy for acute pneumonitis in nonneutropenic cancer patients. *Ann. Thorac. Surg.* **40**:422–427.

Prakash, U. B. S., Divertie, M. B., and Banks, P. M. (1979). Aggressive therapy in acute respiratory failure from leukemic pulmonary infiltrates. *Chest* **75**:345–350.

Price, T. H., and Dale, D. C. (1978). The selective neutropenias. *Clin. Hematol.* **7**:501–521.

Provisor, A. J., Iacuone, J. J., Chilcote, R. R., Neiburger, R. G., Crussi, F. G., and Baehner, R. L. (1975). Acquired agammaglobulinemia after a life-threatening illness with clinical and laboratory features of infectious mononucleosis in three related male children. *N. Engl. J. Med.* **293**:62–65.

Ramsey, P. G., Rubin, R. H., Tokoff-Rubin, N., Cosimi, A. B., Russell, P. S., and Greene, R. (1980). The renal transplant patient with fever and pulmonary infiltrates: etiology, clinical manifestations and management. *Medicine* **59**:206–222.

Ramsey, P. G., Fife, K. H., Hackman, R. C., and Meyers, J. D. (1982). Herpes simplex virus pneumonia. *Ann. Intern. Med.* **97**:813–820.

Rand, K. H., Pollard, R. B., and Merigan T. C. (1978). Increased pulmonary superinfections in cardiac-transplant patients undergoing primary cytomegalovirus infection. *N. Engl. J. Med.* **298**:951–953.

Randhawa, P. S., Yousem, S. A., Paradis, I. L., Dauber, J. A., Griffith, B. P., and Locker, J. (1989). The clinical spectrum, pathology, and clonal analysis of Epstein-Barr virus-associated lymphoproliferative disorders in heart-lung transplant recipients. *Am. J. Clin. Pathol.* **92**:177–185.

Rausch, P. G., and Herion, J. C. (1980). Pulmonary manifestations of Waldenstrom's macroglobulinemia. *Am. J. Hematol.* **9**:201–209.

Redd, S. C., Schuster, D. M., Quan, J., Plikaytis, B. D., Spika, J. S., and Cohen, M. L. (1988). Legionellosis in cardiac transplant recipients: results of a nationwide survey. *J. Infect. Dis.* **158**:651–656.

Reed, E. C., Dandliker, P. S., and Meyers, J. D. (1986). Treatment of cytomegalovirus pneumonia with 9-[2-hydroxy-1-(hydroxymethyl)ethoxymethyl] guanine and high dose corticosteroids. *Ann. Intern. Med.* **105**:214–215.

Reed, E. C., Bowden, R. A., Dandliker, P. S., Gleaves, C. A., and Meyers, J. D. (1987). Efficacy of cytomegalovirus immunoglobulin in marrow transplant recipients with cytomegalovirus pneumonia. *J. Infect. Dis.* **156**:641–645.

Reed, E. C., Bowden, R. A., Dandliker, P. S., Lilleby, K. E., and Meyers, J. D. (1988). Treatment of cytomegalovirus pneumonia with ganciclovir and intravenous cytomegalovirus immunoglobulin in patients with bone marrow transplants. *Ann. Intern. Med.* **109**:783–788.

Remington, J. S., Gaines, J. D., Griepp, R. B., and Shumway, N. E. (1972). Further experience with infection after cardiac transplantation. *Transplant. Proc.* **4**:699–705.

Remold-O'Donnell, E., Kenney, D. M., Parkman, R., Cainns, L., Savage, B., and Rosen, F. S. (1984). Characterization of a human lymphocyte surface sialoglycoprotein that is defective in Wiskott-Aldrich syndrome. *J. Exp. Med.* **159**:1705–1723.

Reusser, P., Fisher, L. D., Buckner, C. D., Thomas, E. D., and Meyers, J. D. (1990). Cytomegalovirus infection after autologous bone marrow transplantation: occurrence of cytomegalovirus disease and effect on engraftment. *Blood* **75**:1888–1894.

Reynolds, H. Y. (1987). Mechanisms of inflammation in the lungs. *Annu. Rev. Med.* **38**:295–323.

Reynolds, H. Y. (1988). Immunoglobulin G and its function in the human respiratory tract. *Mayo Clin. Proc.* **63**:161–174.

Rimm, I. J., and Rappeport, J. M. (1990). Bone marrow transplantation for the Wiskott-Aldrich syndrome. Long-term follow-up. *Transplantation* **50**:617–620.

Riska, H., Gronhagen-Riska, C., and Ahonen, J. (1987). Tuberculosis and renal allograft transplantation. *Transplant. Proc.* **19**:4096–4097.

Robbins, R. A., Linder, J., Stahl, M. G., Thompson, A. B., Haire, W., Kessinger, A., Armitage, J. O., Arneson, M., Woods, G., Vaughan, W. P., and Rennard, S. I. (1989). Diffuse alveolar hemorrhage in autologous bone marrow transplant recipients. *Am. J. Med.* **87**:511–518.

Roifman, C., Pandu Rao, C., Lederman, H., Lavi, S., Quinn, P., and Gelfand, E. W. (1986). Increased susceptibility to *Mycoplasma* infection in patients with hypogammaglobulinemia. *Am. J. Med.* **80**:590–594.

Roifman, C. M., and Gelfand, E. W. (1988). Replacement therapy with high dose intravenous gamma-globulin improves chronic sinopulmonary disease in patients with hypogammaglobulinemia. *Pediatr. Infect. Dis. J.* **7**(suppl 5):S92–S96.

Root, R. K., Rosenthal, A. S., and Balestra, D. J. (1972). Abnormal bactericidal, metabolic, and lysosomal functions of Chediak-Higashi syndrome leukocytes. *J. Clin. Invest.* **51**:649–665.

Rosen, F. S., Cooper, M. D., and Wedgwood, R. J. P. (1984a). The primary immunodeficiencies. I. *N. Engl. J. Med.* **311**:235–242.

Rosen, F. S., Cooper, M. D., and Wedgwood, R. J. P. (1984b). The primary immunodeficiencies. II. *N. Engl. J. Med.* **311**:300–309.

Rosenow, E. C., and Hurley, B. T. (1984). Disorders of the thymus: a review. *Arch. Intern. Med.* **144**:763–770.

Rosenow, E. C., Wilson, W. R., and Cockerill, F. R. (1985). Pulmonary disease in the immunocompromised host. Part 1. *Mayo Clin. Proc.* **60**:473–487.

Rosenthal, C. J., and Franklin, E. C. (1975). Depression of cellular-mediated immunity in systemic lupus erythematosus. *Arthritis Rheum.* **18**:207–217.

Rosner, S., Ginzler, E., Diamond, H., Weiner, M., Schlesinger, M., Fries, J. F., Wasner, C., Medsger, T. A., Ziegler, G., Klippel, J. H., Hadler, N. M., Albert, D. A., Hess, E. V., Spencer-Green, G., Grayzel, A., Worth, D., Hahn, B. H., and Barnett, E. V. (1982). A multicenter study of outcome in systemic lupus erythematosus. II. Causes of death. *Arthritis Rheum.* **25**:612–617.

Ross, S. C., and Densen, P. (1984). Complement deficiency states and infection: epidemiology, pathogenesis, and consequences of neisserial and other infections in a immune deficiency. *Medicine* **62**:243–273.

Royston, D., Minty, B. D., Higenbottam, T. W., Wallwork, J., and Jones, G. J. (1985). The effect of surgery with cardiopulmonary bypass on alveolar-capillary barrier function in human beings. *Ann. Thorac. Surg.* **40**:139–143.

Rubin, R. H. (1988). Infection in the renal and liver transplant recipient. In *Clinical Approach to Infection in the Compromised Host*. Edited by R. Rubin and L. Young. Plenum Press, New York, pp. 657–682.

Rubin, R. H. (1989). The indirect effects of cytomegalovirus infection on the outcome of organ transplantation. *JAMA* **261**:3607–3609.

Rubin, R. H., and Greene, R. (1981). Etiology and management of the compromised patient with fever and pulmonary infiltrates. In *Clinical Approach to Infection in the Compromised Host*. Edited by R. H. Rubin and L. S. Young. Plenum Press, New York, pp. 123–161.

Rubin, R. H., Cosimi, A. B., Tolkoff-Rubin, N. E., Russell, K. P. S., and Hirsch, M. S. (1977). Infectious disease syndromes attributable to cytomegalovirus and their significance among renal transplantation recipients. *Transplantation* **24**:458–464.

Rubin, R. H., Cosimi, A. B., Hirsch, M. S., Herrin, J. T., Russell, P. S., and Tolkoff-Rubin, N. E. (1981). Effects of anti-thymocyte globulin on cytomegalovirus infection in renal transplant recipients. *Transplantation* **31**:143–145.

Ruutu, P., Ruutu, R., Volin, L., Tukiainen, P., Ukkonen, P., and Hovi, T. (1990). Cytomegalovirus is frequently isolated in bronchoalveolar lavage fluid of bone marrow transplant recipients with pneumonia. *Ann. Intern. Med.* **112**:913–916.

Saiki, O., Ralph, P., Cunningham-Rundles, C., and Good, R. A. (1982). Three distinct stages of B cell defects in common varied immunodeficiency. *Proc. Natl. Acad. Sci. USA* **79**:6008–6012.

Saito, H., Anaissie, E. J., Morice, R. C., Dekmezian, R., and Bodey, G. P. (1988). Bronchoalveolar lavage in the diagnosis of pulmonary infiltrates in patients with acute leukemia. *Chest* **94**:745–749.

Saulsbury, F. T., Bernstein, M. T., and Winkelstein, J. A. (1979). *Pneumocystis carinii* pneumonia as the presenting infection in congenital hypogammaglobulinemia. *J. Pediatr.* **95**:559–561.

Savage, D. J., Lindenbaum, J., and Garrett, T. J. (1982). Biphasic pattern of bacterial infection in multiple nyeloma. *Ann. Intern. Med.* **96**:47–50.

Schedel, I. (1986). Application of immunoglobulin preparations in multiple myeloma. In *Clinical Use of Intravenous Immunoglobulins*. Edited by A. Morrell and U. E. Nydegger. Academic Press, London, pp. 123–132.

Schmidt, G. M., Horak, D. A., Niland, J. C., Duncan, S. R., Forman, S. J., and Zaia, J. A. (1991). A randomized, controlled trial of prophylactic ganciclovir for cytomegalovirus pulmonary infection in recipients of allogeneic bone marrow transplants. *N. Engl. J. Med.* **324**:1005–1011.

Schooley, R. T., Hirsch, M. S., Colvin, R. B., Cosimi, B., Tolkoff-Rubin, N. E., McCluskey, R. T., Burton, R. C., Russell, P. S., Herrin, J. T., Delmonico, F. L., Giorgi, J. V., Henle, W., and Rubin, R. H. (1983). Association of herpesvirus infection with T-lymphocyte subset alterations, glomerulopath, and opportunistic infections after renal transplantation. *N. Engl. J. Med.* **308**:307–313.

Schroter, G. P., Hoelscher, M., Putman, C. W., Portor, K. A., Hansbrough, J. F., and Starzl, T. E. (1976). Infections complicating orthotopic liver transplantation: a study emphasizing graft-related septicemia. *Arch. Surg.* **111**:1337–1347.

Schulman, L. L. (1987). Cytomegalovirus pneumonitis and lobar consolidation. *Chest* **91**:558–561.

Schulman, L. L., Smith, C. R., Drusin, R., Rose, E. A., Enson, Y., and Reemtsma, K. (1988). Utility of airway endoscopy in the diagnosis of respiratory complications of cardiac transplantation. *Chest* **93**:960–967.

Schwaber, J. F., Lazarus, H., and Rosen, F. S. (1981). IgM-restricted production of immunoglobulin by lymphoid cell lines from patients with immunodeficiency with hyper IgM (dysgammaglobulinemia). *Clin. Immunol. Immunopathol.* **19**:91–97.

Segal, R., Dayan, M., Epstein, N., Zecler, E., Peller, S., and Michalevitch, R. (1989). Common variable immunodeficiency: a family study and therapeutic trial with cimetidine. *J. Allergy Clin. Immunol.* **84**:753–761.

Siegal, F. P., Siegal, M. A., and Good, R. A. (1978). Role of helper, suppressor and B cell defects in the pathogenesis of the hypogammaglobulinemias. *N. Engl. J. Med.* **299**:172–178.

Shackelford, P. G., Polmar, S., Mayus, J., Johnson, W. L., Corry, J. M., and Nahm, M. H. (1986). Spectrum of IgG2 subclass deficiency in children with recurrent infections: prospective study. *J. Pediatr.* **108**:647–653.

Shackelford, P. G., Granoff, D. M., Madassery, J. V., Scott, M. G., and Nahm, M. H. (1990). Clinical and immunologic characteristics of healthy children with subnormal serum concentrations of IgG2. *Pediatr. Res.* **27**:16–21.

Shea, S. A., Horner, R., Banner, N. R., McKenzie, E., Heaton, R., Yacoub, M. H., and Guz, A. (1988). The effect of human heart-lung transplantation upon breathing at rest and during sleep. *Respir. Physiol.* **72**:131–150.

Shepp, D. H., Dandliker, P. S., de Miranda, P., Burnette, T. C., Cederberg, D. M., Kirk, E., and Meyers, J. D. (1985). Activity of 9-[2-hydroxy-1-(hydroxymethyl)ethoxymethyl] guanine in the treatment of cytomegalovirus pneumonia. *Ann. Intern. Med.* **103**:368–373.

Sherertz, R. J., Belani, A., Kramer, B. S., Elfenbein, G. J., Weiner, R. S., Sullivan, M. L., and Thomas, R. G. (1987). Impact of air filtration on nosocomial *Aspergillus* infections. *Am. J. Med.* **83**:709–718.

Shirazi, K. K., Amendola, A., Tisnado, J., Cho, S. R., Beachley, M. C., and Lower, R. R. (1983). Radiographic findings in the chest of patients following cardiac transplantation. *Cardiovasc. Intervent. Radiol.* **6**:1.

Sciurba, F. C., Owens, G. R., Sanders, M. H., Griffith, B. P., Hardesty, R. L., Paradis, I. L., and Costantino, J. P. (1988). Evidence of an altered pattern of breathing during exercise in recipients of heart-lung transplants. *N. Engl. J. Med.* **319**:1186–1192.

Shapiro, R. S., Chauvenet, A., McGuire, W., Pearson, A., Craft, A. W., McGlave, P., and Filipovich, A. (1988). Treatment of B-cell lymphoproliferative disorders with interferon alpha and intravenous gamma globulin. *N. Engl. J. Med.* **318**:1334.

Sickles, E. A., Greene, W. H., and Wiernik, P. H. (1975). Clinical presentation of infection in granulocytopenic patients. *Arch. Intern. Med.* **135**:715–719.

Siegal, F. P., Siegal, M. A., and Good, R. A. (1978). Role of helper, suppressor and B cell defects in the pathogenesis of the hypogammaglobulinemias. *N. Engl. J. Med.* **299**:172–178.

Simmons, R. L., Uranga, V. M., LaPlante, E. S., Buselmeier, T. J., Kjellstrand, C. M., and Najarian, J. S. (1972). Pulmonary complications in transplant recipients. *Arch. Surg.* **105**:260–268.

Simmons, R. L., Matas, A. J., Rattazzi, L. C., Balfour, H. H., Howard, R. J., and Najarian, J. S. (1977). Clinical characteristics of the lethal cytomegalovirus infection following renal transplantation. *Surgery* **82**:537–546.

Singer, C., Kaplan, M. H., and Armstrong, D. (1977). Bacteremia and fungemia complicating neoplastic disease. *Am. J. Med.* **62**:731–742.

Sloane, J. P., Depledge, M. H., Powles, R. L., Morgenstern, G. R., Trickey, B. S., and Dady, P. J. (1983). Histopathology of the lung after bone marrow transplantation. *J. Clin. Pathol.* **36**:546–554.

Smith, R. M., and Curnutte, J. T. (1991). Molecular basis of chronic granulomatous disease. *Blood* **77**:673–686.

Snydman, D. R., Werner, B. G., Heinze-Lacey, B., Berardi, V. P., Tilney, N. L., Kirkman, R. L., Milford, E. L., Cho, S. I., Bush, H. L., Leavey, R. H., Harmon, W. E., Zimmerman, C. E., Shapiro, M. E., Steinman, T., LoGerfo, F., Idelson, B., Schröter, G. P. J., Levin, M. J., McIver, J., Leszczynski, J., and Grady, G. F. (1987). Use of cytomegalovirus immune globulin to prevent cytomegalovirus disease in renal transplant recipients. *N. Engl. J. Med.* **317**:1049–1054.

Springmeyer, S. C., Silvestri, R. C., Sale, G. E., Peterson, D. L., Weems, C. E., Huseby, J. S., Hudson, L. D., and Thomas, E. D. (1982). The role of transbronchial biopsy for the diagnosis of diffuse pneumonias in immunocompromised marrow transplant recipients. *Am. Rev. Respir. Dis.* **126**:763–765.

Springmeyer, S. C., Flournoy, N., Sullivan, K. M., Storb, R., and Thomas, E. D. (1983). Pulmonary function changes in long-term survivors of allogeneic marrow transplantation. In *Recent Advances in Bone Marrow Transplantation*. Edited by R. P. Gale. Alan R. Liss, New York, pp. 343–353.

Springmeyer, S. C., Silvestri, R. C., Flournoy, N., Kosanke, C. W., Peterson, D. L., Huseby, J. S., Hudson, L. D., Storb, R., and Thomas, E. D. (1984). Pulmonary function of marrow transplant patients. I. Effects of marrow infusion, acute, graft-vs-host disease and interstitial pneumonitis. *Exp. Hematol.* **12**:805–810.

Staples, P. J., Gerding, D. N., and Decker, J. L. (1974). Incidence of infection in systemic lupus erythematosus. *Arthritis Rheum.* **77**:1–10.

Starnes, V., Theodore, J., Oyer, P., Billingham, M. E., Sibley, R. K., Berry, G., Shumway, N. E., and Stinson, E. B. (1989). Evaluation of heart-lung transplant recipients with prospective serial transmural biopsies and pulmonary function studies. *J. Thorac. Cardiovasc. Surg.* **98**:683–690.

Stewart, D. J., and Bodey, G. P. (1981). Infection in hairy cell leukemia (leukemic reticuloendotheliosis). *Cancer* **47**:801–805.

Stinson, E. B., Bieber, C. P., Griepp, R. B., Clark, D. A., Shumway, N. E., and Remington, J. S. (1971). Infectious complications after cardiac transplantation in man. *Ann. Intern. Med.* **74**:22–36.

St. John, R. C., Gadek, J. E., Tutschka, P. J., Kapoor, N., and Dorinsky, P. M. (1990). Analysis of airflow obstruction by bronchoalveolar lavage following bone marrow transplantation. *Chest* **98**:600–607.

Stover, D. E., Zaman, M. B., Hajdu, S. I., Lange, M., Gold, J., and Armstrong, D. (1984). Bronchoalveolar lavage in the diagnosis of diffuse pulmonary infiltrates in the immunosuppressed host. *Ann. Intern. Med.* **101**:1–7.

Sullivan, K. M. (1989). Intravenous immune globulin prophylaxis in recipients of a marrow transplant. *J. Allergy Clin. Immunol.* **84**:632–639.

Sullivan, K. M., Deeg, H. J., Sanders, J. E., Shulman, H. M., Witherspoon, R. P., Doney, K., Appelbaum, F. R., Schubert, M., Stewart, P., Springmeyer, S., McDonald, G. B., and Thomas, E. D. (1984). Late complications after marrow transplantation. *Semin. Hematol.* **21**:53–63.

Sullivan, K. M., Witherspoon, R. P., Storb, R., Weiden, P., Flournoy, N., Dahlberg, S., Deeg, H., Sanders, J. E., Doney, K. C., Appelbaum, F. R., McGuffin, R., McDonald, G. B., Meyers, J., Schubert M. M., Gauvreau, J., Shulman, H. M., Sale, G. E., Anasetti, C., Loughran, T. P., Strom, S., Nims, J., and Thomas E. D. (1988). Prednisone and azathioprine compared to prednisone and placebo for treatment of chronic graft-versus-host disease: prognostic influence of prolonged thrombocytopenia after allogeneic marrow transplantation. *Blood* **72**:546–554.

Sullivan, K. M., Kopecky, K. J., Jocom, J., Fisher, L., Buckner, C. D., Meyers, J. D., Counts, G. W., Bowden, R. A., Petersen, F. B., Witherspoon, R. P., Budinger, M. D., Schwartz, R. S., Appelbaum, F. R., Clint, R. A., Hansen, J. A., Sanders, J. E., Thomas, E. D., and Storb, R. (1990). Immunomodulator and antimicrobial efficacy of intravenous immunoglobulin in bone marrow transplantation. *N. Engl. J. Med.* **323**:705–712.

Swift, M., Sholman, L., Perry, M., and Chase, C. (1976). Malignant neoplasms in the families of patients with ataxia-telangiectasia. *Cancer Res.* **36**:209–215.

Swinnen, L. J., Costanzo-Nordin, M. R., Fisher, S. G., O'Sullivan, E. J., Johnson, M. R., Heroux, A. L., Dizikes, G. J., Pifarre, R., and Fisher, R. I. (1990). Increased incidence of lymphoproliferative disorder after immunosuppression with the monoclonal antibody OKT3 in cardiac transplant recipients. *N. Engl. J. Med.* **323**:1723–1728.

Takaoka, F., Brown, M. R., Paulsen, W., Ramsay, M. A. E., and Lintmalm, G. B. (1989). Adult respiratory distress syndrome following orthotopic liver transplantation. *Clin. Transplant.* **3**:294–299.

Tapper, D. P., Kagawa, F. T., Theodore, J., and Duncan, S. R. (1992). Detection of inspiratory resistive loads by heart-lung transplant recipients. *Am. Rev. Respir. Dis.* (in press).

Tazelaar, H., and Yousem, S. (1988). The pathology of combined heart-lung transplantation: an autopsy study. *Hum. Pathol.* **19**:1403–1416.

Taylor, A. M. R., Harnden, D. G., Arlett, C. V., Harcourt, S. A., Lehman, A. R., Stevens, S., and Bridges, B. A. (1975). Ataxia telangiectasia: a human mutation with abnormal radiation sensitivity. *Nature* **258**:427–429.

Tenholder, M. F., and Hooper, R. G. (1980). Pulmonary infiltrates in leukemia. *Chest* **78**:468–473.

Theodore, J., and Lewiston, N. (1990). Lung transplantation comes of age. *N. Engl. J. Med.* **322**:772–774.

Theodore, J., Jamieson, S. W., Burke, C. M., Reitx, B. A., Stinson, E. B., Kessel, A. V., Dawkins, K. D., Herran, J. J., Oyer, P. E., Hunt, S. A., Shumway, N. E., and Robin, E. D. (1984). Physiologic aspects of human heart-lung transplantation: pulmonary function status of the post-transplanted lung. *Chest* **86**:349–357.

Theodore, J., Starnes, V. A., and Lewiston, N. J. (1990). Obliterative bronchiolitis. *Clin. Chest Med.* **11**:309–321.

Thompson, A. B., Rickard, K. A., Shaw, B. W., Wood, R. P., Williams, L., Burnett, D. A., Robbins, R. A., Stahl, M. G., Sorrell, M. F., and Rennard, S. I. (1988). Pulmonary complications and disease severity in adult liver transplant recipients. *Transplant. Proc.* **20**:646S–649S.

Thompson, R. A., and Kummararatne, D. S. (1989). Hyper-IgE syndrome and H2-receptor blockade. *Lancet* **2**:630.

Thorpe, J. E., Baughman, R. P., Frame, P. T., Wesseler, T. A., and Staneck, J. L. (1987). Bronchoalveolar lavage for diagnosing acute bacterial pneumonia. *J. Infect. Dis.* **155**:855–861.

Tisi, G. M. (1979). Preoperative evaluation of pulmonary function: validity, indications, and benefits. *Am. Rev. Respir. Dis.* **119**:293–310.

Trento, A., Dummer, J. S., Hardesty, R. L., Bahnson, H. T., and Griffith, B. P. (1984). Mediastinitis following heart transplantation: incidence, treatment, and results. *Heart Transplant.* **3**:336–340.

Umetsu, D., Ambosino, D., Quinti, I., Siber, G. R., and Geha, R. S. (1985). Recurrent sinopulmonary infection and impaired antibody response to bacterial capsular polysaccharide antigen in children with selective IgG subclass deficiency. *N. Engl. J. Med.* **313**:1247–1251.

Vandenbroucke, J. P., Kaaks, R., Valkenburgh, H. A., Boersma, J. W., Cats, A., Gesten, J. J. M., Hartman, A. P., Huber-Bruning, O., Rasker, J. J., and Weber, J. (1987). Frequency of infections among rheumatoid arthritis patients, before, and after disease onset. *Arthritis Rheum.* **30**:810–813.

Van Scoy, R. E., Hill, H. R., Ritts, R. E., and Quie, P. G. (1975). Familial neutrophil chemotaxis defect, recurrent bacterial infections, mucocutaneous condidiasis and hyperimmunoglobulin E. *Ann. Intern. Med.* **82**:766–771.

Vernant, J. P., Brun, B., Mannoni, P., and Dreyfus, B. (1979). Respiratory distress of hyperleukocytic granulocytic leukemias. *Cancer* **44**:264–268.

Wade, J. C., Schimpff, S. C., Newman, K. A., and Wiernik, P. H. (1982). *Staphylococcus epidermidis*: an increasing cause of infection in patients with granulocytopenia. *Ann. Intern. Med.* **97**:503–508.

Waldmann, T. A., Broder, S., Blaese, R. M., Durm, M., Blackman, M., and Strober, W. (1974). Role of suppressor T cells in pathogenesis of common variable hypogammaglobulinemia. *Lancet* **2**:609–613.

Waldmann, T. A., Broder, S., Goldman, C. K., Frost, K., Korsmeyer, S. J., and Medici, M. A. (1983). Disorders of B cells and helper T cells in the pathogenesis of the immunoglobulin deficiency of patients with ataxia-telangiectasia. *J. Clin. Invest.* **71**:282–295.

Walsh, T. J., and Pizzo, P. A. (1988). Nosocomial fungal infections: a classification for hospital-acquired fungal infections and mycoses arising from endogenous flora or reactivation. *Annu. Rev. Microbiol.* **42**:517–545.

Walsh, T. J., Rubin, M., and Pizzo, P. A. (1991). Respiratory diseases in patients with malignant neoplasms. In *Respiratory Disease in the Immunosuppressed Host*. Edited by J. Shelhamer, P. A. Pizzo, J. E. Parrillo, and H. Masur. Lippincott, Philadelphia, pp. 640–663.

Wardman, A. G., and Cooke, N. J. (1984). Pulmonary infiltrates in adult acute leukaemia: empirical treatment or lung biopsy? *Thorax* **39**:647–650.

Watson, F. S., O'Connell, J. B., Amber, I. J., Renlund, D. G., Classen, D., Johnston, J. M., Smith, C. B., Bristow, M. R., and Utah Cardiac Transplant Program (1988). Treatment of cytomegalovirus pneumonia in heart transplant recipients with 9(1,3-dihydroxy-2-proproxymethyl)-guanine (DHPG). *J. Heart Transplant.* **7**:102–105.

Weening, R., Corbell, L., de Boer, M., Lutter, R., Van Zwieten, R., Hamers, M. N., and Roos, D. (1985). Cytochrome b deficiency in an autosomal form of chronic granulomatous disease of childhood. *J. Clin. Invest.* **75**:915–920.

Weiner, R. S., Bortin, M. M., Gale, R. P., Gluckman, E., Kay, H. E. M., Hans-Jochem, K., Hartz, A. J., and Rimm, A. A. (1986). Interstitial pneumonitis after bone marrow transplantation. *Ann. Intern. Med.* **104**:168–175.

Weiner, R. S., Horowitz, M. M., Gale, R. P., Dicke, K. A., VanBekkum, D. W., Masaoka, T., Ramsay, N. K. C., Rimm, A. A., Rozman, C., and Bortin, M. M. (1989). Risk factors for interstitial pneumonia following bone marrow transplantation for severe aplastic anaemia. *Br. J. Haematol.* **71**:535–543.

Welte, K., and Mertelsmann, R. (1985). Human interleukin 2: biochemistry, physiology, and possible pathogenetic role in immunodeficiency syndromes. *Cancer Invest.* **3**:35–49.

Wheat, L. J., Smith, E. J., Sathapatayavongs, B., Batteiger, B., Filo, R. S., Leapman, S. B., and French, M. V. (1983). Histoplasmosis in renal allograft recipients: two large urban outbreaks. *Arch. Intern. Med.* **143**:703–707.

Wheeler, E. W., Rubis, L. J., Jones, C. W., and Harrah, J. D. (1985). Etiology and prevention of topical cardiac hypothermia-induced phrenic nerve injury and left lower lobe atelectasis during cardiac surgery. *Chest* **88**:680–683.

White, W. B., and Ballow, M. (1985). Modulation of suppressor-cell activity by cimetidine in patients with common variable hypogammaglobulinemia. *N. Engl. J. Med.* **312**:198–202.

Wingard, J. R., Mellits, E. D., Sostrin, M. B., Chen, D. Y., Burns, W. H., Santos, G. W., Vriesendorp, H. M., Beschorner, W. E., and Saral, R. (1988). Interstitial pneumonitis after allogeneic bone marrow transplantation. *Medicine* **67**:175–186.

Winston, D. J., Gale, R. P., Meyer, D. V., and Young, L. S. (1979). Infectious complications of human bone marrow transplantation. *Medicine* **58**:1–31.

Winston, D. J., Ho, W. G., Lin, C-H., Barrtoni, K., Budinger, M. D., Gale, R. P., and Champlin, R. E. (1987). Intravenous immune globulin for prevention of cytomegalovirus infection and interstitial pneumonia after bone marrow transplantation. *Ann. Intern. Med.* **106**:12–18.

Wolk, P. J., and Apicell, M. A. (1978). The effect of renal function on the febrile response to bacteremia. *Arch. Intern. Med.* **138**:1085–1085.

Wollner, A., Mohle-Boetanti, J., Lambert, R. E., Perruquet, J. L., Raffin, T. A., and McGuire, J. L. (1991). *Pneumocystis carinii* pneumonia complicating low dose methotrexate for rheumatoid arthritis. *Thorax* **46**:205–207.

Wong, T., Toupance, O., and Chanard, J. (1991). Acyclovir to prevent cytomegagalovirus infection after renal transplantation. *Ann. Intern. Med.* **115**:68.

Wright, D. G., Fauci, A. S., Dale, D. C., and Wolff, S. M. (1978). Correction of human cyclic neuropenia with prednisolone. *N. Engl. J. Med.* **298**:295–300.

Wright, D. G., Robichaud, K. J., Pisso, P. A., and Deisseroth, A. B. (1981). Lethal pulmonary reactions associated with the combined use of amphotericin B and leukocyte transfusion. *N. Engl. J. Med.* **304**:1185–1189.

Wright, P. F., Hatch, M. H., Kasselbert, A. J., Lowry, S. P., Wadlington, W. B., and Karzon, D. T. (1977). Vaccine-associated poliomyelitis in a child with sex-linked agammaglobulinemia. *J. Pediatr.* **91**:408–412.

Yam, L. T., Caudhry, A. A., and Janckila, A. J. (1977). Impaired marrow granulocyte reserve and leukocyte mobilization in leukemic reticuloendotheliosis. *Ann. Intern. Med.* **87**:444.

Young, R. C., Bennett, J. E., Vogel, C. L., Carbone, P. P., and De Vita, V. T. (1970). Aspergillosis: the spectrum of the disease in 98 patients. *Medicine* **49**:147–173.

Yousem, S., Burke, C., and Billingham, M. (1985). Pathologic pulmonary alterations in long-term human heart-lung transplantation. *Hum. Pathol.* **16**:911–923.

Yu, V. L., Mader, R. R., and Poorsatter, A. (1986). Significance of isolation of *Aspergillus* from the respiratory tract in diagnosis of invasive pulmonary aspergillosis: results from a three-year prospective study. *Am. J. Med.* **81**:249–254.

Zenati, M., Dowling, R. D., Dummer, J. S., Paradis, I. L., Arena, V. C., Armitage, J. M., Kormos, R. L., Hardesty, R. L., and Griffith, B. P. (1990). Influence of the donor lung on the development of early infections in lung transplant recipients. *J. Heart Transplant.* **9**:502–509.

3

Cardiac Diseases

V. COURTNEY BROADDUS

University of California, San Francisco
and San Francisco General Hospital
San Francisco, California

I. Introduction

The lungs are inextricably linked to the heart by the pulmonary circulation, through which the entire cardiac output normally flows. In addition, the lungs are nourished by the heart through the smaller bronchial circulation. The function of the heart as a pump is therefore critical for the proper functioning of the lungs. In this chapter, I will discuss the ways in which abnormalities of the heart in its major role as a pump leads to lung disease, which includes abnormalities of the blood vessels, airways, interstitium, alveoli, and adjacent pleura.

In general, the heart may malfunction to cause either an increase or a decrease in pressure in the pulmonary circulation. These changes may be either acute or chronic; each of them will be discussed in turn.

II. Circulations Linking Heart and Lung

A. Pulmonary Circulation

The pulmonary circulation is distinguished from the systemic circulation by its low resistance to blood flow (Table 1). As a result, despite the identical flow of

Table 1 Comparison of Normal Pulmonary and Systemic Hemodynamic and Vascular Variables

	Circulation	
	Pulmonary	Systemic
Blood flow	6.3 L/min	6.3 L/min
Arterial pressure	20/10 mmHg	120/70 mmHg
Mean	14 mmHg	88 mmHg
Venous pressure, mean	5 mmHg	3 mmHg
Vascular resistance	1.4 units[a]	13.5 units[a]
	114 dyn s/cm^5 [b]	1080 dyn s/cm^5 [b]
Media to external diameter		
Artery	3–8%	15–25%
Vein	2–5%	3–6%

Source: Adapted from (Murray, 1986) and (Edwards, 1988).
[a]Units = mmHg/L/min.
[b]To convert units to dyn s/cm^5, multiply by 80.

blood through both circulations, the pulmonary artery pressure is approximately only 20% of the systemic. There is some basal tone to the pulmonary circulation and some regional regulation, mainly by hypoxic pulmonary vasoconstriction, but normal pulmonary vascular tone is clearly less than systemic vascular tone. The distensibility of the circulation is evident by the further decrease in pulmonary vascular resistance with exercise, which allows an increase in cardiac output of 3–4 times with only a small increase in pulmonary artery pressure (Murray, 1986). Pulmonary vascular resistance decreases with increases in flow for two main reasons: the thin-walled pulmonary vessels distend with slight increases in transmural pressure which increases vessel radius, and previously unperfused vessels are passively recruited; both factors contribute to an increase in overall cross-sectional area. Presumably, low resistance and distensibility of the pulmonary circulation permit the lungs to accommodate the entire cardiac output at a low cost to the right ventricle in work.

In the fetus, however, the resistance of the pulmonary circulation exceeds that of the systemic and leads to shunting of blood from the systemic venous to the systemic arterial circulations through the ductus arteriosus and foramen ovale. The high resistance of the pulmonary circulation is in part due to the greater muscular thickness of fetal pulmonary arteries than adult arteries of the same external diameter (Reid, 1979), the collapsed state of the lungs, and the active vasoconstriction induced by the hypoxic intrauterine environment. During fetal life, pulmonary resistance gradually decreases with the growth of new vessels. With birth and air breathing, pulmonary resistance falls further owing to the expansion of the lungs and their vessels, the loss of vasoconstrictive tone due to removal of the hypoxic stimulus to vasoconstriction (Cassin et al., 1964), and perhaps release of prostacyclin (Leffler et al., 1984). For the next 3 days, resistance continues to fall owing to the involution of arterial muscle (Reid, 1979). For the next 4 months, normal remodeling consists of continued thinning of the arterial muscular wall with development of a muscular layer in more distal arteries, and the branching of the arterial tree along with the proliferation of alveoli and alveolar ducts (Reid, 1979; Rabinovitch and Reid, 1980) (Fig. 1). At 4 months of age, the pulmonary circulation has already reached adult values of proportionate muscular thickness. The plasticity of the pulmonary circulation is a feature that also characterizes its response to disease states. Abnormal pulmonary flows and pressures that result from cardiac disease can interrupt normal remodeling.

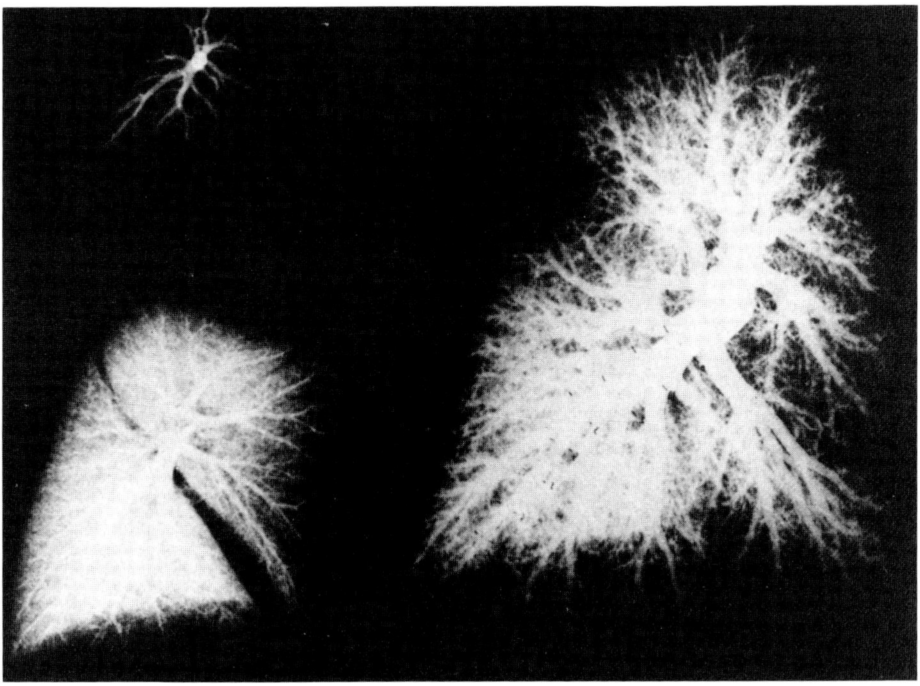

Figure 1 Arteriograms of human lungs at three ages: top left, newborn; bottom left, 18 months; right, adult. After birth, there is a multiplication of intralobular arteries that can be seen as a background "haze" by 18 months. (From Reid, 1979.)

At birth, the balance of resistances that caused blood to bypass the lungs during fetal development reverses. Pulmonary resistance falls with the first breath, and systemic resistance rises with the removal of the placental circulation. The entire cardiac output is then directed into the lungs. As pressure in the right atrium decreases and that in the left atrium increases, there is a functional closure of the foramen ovale that becomes fixed in several days. With an increase in arterial P_{O_2}, the hypoxic stimulus that maintained the ductus patent is removed thereby allowing the ductus to constrict. Hypoxia mediates its dilating effect on the ductus arteriosus in part via the release of prostaglandins that relax the smooth muscle of the ductus. In fact, prostaglandin E_2 has been used to reopen the ductus in newborns with congenital heart disease who are dependent on ductal flow to supply either the lungs (in right heart outflow obstruction) or the systemic circulation (in left heart outflow obstruction) (Olley et al., 1976). The fetal circulation, characterized by the shunting of blood away from the lungs, may persist after birth if the pulmonary vascular resistance does not decrease. Such a persistent fetal circulation can result from a variety of causes, including cardiac (pulmonary venous hypertension or left-to-right shunt) and noncardiac causes (hypoxia, lung disease, or unexplained vasoconstriction) (Gersony, 1984).

In the adult, the pulmonary arterial circulation consists of three types of arteries, the elastic (greater than 1000 μm in diameter), the muscular arteries (100–1000 μm in diameter), and the arterioles ($<$ 100μm) (Murray, 1986). Elastic arteries extend from the heart to the parenchyma of the lungs at the level of the lobule (the cluster of terminal respiratory units separated from adjacent ones by connective tissue septa), muscular arteries course through the lobules alongside the bronchioles to the level of the terminal bronchioles, and the arterioles extend from the terminal bronchioles to supply the alveolar capillary bed. It is only the muscular arteries that consistently contain a media of smooth muscle, although even here the muscle thickness should normally constitute less than 5% of the external diameter of the vessel. These muscular arteries appear to lie in an advantageous position where they can respond to the gas tensions in the alveoli supplied by the adjacent bronchiole and regulate blood flow to the respiratory lobule ventilated by that bronchiole (Murray, 1986). The capillaries lie in close proximity to the alveolar ducts and alveoli; it is here that gas exchange and liquid filtration takes place. Veins are more numerous and thin walled than arteries, which makes the venous system a low-resistance pathway for blood flow from the lungs. Nevertheless, veins do contain a muscular layer and can respond to pressure changes with medial hypertrophy as do the arteries.

The liquid and protein that continuously filter into the lungs owing to the slight imbalance of osmotic and hydrostatic pressures in the microcirculation is removed by the pulmonary lymphatics. Lymphatics lie in connective tissue of the lungs and extend as far as the terminal and respiratory bronchioles (Lauweryns, 1970). Liquid reaches the openings of lymphatic capillaries by passive flow along a pressure gradient and is returned to the systemic circulation by the actively pumping lymphatics. By cannulating the lymph node that drains much of the sheep lungs, Staub (1971) was able to show that liquid and protein are continuously filtered across the lungs' microcirculation, even during steady-state conditions. This model has provided extensive understanding of the effects on filtration of hemodynamic events in the microcirculation of the lungs.

B. Bronchial Circulation

The bronchial circulation is very different from the pulmonary (Deffebach et al., 1987). The bronchial circulation is small, carrying only 1% of the cardiac output. As part of the systemic circulation, it carries oxygenated blood into the lungs and responds to stimuli as do other systemic arteries; for example, bronchial arteries dilate in response to hypoxia (Warren and Powell, 1986) instead of constricting as do the pulmonary arteries. Despite these differences, the circulations are richly interconnected in a complex way and are able to assume some functions of the other.

The two unique features of the bronchial circulation are its connections with the pulmonary circulation and its variable venous drainage. After their origin from the aorta and intercostal arteries, the bronchial arteries reach the hila and course along the bronchi, dividing with the bronchial divisions as far as the terminal bronchioles. From the bronchial arteries, there are described connections to the pulmonary arterioles, through anastomotic vessels that may contain muscle and regulate anastomotic flow, and to the pulmonary veins. The interconnections provide for flexibility of flow from pulmonary to bronchial vessels, and vice versa. From the bronchial arteries, blood flows to a vascular plexus both outside the bronchus and in the submucosa and then drains to veins (Fig. 2). Of great interest, the venous drainage takes one of two routes, either to the right heart or to the left. The extrapulmonary bronchial vessels supplying large airways drain to the right atrium through the azygous and hemiazygous veins; the intrapulmonary vessels drain to the pulmonary veins and into the left atrium (Deffebach et al., 1987). The continuity of the venous plexus suggests that bronchial venous drainage can be redirected depending on downstream pressures or resistances. A flexible drainage route could be an advantage with changing hemodynamic conditions. In addition, this route provides another possible connection between the pulmonary and bronchial circulation, because pulmonary venous blood can shunt through these bronchial venous plexuses to the right atrium (Auld et al., 1960; Ohmichi et al., 1988).

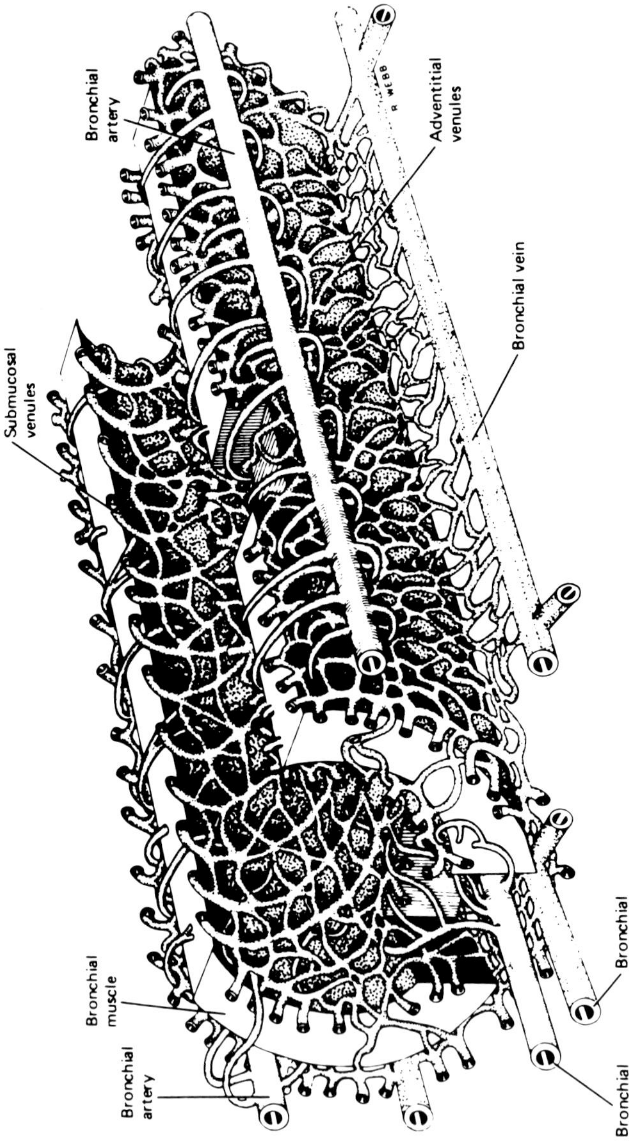

Figure 2 Diagram of the bronchial arteries and veins and the interconnections between them. (From Deffebach et al., 1987.)

III. Increased Pulmonary Venous Pressure

A. Acute

Physiological Changes

Formation of Edema

Normally, pulmonary venous pressure is low and falls only slightly with flow of blood from the lungs into the left ventricle. In many conditions (Table 2), however, pulmonary venous pressure can be acutely increased. Increases in left ventricular end-diastolic or left atrial pressure are transmitted back through the pulmonary veins into the microcirculation and the pulmonary arteries. Following mild increases in pressure, there is an increase in distension of the capillaries, an increased number of capillaries through recruitment, and an increase in blood flow to the uppermost regions of the lungs. More of the lungs function in zone III conditions, in which pulmonary venous pressure exceeds alveolar pressure, and blood flow becomes more homogeneously distributed within the lungs than before. As pressure increases, so does filtration of fluid; lymph flow increases to drain the excess filtrate from the lungs (Erdmann et al., 1975). Microvascular filtrate enters the interstitial spaces of the lungs (Staub et al., 1967), including the loose interstitial tissue around bronchovascular bundles (Fig. 3); in the bronchovascular bundles, liquid can sometimes be seen in chest radiographs

Table 2 Causes of Acutely Increased Pulmonary Venous Pressure

Left atrium
Mitral regurgitation
Endocarditis
Disruption of papillary muscle or chordae tendineae
Degeneration (prolapse)
Mitral stenosis or obstruction
Early presentation
Chronic stenosis with acute increase in flow
Atrial myxoma
Left ventricle
Acute myocardial ischemia
Myocarditis
Tachyarrhythmia
Pericardial tamponade
Aorta
Aortic regurgitation

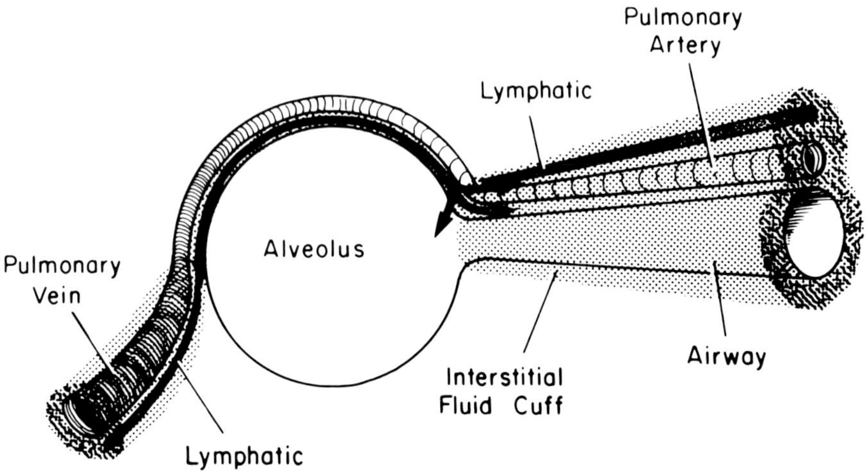

Figure 3 Anatomy of interstitial edema. As microvascular filtration increases above normal, some of the filtrate begins to collect in loose binding connective tissue and be recognized on frozen sections as "cuffs." Once in these interstitial spaces, edema liquid is not cleared by the lung lymphatics but drains to the pleural space and perhaps to the mediastinum. (From Staub, 1983, with permission.)

as an early feature of pulmonary edema. It is estimated that the lungs can accommodate a 100% increase in their water content in the interstitial spaces. When liquid increases beyond this capacity in the lungs, the excess microvascular filtrate suddenly enters the alveolar airspaces; this implies a dramatic decrease in the normally tight barrier of the alveolar membrane (Staub, 1983). Once alveoli are flooded, they fill completely with liquid, which creates a nonaerated portion of the lungs.

Clearance of Edema

Interstitial. Once in the peribronchovascular and subpleural interstitial spaces, edema does not clear the lungs via the lung lymphatics (Gee and Havill, 1980; Mackersie et al., 1987) and must leave via other routes, which have recently been explored. One important route of clearance is into the pleural space, presumably along interlobular septa that become distended with liquid (Fig. 4) (Broaddus et al., 1990). In a study of hydrostatic edema in sheep, 23% of measured edema entered the pleural space, while 34% cleared by the lymphatics with the rest remaining in the lungs (Broaddus et al., 1990). Because the pleural liquid protein concentration was the same as that of the interstitial liquid measured in peribronchial cuffs and lymph, the results suggest that transudative pleural effusions consist mostly of the edema liquid that formed in and then left

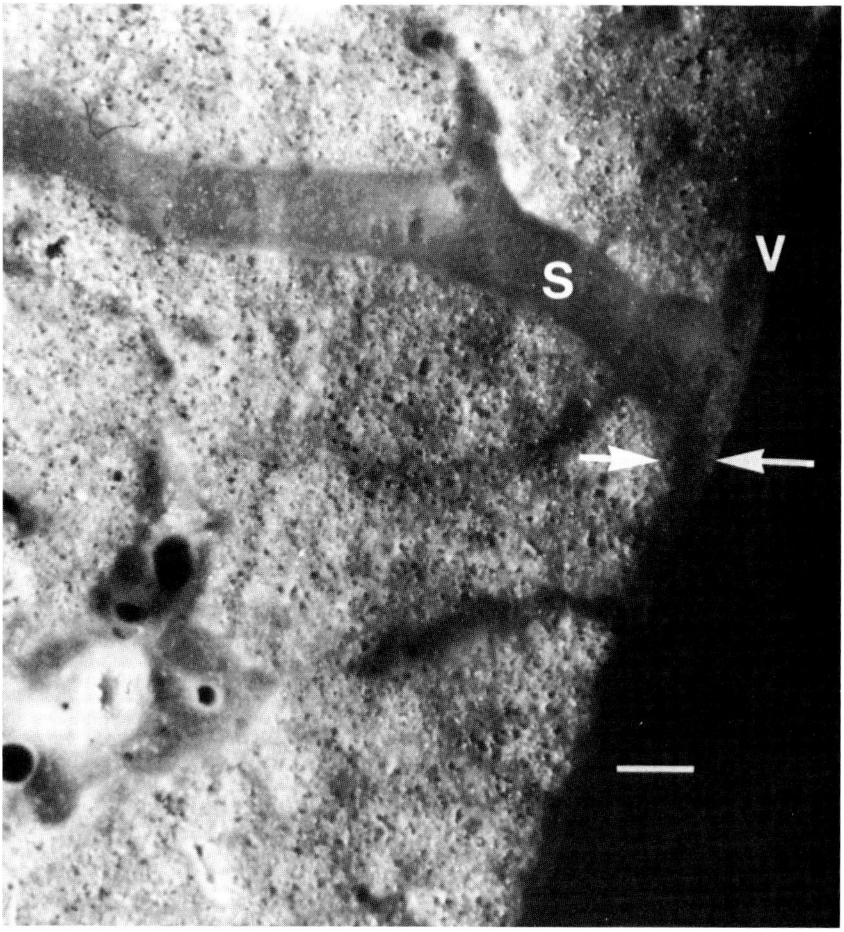

Figure 4 Section of a frozen sheep lung after volume loading to induce interstitial edema. Edema liquid has collected in interlobular septa (S) and the subpleural interstitium (between arrows), from where it can leak across the visceral pleura (V) into the pleural space. (From Broaddus et al., 1990, with permission.)

the lungs. Accordingly, the pleural space appears to serve as an important safety factor to reduce the likelihood of alveolar edema with its attendant abnormalities of gas exchange and pulmonary mechanics. Liquid in the pleural space is absorbed into a different lymphatic system, the parietal pleural lymphatics (Broaddus et al., 1988), and excess liquid in the pleural space has little effect on pulmonary function (Estenne et al., 1983). Additional interstitial liquid may clear the lungs by moving along the peribronchial interstitial tissue into the mediastinum, where it enters lymphatics and is removed (Jerome et al., 1989).

Alveolar. Alveolar liquid is most likely cleared by active transport across the alveolar epithelium. In awake sheep, Matthay and co-workers (1982) described a progressive increase in protein concentration of a protein solution instilled into one lung, which indicates a more rapid clearance of liquid than of protein despite progressively increasing osmotic forces opposing liquid clearance; this phenomenon provides strong evidence for an active, not passive, process. More recently, increase in protein concentration of edema liquid has been described in humans with pulmonary edema (Matthay and Wiener-Kronish, 1990). In those patients whose pulmonary edema specimens could be studied serially, an increase in protein concentration correlated with improvement in oxygenation and radiographic evidence of edema clearance.

Abnormalities of Lung Function

During vascular congestion and recruitment, there are no consistent abnormalities of pulmonary function. Even with interstitial edema, pulmonary function changes little. In some human studies, an increase in Pao_2, a decrease in A-ao_2 difference, and a decrease in dead space ventilation has been described and attributed to improved ventilation-perfusion matching (Noble et al., 1975; Muir et al., 1975). In studies in which experimental animals and humans are acutely volume-loaded, the most consistent finding is a mild increase in resistance of the small airways (Muir et al., 1975). This change may only be detected with sensitive tests for small-airway function, such as closing volume or dynamic compliance in humans (Noble et al., 1975), or by partitioning the resistance of airways distal to a wedged catheter in animals (Hogg et al., 1972). This may explain the absence of detectable abnormalities in interstitial edema when tests sensitive to resistance in larger airways, such as FEV_1 or total pulmonary resistance, are used (Noble et al., 1975). By morphological studies, small (< 2 mm) airways have not been shown to have a decrease in lumen with interstitial edema, but larger ones (6–9 mm) have (Lai-Fook et al., 1984). The change in resistance may be related either to formation of large cuffs of interstitial liquid around the airways greater than 2 mm, to dilation of bronchial vessels with encroachment on the airway lumen (Csete et al., 1990), and/or to airway edema. In patients with established interstitial edema, such as those with congestive heart failure or with a recent myocardial infarction, decreases in expiratory air flows are variably found, whether measured by FEV_1 or by more sensitive measures. In some studies, these flow rates have increased after diuretic therapy (Light and George, 1983; Hales and Kazemi, 1974).

Cardiac asthma is a term used to describe the sudden shortness of breath associated with wheezing experienced by some patients with congestive heart disease. Historically, the use of the term "asthma" indicated wheezing and did not imply airway hyperresponsiveness, which is the meaning of asthma today. Recently, however, investigators have explored the possibility that the airways of patients with heart failure are truly hyperresponsive. Proposed mechanisms include a reflex increase in vagal tone of airways (Kikuchi et al., 1984; Jones et al., 1978) or a susceptibility to bronchoconstrictors by an increased permeability of the edematous bronchial wall (Rolla et al., 1986). Other investigators have not found an important role for vagal reflexes in edema (Lloyd, 1980). Hyperresponsiveness, however, can also be caused by mechanical effects, for instance a decrease of the airway lumen by wall edema or vascular engorgement. In a mathematical model of airway geometry and flow, Moreno and co-workers (1986) calculated that a 20% increase in wall thickness (the percentage of the cross-sectional area of the airway occupied by the wall) would cause a baseline increase in airway resistance (Raw) to only 1.3 times normal, but with a maximal response to agonist airway resistance would increase to 180 times normal. Thus, no increase in muscle response or sensitivity is required to explain an exponential increase in resistance, merely the greater degree of airway narrowing with the same degree of bronchial smooth muscle constriction. A thickened airway wall, therefore, can cause a small increase in baseline airway resistance but a large increase in resistance when challenged with agonists. This mechanical cause of airway narrowing may explain the observed abnormal methacholine "hyperresponsiveness" observed in patients with heart failure (Cabanes et al., 1989; Pison et al., 1989) or after rapid saline infusion (Rolla et al., 1986). In one study of patients in heart failure (Cabanes et al., 1989), the administration of various vasoconstrictive aerosols prevented hyperresponsiveness, which led the authors to conclude that bronchial arterial congestion contributed most to hyperresponsiveness. However, abnormal methacholine tests have not been found universally in patients with congestive failure (Eichacker et al., 1988; Seibert et al., 1989). More studies, including those with morphometric data to document whether hyperresponsiveness correlates with anatomical changes of the airways, are necessary to resolve this confusing area.

Besides changes in airway mechanics, there may be small changes in lung volume (Light and George, 1983; Muir et al., 1975), but this has not been consistently found (Hales and Kazemi, 1974). The explanation of a decrease appears to be a decrease in compliance, although this has also not been invariably found.

Pleural effusions that form in association with interstitial edema have similar minimal effects on pulmonary function. A pleural effusion decreases lung volume by less than one-half the volume of the effusion (Estenne et al., 1983; Krell and Rodarte, 1985). The chest wall expands outward, accommodating the rest of the volume, and it is this expansion and the mechanical disadvantage of the respiratory muscles that may explain the dyspnea associated with pleural effusions (Estenne et al., 1983). Gas exchange abnormalities have not been described, although transient hypoxemia has been reported following thoracentesis, perhaps because perfusion is restored to areas of the lung that are still atelectatic (Brandstetter and Cohen, 1979).

In contrast to interstitial edema and pleural effusion, alveolar edema induces profound decrements in lung function. The flooding of alveoli is indicated by a decrease in Pa_{O_2} as poorly oxygenated venous blood shunts past the flooded alveoli. With the filling of alveoli, lung volume and compliance fall. Airway resistance increases, in one study by 40% (Noble et al., 1975), owing to a decrease in lung volume and to the presence of edema liquid within the airway lumen.

Clinical presentation

With mild increases in pulmonary venous pressure and the resultant pulmonary vascular recruitment, the patient is asymptomatic. Even during interstitial edema, few symptoms may be perceived in a patient with otherwise normal lungs. The signs are also subtle, and lung sounds are normal, although wheezing may be heard, especially at end-expiratory low lung volumes. The safety factors of the lungs that prevent alveolar flooding are remarkably effective in protecting lung function. It is mainly with alveolar edema that the patient will experience dyspnea. The patient may cough up foamy edema liquid, and physical examination at this time often demonstrates tachypnea, pulmonary rales, and cyanosis.

The chest radiograph during the initial vascular engorgement may show few abnormalities except increased vascular markings at the apex and, of course, the changes in heart size characteristic of the underlying disease. With interstitial edema, interstitial markings become more visible in the lungs with peribronchial cuffing, a loss of distinct vascular borders, and Kerley B lines, which are horizontal lines at the periphery of the lungs that represent sequestered liquid in the interlobular septa (Fraser and Paré, 1977). Pleural effusions may be present, although their appearance may lag several hours after the acute interstitial edema develops (Broaddus et al., 1990). Alveolar edema causes fluffy opacities, presumably due to the filling of terminal respiratory units by edema liquid.

Diagnosis

To recognize mild acute elevations of pulmonary venous pressure, the chest radiograph is more sensitive than the history or physical examination. The cause of the cardiac disease may be apparent from the radiograph as well, whether there is an enlarged silhouette of cardiac failure or pericardial effusion or a smaller heart from acute valve disruption. If lung function was normal initially, the PaO_2 will remain nearly normal unless alveolar edema develops.

The cause of the cardiac disease may be suggested by the history, physical examination, or chest radiograph. Often, the electrocardiogram (myocardial ischemia) or echocardiogram (pericardial disease, mitral or aortic disease) is diagnostic. Confirmation and monitoring may be accomplished by pulmonary artery catheterization with wedged measurement of the pulmonary venous pressure. Once alveolar edema occurs, measurement of the edema protein concentration in comparison with that in a simultaneous serum specimen, if obtained early (in the first hour) before significant liquid has been absorbed, can reliably distinguish high-pressure edema from acute lung injury edema (Fein et al., 1984), and repeated measurements can confirm resolution of edema (Matthay and Wiener-Kronish, 1990).

Therapy

Specific therapy is directed to the underlying cardiac disease. General therapy is directed to decreasing the pulmonary venous pressure, by diuretic or vasodilator therapy. Oxygen can be helpful, but when alveolar edema is present, the large shunt limits the benefit from oxygen. In patients with severe hypoxemia from alveolar edema, intubation and positive end-expiratory pressure are indicated; the end-expiratory pressure increases end-expiratory lung volume thereby redistributing liquid, reopening alveoli, and reducing shunt (Malo et al., 1984).

B. Chronic

With a long-standing increase in pulmonary venous pressure, the lung adapts in characteristic ways. Causes of increased pulmonary venous pressure are several (Table 3), but the most well-studied condition is mitral stenosis. Mitral stenosis serves as a model for diseases causing chronically elevated pulmonary venous pressures, because it progresses gradually over decades, which allows the lungs to adapt, and it can be treated with or without surgery (percutaneous balloon commissurotomy), which permits recognition of abnormalities due to the disease.

Physiology

Introduction

The mitral valve, normally 4–6 cm^2 in area, offers almost no resistance to blood flow and there is no pressure gradient across it. In response to the inflammation and then scarring induced by rheumatic fever, the mitral valve orifice narrows and a pressure gradient becomes necessary to cause blood to flow across the valve. When 1 cm^2 in area, the mitral valve requires a gradient of approximately 25 mmHg to maintain a normal cardiac output (Arnott and Withering, 1964).

Table 3 Causes of Chronically Increased Pulmonary Venous Pressure

Pulmonary veins
Mediastinitis
Mediastinal neoplasms
Mediastinal fibrosis
Congenital pulmonary vein stenosis
Veno-occlusive disease
Left atrium
Atrial myxoma
Ball-valve thrombus
Cor triatriatum
Mitral valve
Mitral stenosis
Mitral regurgitation
Left ventricle
Chronic heart failure
Constrictive pericarditis
Restrictive cardiomyopathy
Hypertrophic cardiomyopathy
Congenital subaortic stenosis
Aortic valve
Aortic stenosis
Aortic regurgitation
Thoracic aorta
Supravalvular aortic stenosis
Coarctation of aorta

Source: Taken from (Edwards, 1988).

During the 2–3 decades in which the valve orifice is progressively narrowing, the lungs adapt in response to the gradually increasing pulmonary venous pressures. With the elevated pulmonary venous and capillary pressures, filtration increases and causes a state of chronic interstitial edema. The capacity of the lungs to clear microvascular filtrate by lymphatics increases with the gradual increase in load; the capacity to clear interstitial edema by extralymphatic routes may also increase. It is interesting that pleural effusions are unusual in mitral disease; possible explanations are that other interstitial routes take precedence or that liquid entering the pleural space is removed more rapidly than usual by expanded lymphatic clearance capacity. Alveolar flooding can occur, usually the result of a sudden increase in left atrial pressure brought on either by an increase in cardiac output during exercise or pregnancy, or by the development of atrial fibrillation.

Because of chronic interstitial edema, lymphatic distention, and, perhaps, the intermittent extravasation of blood into the interstitium, interstitial fibrosis develops around septa and blood vessels (Fig. 5). The extreme chronic changes, seen only in long-standing mitral stenosis, include calcium deposition and even ossification.

Vascular Changes

The most characteristic abnormalities are seen in the pulmonary veins, which undergo medial hypertrophy (see Fig. 5). Later venous changes include intimal thickening and fibrosis. An external elastic membrane characteristic of arteries may form; with this so-called ''arterialization'' of veins, the histological distinction of veins from arteries depends on their location in the interlobular septa (Edwards, 1988). Such venous changes are pathognomonic of pulmonary

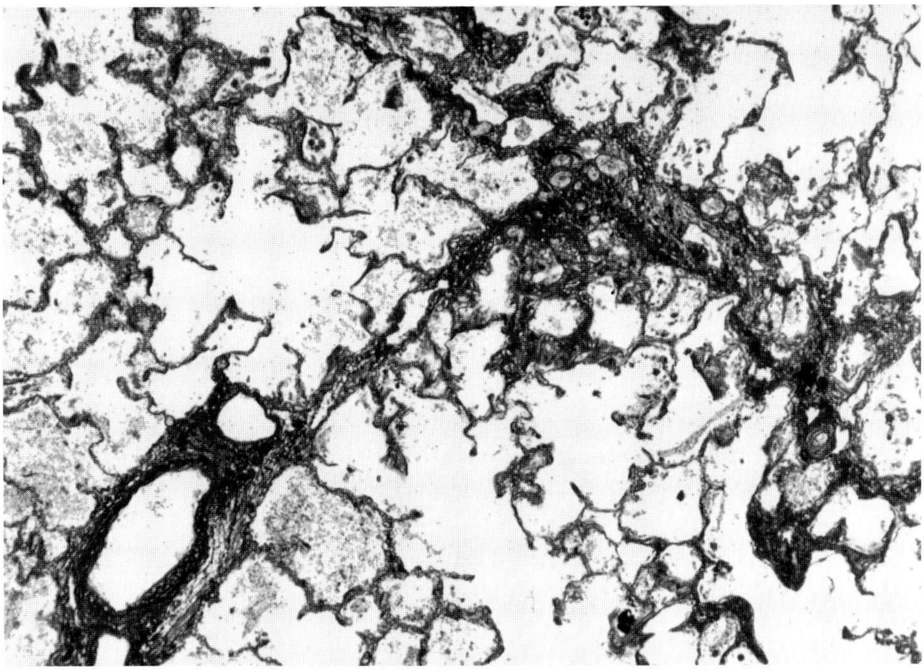

Figure 5 Section of lung from a 60-year-old man with severe mitral stenosis. Note the perivenous fibrosis, which follows long-standing elevations in pulmonary venous pressure. Dilated lymphatics can also be seen. (Courtesy of Martha Warnock, M.D.)

venous hypertension, but nonspecific as to its cause. As venous pressure increases, pressure rises passively in the capillaries and pulmonary arteries. Pulmonary arteries may respond along a continuum from vasoconstriction to severe anatomical vascular lesions (Fig. 6). With elevation of venous pressure to approximately 25 mmHg, reflex vasoconstriction develops (Walston et al., 1973) and causes most of the elevation of pulmonary vascular resistance in some patients as determined by the vasodilator responsiveness of the resistance to acetylcholine (Wood et al., 1957). In other patients, arteries undergo structural changes, with medial hypertrophy and intimal thickening (Selzer and Malmborg, 1962). Because of this arterial narrowing, pulmonary vascular resistance may increase dramatically, reaching almost systemic levels [mean 7.9 units (max. 30.5 units) (Levine et al., 1989), mean 11.6 units (max. 46 units) (Cámara

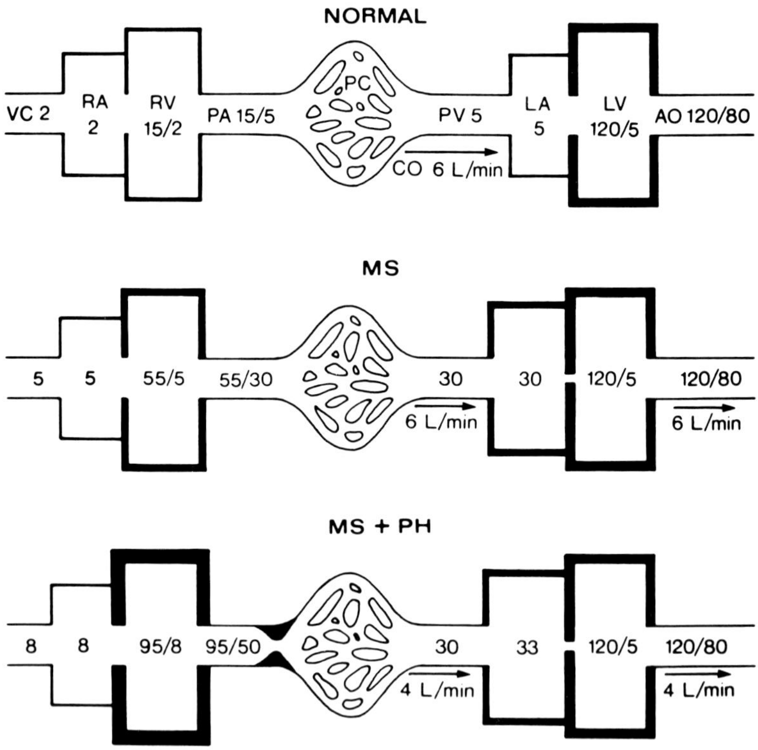

Figure 6 Schema of hemodynamics in normal circulation, severe mitral stenosis (MS) with passive pulmonary hypertension, and severe mitral stenosis with reactive pulmonary hypertension (MS + PH) due to both vasoconstriction and anatomical changes. Note that only in the latter case of reactive pulmonary hypertension is the pulmonary vascular resistance elevated. The units of pressure are mmHg.(From Selzer, 1975, with permission.)

et al., 1988), mean 14.4 units (max. 29.0 units) (Zener et al., 1972)]. It is not possible to predict which patients will develop this excessive structural response, which has been estimated to develop in 40% of those with valve orifices less than 0.7 cm^2 (Selzer and Malmborg, 1962). Of note, pulmonary artery abnormalities do not include necrotizing changes or plexiform lesions characteristic of severe pulmonary hypertension due to congenital heart disease and left-to-right shunts. Although the reason for this key difference is not known, it is significant that pulmonary artery changes due to venous hypertension are mostly reversible after corrective valve repair.

Due to elevated left atrial pressure, bronchial veins that drain into the left atrium are probably rerouted to drain into the right atrium through the interconnected venous plexus. It is also likely that pulmonary venous blood uses this route to shunt from the high-pressure left atrium to the lower-pressure right atrium. Such chronic shunting may explain the dilated vessels that have been noted in large bronchi during bronchoscopy and that resolve after mitral valve surgery (Ohmichi et al., 1988). These vessels are the likely source of hemoptysis in patients with mitral stenosis (Ferguson et al., 1944) (Fig. 7).

After correction of the cause of venous hypertension, most abnormalities in the pulmonary circulation have been shown to improve. This finding is not limited to the surgical or nonsurgical repair of mitral stenosis, but applies also to treatment of severe cardiac failure with heart transplantation (Villanueva et al., 1989; Kawaguchi et al., 1989). Pulmonary vascular resistance decreases rapidly after mitral valve replacement (Dalen et al., 1967); for example, pulmonary vascular resistance was shown to decrease from 15.4 units to 9.2 units in 24 hr and to 7.9 units in 2 days following surgery. More recently it has been recognized that there is an abrupt early decrease followed by a progressive later decrease (Levine et al., 1989). The results of a study of percutaneous valvuloplasty, in which mean valve area increased from 0.7 to 1.6 cm^2, showed an immediate fall in pulmonary vascular resistance from 7.9 to 5.6 units, and after 7 months, pulmonary vascular resistance was 3.5 units, although mean valve area had not increased further. In a study of patients with severe pulmonary hypertension with an average pulmonary arterial systolic pressure of 115 mmHg, 2 years after mitral valve surgery, the pulmonary systolic pressure had decreased to 50 mmHg, and the pulmonary vascular resistance had decreased from 14.4 units to 3.8 units (Zener et al., 1972). Although these resistances have not returned to normal, the improvement seen in pulmonary vascular resistance has encouraged clinicians to send patients with pulmonary hypertension for surgical repair who would not previously have been considered candidates (Cámara et al., 1988; Villanueva et al., 1989).

Abnormalities of Lung Function

Well-documented abnormalities of lung function in patients with mitral stenosis include decreases in lung volume, decreases in lung compliance, and increases

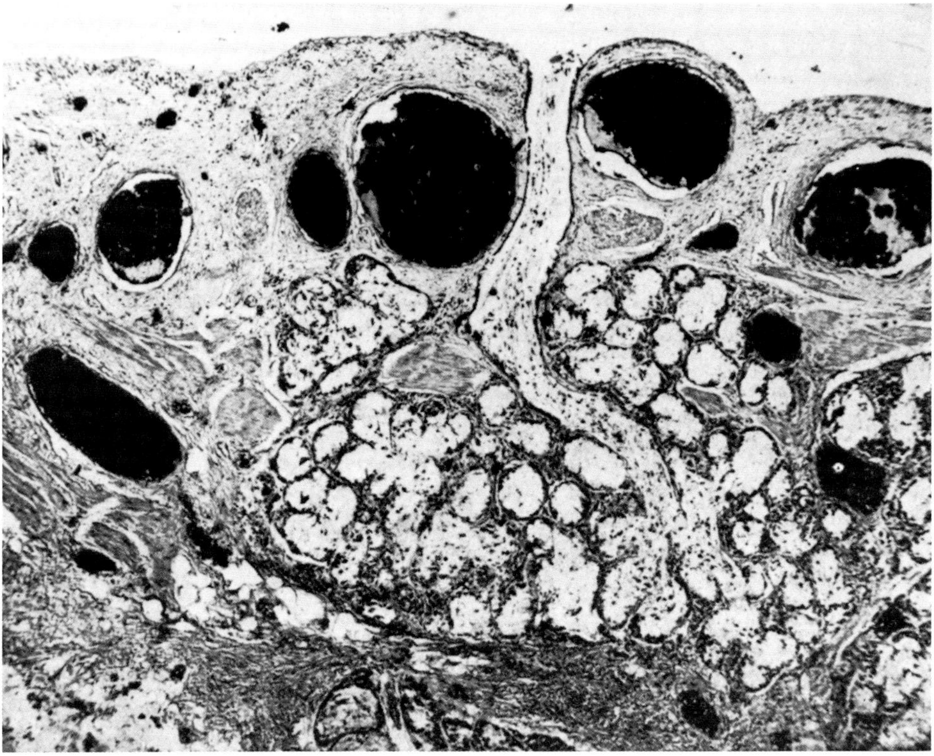

Figure 7 Section of a large bronchus from a 16-year-old girl with severe mitral stenosis. The dilated bronchial veins in the submucosa are a route by which some pulmonary venous blood flows into a lower-pressure right atrium, instead of into a high-pressure left atrium. These varices are the likely source of hemoptysis in patients with severe mitral stenosis. (From Ferguson et al., 1944, with permission.)

in airway resistance. Initial changes due to the congestion of the lungs and interstitial edema may be few, as were discussed; congestion and interstitial edema may lead to decreases in airway caliber. Blood flow to the apex of the lungs increases (Dawson et al., 1976). With increasing years, chronic changes including interlobular fibrosis develop and begin to cause a decrease in lung recoil and volume. Blood flow now may be higher to the apex than to the base, leading to a reversal of the normal gradient (Dawson et al., 1976; Ohno et al., 1987). The recoil of the lungs increases at high lung volumes due to the fibrosis of the parenchyma, but is less than normal at low lung volumes, perhaps because of the support of congested or stiff blood vessels (Wood et al., 1971; De Troyer et al., 1980). With chronic hemodynamic and pulmonary functional limitation, respiratory muscle function may become affected, leading to decreases in maximal strength (De Troyer et al., 1980).

Following correction of the mitral stenosis, most pulmonary function abnormalities in the mild to moderate stages of severity are reversible, but after severe long-standing mitral stenosis, pulmonary function may be permanently abnormal. In one study of patients with mild elevation of venous pressures undergoing transcutaneous balloon commissurotomy, even though lung function prior to commissurotomy was in the normal range, after relief of mitral obstruction and decrease of mean left atrial pressure from 15 to 8 mmHg, there was an increase in vital capacity, FEV_1, and maximal voluntary ventilation (Yoshioka et al., 1990). In another study involving valvular surgery of patients with different degrees of mitral stenosis, the mildest group (pulmonary artery pressure < 25 mmHg) showed no pulmonary abnormalities before and no change after surgery. The moderately severe group (pulmonary artery pressures > 25 mmHg but no tricuspid regurgitation) showed normal pulmonary function, but nonetheless had improvement in lung volumes postoperatively. The most severe group (pulmonary artery pressure > 25 mmHg with moderate to severe tricuspid regurgitation) had abnormal lung volumes and flows prior to surgery, with no improvement more than 1 year after surgery. It appears that long-standing mitral stenosis induces permanent changes in the lung parenchyma. For reasons not understood, interstitial fibrosis appears to characterize the pulmonary response to chronically elevated pulmonary venous pressure, whereas little fibrosis is found in patients with elevated pulmonary arterial pressure alone.

Clinical Presentation

The gradual changes in pulmonary circulatory and lung function lead to the slow and almost imperceptible onset of symptoms in patients with mitral stenosis. Dyspnea, fatigue, and decrease in exercise tolerance are the first noticeable abnormalities. The causes of dyspnea, as in most cases of heart and lung disease, are probably myriad, including the increases in parenchymal stiffness and airway resistance that lead to an increase in work of breathing and stimulation of J receptors in the interstitium of the lungs. Improvement in dyspnea has been associated with an improvement in exercise function after mitral valve surgery (Rhodes et al., 1985). With increases in cardiac output, as from fever, pregnancy, exercise, or decreases in filling time, as with tachyarrhythmias, pulmonary venous pressures can acutely increase and lead to a sudden worsening of the dyspnea, perhaps associated with alveolar edema. As the mitral valve orifice stenoses further, critical elevations in pressures occur with less provocation, and the patient progressively limits his or her activities. Late symptoms include hemoptysis, due to rupture of the dilated bronchial anastomotic vessels (Ferguson et al., 1944).

Pulmonary venous hypertension may initially be recognized on a chest radiograph, as discussed for acute elevations of pressure. With chronic elevations, pulmonary arteries become attenuated, first at the base and then toward the apex. Kerley-B lines now consist of interlobular fibrosis and dilated lymphatics, not interstitial edema as in the acute interstitial edema. Hemosiderin-laden macrophages can fill the lower lobe alveoli and produce a diffuse nodularity. Ossified nodules may also rarely be found at the bases.

Diagnosis

The diagnosis of the cause of pulmonary venous hypertension begins with ascertaining the level of obstruction, initially by chest radiograph. If the level of obstruction is preventricular, i.e., at the atrial level due to mitral stenosis, atrial myxoma or cor triatriatum (a congenital web obstructing flow within the left atrium), the left ventricular silhouette may be normal, although the left atrium may show an enlarged shadow. If the level of impairment lies in the ventricle, due either to myocardial disease or to valvular disease, the heart will likely be enlarged on the chest radiograph. Auscultation of the heart can distinguish mitral stenosis (opening snap, diastolic rumble) from mitral regurgitation (holosystolic murmur). Echocardiography in its M-mode and two-dimensional modes can evaluate cardiac dimensions, identify left atrial myxoma or hypertrophic cardiomyopathy, and describe mitral valve excursion; now, with the Doppler mode for measuring flows, echocardiography can reach a clinically useful measure of the pressure gradient and mitral valve cross-sectional area (Hatle, 1990) and pulmonary artery pressure (Schiller, 1990). Nuclear magnetic resonance imaging is an important additional noninvasive diagnostic technique, which either complements echocardiography or supplants it (Bisset, 1991; Parsons and Baker, 1990). For example, because of the limited penetration of the ultrasound beam, nuclear magnetic resonance imaging is the best noninvasive technique available for examination deep in the thorax, i.e., for the aorta (aortic coarctation), for the posterior cardiac structures (cor triatriatum, pulmonary vein stenosis), or for general examination in patients with abnormal body habitus (obesity, pectus excavatum) (Bisset, 1991). Cardiac catheterization may be necessary to measure flows and pressures to allow accurate calculation of valve area, and to assess coronary perfusion or other abnormalities in complex valvular disease.

Therapy

The inherent reversibility of the underlying pulmonary vascular structural abnormalities highlights the importance of corrective therapy. Whether percutaneous mitral commissurotomy or closed (no cardiac bypass) or open (cardiac bypass) surgery is chosen, the goal in correcting mitral stenosis is to cause a significant ($> 50\%$) increase in valve area without causing significant mitral regurgitation. Either repair or replacement of a regurgitant mitral valve is considered when the patient is symptomatically limited. Removal of an atrial myxoma will cure the patient of the pulmonary venous obstruction, as well as the constitutional symptoms and systemic embolization. In patients with chronic heart failure, management can include therapy to lower systemic vascular resistance and left ventricular diastolic pressures and to control arrhythmias. Recently, heart transplantation has become a viable therapy for patients with end-stage cardiac failure, even for those with severe elevations in pulmonary vascular resistance (Villanueva et al., 1989; Kawaguchi et al., 1989).

IV. Increased Pulmonary Blood Flow and Pressure

A. Introduction

With the normal decrease in pulmonary artery pressure and pulmonary vascular resistance after birth, left-to-right shunts become possible. Sites for these shunts are either intracardiac, at the atrial or ventricular level, or extracardiac, at the ductus arteriosus. Interatrial shunts are generally associated with increased pulmonary blood flow, without an early increase in pressure. Ventricular and ductal shunts, however, depending on their size, may expose the pulmonary vascular tree to systemic pressures and cause earlier vascular changes.

B. Physiology

Circulatory Changes

Pulmonary vascular abnormalities in response to increases in flow and, especially, to pressure are the single most important determinant of the pathophysiology, clinical presentation, and operability for patients with left-to-right shunts. Along a continuum of change, the arteries respond to pressure increases with an increase in medial layer of muscle (medial thickening), an increase in the intimal layer (intimal thickening), and finally by irreversible anatomical changes resulting in plexiform lesions. Heath and Edwards (1958) first categorized these lesions by organizing them into a system for comparison with clinical outcomes. Their system was as follows: grade 1 (medial thickening), 2 (cellular intimal thickening), 3 (fibrous intimal thickening), 4 (plexiform lesion), 5 (hemosiderosis), and 6 (necrotizing arteritis). Virmani and Roberts (1979) clarified and simplified the categories by eliminating features not unique to pulmonary hypertension (hemosiderosis and necrotizing arteritis) and combining the two types of intimal lesions. Their system of three grades, is as follows: grade 1 (medial thickening), 2 (plus intimal thickening), and 3 (plus plexiform lesions) (Fig. 8). Additional grading schemes have categorized the peripheral extension of

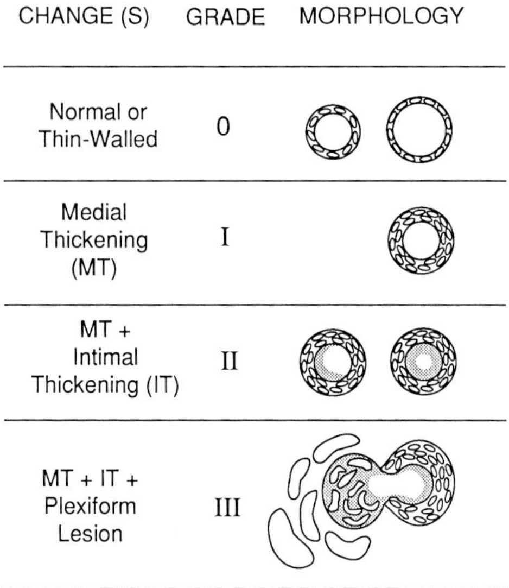

Figure 8 Simplified grading scheme of pulmonary vascular changes due to elevated pulmonary artery pressure and flow from left-to right shunting. (From Virmani and Roberts, 1979, with permission.)

muscle and decrease in number of vessels (Rabinovitch and Reid, 1980), although some argue that a decrease in vessels is an artifact of perfusion (Edwards, 1988). Medial thickening is the earliest response to increased transmural vascular pressure and may come about from hypertrophy of smooth muscle cells or by both hypertrophy and hyperplasia. Intimal thickening can be due to an increase in the number of cells or an accumulation of dense fibrous tissue (Fig. 9). Some investigators have distinguished between cellular and acellular causes of intimal thickening and consider severe intimal fibrous thickening to be an irreversible lesion (Wagenvoort, 1985). The plexiform lesion, however, is generally accepted as demonstrating irreversible pulmonary vascular disease (Fig. 10). This lesion is an aneurysmal structure, which comes off a muscular pulmonary artery at a right angle and which contains a multitude of channels with walls consisting of fibrous tissue covered by endothelial cells. It feeds into a dilated pulmonary vessel and then into alveolar capillaries. The cause of the lesion is much less clear than its significance. Among the hypotheses are that the lesion results from a jet-flow injury (Kanjuh et al., 1964), from recanalization of a thrombosed artery (Naeye and Vennart, 1960), from healing of a necrotic artery (Wagenvoort and Wagenvoort, 1977), or from aneurysms and subsequent thrombosis with recanalization at a site of congenitally weak media (Virmani and Roberts, 1979).

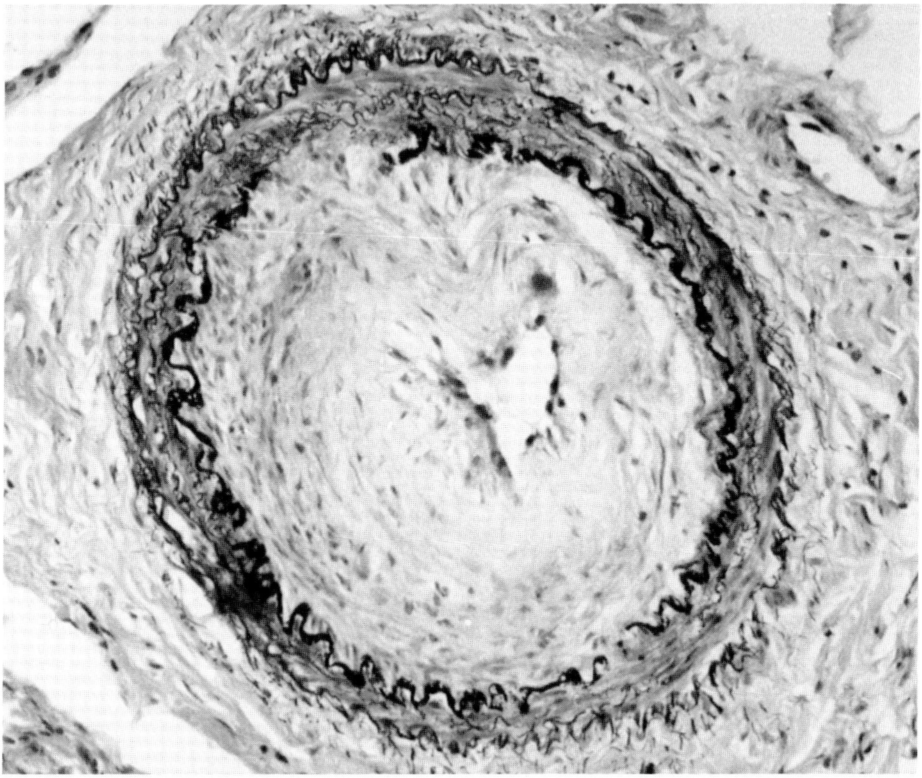

Figure 9 Pulmonary artery from an 11-year-old girl with atrioventricular canal defect and resultant pulmonary hypertension. Mean pulmonary artery pressure (65 mmHg) and pulmonary vascular resistance (17.4 units) were at systemic levels, and the pulmonary flow only slightly exceeded systemic flow (pulmonary:systemic flow ratio 1.2). Note that the thickened media and intima have nearly occluded the vessel lumen. (Courtesy of Martha Warnock, M.D.)

As the pulmonary vascular disease worsens under the stimulus of the abnormally increased pressure, the resulting elevation in pulmonary vascular resistance progressively decreases pulmonary blood flow. When the pulmonary resistance becomes higher than the systemic, the shunt flow then reverses direction, leading to a right-to-left shunt. At this point, regardless of the site of shunt, elevated pulmonary vascular resistance with a right-to-left shunt is defined as Eisenmenger's syndrome. Although Eisenmenger originally described a patient with a large ventricular septal defect, Wood (1958) made the point clearly that, because at least 12 anatomical abnormalities can lead to the identical physiology, the term Eisenmenger's should refer to a syndrome, not a

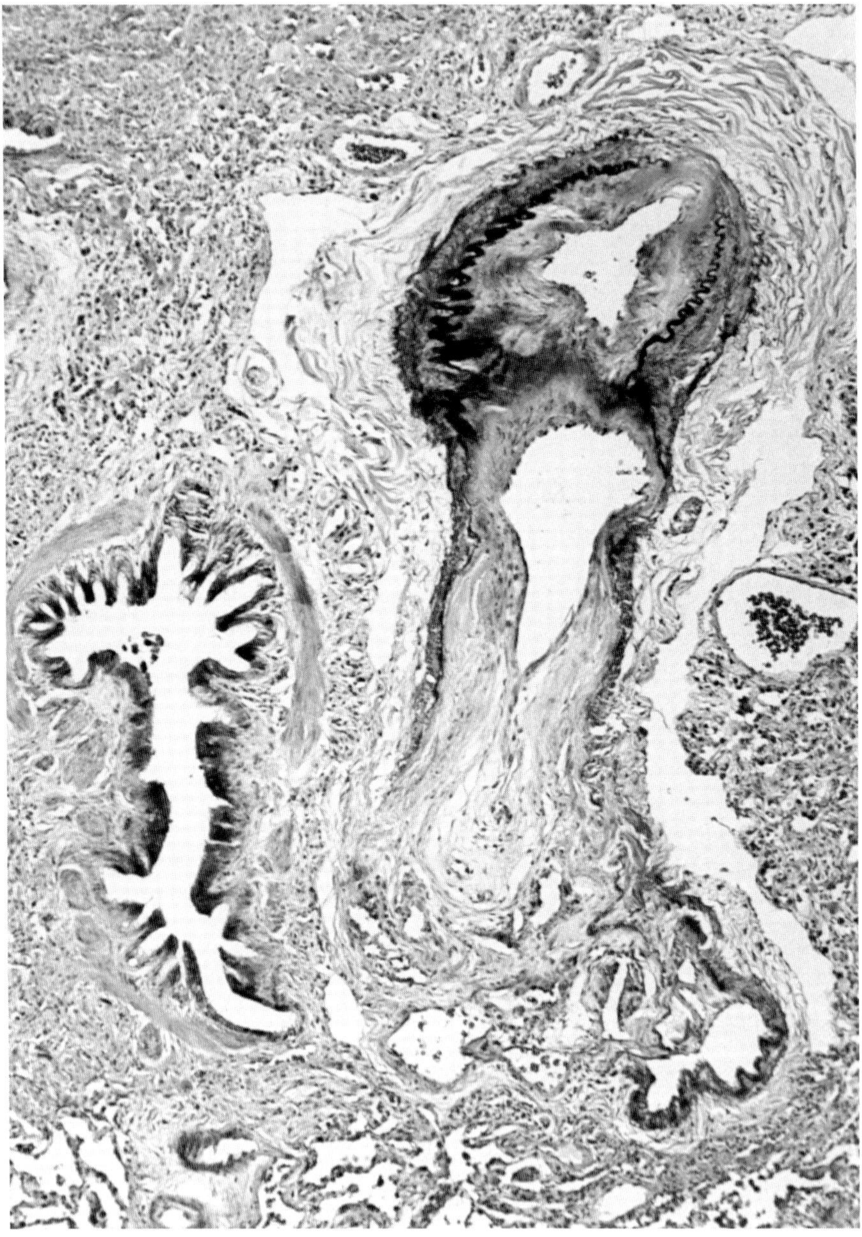

Figure 10 Another section from the same patient as in Figure 9, showing a plexiform lesion (below). A dilated vessel is leaving a muscular pulmonary artery (at right) and demonstrates multiple channels consisting of fibrous tissue without musculature. This lesion signals irreversible pulmonary vascular disease. (Courtesy of Martha Warnock, M.D.)

specific shunt. In Table 4, the possible causes of left-to-right shunt and thus potentially of Eisenmenger's syndrome are basically the same as provided by Wood, with the addition of surgically created left-to-right shunts designed to increase pulmonary blood flow (see Section V, "Decreased Pulmonary Artery Flow and Pressure").

By the time pulmonary vascular resistance has risen to approximately 70% of the systemic level, or when the pulmonary blood flow is less than 1.5 times as much as systemic, it is unlikely that surgical correction of the shunt will reduce the pulmonary flow enough to improve the situation. And, by eliminating a right-to-left shunt through which the right heart can decompress, as in the case of a large ventricular septal defect, corrective surgery may impose more work

Table 4 Causes of Increased Pulmonary Arterial Flow and Pressure

- Atrial
  - Atrial septal defect (ASD)
  - Common atrium (no functional atrial septum)
  - Total or partial anomalous pulmonary venous connection (all or some of the pulmonary veins drain into right atrium)
  - Transposition of the great arteries with ASD
- Ventricle
  - Ventricular septal defect (VSD)
  - Single ventricle
  - Atrioventricular canal (defect in atrial and/or ventricular septum)
  - Associated lesions with VSD
    - Transposition of the great arteries
    - Double-outlet right ventricle
    - Tricuspid atresia without pulmonary stenosis
    - Mitral atresia
- Aortic
  - Patent ductus arteriosus (PDA)
  - Aorticopulmonary window (connection between ascending aorta and pulmonary trunk)
  - Truncus arteriosus (single vessel from both ventricles to systemic and pulmonary circulations)
  - Postsurgical shunts
    - Potts (descending aorta–left pulmonary artery)
    - Waterston (ascending aorta–right pulmonary artery)
    - Blalock-Taussig (subclavian artery to ipsilateral pulmonary artery)

Source: Adapted from Borow and Braunwald, 1988.

on the right heart by forcing its entire output through the restricted pulmonary vascular bed. In addition, by this stage, pulmonary vascular disease can progress independently (Wagenvoort et al., 1984). For all these reasons, for patients with already decreased pulmonary flow, surgery is contraindicated (Nugent et al., 1990).

Although reversibility of certain lesions was originally proposed based on histological appearance, the reversibility of medial thickening and most intimal thickening has been confirmed by following patients with open lung biopsies at the time of pulmonary artery banding and upon corrective surgery 2–10 years later (Wagenvoort et al., 1984) (Fig. 11). In this useful study, severe concentric intimal fibrosis did not regress, and in some cases progressed. The few patients with necrotic and plexiform lesions tended to have progressive pulmonary hypertension. Despite the general association of vascular pathology and pathophysiology, in any one patient there can be a discrepancy. Pulmonary vascular

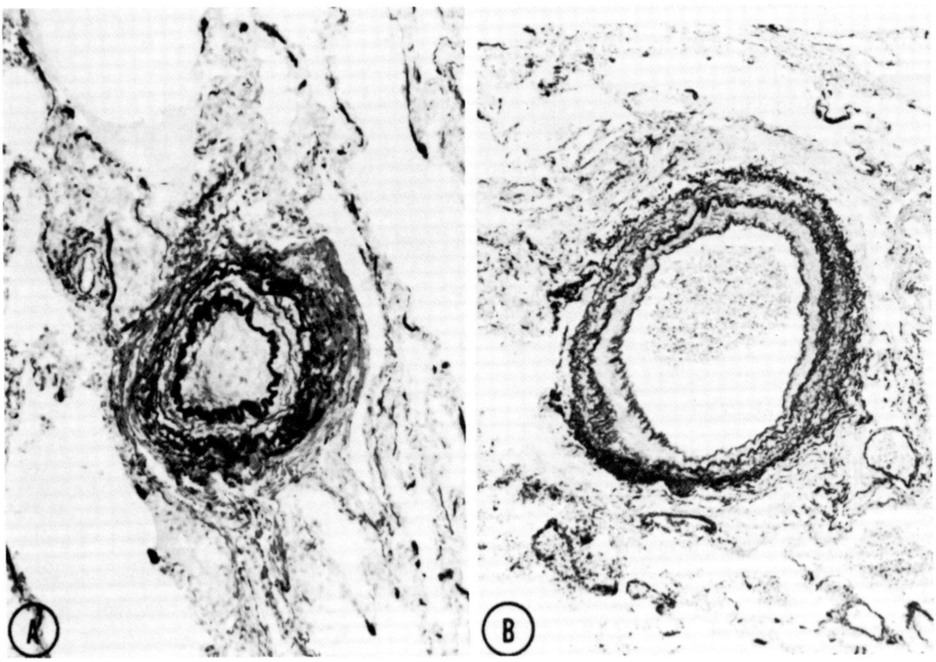

Figure 11 Lung biopsy sections from a boy with ventricular septal defect and patent ductus arteriosus before (A) and 3 years after pulmonary artery banding (B). The medial hypertrophy and intimal thickening (fibrosis with some cellular proliferation) have mostly regressed. (from Wagenvoort et al., 1984, with permission.)

disease can progress after cardiac repair despite apparently reversible lesions on lung biopsy (Haworth et al., 1987).

In experimental studies of animal models and in vitro systems, the primary role of pressure, rather than blood flow per se, in causing pulmonary vascular disease has been supported. Hypoxia is often used as a convenient stimulus for producing pulmonary artery pressure elevations through its vasoconstrictor effect (Stenmark et al., 1987). In young pigs with aortopulmonary shunts, which on average increased pulmonary artery pressure from 9 to 30 mmHg, arterial medial thickening was found after 8 weeks (Rendas et al., 1979). Hypoxia in the rat induced a pulmonary hypertensive response followed by a rapid and reversible increase in collagen and elastin production in the pulmonary artery (Poiani et al., 1990). In another hypoxic rat model, after 2 days of hypoxia, new muscle appeared in nonmuscular pulmonary arteries immediately beneath the endothelium, not as an extension of preexisting muscle but by differentiation of nonmuscular cells into myocytes (Meyrick and Reid, 1978). In studies of pulmonary artery strips, mechanical tension on the strip, to reproduce the effect of a given transmural pressure, caused an increase in connective tissue synthesis, which depended on an intact endothelium (Tozzi et al., 1989). Animal and in vitro models will be invaluable for dissecting the signals for structural changes and devising medical therapies.

Bronchial vessels are known to become enlarged in Eisenmenger's syndrome (Jamieson et al., 1984). Presumably, as pulmonary flow decreases with the development of right-to-left shunting, bronchial vessels dilate to restore pulmonary flow. This bronchial arterial hypertrophy may explain the hemoptysis that may occur with Eisenmenger's syndrome, and it also complicates heart-lung transplantation in these patients because the large, friable bronchial arteries are relatively inaccessible in the posterior mediastinum (Jamieson et al., 1984).

Atrial Septal Defect (ASD)

The defect in the atrium allows left atrial blood to flow into the right atrium and into the right ventricle. The amount of flow through an ASD depends less on the diameter of the defect than on the relative compliances of the right and left ventricles. After birth, the right ventricle normally begins to involute in response to the decreased pressure load in the lungs. As the compliance of the right ventricle increases, blood flow into it from both atria increases, leading to larger and larger pulmonary flows. Generally, these flows are tolerated well, until in some patients, usually in their 4th decade, pulmonary vascular resistance begins to increase and may cause pulmonary arterial hypertension severe enough to lead to heart failure.

The slow progression of pulmonary vascular disease, if it occurs at all, distinguishes atrial shunts from ventricular or aortic shunts, in which the pulmonary vessels are exposed to systemic pressure from birth. Wood (1958) calculated from his experience that only 9% of patients with an interatrial shunt developed Eisenmenger's syndrome, compared with 50% of those with shunts through ventricular or aortic defects. When Eisenmenger's syndrome did occur, it developed in adulthood in almost all patients with interatrial shunts, and in infancy in almost all patients with ventricular or aortic shunts.

Ventricular Septal Defect (VSD)

The major hemodynamic characteristic of a VSD is its size, which determines how much of left ventricular pressure is transmitted into the pulmonary circulation. Large, nonrestrictive defects lead to systemic arterial pressure in the pulmonary artery. When pressures in the two ventricles are equalized, flow through the pulmonary circulation depends on the ratio of pulmonary to systemic vascular resistance.

Patent Ductus Arteriosus (PDA)

This connection leads from the aorta at a site beyond the left subclavian artery to the pulmonary artery and subjects the pulmonary vessels to systemic pressure. In one study (Virmani and Roberts, 1979), pulmonary arterial pressure was reported to be higher in patients with PDA than in those with VSD, although in another study (Heath et al., 1958), this difference was not found.

Abnormalities of Lung Function

In children with increases in pulmonary blood flow, few pulmonary function abnormalities are detectable. Diffusing capacity may be increased due to the distention of capillaries, but even in children with large increases in pulmonary blood flow due to ASD, lung compliance was normal (Griffin et al., 1972). Some investigators have attributed mild to moderate decreases in compliance and increases in airway resistance to elevations in pulmonary artery pressure (Bancalari et al., 1977). The mechanism of alteration in pulmonary mechanics could be by a change in the mechanical properties of the vessels within it, making the lungs stiffer. In contrast to the consequences of chronically elevated pulmonary venous pressure, when pulmonary artery pressures are chronically elevated, the lung parenchyma is generally spared.

C. Clinical Presentation

Patients with atrial shunts tend to be asymptomatic in early life, although the frequency of respiratory infections may be increased. The development of symptoms, chiefly fatigue and dyspnea, signals the onset of increased pulmonary vascular resistance and pulmonary hypertension and usually occurs during adulthood.

Patients with left-to-right shunts at the aortic and ventricular levels may present early in infancy with biventricular congestive heart failure. The infants appear dyspneic, grunt with breathing, and have difficulty with feedings. The consequences of early congestive heart failure include frequent respiratory infections and growth retardation.

After progressing to Eisenmenger's syndrome, all the defects have a similar clinical presentation. Cyanosis is present at rest or with exercise. A pathognomonic finding in PDA is differential cyanosis, in which the upper body is pink and the lower extremities are blue due to right-to-left shunting beyond the left subclavian artery. Clubbing of the fingers (or toes in patients with PDA) is frequent. The most common symptom is breathlessness, followed by chest pain, syncope, and hemoptysis. Hemoptysis may be caused by pulmonary infarction from low pulmonary blood flow and increased viscosity of polycythemic blood (Wood, 1958), or by bronchial arterial bleeding.

Signs of these lesions include the specific auscultatory findings of the fixed splitting of the second sound in ASD, or the systolic murmur of VSD, or the continuous murmur of PDA, and the palpation of right ventricular systolic lifts and thrills. With increases in pulmonary blood flow alone, there may be no physical findings. Once pulmonary pressure increases, the second heart sound may become accentuated. The Eisenmenger's syndrome is announced by the appearance of cyanosis, and the physical findings of pulmonary hypertension and right ventricular hypertrophy will be present. The chest radiograph can document the magnitude of changes in pulmonary blood flow, showing a plethora of vessels when pulmonary blood flow is high and pruning of blood vessels with central pulmonary artery dilation when pulmonary vascular disease has led to decreases in pulmonary blood flow. Similarly, the electrocardiogram can document the development of right ventricular hypertrophy.

D. Diagnosis

The diagnostic evaluation entails finding the site of the shunt and associated abnormalities, deciding on the need for operation, and determining operability. Many of these lesions are not distinguishable on physical examination or initial laboratory tests. The first noninvasive test is echocardiography, with the Doppler mode to recognize shunt directions and quantify shunt velocity. Echocardiography can be used to define the anatomy of both intra- and extracardiac anomalies, to measure the size and function of different chambers, and most recently to measure intracardiac hemodynamics (Child, 1990). Shunt flow can be measured directly at the defect (Hornberger et al., 1989) or inferred by the ratio of pulmonary to systemic blood flow. Nowadays, the next noninvasive test may be nuclear magnetic resonance (MR) imaging. Although its role is currently being defined, MR imaging offers additional useful information for defining the anatomy of complex cardiac anomalies, for visualizing the great vessels, for documenting postoperative changes, and for examining patients with abnormal thoracic anatomy (Parsons and Baker, 1990; Bisset, 1991). Now primarily a technique that provides anatomical information, MR imaging has the potential for ciné and flow imaging that could provide functional information to rival that from cardiac catheterization in the future (Parsons and Baker, 1990). For now, cardiac catheterization is the best method for determining anatomy and hemodynamics and is still required for preoperative evaluation. The level at which an oxygen saturation stepup is detected will identify the level of the shunt, at the atrium, ventricle, or pulmonary artery; associated cardiac anomalies can be detected; and, importantly, the degree of pulmonary vascular resistance can be accurately measured. This is the most crucial determinant of operability, for if pulmonary vascular resistance is more than 70% of systemic, surgery is not indicated (Nugent et al., 1990).

When the criteria for operability are borderline, two other tests may help: lung biopsy and wedge arteriography. Lung biopsy can demonstrate reversible lesions of arteries and thereby clear the way for surgery. It is worth noting that despite documentation of reversible lesions, some patients do not recover and appear to die soon after surgery of intractable pulmonary hypertension (Haworth et al., 1987). The reason may be either that reversibility did not occur rapidly enough to benefit the patient or that irreversible lesions were missed; despite evidence that small (1 cm^2) pieces of lung are representative of the state of the media and intima of the entire pulmonary vascular bed (Haworth and Reid, 1978), plexiform lesions do not develop with every muscular artery and could be overlooked. A qualitative assessment of the lower segmental vascular tree by wedge angiography includes determination of degree of tapering and density of vascular markings "background haze" and tends to correlate with the pulmonary vascular resistance (Rabinovitch et al., 1981).

E. Therapy

Medical management is generally supportive, with attempts to ameliorate symptoms of heart failure and to prevent endocarditis. In one disorder, medical therapy can affect the underlying problem. For PDA in the premature infant, indomethacin may be given to constrict the ductus (Gersony et al., 1983). Otherwise, those infants with left-to-right shunts who are in severe cardiac failure or those who have continuation of elevated pulmonary pressure to more than 50% of systemic by 6 months of age should undergo corrective surgery during their first year of life (Nugent et al., 1990). In patients with early evidence of high pulmonary artery flows and pressures, usually with large ventricular shunts, pulmonary artery banding was a common palliative maneuver to decrease pulmonary artery flow and is sometimes still used to allow further maturation before corrective surgery. Now, because of better success with early correction, banding is mostly undertaken for uncorrectable defects (Nolan, 1987).

Patients with Eisenmenger's syndrome had no curative therapy until recently. Palliative phlebotomy to keep the hematocrit under 70%, digitalis, and diuretics were the main therapies available. With heart-lung transplantation, these patients now have some hope of long-term survival. With the introduction of cyclosporine and the success of heart-lung transplantation in primates, combined heart-lung transplantation was begun in patients at Stanford University Hospital in March 1981. Since then, more than 350 combined heart-lung transplantations have been performed worldwide, mainly for primary pulmonary hypertension and Eisenmenger's syndrome (LeGal, 1990). Recently, 2-month survival has risen from approximately 40–50% to 70%. Long-term benefit is currently limited by a high late incidence of bronchiolitis obliterans (McGregor et al., 1986). Heart-lung transplantation is necessary because both the heart and lungs are diseased. The combined transplantation may offer one interesting advantage over either heart or lung (alone) transplantation; preexisting connections between the coronary and bronchial circulations have been described by which the coronary circulation could supply bronchial blood flow, thereby helping tracheal anastomotic healing (Jamieson et al., 1984).

V. Decreased Pulmonary Artery Flow and Pressure

A. Introduction

Pulmonary blood flow decreases to less than systemic flow when there is both an obstruction to pulmonary outflow and a site of right-to-left shunt (Table 5). The most common anomaly is tetralogy of Fallot, a condition with pulmonary outflow narrowing and a large nonrestrictive ventricular septal defect. The other two components of the "tetralogy" are less important: the biventricular origin of the aorta (overriding) and, secondary to other abnormalities, right ventricular hypertrophy.

B. Physiology

Circulatory Changes

With a large VSD, the ventricles act as a single chamber. Therefore, pulmonary blood flow will be determined by the relative resistances to flow through the

Table 5 Causes of Decreased Pulmonary Arterial Flow and Pressure

Tetralogy of Fallot (large VSD and obstruction to pulmonary outflow)
Pulmonary valvular stenosis with patent foramen ovale
Ebstein's anomaly (malposition of tricuspid valve making the right ventricle functionally smaller and allowing right-to-left shunt across ASD or foramen ovale)

pulmonary and systemic circulations. Without the increased pulmonary outflow resistance offered by the narrowed pulmonary outflow tract in patients with tetralogy of Fallot, pulmonary blood flow would be increased as in simple VSD. The increased resistance to pulmonary outflow, which occurs either at the muscular infundibulum or the pulmonary valve, acts like a pulmonary band designed to protect the pulmonary vasculature from the deleterious effects of systemic blood pressure. However, when the obstruction is too great, pulmonary flow can be seriously limited.

The pulmonary muscular arteries in patients with these disorders exhibit a thinner medial layer and larger diameter than normal (Fig. 12). Other characteristic findings include intraluminal thrombosis, a common complication of polycythemia and low pulmonary blood flow.

In patients with low pulmonary blood flow, the bronchial circulation may assume a prominent role by supplying blood flow to the lungs and by

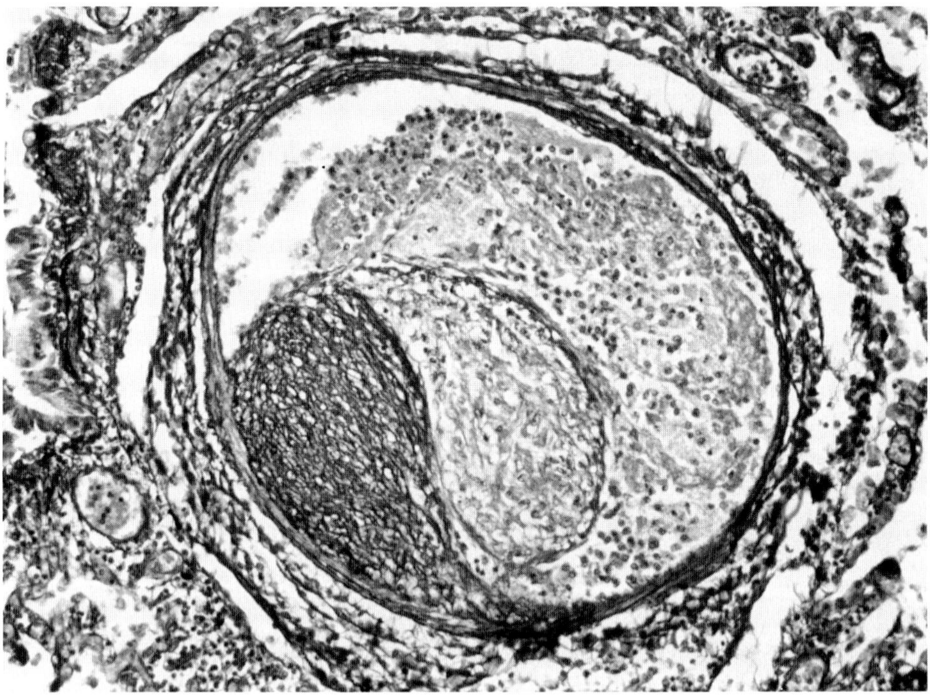

Figure 12 Pulmonary artery from a 28-month-old girl with tetralogy of Fallot. The artery shows a thin muscular layer and intraluminal thrombus associated with decreased pulmonary artery pressure and flow. (Courtesy of Martha Warnock, M.D.)

contributing to gas exchange; in some cases where there is pulmonary atresia and no pulmonary blood supply to the lungs at all, the bronchial arteries together with the ductus arteriosus supply the lungs entirely (Liao et al., 1985). In experimental studies in dogs 3 years after unilateral pulmonary ligation, the ligated lung was able to contribute approximately 10% of total O_2 and 15% of CO_2 exchange, presumably via the bronchial circulation (Lilker and Nagy, 1975). Only if systemic blood is hypoxemic, as in tetralogy of Fallot, will the bronchial blood be able to take up oxygen (Viola and Abbate, 1973). If bronchial blood flow is large enough, shunts designed to increase pulmonary blood flow may not be required (Deffebach et al., 1987).

Abnormalities of Lung Function

Abnormalities in lung function tests are mild; the mechanics of the lungs and their airways appear normal. The diffusing capacity may be decreased, although when expressed per unit of lung volume, this too can be normal (Takkunen, Mattila et al., 1987). In one study of young adults with congenital pulmonic stenosis, lung volumes were significantly reduced compared to normal controls (total lung capacity by body plethysmography, 4.9 L in patients versus 6.2 L in controls). De Troyer and co-workers proposed that low pulmonary blood pressure caused hypoplasia of the lungs (De Troyer et al., 1977). Interestingly, patients with poor hemodynamic results can also have low lung volumes postoperatively (Takkunen et al., 1987). By postoperative exercise testing, many patients are at normal levels, and decreased exercise tolerance is mostly associated with a poor surgical hemodynamic result (Takkunen et al., 1987; Wessel et al., 1980).

C. Clinical Presentation

Patients with severe pulmonary outflow obstruction exhibit cyanosis early in childhood, at first perhaps with crying or straining, which presumably increases pulmonary vascular resistance by a Valsalva-like maneuver. Cyanosis may become severe, with arterial oxygen saturations as low as 50%. These children are usually dyspneic and squat to improve their breathlessness, especially during exercise. Squatting may increase systemic vascular resistance, thereby increasing pulmonary blood flow and improving oxygenation. Periodic attacks of deep cyanosis may relate to pulmonary infundibular muscle contraction and can lead to syncope. Patients with such serious symptoms require palliative or corrective surgery.

Physical findings include cyanosis, clubbing, small stature, right ventricular hypertrophy, and systolic murmur. Laboratory examination will reveal polycythemia and poorly saturated arterial blood. Right ventricular and atrial hypertrophy are demonstrable by electrocardiography. Chest radiographs often show a prominent right ventricle and a small pulmonary artery, which gives a boot shape to the cardiac silhouette, and diminished vascular markings. The vascular pattern may be formed in part or in whole by the bronchial supply.

D. Diagnosis

In case of diminished pulmonary blood flow, cyanosis is an early finding, which clearly points to only a few defects, and which does not signify irreversible disease. The workup with echocardiography, nuclear magnetic resonance imaging, and cardiac catheterization will establish the anatomical abnormalities and the potential for surgical repair. Nuclear magnetic resonance imaging has a potentially important role for defining the pulmonary artery anatomy, which may be difficult with either echocardiography (depth of structures, small echocardiographic window of penetration) or catheterization (overlapping opacification) (Bisset, 1991). In a study comparing the three techniques for their anatomical definition of the pulmonary arteries, nuclear magnetic resonance was superior to echocardiography and similar to angiography (Vick et al., 1990). In cases of pulmonary atresia when catheterization cannot demonstrate whether pulmonary arteries in fact exist, there is another potential route of contrast injection; bronchial arteriography can outline the pulmonary arteries by anastomotic flow (Deffebach et al., 1987).

E. Therapy

There are three approaches to the symptomatic patient with tetralogy of Fallot: medical management of the outflow obstruction with propranolol to delay definitive surgical correction (Ponce et al., 1973), surgical palliation with systemic-pulmonary shunts to delay correction, and surgical correction. The advantages of delay are to allow the child and the pulmonary arteries to grow; the disadvantages are the increased likelihood of death from hypoxic episodes and perhaps failure of normal development of the lungs. By decision analysis of these three options for a 6-month-old with tetralogy of Fallot, Garson and coworkers (1980) suggest that, at their institution, the use of propranolol to delay correction would be the safest choice; if the surgical correction could be performed at less than a 10% mortality, this would become the preferred option. Palliative systemic-pulmonary arterial shunts have become increasingly selective: from the Potts and Waterston shunts connecting the aorta to a pulmonary artery, to the Blalock-Taussig shunt connecting the subclavian artery to the ipsilateral pulmonary artery. With aortic shunts, pulmonary vascular disease due to increased pulmonary vascular pressures is more likely than with a subclavian shunt (Newfeld et al., 1977). Surgical correction is effective, although the operation may still leave the patient with residual pulmonary outflow obstruction, and it may create pulmonary valve insufficiency or a left-to-right shunt (Ruzyllo et al., 1974)

VI. Summary

The interrelationships between the circulations of the heart and lungs are of necessity complex, but essential for normal physiological function. When heart disease occurs, the lungs must adapt to high or low flows and pressures. With acute increases in pulmonary vascular pressure, the lungs do not have sufficient time to adapt and edema develops, first in the parenchyma of the lungs and then in the alveolar and pleural spaces. When the lungs have time to adapt to the slow development of increased pressure, changes are limited mostly to the vasculature, although parenchymal abnormalities may develop after many years of chronic pulmonary venous pressure elevation. To a great degree, chronic vascular abnormalities are reversible if the underlying problem is rectified; only the most severe pulmonary vascular changes due to high pulmonary arterial pressure are self-perpetuating. The structural plasticity of the pulmonary vasculature characterizes the pulmonary response to most cardiac diseases.

References

Arnott, W. M., and Withering, W. (1964). Physiologic problems in mitral stenosis. *Am. Heart J.* **68**:145–148.

Auld, P. A. M., Rudolph, A. M., and Golinko, R. J. (1960). Factors affecting bronchial collateral flow in the dog. *Am. J. Physiol.* **198**(6):1166–1170.

Bancalari, E., Jesse, M. J., Gelband, H., and Garcia, O. (1977). Lung mechanics in congenital heart disease with increased and decreased pulmonary blood flow. *J. Pediatr.* **90**:192–195.

Bisset, G. S., III. (1991). Magnetic resonance imaging of congenital heart disease in the pediatric patient. *Radiol. Clin. North Am.* **29**:279–291.

Borow, K. M., and Braunwald, E. (1988). Congenital heart disease in the adult. In *Heart Disease: A Textbook of Cardiovascular Medicine*. Saunders, Philadelphia.

Brandstetter, R. D., and Cohen, R. P. (1979). Hypoxemia after thoracentesis: a predictable and treatable condition. *JAMA* **242**(10):1060–1061.

Broaddus, V. C., Wiener-Kronish, J. P., Berthiaume, Y., and Staub, N. C. (1988). Removal of pleural liquid and protein by lymphatics in awake sheep. *J. Appl. Physiol.* **64**(1):384–390.

Broaddus, V. C., Wiener-Kronish, J. P., and Staub, N. C. (1990). Clearance of lung edema into the pleural space of volume-loaded anesthetized sheep. *J. Appl. Physiol.* **68**(6):2623–2630.

Cabanes, L. R., Weber, S. N., Matran, R., Regnard, J., Richard, M. O., Degeorges, M. E., and Lockhart, A. (1989). Bronchial hyperresponsiveness to methacholine in patients with impaired left ventricular function. *N. Engl. J. Med.* **320**:1317–1322.

Cámara, M. L., Aris, A., Padró, J. M., and Caralps, J. M. (1988). Long-term results of mitral valve surgery in patients with severe pulmonary hypertension. *Ann. Thorac. Surg.* **45**:133–136.

Cassin, S., Dawes, G. S., Mott, J. C., Ross, B. B., and Strang, L. B. (1964). The vascular resistance of the foetal and newly ventilated lung of the lamb. *J. Physiol.* **171**:61–79.

Child, J. S. (1990). Echo-Doppler and color-flow imaging in congenital heart disease. In *Doppler Echocardiography*. Saunders, Philadelphia.

Csete, M. E., Abraham, W. M., and Wanner, A. (1990). Vasomotion influences airflow in peripheral airways. *Am. Rev. Resp. Dis.* **141**:1409–1413.

Dalen, J. E., Matloff, J. M., Evans, G. L., Hoppin, F. G., Bhardwaj, P., Harken, D. E., and Dexter, L. (1967). Early reduction of pulmonary vascular resistance after mitral valve replacement. *N. Engl. J. Med.* **277**:387–394.

Dawson, A., Rocamora, J. M., and Morgan, J. R. (1976). Regional lung function in chronic pulmonary congestion with and without mitral stenosis. *Am. Rev. Respir. Dis.* **113**:51–59.

Deffebach, M. E., Charan, N. B., Lakshminarayan, S., and Butler, J. (1987). The bronchial circulation: small, but a vital attribute of the lung. *Am. Rev. Respir. Dis.* **135**:463–481.

De Troyer, A., Yernault, J-C., and Englert, M. (1977). Lung hypoplasia in congenital pulmonary valve stenosis. *Circulation* **56**(4):647–651.

De Troyer, A., Estenne, M., and Yernault, J. C. (1980). Disturbance of respiratory muscle function in patients with mitral valve disease. *Am. J. Med.* **69**:867–873.

Edwards, W. D. (1988). Pathology of pulmonary hypertension. *Cardiovasc. Clin.* **18**:321–359.

Eichacker, P. Q., Seidelman, M. J., Rothstein, M. S., and Lejemtel, T. (1988). Methacholine bronchial reactivity testing in patients with chronic congestive heart failure. *Chest* **93**:336–338.

Erdmann, A. J. I., Vaughan, T. R., Brigham, K. L., Woolverton, W. C., and Staub, N. C. (1975). Effect of increased vascular pressure on lung fluid balance in unanesthetized sheep. *Circ. Res.* **37**:271–284.

Estenne, M., Yernault, J.-C., and De Troyer, A. (1983). Mechanism of relief of dyspnea after thoracocentesis in patients with large pleural effusions. *Am. J. Med.* **74**:813–819.

Fein, A. M., Grossman, R. F., Jones, J. G., et al. (1984). The value of edema fluid protein measurements in patients with pulmonary edema. *Am. J. Med.* **67**:32–39.

Ferguson, F. C., Kobilak, R. E., and Deitrick, J. E. (1944). Varices of the bronchial veins as a source of hemoptysis in mitral stenosis. *Am. Heart J.* **28**:445–456.

Fraser, R. G., and Paré, J. A. P. (1977). *Diagnosis of Diseases of the Chest.* Saunders, Philadelphia.

Garson, A., Jr., Gorry, G. A., McNamara, D. G., and Cooley, D. A. (1980). The surgical decision in tetralogy of Fallot: weighing risks and benefits with decision analysis. *Am. J. Cardio.* **45**:108–116.

Gee, M. H., and Havill, A. M. (1980). The relationship between pulmonary perivascular cuff fluid and lung lymph in dogs with edema. *Microvasc.* Res. **19**:209–216.

Gersony, W. M. (1984). Neonatal pulmonary hypertension: pathophysiology, classification, and etiology. *Clin. Perinatol.* **11**(3):517–548.

Gersony, W. M., Peckham, G. J., Ellison, R. C., Miettinen, O. S., and Nadas, A. S. (1983). Effects of indomethacin in premature infants with patent ductus arteriosus: Results of a national collaborative study. *J. Pediatr.* **102**:895–906.

Griffin, A. J., Ferrara, J. D., Lax, J. O., and Cassels, D. E. (1972). Pulmonary compliance. An index of cardiovascular status in infancy. *Am. J. Dis. Child.* **123**:89.

Hales, C. A., and Kazemi, H. (1974). Small-airways function in myocardial infarction. *N. Engl. J. Med.* **290**:761–765.

Hatle, L. (1990). Doppler echocardiographic evaluation of mitral stenosis. *Cardiol. Clin.* **8**:233–247.

Haworth, S. G., and Reid, L. (1978). A morphometric study of regional variation in lung structure in infants with pulmonary hypertension and congenital cardiac defect: a justification of lung biopsy. *Br. Heart J.* **40**:825–831.

Haworth, S. G., Radley-Smith, R., and Yacoub, M. (1987). Lung biopsy findings in transposition of the great arteries with ventricular septal defect: potentially reversible pulmonary vascular disease is not always synonymous with operability. *J. Am. Coll. Cardio.* **9**:327–333.

Heath, D., and Edwards, J. E. (1958). The pathology of hypertensive pulmonary vascular disease. *Circulation* **18**:533–547.

Heath, D., Helmholz, H. F., and Burchell, H. B. (1958). Graded pulmonary vascular changes and hemodynamic findings in cases of atrial and ventricular septal defect and patent ductus arteriosus. *Circulation* **18**:1155.

Hogg, J. C., Agarawal, J. B., Gardiner, A. J. S., Palmer, W. H., and Macklem, P. T. (1972). Distribution of airway resistance with developing pulmonary edema in dogs. *J. Appl. Physiol.* **32**:20–24.

Hornberger, L. K., Sahn, D. J., Krabill, K. A., Sherman, F. S., Swensson, R. E., Pesonen, E., Hagen-Ansert, S., and Chung, K. J. (1989). Elucidation of the natural history of ventricular septal defects by serial Doppler color flow mapping studies. *J. Am. Coll. Cardiol.* **13**:1111–1118.

Jamieson, S. W., Stinson, E. B., Oyer, P. E., Reitz, B. A., Baldwin, J., Modry, D., Dawkins, K., Theodore, J., Hunt, S., and Shumway, N. E. (1984). Heart-lung transplantation for irreversible pulmonary hypertension. *Ann. Thorac. Surg.* **38**:554–562.

Jerome, E. H., Broaddus, V. C., Arakawa, M., Osorio, O., Neuberger, M., and Staub, N. C. (1989). Evidence for mediastinal clearance of interstitial pulmonary edema (abstract). *FASEB J.* **3**:A374.

Jones, J. G., Lemen, R., and Graf, P. D. (1978). Changes in airway calibre following pulmonary venous congestion. *Br. J. Anaesth.* **50**:743–751.

Kanjuh, V. I., Sellers, R. D., and Edwards, J. E. (1964). Pulmonary vascular plexiform lesion. *Arch. Pathol.* **78**:513.

Kawaguchi, A., Gandjbakhch, I., Pavie, A., Bors, V., Muneretto, C., Leger, P., Mestiri, T., Piazza, C., Cabrol, A., Desruennes, M., and Cabrol., C. (1989). Cardiac transplant recipients with preoperative pulmonary hypertension: evolution of pulmonary hemodynamics and surgical options. *Circulation* **80** (suppl III):III-90-III-96.

Kikuchi, R. K., Sekizawa, K., Sasaki, H., Hirose, Y., Matsumoto, N., Takishima, T., and Hildebrandt, J. (1984). Effects of pulmonary congestion on airway reactivity to histamine aerosol in dogs. *J. Appl. Physiol.* **57**(5):1640–1647.

Krell, W. S., and Rodarte, J. R. (1985). Effects of acute pleural effusion on respiratory system mechanics in dogs. *J. Appl. Physiol.* **59**(5):1458–1463.

Lai-Fook, S. J., Beck, K. C., Sutcliffe, A. M., and Donaldson, J. T. (1984). Effect of edema and height on bronchial diameter and shape in excised dog lung. *Resp. Physiol.* **55**:223–237.

Lauweryns, J. M. (1970). The juxta-alveolar lymphatics in the human lung. *Am. Rev. Respir. Dis.* **102**:877–885.

Leffler, C. W., Hessler, J. R., and Green, R. S. (1984). The onset of breathing at birth stimulates pulmonary vascular prostacyclin synthesis. *Paediatr. Res.* **18**:938–42.

LeGal, Y. M. (1990). Lung and heart-lung transplantation. *Ann. Thorac. Surg.* **49**:840–844.

Levine, M. J., Weinstein, J. S., Diver, D. J., Berman, A. D., Wyman, R. M., Cunningham, M. J., Safian, R. D., Grossman, W., and McKay, R. G. (1989). Progressive improvement in pulmonary vascular resistance after percutaneous mitral valvuloplasty. *Circulation* **79**:1061–1067.

Liao, P-K., Edwards, W. D., Julsrud, P. R., Puga, F. J., Danielson, G. K., and Feldt, R. H. (1985). Pulmonary blood supply in patients with pulmonary atresia and ventricular septal defect. *J. Am. Coll. Cardiol.* **6**(6):1343–1350.

Light, R. W., and George, R. B. (1983). Serial pulmonary function in patients with acute heart failure. *Arch. Intern. Med.* **143**:429–433.

Lilker, E. S., and Nagy, E. J. (1975). Gas exchange in the pulmonary collateral circulation of dogs. *Am. Rev. Respir. Dis.* **112**:615–620.

Lloyd, R. C. (1980). Reflex effects of left heart and pulmonary vascular distension on airways of dogs. *J. Appl. Physiol.* **49**:620–626.

Mackersie, R. C., Christensen, J., and Lewis, F. R. (1987). The role of pulmonary lymphatics in the clearance of hydrostatic pulmonary edema. *J. Surg. Res.* **43**:495–504.

Malo, J., Ali, J., and Wood, L. D. H. (1984). How does positive end-expiratory pressure reduce intrapulmonary shunt in canine pulmonary edema? *J. Appl. Physiol.* **57**:1002–1010.

Matthay, M. A., and Wiener-Kronish, J. P. (1990). Intact epithelial barrier function is critical for the resolution of alveolar edema in humans. *Am. Rev. Respir. Dis.* **142**:1250–1257.

Matthay, M. A., Landolt, C. C., and Staub, N. C. (1982). Differential liquid and protein clearance from the alveoli of anesthetized sheep. *J. Appl. Physiol.* **53**(1):96–104.

McGregor, C. G. A., Jamieson, S. W., Baldwin, J. C., Burke, C. M., Dawkins, K. D., Stinson, E. B., Oyer, P. E., Billingham, M. E., Zusman, D. R., Reitz, B. A., Morris, A., Yousem, S., Hunt, S. A., and Shumway, N. E. (1986). Combined heart-lung transplantation for end-stage Eisenmenger's syndrome. *J. Thorac. Cardiovasc. Surg.* **91**:443–450.

Meyrick, B., and Reid, L. (1978). The effect of continued hypoxia on rat pulmonary arterial circulation: an ultrastructure study. *Lab. Invest.* **38**:188–200.

Moreno, R. H., Hogg, J. C., and Paré, P. D. (1986). Mechanics of airway narrowing. *Am. Rev. Respir. Dis.* **133**:1171–1180.

Muir, A. L., Flenley, C., Kirby, B. J., Sudlow, M. F., Guyatt, A. R., and Brash, H. M. (1975). Cardiorespiratory effects of rapid saline infusion in normal man. *J. Appl. Physiol.* **38**:786–793.

Murray, J. F. (1986). *The Normal Lung*. Saunders, Philadelphia.

Naeye, R. L., and Vennart, G. P. (1960). Structure and significance of pulmonary plexiform structures. *Am. J. Pathol.* **36**:593.

Newfeld, E. A., Waldman, J. D., Paul, M. H., Muster, A. J., Cole, R. B., Idriss, F., and Riker, W. (1977). Pulmonary vascular disease after systemic-pulmonary arterial shunt operations. *Am. J. Cardiol.* **39**:715–720.

Noble, W. H., Kay, J. C., and Obdrzalek, J. (1975). Lung mechanics in hypervolemic pulmonary edema. *J. Appl. Physiol.* **38**:681–687.

Noland, S. P. (1987). The origin of pulmonary artery banding. *J. Thorac. Cardiovasc. Surg.* **44**:427.

Nugent, E. W., Plauth, J., W. H., Edwards, J. E., and Williams, W. H. (1990). The pathology, abnormal physiology, clinical recognition, and medical and surgical treatment of congenital heart disease. In *The Heart, Arteries and Veins*. McGraw-Hill, New York.

Ohmichi, M., Tagaki, S., Nomura, N., Tsunematsu K., and Suzuki, A. (1988). Endobronchial changes in chronic pulmonary venous hypertension. *Chest* **94**:1127–1132.

Ohno, K., Nakahara, K., Hirose, H., Nahano, S., and Kawashima, Y. (1987). Effects of valvular surgery on overall and regional lung function in patients with mitral stenosis. *Chest* **92**(2):224–228.

Olley, P. M., Coceani, F., and Badach, E. (1976). E-type prostaglandins: a new emergency therapy for certain cyanotic congenital heart malformations. *Circulation* **53**(4):728–731.

Parsons, J. M., and Baker, E. J. (1990). The use of magnetic resonance imaging in the investigation of infants and children with congenital heart disease: current status and future prospects. *Int. J. Cardiol.* **29**:263–275.

Pison, C., Malo, J-L., Rouleau, J-L., Chalaoui, J., Ghezzo, H., and Malo, J. (1989). Bronchial hyperresponsiveness to inhaled methacholine in subjects with chronic left heart failure at a time of exacerbation and after increasing diuretic therapy. *Chest* **96**:230–235.

Poiani, G. J., Tozzi, C. A., Yohn, S. E., Pierce, R. A., Belsky, S. A., Berg, R. A., Yu, S. Y., Deak, S. B., and Riley, D. J. (1990). Collagen and elastin metabolism in hypertensive pulmonary arteries of rats. *Circ. Res.* **66**:968–978.

Ponce, F. E., Williams, L. C., Webb, H. M., Riopel, D. A., and Hohn, A. R. (1973). Propranolol palliation of tetralogy of Fallot: experience with long-term drug treatment in pediatric patients. *Pediatrics* **52**:100–108.

Rabinovitch, M., and Reid, L. M. (1980). Quantitative structural analysis of the pulmonary vascular bed in congenital heart defects. *Cardiovasc. Clin.* **11**:149–169.

Rabinovitch, M., Keane, J. F., Fellows, K. E., Castaneda, A. R., and Reid, L. (1981). Quantitative analysis of the pulmonary wedge angiogram in congenital heart defects. *Circulation* **63**:152–164.

Reid, L. M. (1979). The pulmonary circulation: Remodeling in growth and disease. *Am. Rev. Respir. Dis.* **119**:531–546.

Rendas, A., Lennox, S., and Reid, L. (1979). Aorta-pulmonary shunts in growing pigs: functional and structural assessment of the changes in the pulmonary circulation. *J. Thorac. Cardiovasc. Surg.* **77**:109–118.

Rhodes, K. M., Evemy, K., Nariman, S., and Gibson, G. J. (1985). Effects of mitral valve surgery on static lung function and exercise performance. *Thorax* **40**:107–112.

Rolla, G., Scappaticci, E., Baldi, S., and Bucca, C. (1986). Methacholine inhalation challenge after rapid saline infusion in healthy subjects. *Respiration* **50**:18–22.

Ruzyllo, W., Nihill, M. R., Mullins, C. E., and McNamara, D. G. (1974). Hemodynamic evaluation of 221 patients after intracardiac repair of tetralogy of Fallot. *Am. J. Cardiol.* **34**:565–576.

Schiller, N. B. (1990). Pulmonary artery pressure estimation by Doppler and two-dimensional echocardiography. *Cardiol. Clin.* **8**:277–287.

Seibert, A. F., Allison, R. C., Bryars, C. H., and Kirkpatrick, M. B. (1989). Normal airway responsiveness to methacholine in cardiac asthma. *Am. Rev. Respir. Dis.* **140**:1805–1806.

Selzer, A. (1975) *Principles of Clinical Cardiology: An Analytical Approach.* Saunders, Philadelphia.

Selzer, A., and Malmborg, R. O. (1962). Some factors influencing changes in pulmonary vascular resistance in mitral valvular disease. *Am. J. Med.* **32**:532–544.

Staub, N. C. (1971). Steady-state pulmonary transvascular water filtration in unanesthetized sheep. *Circ. Res.* **28**(suppl I):I-135–I-139.

Staub, N. C. (1983). Alveolar flooding and clearance. *Am. Rev. Respir. Dis.* **127**:S44–S50.

Staub, N. C., Nagano, H., and Pearce, M. L. (1967). Pulmonary edema in dogs, especially the sequence of fluid accumulation in lungs. *J. Appl. Physiol.* **22**(2):227–240.

Stenmark, K. R., Fasules, J., Hyde, D. M. Voelkel, N. F., Henson, J., Tucker, A., Wilson, H., and Reeves, J. T. (1987). Severe pulmonary hypertension and arterial adventitial changes in newborn calves at 4300 m. *J. Appl. Physiol.* **62**:821–830.

Takkunen, O., Mattila, S., Nieminen, M. S., Sovijärvi, A. R. A., Luosto, R., and Merikallio, E. (1987). Cardiorespiratory function after correction of tetralogy of Fallot. *Scand. J. Thorac. Cardiovasc. Surg.* **21**:21–26.

Tozzi, C. A., Poiani, G. J., Harangozo, A. M., Boyd, C. D., and Riley, D. J. (1989). Pressure-induced connective tissue synthesis in pulmonary artery segments is dependent on intact endothelium. *J. Clin. Invest.* **84**: 1005–1012.

Vick, G. W., Rokey, R., Huhta, J. C., Mulvagh, S. L., and Johnston, D. L. (1990). Nuclear magnetic resonance imaging of the pulmonary arteries, subpulmonary region, and aorticopulmonary shunts: a comparative study with two-dimensional echocardiography and angiography. *Am. Heart J.* **119**:1103–1110.

Villanueva, F. S., Murali, S., Uretsky, B. F., Reddy, P. S., Griffith, B. P., Hardesty, R. L., and Kormos, R. L. (1989). Resolution of severe pulmonary hypertension after heterotopic cardiac tranplantation. *J. Am. Coll. Cardiol.* **14**(5):1239–1243.

Viola, A. R., and Abbate, E. H. (1973). Respiratory function and effective collateral flow 8 years after ligation of the left pulmonary artery. *Am. Rev. Respir. Dis.* **108**:1216–1220.

Virmani, R., and Roberts, W. C. (1979). Pulmonary arteries in congenital heart disease: a structure-function analysis. *Cardiovasc. Clin.* **10**:455–499.

Wagenvoort, C. A. (1985). Open lung biopsies in congenital heart disease for evaluation of pulmonary vascular disease. Predictive value with regard to corrective operability. *Histopathology* **9**:417–436.

Wagenvoort, C. A., and Wagenvoort, N. (1977). *Pathology of Pulmonary Hypertension*. Wiley, New York.

Wagenvoort, C. A., Wagenvoort, N., and Draulans-Noë, Y. (1984). Reversibility of plexogenic pulmonary arteriopathy following banding of the pulmonary artery. *J. Thorac. Cardiovasc. Surg.* **87**:876–886.

Walson, A., Peter, R. H., Morris, J. J., Kong, Y., and Behar, V. S. (1973). Clinical implications of pulmonary hypertension in mitral stenosis. *Am. J. Cardiol.* **32**:650–655.

Warren, R. L., and Powell, W. J. (1986). Acute alveolar hypoxia increases bronchopulmonary shunt flow in the dog. *J. Clin. Invest.* **77**:1515–1524.

Wessel, H. U., Cunningham, W. J., Paul, M. H., Bastanier, C. K., Muster, A. J., and Idriss, F. S. (1980). Exercise performance in tetralogy of Fallot after intracardiac repair. *J. Thorac. Cardiovasc. Surg.* **80**:582–593.

Wood, P. (1958). The Eisenmenger syndrome or pulmonary hypertension with reversed central shunt. *Br. Med. J.* 701–762.

Wood, P., Besterman, E. M., Towers, M. K., and McIlroy, M. B. (1957). The effect of acetylcholine on pulmonary vascular resistance and left atrial pressure in mitral stenosis. *Br. Heart J.* **19**:279–286.

Wood, T. E., McLeod, P., Anthonisen, N. R., and Macklem, P. T. (1971). Mechanics of breathing in mitral stenosis. *Am. Rev. Respir. Dis.* **104**:52–60.

Yoshioka, T., Nakanishi, N., Okubo, S., Kunieda, T., Ishikura, F., and Nagata, S. (1990). Improvement in pulmonary function in mitral stenosis after percutaneous transvenous mitral commissurotomy. *Chest* **98**:290–294.

Zener, J. C., Hancock, E. W., Shumway, N. E., and Harrison, D. C. (1972). Regression of extreme pulmonary hypertension after mitral valve surgery. *Am. J. Cardiol.* **30**:820–826.

4

Pancreatic, Liver, Gastrointestinal, and Renal Diseases

NEIL A. ETTINGER

Washington University School of Medicine
St. Louis, Missouri

ROBERT M. SENIOR

Washington University School of Medicine and
Jewish Hospital at Washington University Medical Center
St. Louis, Missouri

I. Introduction

Abdominal disease processes often produce intrathoracic complications, which may at times be the first clinical manifestation of the abdominal problem (Senior and Lefrak, 1988). Depending on the nature of the abdominal problem, the intrathoracic complication can vary widely (Table 1). The purpose of this chapter is to summarize the main intrathoracic manifestations of several common abdominal problems: acute pancreatitis, chronic liver disease, gastrointestinal disease, and chronic renal disease.

II. Acute Pancreatitis

As noted in a recent review, acute pancreatitis has an annual incidence of approximately 43 cases per 100,000 population in the United States and accounts for more than 2200 deaths (Shapiro et al., 1989). Pulmonary complications are common in acute pancreatitis and are among the most serious features of this disorder (Buggy and Nostrant, 1983; Lankisch et al., 1983; Renner, et al., 1985). Indeed, the gravity of developing pulmonary dysfunction is reflected by the inclusion of arterial hypoxemia ($Pao_2 < 60$ mmHg) as one of four indicators of a

Table 1 Thoracic Manifestations of Abdominal Processes

	Pleural	Pulmonary infiltrates			Pulmonary
Abdominal organ	effusion	ARDS	Pneumonia	Fibrosis	hypertension
Pancreas					
Pancreatitis	•	•			
Abscess	•				
Pseudocyst	•				
Carcinoma	•				
Kidney					
Renal failure	•			•	•
Nephrotic syndrome	• (T)				
Hypernephroma	•				•
Ureteral obstruction	• (T)				
Vasculitis					
Transplantation	•	•	•		
Peritoneal dialysis	• (T)				
Liver					
Cirrhosis	• (T)			•	•
Amebic abscess	•				
Hepatoma	•				
Hepatic resection	•	•	•		
Transplantation	• (T)	•	•		
Schistosomiasis					•
Gastrointestinal					
Aspiration		•	•		
Colitis/Crohn's			•		
Abdominal Abscess	•	•	•		
Peritonitis	•	•			
Abdominal tumor	•				

(T) = transudate

severe episode, along with a fall of > 10 percentage points in hemotocrit, a decrease in serum calcium to < 8 mg/dl, and fluid sequestration of > 6000 mL (Pitchumoni et al., 1988).

For convenience of discussion, the pulmonary manifestations of acute pancreatitis have been divided into three categories based on the chest radiograph and arterial oxygenation: (1) hypoxemia with a normal chest radiograph; (2) hypoxemia with pleural effusion and, often, nonspecific chest radiographic

Pulmonary emboli	Alveolar hemorrhage	Pulmonary calcification	Pulmonary nodules	Mediastinal adenopathy
•			•	
	•	•		
•				
•			•	•
	•			
•		•	•	•
•			•	
•		•	•	
•			•	

findings such as basilar atelectasis and elevated hemidiaphragm; and (3) severe hypoxemia with widespread alveolar infiltrates on the radiograph and a picture indistinguishable from other causes of the adult respiratory distress syndrome (ARDS) (Basran et al., 1987; Shapiro et al., 1989). Patients can progress rapidly from category 1 to category 2 or 3, so any evidence of pulmonary dysfunction early in acute pancreatitis needs to be viewed as heralding the possibility of eventual ARDS.

A. Hypoxemia

Arterial hypoxemia with a normal chest radiograph is common in acute pancreatitis (Levine et al., 1990). Of 116 patients, 69% had a Pao_2 below 76 mmHg during the initial 48 h and in 38% the Pao_2 was below 66 mmHg (Ranson et al., 1973). Hypoxemia is observed even among individuals in whom there is no underlying cardiopulmonary disease and in whom a normal Pao_2 is found after recovery. Ventilation-perfusion imbalance appears to be the predominant mechanism for hypoxemia, because there are only minor reductions in diffusing capacity and alveolar hypoventilation is rarely present, even though breathing may be impaired due to abdominal distention and pain (Murphy et al., 1980). A leftward shift of the oxyhemoglobin dissociation curve has also been observed in acute pancreatitis (Greenburg et al., 1977). but this abnormality alone cannot explain the observed reductions in Pao_2 without concurrent disturbances of alveolar gas exchange. From a clinical standpoint, it is well to appreciate that a normal chest radiograph during a bout of acute pancreatitis does not exclude the possibility of severe arterial hypoxemia.

Acute pancreatitis appears to be distinct from other acute intra-abdominal inflammatory processes with regard to the high incidence of arterial hypoxemia it causes. A comparison of 84 patients with acute pancreatitis and 68 other hospitalized patients with acute abdominal pain that was not due to pancreatitis, of similar age and sex, revealed that hypoxemia was substantially more common and longer lasting among those with acute pancreatitis (Imrie et al., 1977).

B. Pleural Effusion

Chest radiographic abnormalities are also common during acute pancreatitis. The typical findings are small pleural effusions, atelectasis, and elevations of a hemidiaphragm. In one recent study involving 89 patients, pleural effusions were found in 24% and atelectatic changes or an elevated hemidiaphragm was observed in 9% and 5%, respectively (Glasser et al., 1987).

Three mechanisms appear to be involved in the production of pleural effusions associated with acute pancreatitis: (1) leakage of peripancreatic exudates from inflamed lymphatics on the thoracic side of the diaphragm that communicate with peritoneal lymphtics that drain the pancreatic space; (2) extravasation of protein-rich liquid from diaphragmatic capillaries whose permeability is increased because of inflammation in the adjacent pancreas; and (3) movement of peripancreatic exudates directly into the thorax through sinus tracts in the diaphragm (created by the episode of pancreatitis) or through the esophageal or aortic hiatus (Light, 1985). Sinus tract formation is most characteristic of pancreatic pseudocyst. However, when pancreatitis causes the accumulation of a large volume of ascites and there are preexisting defects in the diaphragm, abdominal fluid moves directly from the abdomen into the pleural space in a manner analogous to hepatic hydrothorax (described later). Pleural effusions associated with acute pancreatitis are typically asymptomatic and resolve spontaneously coincident with resolution of the abdominal problems (Table 2).

Besides transient pleural effusions, acute pancreatitis can lead to chronic intrathoracic fluid accumulations (Table 2) that localize in one or both pleural cavities. Occasionally, the fluid is found in both the mediastinum and the pleural space or even exclusively in the mediastinum. These chronic effusions may be massive, and they typically have extraordinarily high amylase values. In contrast to the transient, asymptomatic effusions that are typical of the acute phase of pancreatitis, chronic effusions may produce symptoms that dominate the clinical picture (Dewan et al., 1984; Rockey and Cello, 1990). Interestingly, the episode of acute pancreatitis that triggered the development of a chronic effusion may have been unrecognized (Shapiro et al., 1989). Chronic intrathoracic pancreatitic effusions usually indicate ongoing pancreatic disease, particularly the formation of a pancreatic pseudocyst, but in some cases there is no evidence of a pancreatic abnormality (Dewan et al., 1984). The management of chronic pancreatic intrathoracic effusions will depend on a variety of factors. A 2- to 4-week trial of medical therapy, including no oral intake, total parenteral nutrition,

Table 2 Features of Pleural Effusions Associated with Pancreatitis

	Acute effusions	Chronic effusions
Onset	Occur coincident with acute abdominal symptoms	May occur months after resolution of abdominal symptoms
Symptoms	Abdominal complaints dominant	Chest symptoms prominent, abdominal complaints may be absent
Size	Small to moderate	Large to massive
Appearance	Serosanguineous	Bloody, serosanguineous, or purulent
Characteristics	Exudate, pleural fluid amylase greater than serum amylase	Exudate, pleural fluid amylase much greater than serum amylase
Course	Resolve coincident with abdominal symptoms	Can be recurrent
Treatment	Usually none required	Serial thoracentesis, tube drainage, or operative treatment of fistula

Source: Adapted with permission from Shapiro et al., 1989.

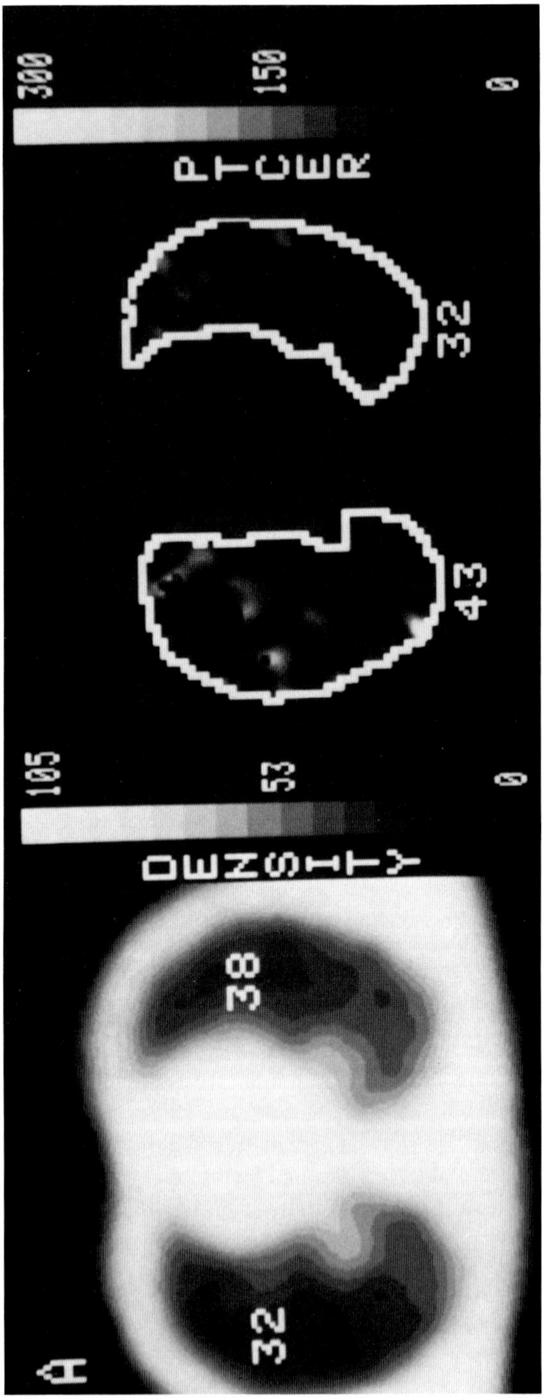
A
32
38
DENSITY
105
53
0
43
32
300
150
0

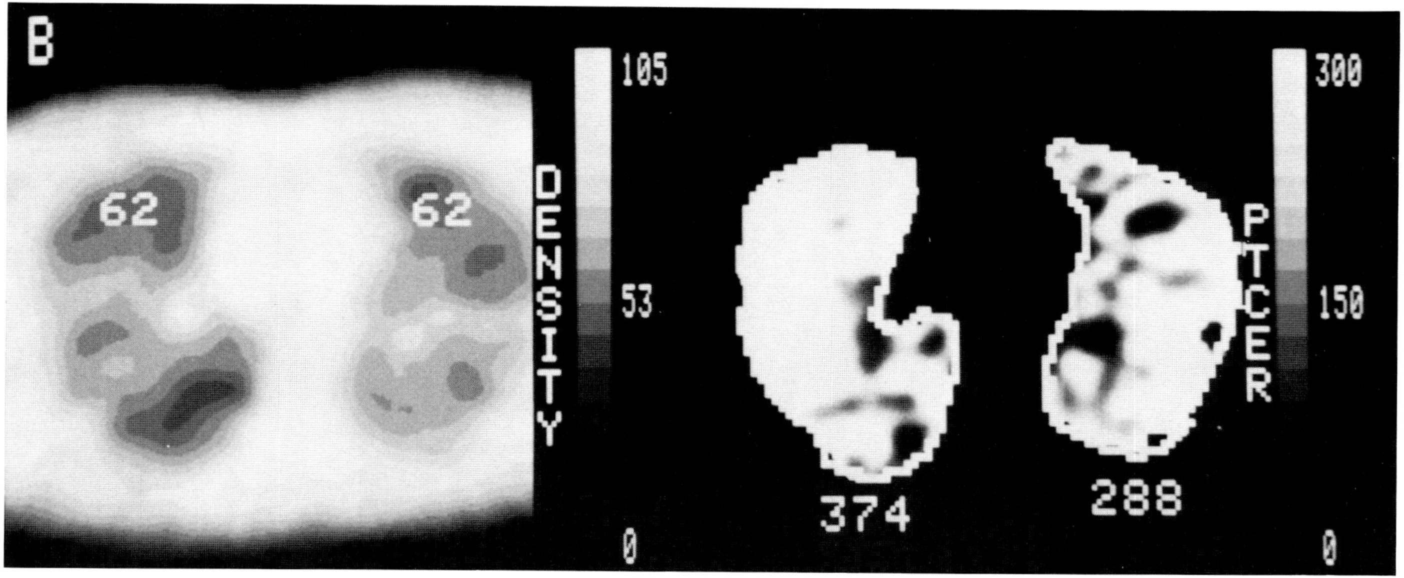

Figure 1 Representative positron emission tomographic (PET) images for a normal subject (A) and a 53-year-old woman with the adult respiratory distress syndrome 3 days after the onset of acute pancreatitis (B). Average values are indicated for each lung region for total lung density (g/100 ml tissue) and pulmonary transcapillary escape rate (PTCER, 10^{-4} min^{-1}) for radiolabeled transferrin, an index of protein permeability. Normal density values are 39 ± 4.7 g/100 ml lung and PTCER values are 21 ± 11 × 10^{-4} min^{-1} for normals and 170 ± 79 during acute ARDS. (Kindly provided by Dr. James D. Kaplan, Washington University Medical Center.) (See Schuster, 1989, for details regarding PET techniques).

repeated thoracentesis or tube thoracostomy, and agents to suppress pancreatic secretion, was recently recommended (Rockey and Cello, 1990). Percutanous drainage is another approach that has been successful (Faling et al., 1984). If these measures fail, surgery is indicated to eliminate the pancreaticopleural fistula. Rarely, thoracic surgery for pleural decortication has been required (Shapiro et al., 1970).

C. Adult Respiratory Distress Syndrome

As with some other situations that do not originate in the lungs, such as sepsis, massive blood transfusions, and disseminated intravascular coagulation, acute pancreatitis can be associated with parenchymal lung injury and multiorgan failure (Murray et al., 1988). Although pulmonary complications of pancreatitis were recognized earlier, the first clear-cut description of the adult respiratory distress syndrome of (ARDS) complicating pancreatitis was in 1972 (Interiano et al., 1972). In that report, 9 (18%) of 50 consecutive patients with acute pancreatitis developed an ARDS picture and five of these patients died. ARDS remains a common, potentially lethal complication of acute pancreatitis (Robertson et al., 1988), but as a cause of ARDS, pancreatitis is infrequent, accounting for perhaps 1% of cases (Fowler et al., 1983).

Considering the high incidence of arterial hypoxemia that accompanies acute pancreatitis, one would speculate that direct evidence of lung injury should be demonstrable in most patients with acute pancreatitis. Indeed, increased pulmonary vascular permeability is a regular finding in experimental acute pancreatitis (Burnweit and Horton, 1988; Garcia-Szabo and Malik, 1984; Guice et al., 1988; Tahamont et al., 1982). However, using indium-113m labeled transferrin to quantify pulmonary vascular permeability in 16 patients with pancreatitis, Robertson and co-workers (1988) observed increased permeability only in those with ARDS and normal permeability in patients without ARDS. Positron emission tomography, another means of examining pulmonary vascular permeability in humans (Schuster, 1989), may also find application in the study of lung involvement in pancreatitis (Fig. 1).

Several mechanisms may be involved in producing the pulmonary injury and dysfunction associated with acute pancreatitis: (1) direct toxic effects of pancreatic enzymes (Garcia-Szabo and Malik, 1984) and/or triglycerides (Kimura et al., 1979) on the pulmonary microvasculature; (2) diminished pulmonary surfactant due to destruction by phospholipases or impaired surfactant synthesis (Das et al., 1987; Guice et al., 1987); and (3) pulmonary microvascular damage secondary to neutrophil-generated oxygen products (Guice et al., 1989a). It is important to recognize that these possibilities are not mutually exclusive, nor are these the only possibilities. As emphasized recently, the production of ARDS is complex (Rinaldo and Christman, 1990).

A number of animal models have been developed to study the basis for lung injury associated with acute pancreatitis. Among these are injections of trypsin and bile acids into the pancreatic ducts of sheep (Tahamont et al., 1982) and intravenous infusions of cerulein, a cholecystokinin analog, in rats (Guice et al., 1988). In both these models the animals develop increased pulmonary vascular permeability with thickening of alveolar septa and congestion of pulmonary capillaries with large numbers of leukocytes (Fig. 2). Although given intravenously, cerulein appears to produce its effects indirectly via pancreatitis since it has no demonstrable direct effect on lung parenchyma in isolated perfused lung preparations or in cultures of pulmonary artery endothelial cells and alveolar type 2 cells.

In these animal models of acute pancreatitis, neutrophil depletion protects against lung injury even though the severity of pancreatitis is similar to that in animals with normal neutrophil counts (Barie et al., 1982; Guice et al., 1989a). The lungs are also protected by interruption of the complement pathway with cobra venom factor (Guice et al., 1989b), by infusions of aprotinin to inhibit pancreatic proteinases (Garcia-Szabo and Malik, 1984), or by infusions of antioxidants such as superoxide dismutase and catalase (Guice et al., 1989b) (Fig. 2). These results, together with the findings of elevated circulating concentrations of C5a in patients with acute pancreatitis (Perez et al., 1983), suggest that neutrophil activation and sequestration in the lungs with release of toxic oxygen products play a central role in causing lung injury associated with acute pancreatitis.

III. Chronic Liver Disease

Patients with chronic liver disease can develop a number of pulmonary problems that may be a direct result of the underlying liver disorder. Severe arterial hypoxemia and pulmonary hypertension are two examples of important hepatopulmonary complications; however, a variety of other thoracic abnormalities occur (Table 3). Liver disease may also affect the lungs indirectly. Massive ascites, for example, can reduce lung volumes and disturb V_A/Q relationships (Ruff et al., 1971). The association between lung disorders and liver disease has taken on new importance with the recent success of orthotopic liver transplantation (OLT) (Busuttil et al., 1986). Substantial numbers of patients with chronic liver disease now require preoperative and postoperative pulmonary assessment (Ettinger and Trulock, 1991). Abnormal pulmonary findings prior to transplantation may, therefore, be relevant to the patient's intraoperative and postoperative course.

A. Types Implicated

Cirrhosis represents the end-stage of a large number of liver disorders, and the majority of patients with pulmonary complications of liver disease have "cirrhosis." Alcohol-related liver disease and chronic active hepatitis (either viral or

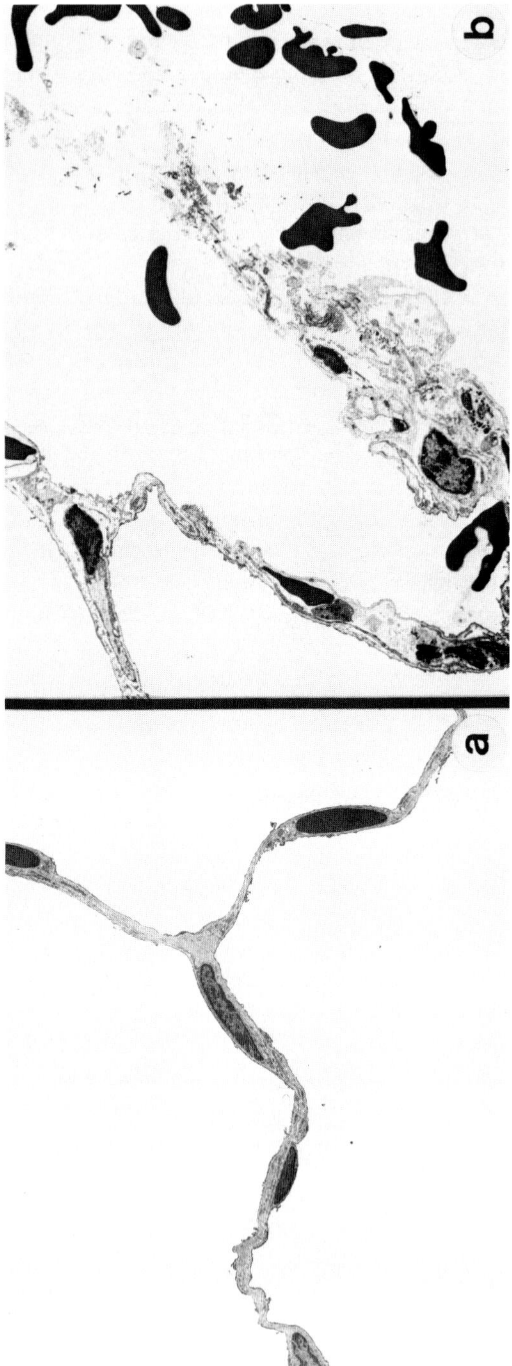
b
a

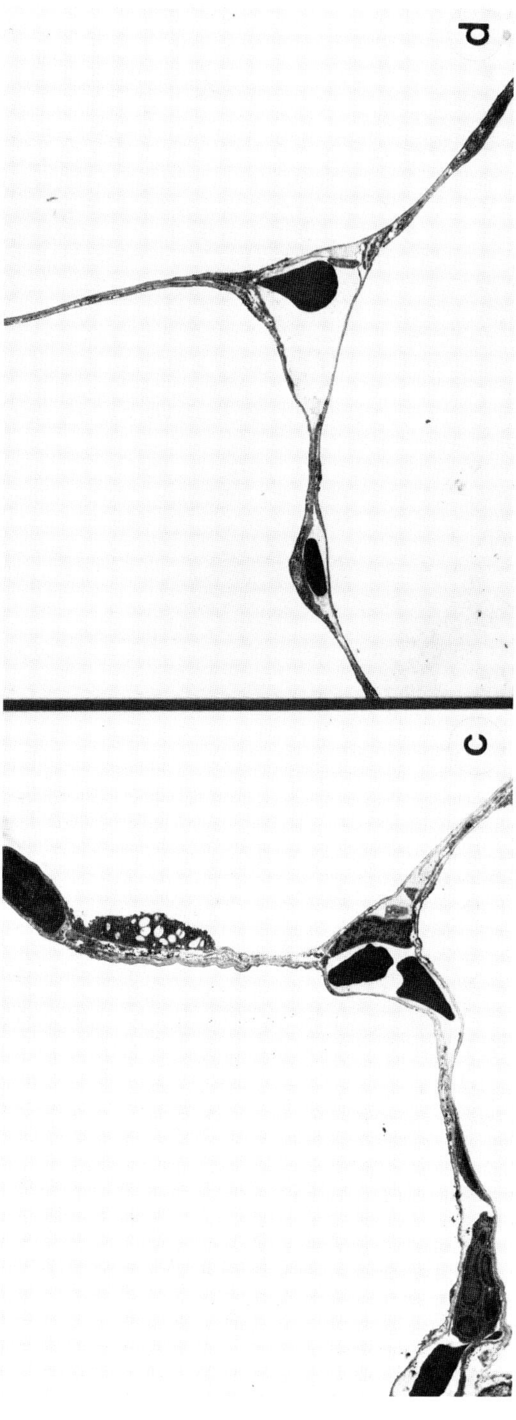

Figure 2 (a–d.) Photomicrographs (×2200) shown from a normal saline-infused rat lung (a) compared to a lung from an animal with cerulein-induced pancreatitis (b). (c) and (d) are lung samples taken from rats with cerulein-induced pancreatitis treated with superoxide dismutase or neutrophil depletion, respectively. Extensive endothelial damage, intra-alveolar hemorrhage, and interstitial edema are present in the cerulein-infused rat lung (b). These features of injury are absent in the SOD-treated, neutrophil-depleted, and normal lungs (c, d, and a). (Reproduced with permission from Guice et al., 1989a.)

Table 3 Liver Disorders and Their Most Common Associated Pulmonary Manifestations

	Type of Chronic Liver Disease				
Pulmonary Abnormality	Cirrhosis[a]	Primary biliary cirrhosis	α_1-antitrypsin deficiency	Chronic active hepatitis	Primary sclerosing cholangitis
Intrapulmonary vascular dilatation with and without shunt	+	+	+	+	
Pulmonary hypertension	+	+	+	+	
Expiratory airflow obstruction		+	+		
Chest wall deformity		+			
Pleural effusions	+	+			
Panacinar emphysema			+		
Pleuritis				+	
Bronchitis/bronchiectasis					+
Impaired hypoxic vasoconstriction	+				
Interstitial pneumonitis/fibrosis		+		+	

[a]Cryptogenic, alcoholic, and/or postnecrotic.
Source: Reproduced with permission from Krowka and Cortese, 1989.

autoimmune in etiology) are the most common causes of cirrhosis in North America. Differences in pathogenesis may account for the fact that specific liver diseases are associated with specific pulmonary complications (Table 3).

Primary Biliary Cirrhosis

Primary biliary cirrhosis (PBC) is caused by chronic inflammation of the intrahepatic bile ducts that ultimately leads to cholestasis, cirrhosis, and hepatic failure (Kaplan, 1987). PBC appears to be a systemic autoimmune disorder because it is strongly associated with immunological abnormalities, such as depressed T-suppressor cell function, hypergammaglobulinema, and the presence of antimitochondial antibodies (Culp et al., 1982). Moreover, Sjögren's syndrome (keratoconjunctivitis sicca and xerostomia) and scleroderma, presumably of autoimmune origin, occur in 66% and 20% of PBC patients, respectively (Krowka and Cortese, 1989; Rodriguez-Roisin et al., 1981).

PBC is rarely associated with clinical lung disease (Wallace et al., 1987; Wallaert et al., 1986), and it is the subset of PBC patients with Sjögren's syndrome that accounts for the majority of PBC patients with pulmonary findings. Dyspnea and a chronic, productive cough are the most frequent respiratory symptoms (Rodriguez-Roisin et al., 1981). Pulmonary function abnormalities, when present, are usually obstructive (Rodriguez-Roisin et al., 1981; Uddenfeldt et al., 1988), although a reduction in DLco occurs in over 50% of patients (Krowka and Cortese, 1989). Rapidly progressive interstitial disease resulting in death has been reported in four patients with the Sjögren's variant of PBC (Wallace et al., 1987). Patients with the scleroderma variant of PBC may also have pulmonary symptoms; however, as with the Sjögren's variant, a reduction in DLco is the most common, abnormal pulmonary finding (Clarke et al., 1978). Severe restrictive abnormalities or advanced pulmonary vascular disease, which are characteristic of scleroderma (Hunninghake and Fauci, 1979), have not been described in the PBC-scleroderma subset.

PBC has been associated with pulmonary fibrosis (Izdebeska-Makosa and Zeilinski, 1987), but this finding is rare (Wallaert et al., 1986). When interstitial lung disease is present, the most typical biopsy finding is lymphocytic interstitial pneumonitis (Krowka and Cortese, 1989), which may be recurrent and may progress to respiratory failure. Occasionally, granulomatous inflammation resembling sarcoidosis is described (Fagan et al., 1983; Maddrey, 1983). The actual incidence of lung involvement in PBC may be underestimated, however, because of the low level of pulmonary symptoms.

Wallaert and co-workers (1986) found evidence of lymphocytic alveolitis in bronchoalveolar lavage fluid in the majority of patients in the early stages of PBC, irrespective of the presence of the Sjögren's variant. The lavage fluid findings and the occasional overlapping clinical and histological features (Table

4) suggest that PBC and sarcoidosis may be etiologically related. However, the fact that patients with sarcoidosis rarely develop symptomatic liver disease and, conversely, that patients with PBC rarely develop the typical features of sarcoidosis argues against this hypothesis (Maddrey 1983). The question of whether these two disease entities are related awaits improvement in our understanding of the pathogenesis of these disorders.

An important thoracic complication of PBC is the development of chest wall deformity due to severe osteopenia. Patients with PBC often have abnormal vitamin D metabolism due to poor absorption of fat-soluble vitamins (vitamin D) and failure of hydroxylation of 25-hydroxy-vitamin D in the failing liver (Vierling, 1982). Vertebral compression fractures and rib fractures may occur, causing progressive loss of lung volume (Krowka and Cortese, 1989).

Chronic Active Hepatitis

Chronic active hepatitis (CAH) is characterized by inflammation of the hepatic parenchyma with associated hepatocyte necrosis. It may result in fulminant hepatic failure or may culminate in cirrhosis, and it is the most common indication for OLT in many transplant centers. The principal causes of CAH are viral hepatitis, autoimmune disorders, and drug-related injury (Tong, 1982).

The majority of pulmonary problems in patients with CAH probably have an autoimmune basis, particularly the development of pleural effusions and pleuritic chest pain (Golding et al., 1973). Reports of lung biopsies have described pulmonary fibrosis (Turner-Warwick, 1968) and lymphoid interstitial pneumonitis (Helman et al., 1977), but these associations are rare. Significant

Table 4 Pulmonary Comparisons Between Sarcoidosis and Primary Biliary Cirrhosis (PBC)

Similarities
BAL T4 lymphocytosis
Interstitial lung disease
Granulomas on transbronchial lung biopsy
Isolated reduction in DLco
Obstructive ventilatory pattern (rare)
Differences
Vertebral osteopenia (PBC)
Bilateral hilar adenopathy (sarcoidosis)
Granulomas on bronchial biopsy (sarcoidosis)
Restrictive lung disease (sarcoidosis)
Steroid responsive lung disease (sarcoidosis)

Source: Adapted with permission from Krowka and Cortese, 1989.

pulmonary function abnormalities that can clearly be attributed to CAH are also infrequent. In a review of 35 OLT candidates with CAH at the Mayo Clinic, obstructive defects were observed in a single patient, restrictive defects were found in one-third, and half were observed to have a reduction in DLco (Krowka and Cortese, 1989). The importance of these findings and their specific relationship to CAH were not established.

Alpha-1-Antitrypsin Deficiency

Individuals having the PiZ antitrypsin phenotype have both a quantitative reduction in serum alpha-1-antitrypsin concentration and an abnormal form of the protein (Pierce, 1988). The abnormal PiZ protein is not secreted properly from the hepatocyte, so it accumulates intracellularly (Bathhurst et al., 1985). Approximately 50% of PiZZ neonates have biochemical evidence of liver abnormalities, but symptomatic hepatic disease develops in only 15% (Sveger 1976); in contrast, approximately one-third of afflicted adults have morphological evidence of cirrhosis (Eriksson, 1987). Viewed from the hepatic perspective, up to 50% of patients with symptomatic liver disease have been observed to have obstructive lung disease (Rakela et al., 1987), although children rarely develop coexistent hepatic and pulmonary dysfunction (Buist et al., 1980).

The most common pulmonary manifestation of the PiZZ phenotype is COPD due to panacinar emphysema. Cigarette smoking may accelerate its development, although nonsmokers develop symptomatic obstructive disease as well (Pierce, 1988). Common pulmonary complaints include dyspnea, bronchitis, and nonproductive cough, and the risk for pneumonia and pneumothorax is increased (Brantly et al., 1988). Although for a number of years it was widely accepted that emphysema is almost universal in PiZ individuals especially among smokers, recent studies show that some PiZ individuals do not develop obstructive lung disease despite smoking (Silverman et al., 1989).

Sclerosing Cholangitis

Sclerosing cholangitis is a rare disorder caused by chronic inflammation of the intrahepatic and extrahepatic bile ducts. The inflammatory process leads to severe cholestasis that ultimately results in cirrhosis and hepatic failure (Wiesner and LaRusso, 1980). Bronchitis and bronchiectasis have been associated with this disorder, but it is unclear whether the pulmonary symptoms correlate with coexistent inflammatory bowel disease such as ulcerative colitis, which is associated with sclerosing cholangitis and has pulmonary manifestations (see below).

B. Cardiopulmonary Abnormalities in Cirrhosis

Cardiopulmonary abnormalities occur regularly in patients with end-stage liver disease. Prominent findings include a markedly elevated cardiac index with decreased systemic vascular resistance and abnormally low pulmonary vascular resistance. A chronic increase in alveolar ventilation with resulting compensated, respiratory alkalosis is also common (Agusti et al., 1990). Less often, these patients demonstrate hypoxemia and pulmonary hypertension, the mechanisms of which are not completely known.

Hypoxemia

The clinical syndrome of clubbing and cyanosis in cirrhotic patients was first described by Fluckinger in 1884, but it was not until 1935 that Snell documented arterial desaturation. Presently, it is estimated that 30–50% of cirrhotic patients have some degree of arterial hypoxemia (Furukawa et al., 1984; Silverman et al., 1968).

Patients with liver disease and hypoxemia can be separated into two groups based on the severity of hypoxemia and the presence or absence of clinical signs and symptoms or radiographic abnormalities. Most patients have mild hypoxemia with minimal or no pulmonary symptoms, normal pulmonary function, and a normal chest radiograph (Furukawa et al., 1984; Krowka and Cortese, 1990). A small percentage, however, have severe hypoxemia that is associated with profound dyspnea, cyanosis, and clubbing and that worsens with exercise and when changing from the supine to the standing position (orthodeoxia) (Krowka and Cortese, 1987). The chest radiograph in these patients may reveal pulmonary infiltrates that are predominantly in the lower lobes (Stanley and Woodgate, 1972).

Several mechanisms have been proposed for arterial hypoxemia due to cirrhosis, but until recently, none seemed plausible (Agusti et al., 1990). Three early speculations included: (1) A rightward shift of the oxyhemoglobin dissociation curve, caused by cirrhosis-associated increased erythrocyte levels of 2,3-diphosphoglycerate; against this idea is that the shift is equivalent in hypoxemic and normoxemic cirrhotics. (2) Venous admixture from portopulmonary anastomoses that carry portal venous blood directly into the pulmonary veins, a notion that is not supported by postmortem studies; moreover, the portal veins carry venous blood with a relatively high PO_2 so that a large amount of blood would have to flow through these vessels to account for the observed degree of hypoxemia. Finally, (3) anatomical shunting through intrapulmonary arteriovenous malformations; as with portopulmonary shunts, however, these vascular connections are virtually never found postmortem (Berthelot et al., 1966).

Recent investigations into the mechanisms of hypoxemia in liver disease have uncovered abnormal hypoxic pulmonary vasoconstriction (HPV), disturbed V_A/Q relationships, and intrapulmonary vascular dilatations (IPVD) in hypoxemic patients. The relative contribution of these abnormalities to hypoxemia is not known and, as noted below, may vary not only among patients, but also at different stages of cirrhosis in the same individual.

Daoud and co-workers (1972) observed the complete loss of HPV in 10 patients with chronic liver disease and concluded that the absence of this vasoregulatory mechanism resulted in the chronic loss of pulmonary arteriolar tone, microvascular dilatation, abnormal VA/Q relationships, and hypoxemia (Fig 3A). In contrast, Naeije and co-workers (1981) observed normal HPV (Fig. 3B) and concluded that impaired HPV was probably not responsible for hypoxemia. There were, however, important differences in patient selection between these two studies. Most of Daoud's patients had advanced liver disease and hyperdynamic circulatory findings, whereas the majority of subjects studied by Naeije had relatively mild liver disease and normal systemic hemodynamics.

The role of VA/Q imbalance in hypoxemia of liver disease has been studied using the multiple inert gas elimination technique. Rodriguez-Roisin and colleagues (1987) found that subjects with normal HPV tended to have normal systemic and pulmonary hemodynamics and gas exchange, whereas subjects with abnormal HPV often had pulmonary and systemic vasodilation, worse hepatocellular function, increased VA/Q mismatching, and cutaneous spider nevi.

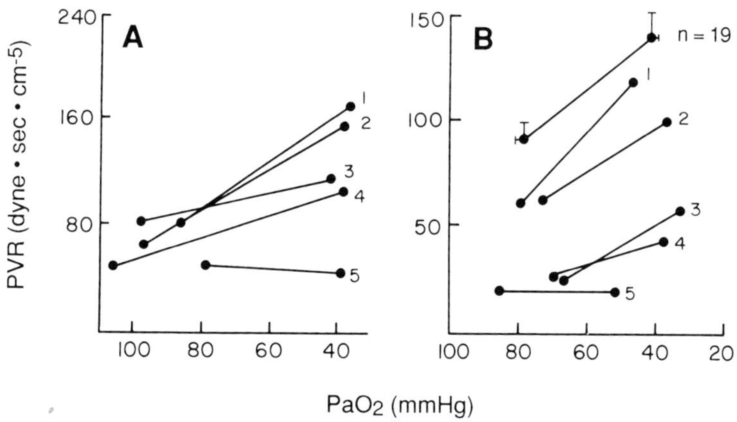

Figure 3 Pulmonary vascular reactivity in cirrhosis. (A) Study by Daoud and coworkers (1972) examining the effect of hypoxia on pulmonary vascular resistance in groups of patients with (1) normal subjects, (2) intracardiac left-to-right shunts, (3) renal failure, (4) hyperkinetic syndrome, and (5) cirrhosis. These authors concluded that hypoxic pulmonary vasoconstriction (HPV) was abolished in cirrhosis. (B) Similar study by Naeije et al. (1981) in which patients with cirrhosis who had normal pulmonary and systemic hemodynamics ($n = 19$) were observed to have normal HPV. Four of five patients (1–5) with a hyperkinetic circulatory state had intact, although diminished HPV. These authors concluded that HPV was preserved in the majority of individuals with cirrhosis. (Adapted by copyright permission of the American Society of Clinical Investigation from Daoud et al., 1972, and Naeije et al., 1981).

These investigators also demonstrated a shift in pulmonary perfusion to low VA/Q lung units in hypoxemic patients. In contrast, Melot and co-workers (1989) failed to find a relationship between the severity of liver disease, HPV, or VA/Q distribution, although they confirmed increased perfusion of low VA/Q lung units (Fig. 4).

There are a number of explanations for abnormal VA/Q relationships in patients with chronic liver disease, including pleural effusions, massive ascites, thoracic cage abnormalities, interstitial edema, and pneumonitis (Krowka and Cortese, 1990). Intrapulmonary vascular dilatations, involving the pulmonary capillaries, appear to provide the most comprehensive explanation for hypoxemia in cirrhotic patients. These abnormal vessels, which range up to 160 μ in diameter (normal capillaries = 8–15 μ), are found in patients with or without hypoxemia (Williams et al., 1979); right-to-left shunts, when present, can be easily detected in vivo by contrast echocardiography (Fig. 5). The typical location of these vessels in the lung bases accounts for orthodeoxia (Seward et al., 1984). It is suggested that these dilated vessels increase the alveolar-capillary diffusion distance (Fig. 6) which results in inadequate transfer of oxygen from the alveolus to the red cells flowing through the center of the dilated vessels (Krowka and Cortese, 1990). The shortened pulmonary capillary transit time that is characteristic of patients with hyperdynamic circulatory states further aggrevates the degree of alveolocapillary "diffusion dysequilibrium" (Wolfe et al., 1977). Whether these dilated vessels arise as a result of chronic loss of HPV

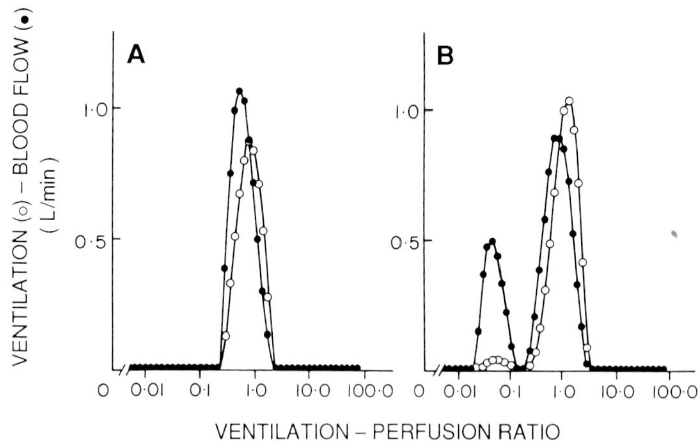

Figure 4 Distribution of ventilation and perfusion in cirrhosis. The Va/Q ratio is plotted against ventilation (○) or blood flow (•). Distribution of ventilation-perfusion ratios (A) in a cirrhotic patient with normal arterial Pao_2, and (B) in a cirrhotic patient with arterial hypoxemia. Increased perfusion of low VA/Q lung units is seen in the patient with hypoxemia. (Adapted with permission from Melot et al., 1989).

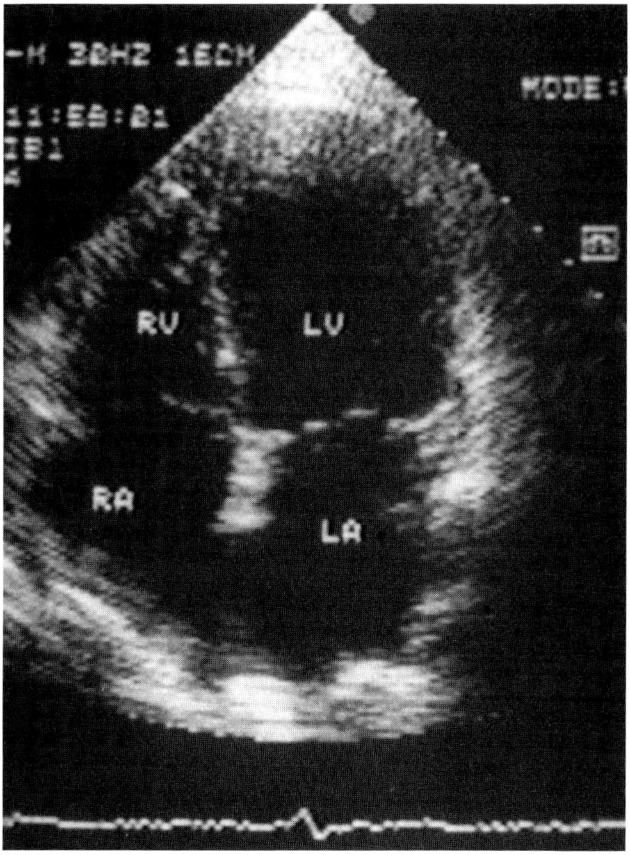

(A)

Figure 5 (A) Contrast 2-D echocardiography of a 51-year-old woman with primary biliary cirrhosis evaluated for arterial hypoxemia prior to orthotopic liver transplantation. Arterial blood gas: pH = 7.42, Pco_2 = 27 mmHg, Po_2 = 62 mmHg breathing room air. (a) Normal cardiac anatomy seen from the apical four-chamber view. (B) Same view immediately following injection of contrast (saline microbubbles) demonstrating the normal appearance of the microbubbles in the right atrium and right ventricle. (C) Subsequent appearance of microbubbles in the left-sided chambers within three to four cardiac cycles indicating the presence of an intrapulmonary shunt. RV = right ventricle; RA = right atrium; LV = left ventricle; LA = left atrium. (Reproduced with permission from Ettinger and Trulock, 1991.)

(B)

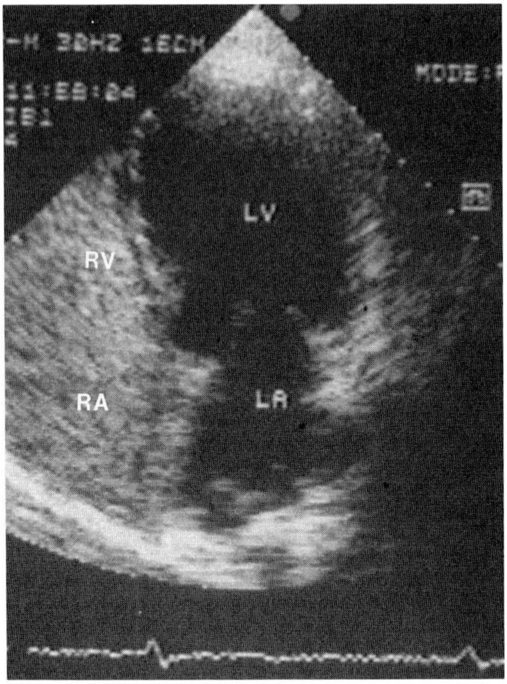

Figure 5 *(continued)*

or whether they represent a direct structural effect of a humoral mediator, or both, is unknown. In effect, the vessels result in intrapulmonary shunting of pulmonary arterial blood, although unlike most true anatomical intrapulmonary shunts, Pa_{O_2} may reach normal values when the patient breathes 100% oxygen (> 550 mmHg) (Wolfe et al., 1977).

Whether hypoxemia in cirrhosis reflects an evolutionary process characterized by the loss of pulmonary vascular reactivity in parallel with the decline in hepatic function is unknown. The conflicting findings of Daoud, on the one hand, and Naeije and Rodriguez-Roisin and Melot, on the other, are probably explained by differences in patient selection. Measurements of HPV and multiple inert gas studies were performed in various permutations of both hypoxemic and nonhypoxemic patients, who were either clinically stable or profoundly ill, some of whom had a hyperdynamic circulation. When these studies are considered together, there is sufficient evidence to conclude that early in the evolution of cirrhosis, there may be little, if any, abnormality in V_A/Q relationships or HPV. It is tempting to speculate that as the disease progresses, substantial loss or impairment of HPV may occur in some patients, along with the appearance of intrapulmonary vascular dilatations, both of which may be related

(C)

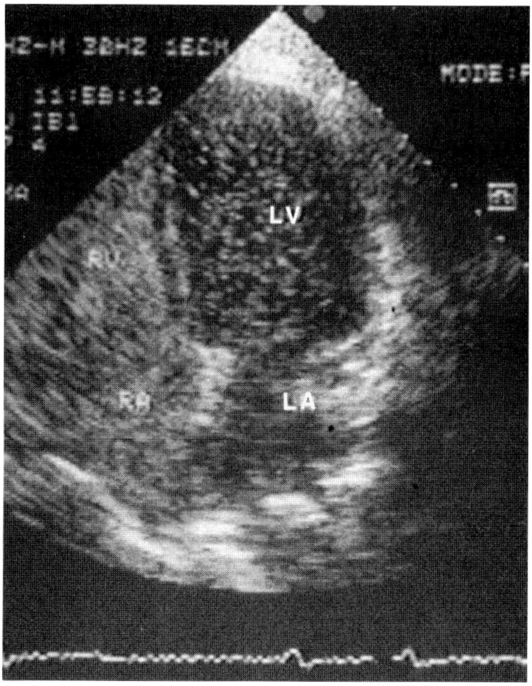

Figure 5 (*continued*)

(Agusti et al., 1990). However, not all patients with intrapulmonary vascular dilatations are hypoxemic (Krowka and Cortese, 1990), which demonstrates the existence of compensatory mechanisms that preserve Pao_2 in cirrhosis (Melot, et al., 1989). In the final stages of progressive liver disease, right-to-left shunting of blood may become prominent, compensatory mechanisms may become inadequate, and severe hypoxemia results.

Until recently, severe hypoxemia ($Pao_2 < 50$ mmHg) was considered an absolute contraindication to liver transplantation, based largely on unfavorable experience in a few patients who had severe hypoxemia and required prolonged ventilatory support posttransplant (Krowka and Cortese, 1990; Van Thiel et al., 1984). Now, however, there is evidence that these patients can withstand liver transplantation and that intrapulmonary shunting may even reverse after the procedure. Stoller and colleagues (1990) recently described resolution of clubbing and hypoxemia in a patient following OLT and verified the reversal of intrapulmonary shunt previously detected by contrast echocardiography. Although these findings suggest that intrapulmonary shunting may disappear following OLT, there are currently no methods of predicting which patients will benefit. Pharmacological closure of intrapulmonary vascular dilatations with pulmonary

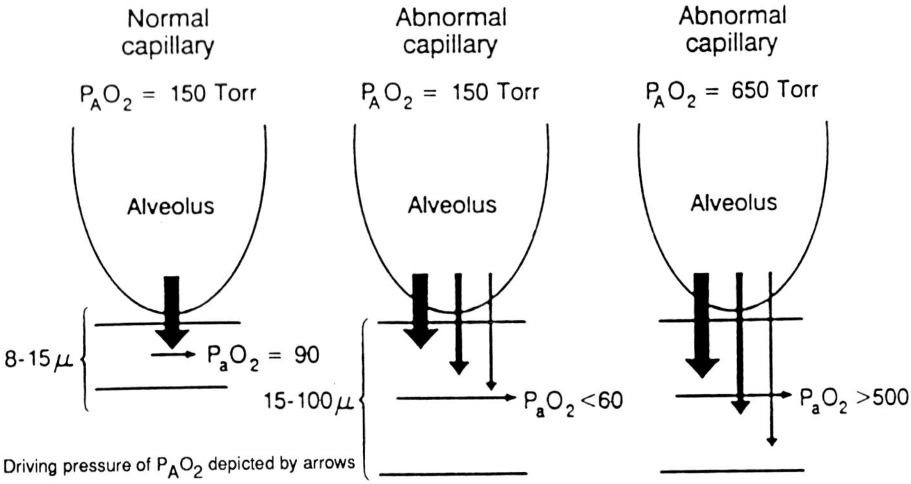

Figure 6 Schematic diagram of intrapulmonary vascular dilatations that are seen in both acute and chronic liver disease. In contrast to the normal capillary on the left, the increased diameter of the abnormal pulmonary capillary, shown in the middle, increases the diffusion distance and results in inadequate oxygen saturation of hemoglobin within red blood cells flowing in the center of the dilated vessel. The oxygenation gradient in the abnormal vessel is easily overcome by the administration of high concentrations of inspired oxygen, as shown on the right. (Reproduced with permission from Krowka and Cortese, 1987.)

vasoconstrictors, such as almitrine bismylate, has been largely unsuccessful (Krowka and Cortese, 1987), although a recent report of successful closure with a somatostatin analog is intriguing (Salem et al., 1989) and may have application in predicting reversibility posttransplant.

Pulmonary Hypertension

Pulmonary hypertension occurs in 0.25–0.75% of cirrhotic patients. This prevalence is much higher than the prevalence of primary pulmonary hypertension in the general population, which suggests that pulmonary hypertension in chronic liver disease is a distinct clinical association, not the coincidental occurrence of two diseases (McDonnell et al., 1983).

The diagnosis of pulmonary hypertension is usually made after the onset of clinical hepatic disease, although rare exceptions have been reported (Lebrec et al, 1979; Lockhart, 1985). The insidious development of exertional dyspnea is described in nearly all reported cases and is usually the predominant clinical symptom. The physical examination and the electrocardiogram reveal the typical features of right ventricular dysfunction, and the chest radiograph shows enlargement of the main pulmonary arteries. Most of these patients die of progressive right ventricular failure (Lebrec et al., 1979).

Although cirrhosis is usually present, parenchymal hepatic disease does not appear to be necessary for the development of pulmonary hypertension. Rather, the development of pulmonary hypertension is strongly associated with portal hypertension (Edwards et al., 1987; Lockhart, 1985), regardless of its cause, and review of published cases reveals a strong association between surgical portacaval shunt procedures and the subsequent development of pulmonary hypertension. Overall, nearly one-third of all published cases are associated with such a procedure (Robalino and Moodie, 1991).

The mechanism of pulmonary hypertension associated with liver disease is unknown. The histopathological features resemble those of primary pulmonary hypertension, namely, medial hypertrophy, intimal hyperplasia, and plexogenic arteriopathy (Lockhart, 1985). At autopsy studies performed in the 1960s, recanalizing intravascular thrombi in the small pulmonary arteries of these patients were identified (Naeye, 1960; Senior et al., 1968), which suggested that thromboemboli arising from the portal vein could be causative; however, portal vein thrombi are rarely present, and it is likely that the pathological abnormalities observed in the pulmonary arteries were plexiform lesions, which are commonly associated with thrombosis and fibrin deposition (Edwards et al., 1987). As such, there is little evidence to support thromboembolization in the pathogenesis of this disorder in most patients.

The strong association between the functional or surgical bypass of the liver, increased collateral circulation, or portacaval anastomosis, suggests that a humoral mediator(s), normally inactivated by the liver, constricts or injures the pulmonary vasculature directly (Lockhart, 1985). Individual susceptibility must exist, however, since pulmonary hypertension develops in an extremely small percentage of all patients with portal hypertension.

Pleural Effusions

Pleural effusions occur in 5% of patients with cirrhosis and, in the absence of other cardiopulmonary causes of pleural fluid accumulation, are referred to as hepatic hydrothorax (Johnston and Loo, 1964). The effusions are transudative in uncomplicated cases, are frequently right-sided in location, and are nearly always associated with ascites (Lieberman et al., 1966). Although usually small to moderate in size, they may be massive and cause respiratory embarrassment.

The pathogenesis of hepatic hydrothorax is related to diaphragmatic defects that permit one-way pleuroperitoneal transfer of ascitic fluid with the normal fluctuation of intrathoracic pressure (Lieberman et al., 1966). Transfer of ascitic fluid via lymphatics in the diaphragm, although possible, occurs in a minority of patients (Light 1990) and is not considered a major mechanism of fluid accumulation. Rarely, patients with hepatic hydrothorax have no clinical evidence of ascites, which leads to the suspicion that the patient has a primary intrathoracic process. These patients do have ascites, however, as shown by careful studies with ultrasonography or peritoneal-pleural transfer of fluid after intraperitoneal injection of Tc99m-DTPA (Albin and Johnston, 1989; Light, 1990).

Treatment of hepatic hydrothorax is often difficult. Thoracentesis is usually ineffective owing to the rapid reaccumulation of fluid and the considerable potential for severe protein malnutrition from repeated removal of fluid (Light, 1990). In general, treatment should be directed at minimizing ascites formation. Salt restriction and diuretics are useful in some patients, although many become refractory to this approach. Tube thoracostomy with tetracycline pleurodesis may be effective but is not without risk, because it may result in continuous drainage of ascites that leads to loss of protein, electrolytes, and intravascular volume; there is also risk of hypotension, particularly in patients with massive ascites. Therefore, the procedure should be performed in a monitored setting (Light, 1990).

Other surgical options for the management of symptomatic hepatic hydrothorax include the placement of a peritoneojugular shunt to transfer ascites directly into the circulation. While theoretically attractive, this procedure is often ineffective because transfer of fluid across the diaphragm may continue. The most definitive therapy is repair of the diaphragmatic defects along with surgical pleurodesis. However, this procedure is not without risk in patients with multiple medical problems (Light, 1990).

Effects of Ascites

Ascites can diminish ventilatory function and produce respiratory symptoms in patients with chronic liver disease. Abelmann and colleagues (1954) observed reductions in lung volumes, TLC, FRC, and VC in patients with massive ascites and detected improvement in these measurements as well as relief of dyspnea following paracentesis. They proposed that transmission of increased intraperitoneal pressure into the chest reduces lung volumes by elevating and fixing the diaphragm and by decreasing abdominal wall compliance. Chest wall compliance also falls, presumably because of the interdependent relationship between the abdomen and thoracic cage. These mechanical changes can cause dyspnea, tachypnea, and increased work of breathing.

The effect of ascites on lung volume was recently studied by Hanson and colleagues (1990), who also found that static lung volumes varied inversely with intra-abdominal hydrostatic pressure. However, they observed that intra-abdominal pressure decreased negligibly during paracentesis and that FRC did not improve. They postulated that removal of fluid causes both diaphragmatic descent and rib cage deflation, which have offsetting effects on lung volumes.

However, the intra-abdominal pressure-volume relationship that was established in this study was obtained by removing only 300–500 ml of ascites, a quantity far less than the 5–10 L removed by Abelmann and co-workers. Irrespective of the physiological mechanisms, paracentesis provides relief of dyspnea and improvement in lung volumes when a large amount of ascites is removed.

IV. Gastrointestinal Disease

Individual case reports, studies of small series of patients, and the results of surveys of lung function and bronchoalveolar lavage fluid all suggest that lung involvement may occur in patients with inflammatory bowel diseases. However, the certainty and importance of an association between the lungs and inflammatory bowel diseases must be viewed with reservation since the numbers of cases are few and the surveys of lung function and lavageable cells in randomly selected subjects with these bowel disorders reveal only minimal differences from controls or differences that do not appear to have any clinical significance.

A. Ulcerative Colitis

Between 1976 and 1980, three reports appeared describing a total of 23 patients who had ulcerative colitis that was followed by the development of otherwise unexplained airway disease (Butland et al., 1981; Higenbottam et al., 1980; Kraft et al., 1976). Productive cough was the predominant symptom and bronchiectasis developed quickly in a number of patients. There was a variable association between the activity of the ulcerative colitis, other extraintestinal manifestations of ulcerative colitis, and the pulmonary problems. Joint and skin findings were common in two of these studies (Higenbottam et al., 1980; Kraft et al., 1976), and the presence of serological abnormalities characteristic of collagen vascular disease in one study suggested multisystem disease. Pulmonary function testing typically showed features of airflow obstruction and corticosteroids usually produced symptomatic and functional improvements in the airway abnormalities.

Since that small flurry of reports more than a decade ago, relatively little has been reported relating the lungs to ulcerative colitis. There has been at least one case of pulmonary vasculitis (Sargent et al., 1985), two of bronchiolitis obliterans (Swinburn et al., 1988; Wilcox et al., 1987), and one of a patient who developed a fibrotic, obstructive process confined to the lower trachea and a mainstem bronchus (Wilcox et al., 1987). Also, two studies of lung function in ulcerative colitis patients have been performed. In one study of 23 randomly selected patients, forced vital capacity, FEV_1, and diffusing capacity were found to be normal even though some of the patients were taking sulfasalazine, an agent that has occasionally been implicated in the development of alveolitis

(Eade et al., 1980). In the other study, 18 subjects with severe ulcerative colitis were found to have borderline reductions in a few spirometric measurements (Sharma and Kar, 1985). It appears that if there is an association between the lungs and ulcerative colitis, it is most often involves the airways, it affects few patients with ulcerative colitis, and its occurrence is unpredictable with regard to either the severity of ulcerative colitis or other extraintestinal manifestations.

B. Crohn's Disease

In contrast to ulcerative colitis, Crohn's disease often produces detectable changes in the lungs, typically an increase in the number of lymphocytes in bronchoalveolar lavage fluid (Wallaert et al., 1985); this abnormality occurred in 12 of 22 patients in one study (Bonniere et al., 1986) and in 8 of 10 patients in another study (Smiejan et al., 1986). The lymphocytosis, which amounts to about four times the normal number of lymphocytes in bronchoalveolar lavage fluid, is due to an expansion of the T lymphocyte population, principally of the T4+ subset, and it is not observed in other types of inflammatory bowel disease (Smiejan et al., 1986). This finding resembles the lavage results in sarcoidosis and primary biliary cirrhosis (PBC, see above), which raises speculation about overlap between Crohn's disease and sarcoidosis. Despite the frequent occurrence of alveolar lymphocytosis, however, there have been only a few reported cases with otherwise unexplained pulmonary disease and Crohn's disease (Kayser et al., 1990; Lemann et al., 1987). These patients have had granulomatous infiltration of the lungs or airways, but nothing else to support a diagnosis of sarcoidosis in addition to Crohn's disease. Moreover, only minimal alterations in pulmonary function have been found in patients with Crohn's disease (Neilly et al., 1989), and there is no correlation between alveolar lymphocytosis and lung function (Bonniere et al., 1986). The mechanisms leading to alveolar lymphocytosis in Crohn's disease and the relationship of Crohn's disease to sarcoidosis, if any, are interesting areas for future study.

V. Chronic Renal Disease

Chronic renal diseases are associated with a variety of thoracic manifestations that may appear before renal function has declined to the point that dialysis is required. Pulmonary edema, pleuritis, pleural effusions, pulmonary calcification, and pulmonary vascular disease are well-documented findings in patients with chronic renal insufficiency. Renal failure and its treatment also produce alterations in alveolar gas exchange and pulmonary function that may be of clinical importance in patients with underlying cardiopulmonary disorders. These issues are discussed in the following sections. Pulmonary-renal syndromes, such as Wegener's granulomatosis and Goodpasture's syndrome, are considered elsewhere in this volume.

A. Pulmonary Edema

Pulmonary edema is common in patients with acute or chronic renal insufficiency. Although hypervolemia is often the precipitating factor, a number of additional mechanisms may be operative, principally cardiac dysfunction, hypoalbuminemia, and increases in pulmonary microvascular and epithelial permeability.

In the predialysis era, descriptions of pulmonary edema associated with renal failure identified a clinicopathological entity that appeared to be distinct from hypervolemia. Autopsy findings typically revealed diffusely indurated lungs filled with protein-rich edema fluid, hyaline membranes, and alveolar hemorrhage (Henkin et al., 1962; Hopps and Wissler, 1953). Although many workers considered these observations proof that uremic edema represented injury to the lungs as a result of uremic toxins, the findings are nonspecific and do not help identify the most likely causes (Bass et al., 1952; Henkin et al., 1962).

The role of the heart in ''uremic'' pulmonary edema may be difficult to determine but should not be underestimated. Cardiac disorders are common in end-stage renal disease, and a variety of factors, including anemia, surgical arteriovenous fistulas, hypertension, and ischemic heart disease, may coexist to adversely affect left ventricular function (Hung et al., 1980; Scharf et al., 1980). The high incidence of unexplained left ventricular dysfunction in uremic patients that is reversible following dialysis or renal transplantation argues that a specific ''uremic cardiomyopathy'' may exist (Burt et al., 1989; Capelli and Kasparian, 1977; Hung et al., 1980; Lai et al., 1982; Pehrsson et al., 1984). A study by Pehrsson and colleagues (1984) also suggests that left ventricular function may fall in parallel with renal function. These findings are intriguing but require further study in larger numbers of patients before such a direct relationship can be confirmed.

Some experimental evidence supports the hypothesis that increased alveolar epithelial and capillary endothelial permeability occurs in uremic pulmonary edema. Crosbie and co-workers (1972) demonstrated increased sodium permeability across the alveolar-capillary membrane, and Belcher and Rees (1986) observed increased clearance of inhaled ^{99m}Tc-DTPA that was reversible with hemodialysis. Although these findings do not prove that uremic pulmonary edema is related to changes in permeability or elucidate its mechanisms, they do help to reconcile many of the clinical observations and the histopathological findings. The issue remains controversial, however, as others have failed to find increased permeability in patients with renal insufficiency (Rocker et al., 1988). Clinically, the cause of pulmonary edema is probably multifactorial in most patients and involves elevation of intravascular volume, hypertension, and abnormal left ventricular function. Increased permeability of the alveolar-capillary membrane may be important in some patients.

B. Pleural Disease

Transudative pleural effusions are common in patients with end-stage renal disease and are usually caused by hypervolemia or congestive heart failure (Rodelas et al., 1980). However, uremia may also cause pleural inflammation ("uremic pleuritis") and lead to the development of pleuritic pain, pleural friction rubs, and exudative effusions (Nidus et al., 1969). The incidence of uremic pleuritis is probably underestimated as not all patients are symptomatic. Overall, approximately 20–40% of uremic patients have fibrinous pleuritis detected at autopsy (Fairshter et al., 1982; Hopps and Wissler, 1953).

(A)

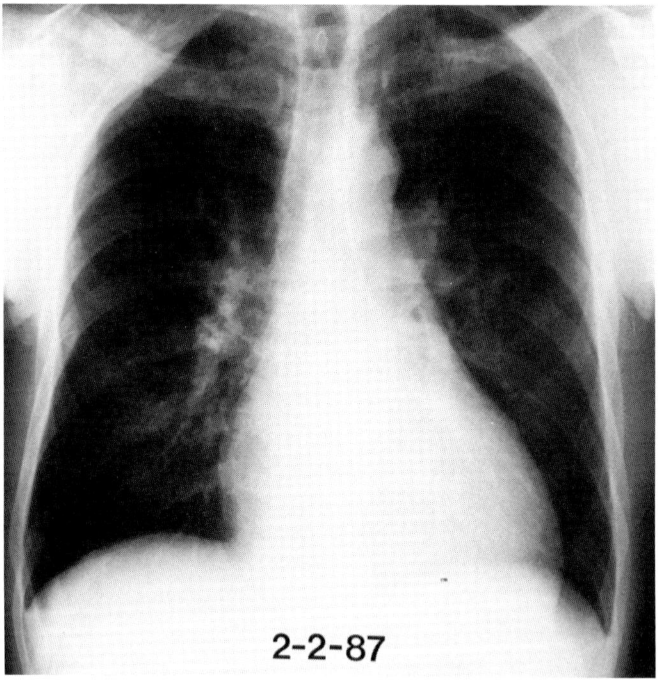

Figure 7 Radiographs of a 47-year-old man with end-stage renal disease. (A) Radiograph taken when the patient presented with low-grade fever and biapical pulmonary infiltrates. A presumptive diagnosis of tuberculosis was made, but subsequent transbronchial lung biopsy showed the presence of pulmonary calcification. (B) Radiograph taken 18 months later when the patient had developed progressive metastatic calcification in the lung parenchyma and soft tissues. (Reproduced with permission from Ettinger and Trulock, 1991).

The development of uremic pleuritis does not appear to be related to the adequacy of dialysis, the duration of dialysis, or the interdialysis interval (Berger et al., 1975; Nidus et al., 1969). Effusions may be bilateral, large, and hemorrhagic. Although the pleural fluid is usually exudative and lymphocytic, peritoneal dialysis may obscure the pleural fluid chemistry by diluting the fluid so that it appears to be a transudate (Berger et al., 1975; Galen et al., 1975; Nidus et al., 1969). Closed pleural biopsy findings are typically nonspecific and reveal an organized fibrinous exudate or granulation tissue in most cases (Berger et al., 1975).

Uremic effusions often resolve spontaneously within weeks of their appearance (Berger et al., 1975). Intensification of dialysis may provide symptomatic relief, but will generally not accelerate the resolution of the effusion. Fibrothorax or empyema may complicate these effusions and require decortication (Galen et al., 1975; Gilbert et al., 1975; McCabe et al., 1982; Rodelas et al., 1980). Restrictive ventilatory changes often signal the development of significant pleural space fibrosis.

(B)

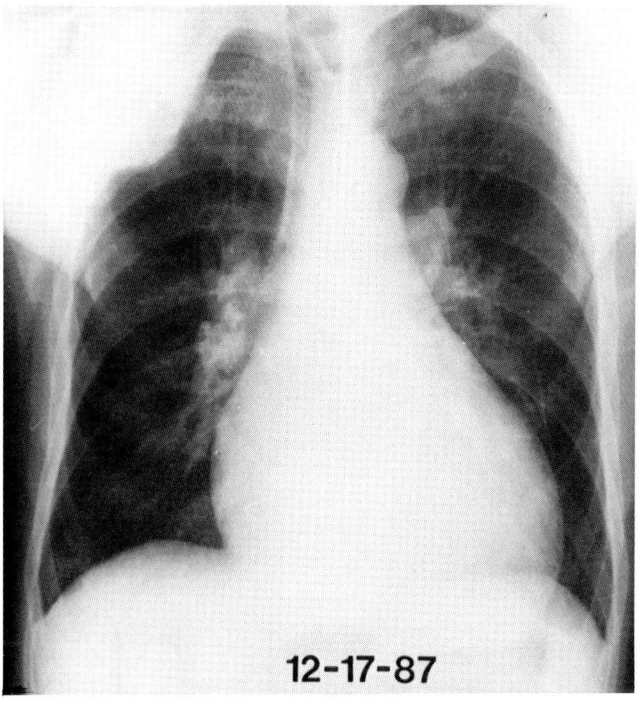

Figure 7 *(continued)*

C. Pulmonary Calcification

Metastatic calcification is a complication of chronic renal failure that affects visceral organs and other sites (Jastrabo et al., 1979). Pulmonary involvement is extremely common, but it is usually asymptomatic. Conger and co-workers (1975) found pulmonary calcification in 60% of hemodialysis patients in a prospective autopsy study. Only one patient had radiographic changes that suggested the pathological findings and none had respiratory symptoms attributable to pulmonary calcification. Rarely, pulmonary calcification may progress to respiratory failure (Jastrabo et al., 1979).

The chest radiograph in metastatic calcification may be misleading as the calcific nature of the pulmonary infiltrates is not always apparent (Mootz et al., 1973). The infiltrates, which can be diffuse or localized, are usually composed of nodular opacities less than 2 mm in diameter, although larger, nodular lesions have also been reported (Fig. 7). The relative stability of these pulmonary infiltrates, in contrast to infectious processes, serves as a clue to the diagnosis. It is not surprising that there are few associated symptoms because measurements of pulmonary function are usually normal; however, restrictive abnormalities or a reduction in DLCO may occur in severe cases. Disturbances of pulmonary function tend to follow the degree of associated pulmonary fibrosis and not the amount of calcium in the tissues (Conger, et al., 1975).

The diagnosis of pulmonary calcification can be made by ^{99m}Tc-diphosphonate scanning (Fig. 8), although the sensitivity and specificity of this approach are controversial (Faubert et al., 1980; Margolin and Addison, 1984). Tissue should be obtained by transbronchial biopsy whenever possible, particularly when infection is suspected. Treatment is generally unsatisfactory. Reduction of vitamin D or calcium intake has occasionally been successful (Evans et al., 1983; Gilman et al., 1980; Smith et al., 1969). Renal transplantation has been suggested as a therapeutic alternative, although rapid progression has been described following transplantation (Alfrey et al., 1968; Justrabo et al., 1979).

A number of mechanisms have been proposed to explain the development of pulmonary calcification, including elevated parathyroid hormone levels or increases in the calcium-phosphate product above the solubility constant for these ions. The most likely mechanism is calciphylaxis, an obscure process whereby soft tissues respond to a variety of chemical sensitizers with calcium deposition (Conger et al., 1975; Gilman et al., 1980). The patient's age, the type of underlying renal disease, and the duration of dialysis do not appear to be important factors in the development of this complication (Conger et al., 1975).

D. Pulmonary Vascular Disease

Pulmonary artery atherosclerosis is a common postmortem finding in dialysis patients. Its presence suggests chronic elevations in pulmonary artery pressure

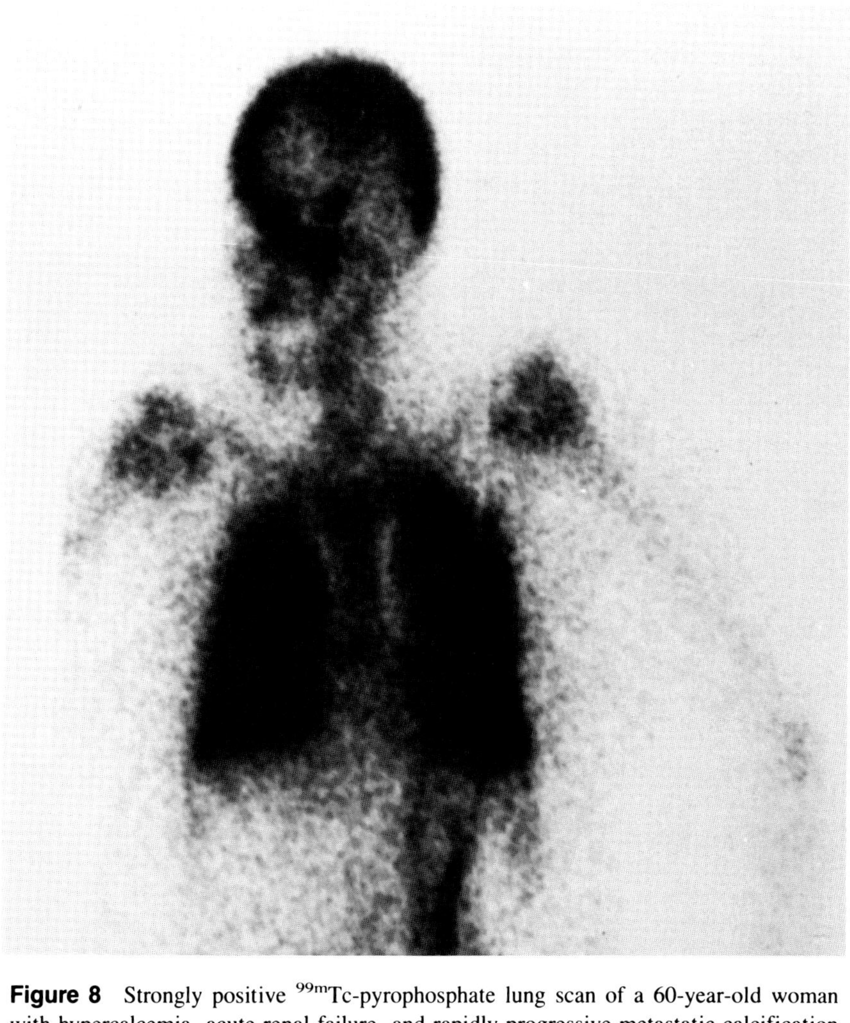

Figure 8 Strongly positive ^{99m}Tc-pyrophosphate lung scan of a 60-year-old woman with hypercalcemia, acute renal failure, and rapidly progressive metastatic calcification of the lungs. The diagnosis was confirmed by transbronchial lung biopsy. (Reproduced with permission from Margolin and Addison, 1984.)

during life. The cause of these changes is unclear; however, it is hypothesized that repetitive insults to the vascular endothelium may occur in association with dialysis (see later) or as part of a systemic disease process (Fairshter et al., 1982). Unlike chronic liver disease, there does not appear to be a syndrome of severe pulmonary arterial hypertension associated with chronic renal insufficiency.

E. Urinothorax

Urinothorax is an uncommon cause of pleural effusion. It develops when urine that has extravasated from the urinary tract because of obstruction flows from the retroperitoneum into the thorax (Salcedo, 1986). A urinothorax can develop quickly (Fig. 9). The pleural fluid in a urinothorax is a transudate with a creatinine concentration that is higher than serum creatinine and a pH < 7.30 (Miller et al., 1988; Stark et al., 1982).

F. Pulmonary Complications of Dialysis

Hemodialysis and peritoneal dialysis are accompanied by changes in lung function and gas exchange that may be clinically important in patients with underlying cardiopulmonary impairment.

Hemodialysis

During hemodialysis, nearly 90% of patients develop some reduction in oxygen tension, usually 5–35 mmHg, below their baseline Pao_2 (Ross et al., 1987). The Pao_2 begins to decline almost immediately after dialysis commences, reaches a minimum value after 30–60 min, and persists for a variable period after the procedure. Except in patients with underlying cardiopulmonary disorders, the Pao_2 usually does not fall below 70 mmHg (Cardoso et al., 1988).

Hemodialysis produces cellular and metabolic changes that vary with the type of dialysis membrane used and with the chemical composition of the dialysate. Exposure of blood to dialysis membranes activates the alternate complement pathway, which generates C3a and C5a within minutes after the procedure is started. It is postulated that these complement fragments become deposited on the membrane surface, where they cause circulating leukocytes and platelets to form aggregates that then occlude the pulmonary capillaries and alter VA/Q relationships (Craddock et al., 1977). Sequestration of leukocytes in the lung coincides temporally with the development of peripheral neutropenia and the fall in Pao_2. However, pulmonary capillary leukostasis is now thought to account for only a small part (< 10%) of dialysis-related hypoxemia, and the magnitude of effect varies with the type of dialysis membrane used. Cuprophane membranes activate complement more than polyacrylonitrile or cellulose membranes and are associated with a larger fall in Pao_2 (Cardoso et al., 1988).

Currently, a decrease in alveolar ventilation, secondary to a decrease in metabolic CO_2 production plus any dialysis-related loss of CO_2, is regarded as the major determinant of hypoxemia during hemodialysis. A number of investigators have proposed that the loss of gaseous CO_2 across the dialysis membrane results in compensatory underventilation in order to maintain a constant $Paco_2$ (Ross et al., 1987). However, the loss of gaseous CO_2 into the dialysate

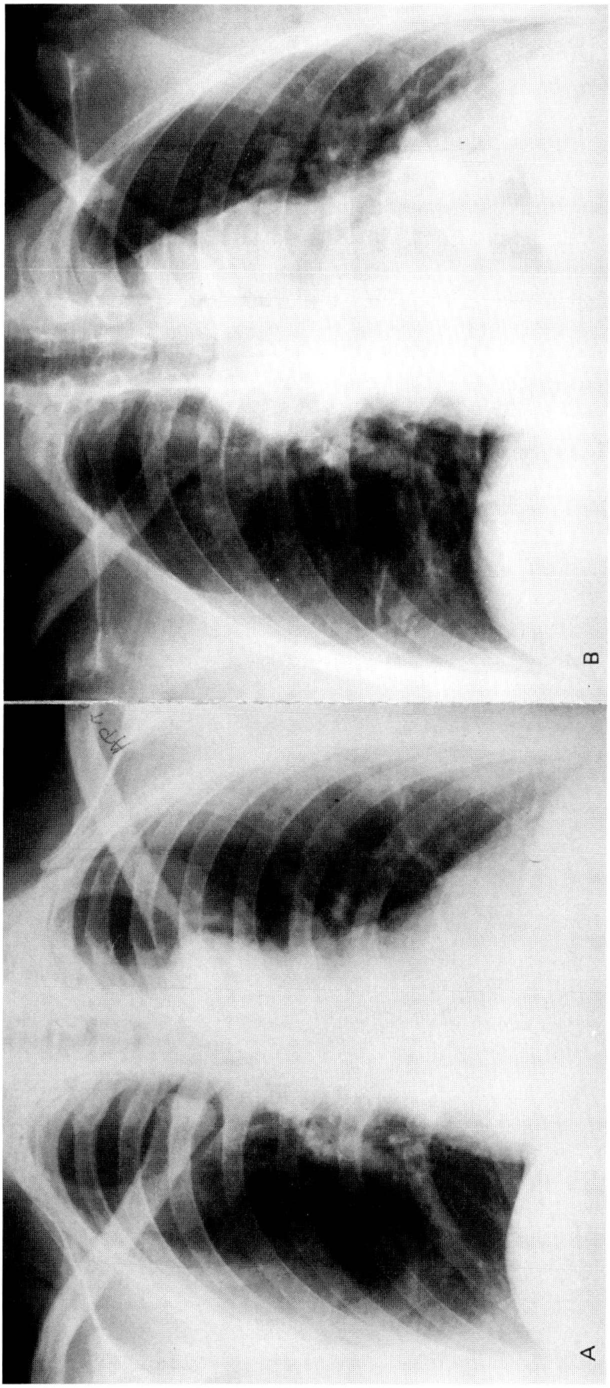

Figure 9 Radiographs showing acute mediastinal widening due to urinthorax in a 52-year-old woman who presented with the sudden onset of left flank pain. The initial chest radiograph was normal (A), but 12 hr later there was mediastinal widening and a left-sided pleural effusion (B). Excretory urography demonstrated extravasation of contrast material into the superior and inferior perirenal spaces and a calculus obstructing the left ureter proximally. At surgery, urine was found throughout the retroperitoneum up to the diaphragm, which appeared intact. After drainage of the retroperitoneal urinoma and removal of the ureteral calculus, the chest radiograph showed rapid resolution to normal. (Reproduced with permission from Baron, 1981).

is quantitatively insufficient to account for the fall in CO_2 production (Vco_2) that is observed, implying that other mechanisms must be operative (Prezant, 1990).

Metabolic studies have demonstrated that during hemodialysis against acetate, endogenous substrates that are normally oxidized to support the energy needs of the body are displaced by acetate. The oxidation of acetate is associated with a marked reduction in CO_2 production, the net effect of which is a decrease in the amount of alveolar ventilation required to maintain $Paco_2$ constant. A slight, concomitant increase in oxygen consumption, in addition to the reduction in ventilation, combines to reduce the arterial oxygen tension (Cardoso et al., 1988). The reduction in CO_2 production is particularly pronounced during acetate dialysis and is minimal during bicarbonate dialysis. Accordingly, hypoxemia is most likely during acetate dialysis, particularly when used in conjunction with a cuprophane membrane (Fig. 10). In contrast, dialysis against a bicarbonate bath is associated with minimal changes in the respiratory quotient or Pao_2 (De Backer et al., 1983).

The clinical importance of these findings is that the composition of the dialysis membrane and the chemical nature of the dialysate should be considered when dialyzing patients with cardiopulmonary impairment. Cellulose or polyacrylonitrile filters and a bicarbonate bath are preferred in situations where

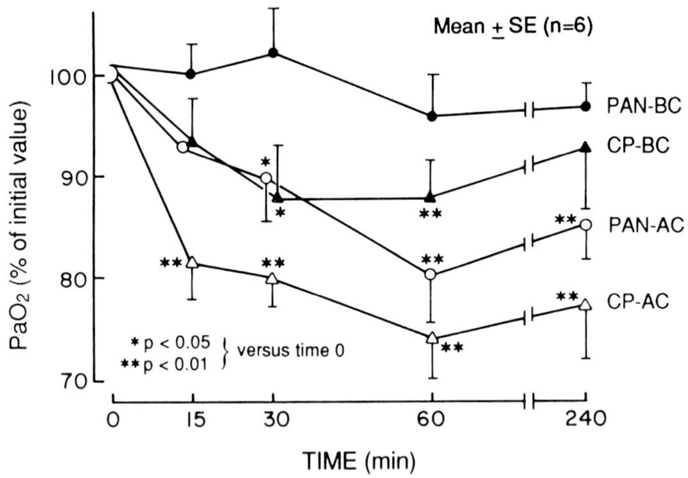

Figure 10 Effect of membrane composition and dialysate on Pao_2 during hemodialysis. The greatest decline in oxygenation occurs when cuprophane membranes are used in conjunction with acetate dialysis. Each data point represents mean ± SEM (n = 6). PAN = polyacrylonitrile membrane; CP = cuprophane membrane; BC = bicarbonate dialysate; AC = acetate dialysate. (Adapted with permission from De backer et al., 1983).

hypoxemia is already present or where its development would be poorly tolerated. It is to be remembered that patients with hypoxemia due to obstructive or other forms of lung disease experience a fall in Pa_{O_2} of similar magnitude to that in persons with normal lungs (Pitcher et al., 1989). Because the fall often begins from a lower baseline Pa_{O_2} in these patients, the resulting Pa_{O_2} may reach dangerously low levels and supplemental oxygen may be required.

Peritoneal dialysis

The major pulmonary complications associated with peritoneal dialysis are pulmonary edema, pleural effusions, atelectasis, and pneumonia (Cohn et al., 1990). In patients who are acutely or intermittently dialyzed, large decreases in vital capacity and Pa_{O_2} may occur (Berlyne et al., 1966; Gotloib et al., 1981). Hypercapnea and acute respiratory acidosis also may develop in patients undergoing acute peritoneal dialysis who have limited ventilatory reserve, apparently owing to the increased carbohydrate load provided by the peritoneal dialysate (Cohn et al., 1990). Disturbances of pulmonary function or gas exchange in patients undergoing acute or intermittent peritoneal dialysis have little relevance to stable patients undergoing chronic ambulatory peritoneal dialysis (CAPD) (Singh et al., 1984).

CAPD is a state of iatrogenic ascites, although the standard 2-L dialysate infusion is considerably less than the 10–20 L of ascites often present in patients with hepatic cirrhosis (Abelmann et al., 1954). A recent study of 13 patients undergoing CAPD revealed significant falls in vital capacity and measurements of static lung volumes (FRC, TLC). Reductions in FEV_1, ERV, and RV were also observed but did not reach statistical significance (Signh et al., 1984). Of interest, all the changes returned to baseline within 2 weeks of initiation of CAPD, possibly as a result of adaptation to the intra-abdominal fluid. The authors suggested that stretching of the abdominal wall could permit the diaphragm to return to its normal position, thereby allowing lung volumes to return to baseline. Beasley and colleagues (1986) performed similar measurements before and after instillation of dialysate in 20 CAPD patients with underlying cardiopulmonary disease and observed a 16% decrease in FRC but no other significant changes in lung volumes. These patients were undergoing maintainence CAPD and may therefore have adapted in a similar fashion.

Overall, CAPD results in minor changes in pulmonary function that appear to reverse over time and appear to pose little threat to the majority of patients with underlying cardiopulmonary disorders.

VI. Summary

Abdominal disorders, from time to time and with varying frequency, produce a variety of intrathoracic complications, which may be life-threatening and which require prompt recognition and treatment. Although most of these complications are not specific for a particular abdominal disease, it is important to remember that they may be the initial manifestation of an intra-abdominal process.

References

Abelmann, W. H., Frank, N. R., Gaensler, E. A., and Cugell, D. W. (1954) Effects of abdominal distention by ascites on lung volumes and ventilation. *Arch. Intern. Med.* **93**:528–540.

Augusti, A. G. N., Roca, J., Boach, J., and Rodriguez-Roisin, R. R. (1990). The lungs in patients with cirrhosis. *J. Hepatol.* **10**:251–257.

Albin, R. J., and Johnston, G. S. (1989). External accumulation of radionuclide in hepatic hydrothorax. *Clin. Nucl. Med.* **14**:341–343.

Alfrey, A. C., Jenkins, D., Groth, C. G., Schorr, W. S., Gecelter, L., and Ogden, D. A. (1968). Resolution of hyperparathyroidism, renal osteodystrophy and metastatic calcification after renal homotransplantation. *N. Engl. J. Med.* **279**:1349–1356.

Barie, P. S., Tahamount, M. V., and Malik, A. B. (1982). Prevention of increased pulmonary vascular permeability after pancreatitis by granulocyte depletion in sheep. *Am. Rev. Respir. Dis.* **126**:904–908.

Basran, G. S., Ramasubramanian, R., and Verma, R. (1987). Intrathoracic complications of acute pancreatitis. *Br. J. Dis. Chest.* **81**:326–331.

Bass, H. E., Greenberg, D., Singer, E., and Miller, M. (1952). Pulmonary changes in uremia. *JAMA* **148**:724–726.

Bathurst, I. C., Errington, D. M., and Foreman, R. C. (1985). Human Z alpha1 antitrypsin accumulates intracellularly and stimulates lysosomal activity when synthesized in the Xenopus oocyte. *FEBS Lett.* **183**:304–308.

Beasley, C. R. W., Ripley, J. M., Smith, D. A., and Neale, T. J. (1986). Pulmonary function in chronic renal failure patients managed by continuous ambulatory peritoneal dialysis. *NZ Med. J.* **99**:313–315.

Belcher, N. G., and Rees, P. J. (1986). Changes in pulmonary clearance of technitium labelled DTPA during hemodialysis. *Thorax* **41**:381–385.

Berger, H. W., Rammohan, G., Neff, M. S., and Buhian, W. J. (1975). Uremic pleural effusion. *Ann. Intern. Med.* **82**:362–364.

Berlyne, G. M., Lee, H. A., Ralston, H. A., and Woolcock, J. A. (1966). Pulmonary complications of peritoneal dialysis. *Lancet* **2**:75–78.

Berthelot, P., Walker, J. G., Sherlock, S., and Reid, L. (1966). Arterial changes in the lungs in cirrhosis of the liver-lung spider nevi. *N. Engl. J. Med.* **274**:291–298.

Bonniere, P., Wallaert, B., Cortot, A., Marchandise, X., Riou, Y., Tonnel, A. B., Colombel, J. F., Voisin, C., and Paris, J. C. (1986). Latent pulmonary involvement in Crohn's disease: biological, functional, bronchoalveolar lavage and scintigraphic studies. *Gut* **27**:919–925.

Brantly, M. L., Paul, L. D., Miller, B. H., Falk, R. T., Wu, M., and Crystal, R. G. (1988). Clinical features and history of destructive lung disease associated with alpha-1-antitrysin deficiency of adults with pulmonary symptoms. *Am. Rev. Respir. Dis.* **138**:327–336.

Buggy, B. P., and Nostrant, T. T. (1983). Lethal pancreatitis. *Am. J. Gastroenterol.* **78**:810–814.

Buist, A. S., Adams, B. E., Azzam, A. H., and Sexton, G. J. (1980). Pulmonary function in young children with alpha1-antitrypsin deficiency: comparison with matched control subjects. *Am. Rev. Respir. Dis.* **122**:817–822.

Burnweit, C. A., and Horton, J. W. (1988). Extravascular lung water as an indicator of pulmonary dysfunction in acute hemorrhagic pancreatitis. *Ann. Surg.* **207**:33–38.

Burt, R. K., Gupta-Burt, S., Suki, W. N., Barcenas, C. G., Ferguson, J. J., and Van Buren, C. T. (1989). Reversal of left ventricular dysfunction after renal transplantation. *Ann. Intern. Med.* **111**:635–640.

Busuttil, R. W., Goldstein, L., Danovitch, G. M., Ament, M. E., and Memsic, L. D. (1986). Liver transplantation today. *Ann. Intern. Med.* **104**:377–389.

Butland, R. J. A., Cole, P., Citron, K. M., and Turner-Warwick, M. (1981). Chronic bronchial suppuration and inflammatory bowel disease. *Q. J. Med.* **197**:63–75.

Capelli, J. P., and Kasparian, H. (1977). Cardiac work demands and left ventricular function in end-stage renal disease. *Ann. Intern. Med.* **86**: 261–267.

Cardoso, M., Vinay, P., Vinet, B., Leveillee, M., Prud'homme, M., Tejedor, A., Courteau, M., Gougoux, A., St.-Louis, G., Laperre, L., and Piette, Y. (1988). Hypoxemia during hemodialysis: a critical review of the facts. *Am. J. Kidney Dis.* **11**:281–297.

Clarke, A. K., Galbraith, R. M., Hamilton, E. R. D., and Williams, R. (1978). Rheumatic disorders in primary biliary cirrhosis. *Ann. Rheum. Dis.* **37**:42–47.

Cohn, J., Balk, R. A., and Bone, R. C. (1990). Dialysis-induced respiratory acidosis. *Chest* **98**:1285–1288.

Conger, J. D., Hammond, W. S., Alfrey, A. C., Contiguglia, S. R., Stanford, R. E., and Huffer, W. E. (1975). Pulmonary calcification in chronic dialysis patients. *Ann. Intern. Med.* **83**:330–336.

Craddock, P. R., Fehr, J., Brigham, K. L., Kronenberg, R. S., and Jacob, H. S. (1977). Complement and leukocyte-mediated pulmonary dysfunction in hemodialysis. *N. Engl. Med.* **296**:769–774.

Crosbie, W. A., Snowden, S., and Parsons, V. (1972). Changes in lung capillary permeability in renal failure. *Bri. Med. J.* **4**:388–390.

Culp, K. S., Fleming, C. R., and Duffy, J. (1982). Auto-immune associations in primary biliary cirrhosis. *Mayo Clin. Proc.* **57**:365–370.

Daoud, F. S., Reeves, J. T., and Schaefer, J. W. (1972). Failure of hypoxic pulmonary vasoconstriction in patients with liver cirrhosis. *J. Clin. Invest.* **51**:1076–1080.

Das, S. K., Scott, M. T., and McCuiston, S. (1987). Effects of experimental acute pancreatitis in dogs on metabolism of lung surfactant phosphatidylcholine. *Biochem. Biophys. Res. Commun.* **145**:612–618.

De Backer, W. A., Verpooten, G. A., Borgonjon, D. J., Vermeire, P. A., Lins, R. R., and DeBroe, M. E. (1983). Hypoxemia during hemodialysis: effects of different membranes and dialysate compositions. *Kidney Int.* **23**:738–743.

Dewan, N. A., Kinney, W. W., and O'Donohue, J., W. J. (1984). Chronic massive pancreatic pleural effusion. *Chest* **85**:497–501.

Eade, O. E., Smith, C. L., Alexander, J. R., and Whorwell, P. J. (1980). Pulmonary function in patients with inflammatory bowel disease. *Am. J. Gastroenterol.* **73**(2):154–156.

Edwards, B. S., Weir, E. K., Edwards, W. D., Ludwig, J., Dykoski, R. K., and Edwards, J. E. (1987). Coexistent pulmonary and portal hypertension: morphologic and clinical features. *J. Am. Coll. Cardiol.* **10**:1233–1238.

Eriksson, S. (1987). Alpha1-antitrypsin deficiency and liver cirrhosis in adults. *Acta Med. Scand.* **221**:461–467.

Ettinger, N. A., and Trulock, N. A. (1991). Pulmonary considerations of organ transplantation. *Am. Rev. Respir. Dis.* (in press).

Evans, T. W., Collins, M., Adams, J. E., Howard, P., Fox, M., Platts, M. M., and Brown, C. B. (1983). Pulmonary calcification in a renal transplant recipient. *Br. J. Dis. Chest.* **77**:202–205.

Fagan, E. A., Moore-Gillon, J. C., and Turner-Warwick, M. (1983). Multiorgan granulomas and mitochrondrial antibodies. *N. Engl. J. Med.* **308**:472–475.

Fairshter, R. D., Vaziri, N. D., and Mirahmadi, M. K. (1982). Lung pathology in chronic hemodialysis patients. *Int. J. Artif. Organs* **5**:97–100.

Faling, I. J., Gerzof, S. G., Daly, B. D. T., Pugatch, R. D., and Snider, G. L. (1984). Treatment of chronic pancreatitic pleural effusion by percutaneous catheter drainage of abdominal pseudocyst. *Am. J. Med.* **76**:329–333.

Faubert, P. F., Shapiro, W. B., Porush, J. G., Chou, S., Gross, J. M., Bondi, E., and Gomez-Leon, G. (1980). Pulmonary calcification in hemodialyzed patients detected by technetium-99m diphosphonate scanning. *idney Int.* **18**:95–102.

Fluckinger, M. (1884). Vorkommen von trommelschagerformigen Fingerendphalangen ohne chronische Veranderungen an der Lunge oder am Herzen. *Wien. Med. Wochnschr.* **34**:1457–1458.

Fowler, A. A., Hamman, R. F., Good, J. T., Benson, K. N., Baird, M., Eberle, D. J., Petty, T. L., and Hyers, T. M. (1983). Adult respiratory distress syndrome: risk with common predispositions. *Ann. Intern. Med.* **98**:593–598.

Furukawa, T., Hara, N., Yasumoto, K., and Inokuchi, K. (1984). Arterial hypoxemia in patients with hepatic cirrhosis. *Am. J. Med. Sci.* **287**:10–13.

Galen, M. A., Steinberg, S. M., Lowrie, E. G., Lazarus, J. M., Hampers, C. L., and Merrill, J. P. (1975). Hemorrhagic pleural effusion in patients undergoing chronic hemodialysis. *Ann. Intern. Med.* **82**:359–361.

Garcia-Szabo, R. R., and Malik, A. B. (1984). Pancreatitis-induced increase in lung vascular permeability: Protective effect of trasylol. *Am. Rev. Respir. Dis.* **129**:580–583.

Gilbert, L., Seymour, R., Frankel, H., Jacobs, M., and Mankowitz, B. J. (1975). Fibrinous uremic pleuritis: a surgical entity. *Chest* **67**:53–56.

Gilman, M., Nissm, J., Terry, P., and Whelton, A. (1980). Metastatic pulmonary calcification in the renal transplant recipient. *Am. Rev. Respir. Dis.* **121**:415–419.

Glasser, F., Feinsilver, S., Niederman, M., and Fein, A. (1987). Hypoxemia but not ARDS is common in pancreatitis. *Chest* **92**:56S.

Golding, P. L., Smith, M., and Williams, R. (1973). Multisystem involvement in chronic liver disease: studies on the incidence and pathogenesis. *Am. J. Med.* **55**:772–782.

Gotloib, L., Garmizo, L., Varak, I., and Mines, M. (1981). Reduction of vital capacity due to increased intra-abdominal pressure during peritoneal dialysis. *Perit. Dial. Bull.* **1**:63–64.

Greenburg, A. G., Terlizzi, L., and Peskin, G. W. (1977). Oxyhemoglobin affinity in acute pancreatitis. *J. Surg. Res.* **22**:561–565.

Guice, K. S., Oldham, K. T., Wolfe, R. R., and Simon, R. H. (1987). Lung injury in acute pancreatitis: primary inhibition of pulmonary phospholipid synthesis. *Am. J. Surg.* **153**:54–61.

Guice, K. S., Oldham, K. T., Johnson, K. J., Kunkel, R. G., Morganroth, M. L., and Ward, P. A. (1988). Pancreatitis-induced acute lung injury: an ARDS model. *Ann. Surg.* **208**:71–77.

Guice, K. S., Oldham, K. T., Caty, M. G., Johnson, K. J., and Ward, P. A. (1989a). Neutrophil-dependent, oxygen-radical mediated lung injury associated with acute pancreatitis. *Ann. Surg.* **210**(6): 740–747.

Guice, K. S., Oldham, K. T., and Johnson, K. J. (1989b). Failure of antioxidant therapy(polyethylene glycol-conjugated catalase) in acute pancreatitis. *Am. J. Surg.* **157**:145–149.

Hanson, C. A., Ritter, A. B., Duran, W., and Lavietes, M. H. (1990). Ascites: its effect upon static inflation of the respiratory system. *Am. Rev. Respir. Dis.* **142**:39–42.

Helman, C. A., Keeton, G. R., and Benatar, S. R. (1977). Lymphoid interstitial pneumonia with associated chronic active hepatitis and renal tubular acidosis. *Am. Rev. Respir. Dis.* **115**:161–164.

Henkin, R. I., Maxwell, M. H., and Murray, J. F. (1962). Uremic pneumonitis: a clinical, physiological study. *Ann. Intern. Med.* **57**:1001–1008.

Higenbottam, T., Cochrane, G. M., Clark, T. J. H., Turner, D., Millis, R., and Seymour, W. (1980). Bronchial disease in ulcerative colitis. *Thorax* **35**:581–585.

Hopps, H. C., and Wissler, R. W. (1953). Uremic pneumonitis. *Am. J. Pathol.* **31**:261–273.

Hung, J., Harris, P. J., Uren, R. F., Tiller, D. J., and Kelly, D. T. (1980). Uremic cardiomyopathy-effect of hemodialysis on left ventricular function in end-stage renal failure. *N. Engl. J. Med.* **302**:547–551.

Hunninghake, G. W., and Fauci, A. S. (1979). Pulmonary involvement in the collagen vascular diseases. *Am. Rev. Respir. Dis.* **119**:471–494.

Imrie, C. W., Ferguson, J. C., Murphy, D., and Blumgart, L. H. (1977). Arterial hypoxia in acute pancreatitis. *Br. J. Surg.* **64**:185–188.

Interiano, B., Stuard, I. D., and Hyde, R. W. (1972). Acute respiratory distress syndrome in pancreatitis. *Ann. Intern. Med.* **77**:923–926.

Izdebeska-Makosa, Z., and Zeilinski, J. (1987). Primary biliary cirrhosis in a patient with interstitial fibrosis. *Chest* **92**:766–767.

Johnston, R. F., and Loo, R. V. (1964). Hepatic hydrothorax: studies to determine the source of the fluid and report of thirteen cases. *Ann. Intern. Med.* **61**:385.

Justrabo, E., Genin, R., and Rifle, G. (1979). Pulmonary metastatic calcification with respiratory insufficiency in patients on maintenance haemodialysis. *Thorax* **34**:384–388.

Kaplan, M. M. (1987). Primary biliary cirrhosis. *N. Engl. J. Med.* **316**:521–528.

Kayser, K., Probst, F., Gabius, H. J., and Muller, K. M. (1990). Are there characteristic alterations of lung tissue associated with Crohn's disease? *Path. Res. Prac.* **186**:485–490.

Kimura, T., Toung, J. K., Margolis, S., Permutt, S., and Cameron, J. L. (1979). Respiratory failure in acute pancreatitis: a possible role of triglycerides. *Ann. Surg.* **189**:509–517.

Kraft, S. C., Earle, R. H., Roesler, M., and Esterly, J. R. (1976). Unexplained bronchopulmonary disease with inflammatory bowel disease. *Arch. Intern. Med.* **136**:454–459.

Krowka, M. J., and Cortese, D. A. (1987) Severe hypoxemia associated with liver disease; Mayo Clinic experience and the experimental use of almitrine bismesylate. *Mayo Clin. Proc.* **62**:164–173.

Krowka, M. J., and Cortese, D. A. (1989). Pulmonary aspects of liver disease and liver transplantation. *Clin. Chest. Med.* **10**(4):593–616.

Krowka, M. J., and Cortese, D. A. (1990). Hepatopulmonary syndrome: an evolving perspective in the era of liver transplantation (editorial). *Hepatology* **11**:138–141.

Lai, K. N., Barneden, L., and Mathew, T. H. (1982). Effect of renal transplantation on left ventricular function in hemodialysis patients. *Clin. Nephrol.* **16**:74–78.

Lankisch, P. G., Rahlf, G., and Koop, H. (1983). Death due to acute pancreatitis: A retrospective analysis of 405 autopsy cases. *Dig. Dis. Sci.* **28**(2):111–116.

Lebrec, D., Capron, J. P., Dhumeaux, D., and Benhamou, J. P. (1979). Pulmonary hypertension complicating portal hypertension. *Am. Rev. Respir. Dis.* **120**:849–856.

Lemann, M., Messing, B., D'Agay, F., and Modigliani, R. (1987). Crohn's disease with respiratory tract involvement. *Gut* **28**:1669–1672.

Levine, S. A., Feinsilver, S. H., and Fein, A. M. (1990). What to do when pancreatitis causes pleuropulmonary complications: occult hypoxemia may be the first sign of acute lung injury. *J. Crit. Illness* **5**(7):715–734.

Lieberman, F., Hidemura, R., Peters, R. L., and Reynolds, T. B. (1966). Pathogenesis and treatment of hydrothorax complicating cirrhosis with ascites. *Ann. Intern. Med.* **64**:341–351.

Light, R. W. (1985). Exudative pleural effusions secondary to gastrointestinal diseases. *Clin. Chest. Med.* **6**:103–111.

Light, R. W. (1990). *Pleural diseases*. Lea & Febiger, Philadelphia.

Lockhart, A. (1985). Pulmonary arterial hypertension in portal hypertension. *Clin. Gastroenterol.* **14**:123–138.

Maddrey, W. C. (1983). Sarcoidosis and primary biliary cirrhosis: associated disorders? *N. Engl. J. Med.* **308**:588–590.

Margolin, R. J., and Addison, T. E. (1984). Hypercalcemia and rapidly progressive respiratory failure. *Chest* **86**:767–769.

McCabe, T. A., Rakowski, T. A., Argy, W. P., and Reilly, M. J. (1982). Fibrosing uremic pleuritis complicated by thoracic empyema. *Arch. Intern. Med.* **142**:1369–1370.

McDonnell, P. J., Toye, P. A., and Hutchins, G. M. (1983). Primary pulmonary hypertension in cirrhosis: are they related? *Am. Rev. Respir. Dis.* **127**:437–441.

Melot, C., Naeije, R., Dechamps, P., Hallemans, R., and Lejeune, P. (1989). Pulmonary and extrapulmonary contributors to hypoxemia in liver cirrhosis. *Am. Rev. Respir. Dis.* **139**:632–640.

Miller, K. S., Wooten, S., and Sahn, S. A. (1988). Urinothorax: a cause of low pH transudative pleural effusions. *Am. J. Med.* **85**:448–449.

Mootz, J. R., Sagel, S. S., and Roberts, T. H. (1973). Roentgenographic manifestations of pulmonary calcifications. *Radiology* **107**:55–60.

Murphy, D., Pack, A. I., and Imrie, C. W. (1980). The mechanism of arterial hypoxia occurring in acute pancreatitis. *Q. J. Med.* **49**(194):151–163.

Murray, J. F., Matthay, M. A., Luce, J. M., and Flick, M. R. (1988). An expanded definition of the adult respiratory distress syndrome. *Am. Rev. Respir. Dis.* **138**:720–723.

Naeije, R., Hallemans, R., Mols, P., and Melot, C. (1981). Hypoxic pulmonary vasoconstriction in liver cirrhosis. *Chest* **80**:570–574.

Naeye, R. L. (1960). "Primary" pulmonary hypertension with co-existing portal hypertension: a retrospective study of six cases. *Circulation* **22**:376–384.

Neilly, J. B., Main, A. N. H., McSharry, C., Murray, J., Russell, R. I., and Moran, F. (1989). Pulmonary abnormalities in Crohn's disease. *Respir. Med.* **83**:487–491.

Nidus, B. D., Matalon, R., Cantacuzino, D., and Eisinger, R. P. (1969). Uremic pleuritis: a clinicopathologic entity. *N. Engl. J. Med.* **281**:255–257.

Pehrsson, S. K., Jonasson, R., and Lins, L. (1984). Cardiac performance in various stages of renal failure. *Br. Heart J.* **52**:667–673.

Perez, H. D., Horn, J. D., Ong, R., and Goldstein, I. M. (1983). Complement (C5)-derived chemotactic activity in serum from patients with pancreatitis. *J. Lab. Clin. Med.* **101**:123–129.

Pierce, J. A. (1988). Antitrypsin and emphysema. *JAMA* **259**:2890–2895.

Pitcher, W. D., Diamond, S. M., and Henrich, W. L. (1989). Pulmonary gas exchange during dialysis in patients with obstructive lung disease. *Chest* **96**:1136–1141.

Pitchumoni, C. S., Agarwal, N., and Jian, N. K. (1988). Systemic complications of pancreatitis. *Am. J. Gastroenterol.* **83**:597–606.

Prezant, D. J. (1990). Effect of uremia and its treatment on pulmonary function. *Lung* **168**:1–14.

Rakela, J., Goldschmier, M., and Ludwig, J. (1987). Late manifestations of chronic liver disease in adults with alpha-1-antitrypsin deficiency. *Dig. Dis. Sci.* **32**:1358–1362.

Ranson, H. C., Roses, D. F., and Fink, S. D. (1973). Early respiratory insufficiency in acute pancreatitis. *Ann. Surg.* **178**:75–79.

Renner, I. G., Fracp, M. D., Savage, W. T., Pantoja, J. L., and Renner, V. J. (1985). Death due to acute pancreatitis: a retrospective analysis of 405 autopsy cases. *Dig. Dis. Sci.* **30**:1005–1018.

Rinaldo, J. E., and Christman, J. W. (1990). Mechanisms and mediators of the adult respiratory distress syndrome. *Clin. Chest Med.* **11**:621–632.

Robalino, B. D., and Moodie, D. S. (1991). Association between primary pulmonary hyptertension and portal hypertension: analysis of its pathophysiology and clinical laboratory and hemodynamic manifestations. *J. Am. Coll. Cardiol.* **17**:492–498.

Robertson, C. S., Basran, G. S., and Hardy, J. G. (1988). Lung vascular permeability in patients with acute pancreatitis. *Pancreas* **3**(2):162–165.

Rocker, G. M., Morgan, A. G., and Shale, D. J. (1988). Pulmonary oedema and renal failure. *Nephrol. Dial. Transplant.* **3**:244–246.

Rockey, D. C., and Cello, J. P. (1990). Pancreaticopleural fistula. *Medicine* **69**:332–344.

Rodelas, P., Rakowski, T. A., Argy, W. P., an Schreiner, G. E. (1980). Fibrosing uremic pleuritis during hemodialysis. *JAMA* **243**:2424–2425.

Rodriguez-Roisin, R., Pares, A., Bruguera, M., Coll, J., Picado, C., Agusti-Vidal, A., Burgos, F., and Rodes, J. (1981). Pulmonary involvement in primary biliary cirrhosis. *Thorax* **36**:208–212.

Rodriguez-Roisin, R., Roca, J., Augsti, A. G., Mastai, R., Wagner, P. D., and Bosch, J. (1987). Gas exchange and pulmonary vascular reactivity in patients with liver cirrhosis. *Am. Rev. Respir. Dis.* **135**:1085–1092.

Ross, E. A., Tashkin, D., Chenoweth, D., Webber, M. M., and Nissenson, A. R. (1987). Pulmonary leukosequestration without hypoxemia during hemodialysis. *Int. J. Artif. Organs.* **10**:367–374.

Ruff, R., Hughes, J. B. M., Stanley, N., McCarthy, D., Greene, R., Aronoff, A., Clayton, L., and Milic-Emili, J. (1971). Regional lung function in patients with hepatic cirrhosis. *J. Clin. Invest.* **50**:2403–2413.

Salcedo, J. E. (1986). Urinothorax: report of 4 cases and review of the literature. *J. Urol.* **134**:805–808.

Salem, O., Dindzans, V., Freeman, J., O'Dorisio, T., Ruthardt, F., and Van Their, D. (1989). Liver transplantation following pre-operative closure of intrapulmonary shunts. *Hepatology* **10**:569.

Sargent, D., Sessions, J. T., and Fairman, R. P. (1985). Pulmonary vasculitis complicating ulcerative colitis. *South Med. J.* **78**:624–625.

Scharf, S., Wexler, J., Longnecker, R. E., and Blaufox, M. D. (1980). Cardiovascular disease in patients on chronic hemodialytic therapy. *Prog. Cardiovasc. Dis.* **22**:343–356.

Schuster, D. P. (1989). Positron emission tomography: theory and its application to the study of lung disease. *Am. Rev. Respir. Dis.* **139**:818–840.

Senior, R. M., and Lefrak, S. S. (1988). The lungs in abdominal disease. In *Textbook of Respiratory Medicine*. Edited by J. F. Murray and J. A. Nadal. Saunders, Philadelphia, pp. 1894–1905.

Senior, R. M., Britton, A. C., Turino, G. M., Wood, J. A. Lauper, G. A., and Fishman, A. P. (1968). Pulmonary hypertension associated with cirrhosis of the liver and with portacaval shunts. *Circulation* **37**:88–96.

Seward, J. B., Hayes, D. L., Smith, H. C., Williams, D. E., Rosenow, E. C., Reeder, G. S., Piehler, J. M., and Tajik, J. (1984). Platypnea-orthodeoxia: clinical profile, diagnostic workup, management, and report of seven cases. *Mayo Clin. Proc.* **59**:221–231.

Shapiro, D. H., Anagnostopoulos, C. E., and, Dineen, J. P. (1970). Decortication and pleurectomy for the pleuropulmonary complications of pancreatitis. *Ann. Thorac. Surg.* **9**:76–80.

Shapiro, M. S., Dobbins, J. W., and Matthay, R. A. (1989). Pulmonary manifestations of gastrointestinal disease. *Clin. Chest Med.* **10**:617–643.

Sharma, M. P., and Kar, P. (1985). Pulmonary functions in ulcerative colitis. *JAPI* **33**:613–614.

Silverman, A., Cooper, M. D., Moller, J. H., and Good, R. A. (1968). Syndrome of cyanosis, digital clubbing, and hepatic disease in siblings. *J. Pediatr.* **72**:70–80.

Silverman, E. K., Pierce, J. A., Province, M. A., Rao, D. C., and Campbell, E. J. (1989). Variability of pulmonary function in alpha-1-antitrypsin deficiency: clinical correlates. *Ann. Intern. Med.* **111**:982–991.

Singh, S., Dale, A., Morgan, B., and Sahebjami, H. (1984). Serial studies of pulmonary function in continuous ambulatory peritoneal dialysis. *Chest* **86**:874–877.

Smiejan, J.-M., Cosnes, J., Chollet-Martin, S., Soler, P., Basset, F. M., Le Quintrec, Y., and Hance, A. J. (1986). Sarcoid-like lymphocytosis of the lower respiratory tract in patients with active Crohn's disease. *Ann. Intern. Med.* **104**:17–21.

Smith, J. C., Stanton, L. W., Kramer, N. C., and Parrish, A. E. (1969). Nodular pulmonary calcification in renal failure. *Am. Rev. Respir. Dis.* **100**:723–728.

Snell, A. M. (1935). The effects of chronic disease of the liver on the composition and the physicochemical properties of the blood: changes in the serum proteins; reduction in the arterial saturation of the arterial blood. *Ann. Intern. Med.* **9**:690–711.

Stanley, N. N., and Woodgate, D. J. (1972). Mottled chest radiograph and gas transfer defect in chronic liver disease. *Thorax* **27**:315–323.

Stark, D. D., Shanes, J. G., Baron, R. L., and Koch, D. D. (1982). Biochemical features of urinothorax. *Arch. Intern. Med.* **142**:1509–1511.

Stoller, J. K., Moodie, D., Schiavone, W. A., Vogt, D., Brougham, T., Winkelmann, E., Rehm, P. K., and Carey, W. D. (1990). Reduction of intrapulmonary shunt and resolution of digital clubbing after liver transplantation. *Hepatology* **11**:138–141.

Sveger, T. (1976). Liver disease in alpha-1 antitrpysin deficiency detected by screening 200,000 infants. *N. Engl. J. Med.* **294**:1316–1321.

Swinburn, C. R., Jackson, G. J., Cobden, I., Ashcroft, T., Morritt, G. N., and Corris, P. A. (1988). Bronchiolitis obliterans organising pneumonia in a patient with ulcerative colitis. *Thorax* **43**:735–736.

Tahamont, M. V., Barie, P. S., Blumenstock, F. A., Hussain, M. H., and Malik, A. B. (1982). Increased lung vascular permeability after pancreatitis and trypsin infusion. *Am. J. Pathol.* **109**:15–26.

Tong, M. J. (1982). Chronic hepatitis. In *Hepatology: A Textbook of Liver Disease*. Edited by D. Zakim and T. D. Boyer. Saunders, Philadelphia, pp. 972–994.

Turner-Warwick, M. (1968). Fibrosing alveolitis and chronic liver disease. *Q. J. Med.* **37**:133–149.

Uddenfeldt, P., Bjerle, P., Danielsson, A., Nystrom, L., and Stjernberg, N. (1988). Lung function abnormalities in patients with primary biliary cirrhosis. *Acta Med. Scand.* **223**:549–555.

Van Thiel, D. H., Schade, R. R., Gavaler, J. S., Shaw, B. W., Iwatsuki, S., and Starzl, T. E. (1984). Medical aspects of liver transplantation. *Hepatology* **4**:79S–83S.

Vierling, J. M. (1982). Primary biliary cirrhosis. In *Hepatology: A Textbook of Liver Disease*. Edited by D. Zakim and T. D. Boyer. Saunders, Philadelphia, pp. 825–861.

Wallace, J. G., Tong, M. J., Ueki, B. H., and Quismorio, F. P. (1987). Pulmonary involvement in primary biliary cirrhosis. *J. Clin. Gastroenterol.* **9**:431–445.

Wallaert, B., Colombel, J. F., Tonnel, A. B., Bonniere, P., Cortot, A., Paris, J. C., and Voisin, C. (1985). Evidence of lymphocyte alveolitis in Crohn's disease. *Chest* **87**(3):363–367.

Wallaert, B., Bonniere, P., Prin, L., Cortot, A., Tonnel, A. B., and Voisin, C. (1986). Primary biliary cirrhosis: subclinical inflammatory alveolitis in patients with normal chest roentgenograms. *Chest* **90**:842–848.

Wiesner, R. H., and La Russo, N. F. (1980). Clinicopatholgic features of the syndrome of primary sclerosing cholangitis. *Gastroenterology* **79**: 200–206.

Wilcox, P., Miller, R., Miller, G., Heath, J., Nelems, B., Muller, N., and Ostrow, D. (1987). Airway involvement in ulcerative colitis. *Chest* **92**(1): 18–22.

Williams, A., Trewby, P., and Williams, R. (1979). Structural alterations to the pulmonary circulation in fulminant hepatic failure. *Thorax* **34**:447–453.

Wolfe, J. D., Tashkin, D. P., Holly, F. E., Brachman, M. B., and Genovesi, M. G. (1977). Hypoxemia in cirrhosis: detection of abnormal small pulmonary vascular channels by a quantitative radionuclide method. *Am. J. Med.* **63**:746–765.

5

Hematological Diseases

LEE R. BERKOWITZ and PHILIP A. BROMBERG

University of North Carolina at Chapel Hill
Chapel Hill, North Carolina

I. Introduction

The vast scope of hematological disease, as well as the complexities associated with the treatment of these illnesses, precludes an exhaustive review of all their associated respiratory problems. We have selected a number of topics of interest that are important to the pulmonary specialist and emhasized their clinical features rather than underlying mechanisms. Certain elements of these diseases that are not related to the respiratory system may not be discussed; the interested reader is referred to hematology texts for further information on these points. Other recent reviews may also be helpful, including those by Bromberg and Ross (1988), Prakash (1989), and Edwards and Matthay (1989). Information about the pulmonary complications of chemotherapeutic drugs and further details concerning leukemias, lymphomas, and bone marrow transplantation may be found in Chapter 2.

II. Sickle Cell Disease

Erythrocytes containing hemoglobin S cause alterations in blood flow that may produce a variety of pulmonary complications, ranging from abnormalities of gas exchange to pulmonary vascular occlusion. These problems may be acute or chronic and can be life-threatening for the patient with homozygous sickle cell (SS) anemia, sickle-beta thalassemia, and hemoglobin SC disease. Patients with sickle cell trait are generally spared. The pulmonologist must be able to recognize these problems and institute appropriate therapy. Table 1 lists known pulmonary complications of sickle hemoglobinopathies, divided into acute and chronic problems. Each will be discussed in terms of pathogenesis, clinical manifestations, and treatment.

A. Acute Syndromes

Acute Chest Syndrome

The acute chest syndrome, defined as chest pain, fever, leukocytosis, and new infiltrates on chest x-ray, is probably the most common pulmonary syndrome seen in patients with significant sickle hemoglobinopathies (Bromberg, 1974). In one series of adults with sickle cell anemia, 14% of sickle-related hospital admissions resulted from this syndrome (Davies et al., 1984). In a population of children with sickle cell anemia, 10% of hospital admissions were caused by the acute chest syndrome (Murtaza et al., 1981). The pathogenesis of the syndrome is complex. Based on histopathological reviews of lung specimens both pre- and postmortem, almost all authorities on this subject state that a major component is caused by microvascular occlusion by rigid sickle cells, with resultant alveolar wall necrosis and scarring (Hasleton et al., 1989; Haupt et al., 1982). Platelets and neutrophils do not appear to contribute to the vessel occlusion and parenchymal damage.

Table 1 Pulmonary Complications of Sickle Hemoglobinopathies

I. Acute syndromes
    A. Acute chest syndrome
    B. Chest syndrome of pregnancy
    C. Bacterial pneumonia
    D. Fat emboli
    E. Cocaine ingestion
II. Chronic syndromes
    A. Sickle cell lung disease
    B. Pulmonary hypertension
    C. Lung cancer
    D. Upper airway obstruction

Bacterial infection seldom contributes to the process, because sputum cultures, even with transtracheal aspiration and bronchoscopy, are positive in only 10–20% of episodes (Kirkpatrick et al., 1991). Several groups have analyzed their experiences with the acute chest syndrome in an attempt to determine the role of infection (Charache et al., 1979; Petch and Serjeant, 1970; Poncz et al., 1985). Short of a positive culture from sputum, blood, needle aspirate of an infiltrate, or bronchoscopically obtained secretions, no physical finding or laboratory test indicates which patients have infection as part of the process, although the general notion is that the sicker the patient, the more likely a pulmonary infection. Management is dictated by the clinical course. In many patients the syndrome resolves in a few days. These patients are usually treated with supportive measures, including supplemental oxygen and intravenous hydration. For the toxic patients with high fever, antibiotics are added to cover gram-positive organisms, the most likely pathogens in these functionally asplenic patients. Some patients with the acute chest syndrome exhibit marked hypoxemia with respiratory and metabolic acidosis. These patients require exchange transfusion to reduce the percentage of hemoglobin S in their blood to 20–30% (Davies et al., 1984). In severely hypoxemic patients, death has been reported (Davies et al., 1984).

Acute Chest Syndrome of Pregnancy

This syndrome has been reported in pregnant women with sickle cell anemia as well as pregnant women with hemoglobin SC disease. In a large multicenter prospective study of pregnant women with sickle cell anemia, acute chest syndrome occurred in 6% of the patients. Comparing patients randomized to receive exchange transfusion therapy versus a control group, no difference was observed in the frequency of the acute chest syndrome. No mortality was reported in the control or transfused group (Koshy et al., 1988). Previous case reports of a small number of patients with hemoglobin SC disease describe a more severe course requiring emergency exchange transfusion (Edwards and Matthay, 1989). Fat embolization from bone marrow infarction was likely responsible for the additional morbidity in these patients.

Bacterial Pneumonia

Although infection may be a component of the acute chest syndrome, some authors call separate attention to bacterial pneumonia in sickle cell patients. This complication is observed mostly in pediatric patients, in whom the incidence of gram-positive infection, particularly with *Streptococcus pneumoniae*, is reported as high as 7–8 per hundred person-years of observation (Gaston et al., 1986). Retrospective reviews of pediatric patients record episodes of bacterial pneumonia in 36–67% of clinic patients followed over a 5- to 10-year period, although positive cultures, either blood or sputum, were documented in only about half these episodes (Poncz et al., Gill, 1985; De Ceulaer et al., 1985). Organisms cultured include *S. pneumoniae*, *Haemophilus influenzae*, alpha-hemolytic *Streptococcus*, and *Salmonella* species. Retrospective analyses of clinical and laboratory data in these series, seeking to identify indicators of a bacterial infection, have been unsuccessful.

Few other pathogens have been reported as causing pulmonary syndromes in sickle cell patients. Included are *Cryptococcus neoformans*, *Mycobacterium tuberculosis*, *Mycoplasma pneumoniae*, and *Legionella* species (Hardy et al., 1986; Prakash, 1989; Bromberg and Ross, 1988).

Fat Emboli

Because intravascular sickling can result in bone marrow necrosis, fat may embolize to the pulmonary arterial system and cause fever, pulmonary symptoms, and hypoxemia. A similar syndrome has been recognized in orthopedic patients with long bone fractures. Fat embolism in sickle cell patients has been largely identified at postmortem examination, with only a few reported cases diagnosed antemortem (Shapiro and Hayes, 1984). The diagnosis is made by finding fat droplets in the sputum or in alveolar macrophages obtained by bronchoalveolar lavage (Kollef et al., 1990). The diagnosis should be entertained in the presence of evidence of fat embolization to other organs. Manifestations of such systemic embolization include petechial hemorrhages, livedo reticularis, renal insufficiency, and retinal embolization (Holtz et al., 1990). Several patients have responded to exchange transfusion (Shapiro and Hayes, 1984); otherwise, care is supportive.

Cocaine Ingestion

The widespread use of cocaine raises the possibility that a patient with sickle cell disease presenting with manifestations of cocaine use may be confused with a problem due to sickling. Alternatively, because cocaine causes pulmonary arterial constriction, cocaine might provoke microvascular occlusion in sickle cell patients, leading to the acute chest syndrome. There is one report of a pulmonary death in a sickle cell patient after ingestion of a large amount of cocaine (Strauss and LaCandia, 1989).

B. Chronic Syndromes

Sickle Cell Chronic Lung Disease

As early as 1936 it was suggested that repeated pulmonary vascular occlusion by sickle erythrocytes led to permanent pulmonary damage (Bromberg, 1974).

Several autopsy series as well as additional case reports have substantiated this idea (Oppenheimer and Esterly, 1971; Haupt et al., 1982). A retrospective longitudinal study of this complication has reviewed the course of 28 patients followed at one comprehensive sickle cell center (Powars et al., 1988). The patients were selected based on the presence of pulmonary symptoms, the results of pulmonary function studies, x-ray abnormalities, hypoxemia, and evidence of cor pulmonale. Minimal criteria for inclusion included chest pain and cough, interstitial markings on a chest x-ray, electrocardiogram and echocardiogram showing left ventricular preponderance, and a 20% reduction in FVC, TLC, FEV_1, and FEV_1/FVC ratio. Patients began to show these abnormalities in the second decade of life and progressed to pulmonary failure, cor pulmonale, and death by the fourth decade. Risk factors included the number of episodes of acute chest syndrome and aseptic necrosis of bone. Often patients had clustering of multiple episodes of the acute chest syndrome immediately before the onset of overt chronic lung disease. Patients with more advanced disease were treated with chronic transfusions, which did not appear to influence outcome.

Pulmonary Hypertension

There are several reports of this complication in patients with sickle hemoglobinopathies (Hammond and Mosesson, 1989; Collins and Orringer, 1982). We have separated these reports from those of sickle cell chronic lung disease for two reasons. First, these reports describe patients who presented with hypertension without antecedent acute chest syndrome; this suggests that progressive evolution of pulmonary involvement from mild to severe did not occur. Second, more than half the patients described had hemoglobin SC disease; this is consistent with the suggestion that the higher hematocrits commonly found in SC disease may be a contributing factor (Collins and Orringer, 1982).

Lung Cancer

There is one report in the literature of a patient with sickle cell anemia who developed alveolar cell carcinoma of the lung (Labi et al., 1989). The patient was a 34-year-old man with a long, complicated pulmonary history, which included empyema, pulmonary embolism, pneumothorax, and several episodes of pneumonia. The patient also had a 15 pack-year history of cigarette smoking. The diagnosis of lung cancer was made by bronchoscopy, which was performed to evaluate progressive infiltrates on the chest x-ray. The authors discuss whether the lung cancer may have been secondary to sickle cell disease associated with chronic inflammation and scarring.

Clearly, more experience is needed to know whether chronic or recurrent pulmonary damage due to erythrocyte sickling is a risk factor for the development of lung cancer. Regardless, as patients with sickle hemoglobinopathies live longer, the possibility of a lung malignancy must be considered in the differential diagnosis of radiological abnormalities.

Upper Airway Obstruction

Two recently reported series document upper airway obstruction in pediatric patients with sickle cell (SC) disease (Davies et al, 1989; Maddern et al., 1989). One series included children who were evaluated for a history of snoring and apnea pauses. A total of 21 patients were evaluated by physical examination and polysomnography; all 21 fulfilled criteria for the obstructive sleep apnea syndrome (Maddern et al., 1989). Thirteen patients underwent adenotonsillectomy and showed improvement in subjective complaints and a statistically significant reduction in end tidal $Paco_2$ during sleep. However, the number of apneas and episodes of arterial desaturation did not change significantly after surgery. The cause of the lymphoid tissue enlargement was not found. The second series was generated by screening 45 children with homozygous sickle cell (SS) disease and 29 with SC disease at one hospital (Davies et al, 1989). If patients had tonsillar hypertrophy with a history of snoring or deterioration in attention span, they underwent a sleep study. Twenty patients with SS disease and three with SC disease were monitored. Eight patients, with all SS disease, fulfilled criteria for upper airway obstruction and underwent adenotonsillectomy, with complete resolution of obstruction in six cases. The authors speculate that the adenotonsillar hypertrophy in SS patients is a compensation for the splenic infarction characteristic of sickle cell disease. This was not seen in their SC patients, perhaps because splenic function is not as impaired in this condition as in hemoglobin SS disease.

III. Gas Exchange in Anemia

Patients with severe anemia partially compensate for their decrease in arterial O_2 content by increasing cardiac output in an effort to maintain systemic O_2 transport. This results in a narrowing of the arterial-mixed venous (a-v) oxygen difference. However, because of the low O_2 capacity of anemic blood, both mixed venous (pulmonary arterial) O_2 saturation and pO_2 are reduced. The limitation of systemic oxygen transport results in a decrease in maximal O_2 consumption and an excessive cardiac output both at rest and during exercise (Bishop et al., 1955; Sproule et al., 1960). Remarkably, the anemic patients attained a mean maximal cardiac output (23.6 L/min) equal to that of the normal controls (Sproule et al., 1960).

Bishop and colleagues (1955) found that $\dot{V}_E$ was excessive in anemic patients and that arterial pCO_2 was decreased. In sickle cell disease, the V_D/V_T ratio does not fall as much as expected during exercise (Pianosi et al., 1991;

Miller et al., 1973), possibly because of the presence of subclinical pulmonary vascular occlusion. The increased $\dot{V}_E$ coupled with somewhat reduced vital capacity and maximum sustainable ventilation may account for exertional dyspnea in sickle cell disease patients who have neither left ventricular compromise nor pulmonary hypertension.

As is true of other types of severe anemia, sickle cell disease patients generally have a widened resting alveolar-arterial pO_2 difference for their age. Because blood O_2 affinity is variably decreased in sickle cell disease (Bromberg and Jensen, 1967; Milner, 1974), arterial O_2 saturation may be depressed in this condition. However, reduced O_2-hemoglobin affinity may be useful in terms of tissue oxygenation by allowing capillary pO_2 to remain at a higher level as O_2 is released by the red cells.

Lung diffusing capacity for CO is reduced in proportion to the degree of anemia, and observed D_L CO measurements must be corrected (upward) according to the hemoglobin level at the time of testing before interpreting what appears to be a reduced value.

IV. Other Hemoglobin Disorders

The scope of clinical problems encountered by the pulmonologist due to abnormalities of hemoglobin extends beyond sickle cell disease. These additional hemoglobinopathies, which may be quantitative or qualitative, are outlined in Table 2. The most common is a quantitative increase in hemoglobin concentration, frequently called erythrocytosis. Erythrocytosis may represent the myeloproliferative disorder polycythemia vera, or it may be secondary to a number of

Table 2 Hemoglobinopathies

- I. Quantitative—erythrocytosis
  - A. Primary—polycythemia vera
  - B. Secondary
    1. Chronic lung disease
    2. High-altitude residence
    3. Chronic carbon monoxide poisoning
    4. Cyanotic congenital heart disease
    5. Various neoplasms
- II. Qualitative
  - A. High-oxygen-affinity hemoglobinemia
  - B. Methemoglobinemia

hypoxemic conditions, including chronic carbon monoxide exposure (DiMarco, 1988). Pathophysiologically, the two types of erythrocytosis are distinct. Polycythemia vera results from clonal proliferation of hematopoietic cells independent of erythropoietin, whereas the secondary conditions are driven by excessive production of erythopoietin. Clinically, patients with the two types of erythrocytosis are not distinct. All present with expansion of their red cell mass and adverse effects may be seen in any patient when the hematocrit is greater than 55% (Editorial, 1987). Cardiac function is impaired on both sides of the heart by increased blood viscosity, and on the right side in addition by hypoxia-induced vasoconstriction in the pulmonary circulation (Editorial, 1989). Treatment is usually begun with phlebotomy to decrease the hemotocrit to 50%. At this level, improvement in both right ventricular and left ventricular function has been demonstrated (Milne, Light, and Chetty, 1990). Patients with polycythemia vera are also often treated with the chemotherapeutic agent hydroxyurea. A report that theophylline decreases erythropoietin production raises the possibility of using this drug in the secondary disorders (Bakris et al., 1990).

Approximately 500 variants of hemoglobin have been identified, most due to single amino acid substitutions in the globin molecule (Zinkham and Winslow, 1989). Two phenotypes should be recognized by the pulmonologist. First are the high-oxygen-affinity hemoglobins with resulting erythrocytosis due to tissue hypoxemia. These patients are treated with phlebotomy when their hematocrits are extremely high.Second are the methemoglobins.Congenital methemoglobinopathies cause cyanosis,which only affects the patient cosmetically and requires no therapy. Congenital methemoglobinemia must be distinguished from the acquired form due to ingestion of oxidant drugs. Acquired methemoglobinemia may be fatal if not treated with methylene blue.

V. Hyperleukocytosis

Patients with peripheral blood leukocyte counts greater than 100,000/μL may develop symptoms due to small vessel occlusion by white cells (Prakash, 1989). This symptom complex, called leukostasis, was first reported in a large group of patients by McKee and Collins (1974). They reviewed autopsy reports on 206 adult patients with acute nonlymphocytic leukemia, chronic granulocytic leukemia (including blast crisis), acute lymphoblastic leukemia, and chronic lymphocytic leukemia. Two pathological patterns were seen: leukemic thrombi, which were defined as leukemic cells plus fibrin filling the vessel lumen; and leukemic aggregates, which were defined as leukemic cells filling the lumen without fibrin. The lungs were the most frequently involved organ and showed pulmonary infarction and hemorrhage from vessel occlusion. Patients with this complication complained chiefly of dyspnea. Leukostasis was seen almost exclusively in the myeloid leukemias, both acute and chronic. No patients with acute lymphatic leukemia had this complication and only three patients with chronic lymphatic leukemia had leukostasis at pathological examination. Analyzing leukostasis with respect to peripheral white blood cell counts showed that when the white blood cell count was greater than 200,000/μL, all patients had leukostasis. When the peripheral white cell count was between 50,000/μL and 200,000μL, 50% of patients had leukostasis, and when the peripheral blood white cell count was less than 50,000/μL, there were no instances of leukostasis.

The observations of McKee and Collins (1974) have been confirmed in subsequent reports, including some of children with acute leukemia (Bunin et al., 1987; Callaghan and Fitzsimons, 1989). Most notable is the reporting of pulmonary leukostasis only in the myeloid leukemias. For example, Maurer et al. (1988) reported on 124 children with acute lymphoblastic leukemia with peripheral white blood cells of greater than 200,000/μL. None of these children had pulmonary leukostasis.

There is some information on radiographic findings in patients with pulmonary leukostasis. McKee and Collins (1974) reported normal chest x-rays, chest x-rays showing congestive heart failure, and chest x-rays with pulmonary infiltrates in those patients whose cause of death was leukostasis. A review of 10 patients with autopsy-confirmed leukostasis and a chest x-ray obtained within 3 days of death describes four patients with normal chest x-rays, four with diffuse alveolar consolidation, one patient with pleural effusion, and one patient with lobar consolidation on chest x-ray (van Buchem et al., 1987). Hug et al. (1983) reported on 46 patients with acute nonlymphocytic leukemia with pretreatment white blood cell counts of greater than 100,000/μL. Twenty-seven patients had abnormal chest x-rays, with parenchymal infiltrates being the most common finding. Adenopathy and pleural effusions were found in a few patients.

In vitro studies have shown that myeloblasts and monoblasts are more rigid and less deformable than lymphoblasts (Snyder et al., 1990; Bromberg and Ross, 1988). This observation may explain the difference in prevalence of leukostasis between myeloid and lymphoid leukemias. An increase in blood viscosity does not appear to contribute to leukostasis, as measurements of blood viscosity in these patients are usually normal, perhaps due to coexisting anemia (Prakash, 1989).

Patients with clinical symptoms of leukostasis need emergent leukapheresis due to the appreciable mortality associated with this syndrome, which may be as high as 50% (Creutzig et al., 1987; Hug et al., 1983). Cytoreduction with conventional chemotherapy is not rapid enough. Transfusion of packed red cells should be done cautiously to avoid increases in blood viscosity that could exacerbate the situation. Patients without clinical symptoms of leukostasis but with peripheral white cell counts greater than 100,000/μL should be monitored carefully for leukostasis during induction therapy. Several reports have described the onset of leukostasis approximately 2 days after starting chemotherapy. The authors of these reports have speculated that lung injury in this situation is due to by-products of the destroyed myeloblasts (Nagler et al., 1988; Hug et al., 1983).

VI. Coagulopathies

Pulmonologists must be able to recognize and manage a number of coagulopathies if bronchoscopy and transbronchial biopsy are to be performed safely. Many, but not all, of these coagulopathies occur in patients with primary hematological disease. Patients who receive aggressive chemotherapy often simultaneously become thrombocytopenic and immunosuppressed and then present with pulmonary infiltrates. The pulmonologist must pay careful attention to the level of the platelet count. With a platelet count greater than 50,000/μL, the patient should be able to tolerate invasive procedures without excessive bleeding and does not require platelet transfusion. Lower platelet counts or evidence of platelet dysfunction (see below) argue for platelet transfusions (Consensus Development Conference, 1987). The immunocompromised patient may also develop disseminated intravascular coagulation from sepsis. The diagnosis is established by laboratory findings that demonstrate excessive activation of thrombin with resultant release of fibrin into the circulation. Common additional abnormalities are prolonged prothrombin and partial thromboplastin times, a low platelet count, decreased fibrinogen, increased fibrin degradation products, and low levels of activity of several clotting factors. Treatment should focus on defining the site and cause of the infection and instituting antibiotic therapy. Adjunctive therapy includes the replacement of antithrombin III and clotting factors by infusions of fresh frozen plasma. Cryoprecipitate is administered when the fibrinogen level is less than 100 mg/dl, and heparin is used only when there is evidence of thrombosis, manifested as digital gangrene.

A qualitative disorder of platelets may also represent an excessive risk for invasive procedure. Patients with uremia, ingestion of aspirin or nonsteroidal anti-inflammatory drugs, and thrombocytopenic patients may have platelet dysfunction and an abnormal bleeding time. The results of measurement of the bleeding time, if obtained, should be coupled with a clinical history of bleeding to assess risk because the bleeding time alone is not an adequate predictor of risk of hemorrhage (Lind, 1991). If all information results in the judgment of increased risk, there are several therapeutic options. Infusion of 1-deamino-8-D-arginine vasopressin (DDAVP) shortens the bleeding time, particularly in the uremic patient. Platelet transfusion may also shorten the bleeding time for the patient who is thrombocytopenic or who has ingested drugs that interfere with platelet function.

The anticoagulated patient requiring invasive procedures needs specific management. For the patient on heparin, discontinuation of heparin 6–12 hr before a procedure should allow the partial thromboplastin time to return to normal. Heparin should be reinstituted as quickly as possible afterward. For the patient on warfarin, the drug may also be discontinued, but a period of 3–5 days will be needed for the prothrombin time to normalize. Rapid reversal can be achieved with fresh frozen plasma, vitamin K, or both. Fresh frozen plasma therapy will need to be repeated frequently owing to the short half-life of factor VII (5 hr). Vitamin K may make the patient refractory to warfarin for days after vitamin K administration. The implications of these factors should be considered for each particular patient.

VII. Bone Marrow Transplantation

Bone marrow transplantation (BMT) is a relatively new, but increasingly widely employed, mode of treatment for patients with malignant hematological diseases, solid tumors, aplastic anemia, and other serious disorders (Bortin and Rimm, 1986). Pulmonary complications of this procedure are common and serious, occurring both early and late after grafting. Apart from graft-versus-host disease (GVHD) and recurrence of the original malignancy, pulmonary disease is the major cause of death in patients with successful engraftment. Older reviews of the pulmonary and infectious complications of BMT by Buckner et al. (1984), Krowka et al. (1985), and Meyers (1985) remain valuable. Chan et al. (1990) have more recently reviewed the pulmonary disorders associated with BMT.

There are three types of BMT. Autografts, using the patient's own marrow, are employed in the radical treatment of neoplastic diseases where the marrow is basically normal. The marrow is cryopreserved pending the completion of the pretransplant cancer erradication regime. These patients are not subject to GVHD and do not require immunosuppressive therapy for its prophylaxis or treatment. After successful engraftment, there should be relatively few complications if the original neoplastic process does not recur. Syngeneic transplants, from an identical twin, are also free of GVHD and immunosuppressive drug-related complications. Allogeneic, HLA-matched BMT, with marrow usually from a sibling, is used in treatment of leukemias and aplastic anemia. Immunosuppression is required to allow engraftment and also for prophylaxis or treatment of GVHD, which is a frequent and severe complication. Nevertheless, despite the absence of GVHD and immune rejection of the transplant in recipients of autografts or syngeneic marrow, the posttransplant period is fraught with many hazards that are shared with the recipients of HLA-matched allografts.

A. General Features

The course of BMT can be divided into three sequential phases. In the first, the patient is "cured" of malignancy with total-body irradiation and/or high-dose chemotherapy appropriate to the malignancy being treated, as well as "conditioned" to receive the transplant. Prevention of rejection of an allogeneic marrow graft requires additional immune suppressive therapy. Even with successful engraftments, regeneration of the formed blood elements by the marrow transplant does not occur for several weeks. During this time the patient is at high risk for bacteremia with gram-positive or gram-negative organisms and for fungal or viral infections. One portal of entry for microorganisms is mucositis induced by the conditioning regime, which breaches the oral-pharyngeal and gastrointestinal barriers, thereby allowing penetration of oral and gut microbial flora. Venous access lines are another portal of entry. Prophylactic therapy with ciprofloxacin and acyclovir, oral nonabsorbable antibiotics, and use of laminar flow rooms, as well as careful attention to prevention of nosocomial infection, have decreased morbidity and mortality in this phase. Transfusions of red cells and platelets are needed, and particular attention is required to avoid infusing latent cytomegalovirus (CMV) or Epstein-Barr (E-B) virus into seronegative recipients who have received marrow from a seronegative donor. Transfusion of viable lymphocytes along with blood may result in GVHD (not due to the marrow transplant itself), because the newly transfused lymphocytes, unopposed by the heavily immune-suppressed host, may destroy the marrow transplant as well.

The second phase begins after several weeks with successful marrow engraftment. There is a release of granulocytes and lymphocytes (as well as other formed blood elements) so that the incidence of the infections encountered in the early phase falls. Unfortunately, the new granulocytes may attack pulmonary capillaries, which were previously damaged by irradiation and high-dose chemotherapy, and cause diffuse infiltrates and hypoxemia with pulmonary edema that may be associated with diffuse pulmonary hemorrhage.

Full reconstitution of host defenses after marrow engraftment is generally complete at 12 months posttransport in syngeneic and autologous transplant recipients. In allogeneic transplants host immunity may never be perfectly reconstituted, and if GVHD occurs, host immunity remains more or less seriously impaired. This important area has been discussed by Witherspoon et al. (1984), Lum (1987), and Sullivan (1987), among others. Impaired antibody production against specific antigens is an important mechanism that contributes to the susceptibility of patients with chronic GVHD to late-onset bacterial infections of the sinuses and lower respiratory tract. It also is a significant feature of the difficulty encountered by the patient with GVHD in coping with CMV infections.

CMV pneumonia is a major problem in the second phase. The infection tends to occur earlier in seronegative than seropositive recipients, and takes the form of a miliary infiltrate with an acute febrile onset and a rapidly progressive course; this form is thought to represent primary CMV infection. In allograft recipients who are seropositive, a more indolent illness occurs, which is associated with bilateral or unilateral alveolar-interstitial infiltrates and which progresses to diffuse interstitial pneumonitis (Beschorner et al., 1980; Smith, 1989). This picture is more likely to develop in the presence of acute GVHD (Cordonnier et al., 1986; Chan et al., 1990) and is responsible for about 40% of the cases of "interstitial pneumonitis" that appear in this phase.

In allogeneic transplant recipients, the reconstitution of immunological competence in the second phase is frequently (30–50%) associated with the development of acute GVHD, despite the use of prophylactic corticosterioids and cyclosporine A, with or without methotrexate. Acute GVHD in BMT recipients is manifested by skin rash of varying severity and extent, by hepatic abnormalities, and by intestinal involvement manifested by diarrhea. The marrow is, of course, spared. The intensive immunosuppressive therapy for acute GVHD (including antithymocyte globulin) and the presence per se of GVHD substantially increase the risk of infection with viruses of the herpes group [HSV-1, HSV-2, CMV, E-B virus, varicella-zoster virus (VZV)] and adenovirus, as well as of organisms like *Pneumocystis carinii* or *Listeria monocytogenes*. The intestinal component of GVHD provides a portal of entry for gut organisms, and continued suppression of phagocytic functions favors fungal invasion.

Acute GVHD is a major risk factor for the subsequent development of chronic GVHD. Chronic GVHD occurs in up to 50% of fully MHC-matched, family-member-donated, allogeneic BMT and is a feature of the third, or late, phase. The skin develops a sclerodermatous appearance but may also show a pattern of papules on a licheniform background. Oral sicca syndrome occurs and may be accompanied by dry cough, as in Sjögren's syndrome. Cholestatic periportal hepatic disease is prominent. VZV infections occur commonly and can become disseminated. Chronic GVHD is primarily managed with corticosteroids, but azathioprine or cyclosporine A may be added.

Table 3 outlines the pulmonary problems associated with each of the phases. The durations of the phases given in the table are approximate. Several of these entities will be discussed in some detail. Others are briefly mentioned.

In the early phase, a new focal pulmonary infiltrate associated with fever is likely to represent bacterial pneumonia and should be treated empirically with broad-spectrum antimicrobial coverage. Acyclovir prophylaxis diminishes the likelihood of pneumonitis or serious airways infection due to HSV. Lack of response to treatment raises the possibility of fungal infection, such as with *Aspergillus* species, which are discussed below.

Bronchoscopy with BAL is usually successful at diagnosing most pulmonary infections that have failed to respond to empirical antibacterial therapy, as well as pulmonary hemorrhage (Stover et al., 1984; Cordonnier et al., 1986;

Table 3 Pulmonary Complications of Bone Marrow Transplantation

I. Phase 1 (−7 to +21 days)
  A. Infection
    1. Bacterial pneumonia
    2. Herpes simplex tracheitis, bronchitis, pneumonia
    3. Respiratory syncytial virus pneumonia
    4. Fungal pneumonia (*Candida, Aspergillus)*
  B. Pulmonary edema
    1. Volume overload
    2. Sepsis/endotoxinemia
    3. Acute lung injury, hemorrhage
    4. Reactions to granulocyte transfusion (rarely used)
    5. Aspiration (esophagitis, vomiting)

II. Phase 2 (+21 to +90 days)
  A. Acute lung injury, hemorrhage
  B. Cytomegalovirus pneumonia, miliary (in seronegative recipients)
  C. Interstitial pneumonitis (nonbacterial, nonfungal)
    1. Cytomegalovirus, other viruses
    2. Idiopathic
  D. Acute GVHD-associated phenomena
    1. *Aspergillus* pneumonia/sinusitis
    2. *Pneumocystis carinii* pneumonia

III. Phase 3 (+90 days →)
  A. Infection
    1. Disseminated varicella-zoster
    2. Encapsulated bacteria
    3. Staphylococcus, gram-negative bacteria
    4. *Toxoplasma*
  B. Chronic GVHD-associated phenomena
    1. Sicca syndrome bronchitis
    2. Obstructive bronchiolitis

Milburn et al., 1987). This includes detection of viruses like RSV (Hertz et al., 1989), CMV, and HSV. The procedure is well tolerated, even by patients who require ventilatory support, and avoids the risks of transbronchial, percutaneous, or open lung biopsy (Milburn et al., 1987). Bronchoscopy and BAL should be undertaken in patients who develop dyspnea, cough, and fever, with or without hypoxemia and decreased D_L CO, even if the chest x-ray is unchanged. As improvements in prophylaxis of nonbacterial as well as bacterial infection occur, the causes of pneumonitis in BMT recipients will shift toward other entities (e.g., idiopathic interstitial pneumonitis; ARDS) that cannot be positively identified by bronchoscopy and BAL; this will result in a decrease in "diagnostic yield" from the reported values of 66% (Cordonnier et al., 1986) and 80% (Milburn et al., 1987). Even in this situation, some diagnoses (e.g., leukemic relapse with pulmonary infiltration by leukemic cells) may be identified by the alert cytologist.

A pulmonary edema picture without fever suggests fluid overload, with or without cardiac dysfunction. It will respond to diuretic therapy and careful fluid management (Dickout et al., 1987). Aspiration secondary to severe esophagitis and nausea and vomiting may occur.

The appearance of fever and a diffuse pulmonary infiltrate as marrow function begins to return suggests diffuse lung injury. Hemorrhagic pulmonary edema with an ARDS-like picture is discussed below. Interstitial pneumonitis (IP) is discussed below in connection with CMV infection, although one-third of the cases of IP are of unknown origin. Later complications such as obstructive bronchiolitis are discussed below in relation to GVHD and to the longer-term effects of BMT on lung function.

B. Invasive Pulmonary Aspergillosis (IPA)

Aspergillus spores are ubiquitous and of respirable size, so IPA is a frequent and serious event in severely granulocytopenic patients. In BMT recipients, the resulting mortality has been in excess of 90%. BMT patients can also develop IPA after engraftment, presumably secondary to immunosuppressive therapy. Evidence of nonpulmonary *Aspergillus* infection (e.g., skin, sinuses) increases the likelihood that a new pulmonary infiltrate associated with fever is attributable to IPA. The standard of diagnosis is both histological demonstration of the typical septate, 45°-angle branching hyphae in tissue, and a positive culture to identify *Aspergillus* and to distinguish it from other fungi (e.g., *Pseudallescheria boydii*). However, if tissue cannot be obtained, a strong presumptive diagnosis can be made from percutaneous aspirate of a suspected lesion. Less certain presumptive diagnosis is made from bronchial brushings and washings or from sputum culture in the appropriate clinical setting.

Following several days of indolence, the original radiographic infiltrate often becomes more confluent and dense and may cavitate. The vasculotropic nature of the organism produces infarctive necrosis. Minor and major hemoptyses are not infrequent despite apparent improvement with therapy.

Early recognition and aggressive therapy are essential to increase the chance of survival. Apart from efforts to hasten return of neutrophils with cytokines [granulocyte transfusions are rarely used (Lazarus, 1990)], the accepted antibiotic treatment remains intravenous amphotericin B in daily doses of 1.0 mg/kg, or even higher if tolerated. The value of liposomes containing amphotericin B is under investigation, because they exhibit different pharmacokinetic features than the parent drug and may succeed where conventional therapy has failed, while offering some renal protection (Denning and Stevens, 1990). Flucytosine has been used in conjunction with amphotericin B (Denning and Stevens, 1990). Newer antifungal triazole drugs include oral or intravenous fluconazole and oral itraconazole, and the role of the latter in the treatment and prophylaxis of *Aspergillus* infection is under active study. Experience with fluconazole has been limited apart from treatment of *Candida* and *Cryptococcus* infections (Morrow, 1991; Galgiani, 1990). Rifampin can serve as an adjunct to amphotericin B therapy, but its use would greatly complicate cyclosporin and corticosteroid management because of hepatic enzyme induction.

Surgical resection of localized IPA has been used successfully in conjunction with amphotericin B in renal transplant patients (Weiland et al., 1983). Successful resectional surgery for severe hemoptysis from cavitary IPA has been reported in cases of leukemia (Albelda et al., 1985). Resection may be an option in comparable cases of IPA complicating BMT. The therapeutic role of bronchial artery embolization in the management of hemoptysis is unclear.

C. Diffuse Alveolar Hemorrhage (DAH)

The technique of bronchoalveolar lavage (BAL), refined by staining of alveolar macrophages for hemosiderin (Drew et al., 1977) and further refined by sequential small-volume lavage, has facilitated the detection of occult lung hemorrhage. Robbins et al. (1989) evaluated the clinical course of 141 autologous BMT patients being treated for lymphoma or solid tumors. In 29 (20%), a syndrome of dyspnea, cough, bilateral consolidation, fever, and hypoxemia developed between 7 days before and 40 days after transplant. Spirometry showed large decreases in FVC and FEV_1. BAL showed progressive increase in the bloodiness of the return of successive aliquots of instilled liquid. The alveolar macrophages recovered in the lavage were laden with hemosiderin. Interestingly, neutrophils ($>2\%$) were found in BAL in 12 patients whose peripheral white blood cell count was $\leq 200/\mu L$. The intrapulmonary hemorrhage could not be ascribed to coagulopathies and the syndrome did not improve with platelet transfusion. Twenty-three of the twenty-nine patients died, accounting for 62% of a total of 37 in-hospital deaths. Fifteen autopsies confirmed the finding of alveolar hemorrhage with diffuse alveolar damage in a proliferative phase. Microorganisms were found in only one case. Robbins et al. (1989) suggest that in at least some patients, the syndrome develops coincident with the reappearance of leukocytes in the circulation, and that previous damage by chemo- and radiation therapy sensitizes the alveolar structures to activated neutrophils. Renal insufficiency may have also played some pathogenic role in the DAH syndrome in these patients.

Chao et al. (1991) confirmed the occurrence of DAH in 4 of 77 patients undergoing autologous BMT for lymphoma. Fever was low grade and peripheral white blood cell count ranged from 0.4 to 4.3 $\times$ $10^3/\mu L$ at the onset of DAH. Interestingly, neither Chao et al. (1991) nor Robbins et al. (1989) appear to have found a sharp decline in peripheral blood hematocrit at the onset of the syndrome. Creatinine levels were borderline elevated and there was no evidence of pulmonary infection. Following prompt bronchoscopy-confirmed diagnosis, high-dose methylprednisolone was administered intravenously. Ventilatory support was required in two cases. All four patients survived and were discharged after resolution of the chest x-ray infiltrates. Chao et al. (1991) point out that the addition of dimethylsulfoxide (DMSO) for autologous marrow cryopreservation may contribute to alveolar toxicity.

D. Cytomegalovirus (CMV) Infection and Interstitial Pneumonitis (IP)

CMV infection after allogeneic BMT has been critically reviewed by Winston and colleagues (1990). CMV infection has occurred in about 50% of all recipients of allogeneic BMT and in about 70% of the CMV-seropositive recipients. However, this incidence appears to be decreasing (Wingard et al., 1988). Many of the signs of CMV infection are nonspecific. These include unexplained fever and malaise, leukopenia, thrombocytopenia, hepatitis, esophagitis, nausea, vomiting, and diarrhea. Rarely, hemorrhagic cystitis, retinitis, and central nervous system disease occur.

Up to 40% of allogeneic BMT patients develop IP, which can vary from fulminant to slowly advancing. Most cases of IP occur between 3 and 12 weeks after BMT, but a few occur earlier or later. Fever, advancing bilateral pulmonary infiltrates, nonproductive cough, and hypoxemia progressing to respiratory failure characterize the clinical picture. Of these cases of IP, about 40% are due to CMV and about one-third are idiopathic. The latter are thought to be due to lung injury by the pretransplantation whole-body irradiation and chemotherapy, which remains quiescent until marrow engraftment begins to repopulate the blood. The remaining cases of IP are associated with other viral infections or with *Pneumocystis carinii*.

The incidence of CMV-related interstitial pneumonia appears to be decreasing while that of idiopathic IP remains constant. Thus, an increasing proportion of the cases of IP are being classified as idiopathic. It is also noteworthy that the Seattle group has reported that idiopathic IP occurred about as frequently in recipients of syngeneic BMT as in allogeneic BMT recipients (Appelbaum et al., 1982). This suggests that the pathogenetic mechanisms of CMV-induced and idiopathic IP are fundamentally different.

CMV pneumonia, although it occurs (Pecego et al., 1986), is much less common in autologous BMT recipients and in syngeneic identical twin BMT recipients (Appelbaum et al., 1982), despite the evidence of a high frequency of active CMV replication in such patients (positive blood and urine cultures), and despite the use of similar conditioning procedures. These findings suggest that GVHD and its treatment are intimately involved in the pathogenesis of CMV pneumonia. Hypotheses to explain these relationships have been proposed by Grundy et al. (1987) and by Zaia et al. (1987). The use of cyclosporine A as prophylaxis against GVHD has been reported to relate significantly to a decreased incidence of CMV pneumonitis in a retrospective analysis of the experience at the Johns Hopkins Hospital (Wingard et al., 1990).

The development of sensitive techniques for CMV detection has enhanced the value of BAL in establishing the diagnosis of CMV pneumonia and reduced the need for biopsy (Cordonnier et al., 1987; Crawford et al., 1988). Routine cytological evaluation of BAL is not very sensitive, however. Polymerase chain-reaction-based techniques may become useful for detecting other viral agents as well as CMV (Jiwa et al., 1989; Spector, 1990).

Early diagnosis of CMV pneumonitis has become particularly important because of the emerging evidence that effective treatment is provided by ganciclovir combined with intravenous CMV–immune globulin or polyvalent immune globulin (IVIG) (Emanuel et al., 1988; Reed et al., 1988; Snydman, 1990; Winston et al., 1990). Ganciclovir alone is efficacious in treatment of other manifestations of CMV disease in BMT patients, but not the pneumonitis. Even though ganciclovir treatment sterilized the respiratory secretions and body fluids, 80% of patients with CMV pneumonitis succumbed (Winston et al., 1990).

Recent work summarized by Winston et al. (1990) indicates that passive immunoprophylaxis with various preparations results in reduced incidence of CMV pneumonitis. IVIG may also have additional benefits. Prophylactic high-dose acyclovir may have some potential for CMV prophylaxis (Meyers et al., 1988), and the value of prophylactic ganciclovir is under active investigation (Winston et al., 1990).

E. Other Viral Infections

Herpes simplex virus (HSV) 1 and 2 can cause severe febrile, painful tracheobronchitis and esophagitis as well as pneumonitis. Mucocutaneous herpetic lesions are generally present as well. Acyclovir prophylaxis has greatly reduced the incidence of serious HSV (and VZV) disease, but must be continued for several months posttransplant to avoid emergence of significant clinical infection and to decrease the risk of development of acyclovir resistance (Meyers, 1985). Adenovirus (epsecially type 34/35) can cause lung infection within the first 3 months post-BMT. Giant cell penumonia can result from measles or parainfluenza 3 infection.

Respiratory syncytial virus (RSV) can cause upper respiratory trace infection and pneumonia in the peritransplant period (Englund et al., 1988; Hertz et al., 1989). RSV can also occur much later, but is then less likely to cause pulmonary infiltrates. The disease is almost invariably associated with fever and usually with coryza, rhinorrhea, and sinusitis. Cough with rales and/or wheezes are common. Otitis media may occur. RSV is characteristically a winter-spring infection. BAL is a very effective diagnostic procedure when coupled with RSV nucleocapsid antigen detection by ELISA (Hertz et al., 1989). Increased neutrophils may be present in BAL liquid, even in patients whose peripheral white blood cell counts are $< 50/\mu L$.

Of six BMT patients with RSV infections occurring in the peritransplant period, all of whom received ribavirin aerosol inhalation therapy, two survived. Two patients with RSV infections that occurred long after engraftment both had chronic GVHD. Both survived with ribavirin therapy (Hertz et al., 1989).

F. Chronic Graft-Versus-Host Disease

Chronic GVHD affects about 40% of long-term survivors of allogeneic BMT. The GVHD and its treatment produce chronic immunosuppression with defective humoral and cellular immunity. The sicca syndrome may cause impaired mucosal surface immunity as well.

Sinusitis, bronchitis, and pneumonia with encapsulated organisms are important long-term problems; disseminated VZV infection may occur; acute fungal infections are also seen; and reactivation of quiescent fungal (e.g., *Histoplasma*) or mycobacterial infections is possible. Chronic antibacterial prophylaxis with trimethoprim/sulfamethoxazole is useful and also prevents PCP, but the changing spectrum of antibiotic resistance of the pneumococcus may pose difficulties. Immunization with nonliving vaccines may be useful, although the antibody response in these patients is problematic.

Chronic GVHD is also associated with a syndrome of progressive obstructive airways disease due to bronchiolitis (Ralph et al., 1984; Chan et al., 1987; Holland et al., 1988). Symptoms of undue exertional dyspnea and cough, and the presence of decreased FEV_1, FVC, and FEV_1/FVC ratio in the absence of chest x-ray infiltrates or fever, accompanied by hypoxemia but not by CO_2 retention, herald the onset of this syndrome. Because obstructive bronchiolitis is seen only in the context of chronic GVHD, it is limited to allogeneic BMT recipients. The onset of symptoms may be as early as 3 months or as late as 2 years posttransplant.

The picture is more confusing when it occurs rather early posttransplant and is associated with bilateral pulmonary infiltrates (diffuse alveolar damage and/or interstitial disease) and, often, with a recoverable infectious agent.

Even late-onset cases should raise the question of infective bronchiolitis, and further diagnostic procedures are warranted. The classical histological picture of bronchiolitis fibrosa obliterans is not always present. Instead there is bronchiolar and peribronchiolar inflammation (neutrophils or mononuclear cells, or both) with focal intraluminal plugs of degenerated epithelium and mucus. The pathology is said (Urbanski et al., 1987) to resemble that of Sjögren's disease with obstructive air-flow impairment (Newball and Brahim, 1977). The precise relationship between GVHD and the small-airways disorder is uncertain. The development of a similar syndrome of airways obstruction in heart-lung transplant patients (Theodore et al., 1990) has been noted.

The Johns Hopkins Hospital experience with BMT (Holland et al., 1988) suggests that reduced serum IgG (and perhaps mucosal sIgA) is an important additional risk factor for the development of classical bronchiolitis obliterans in patients with GVHD. Only those recipients of allogeneic BMT (549 total cases) with *both* chronic GVHD and decreased serum Ig levels (four cases) developed bronchiolitis obliterans. Holland et al. (1988) included in their report three patients with acute GVHD who died early post-BMT from ventilatory failure and interstitial pneumonitis, but who also had bronchiolitis obliterans at autopsy.

Therapy for obstructive bronchiolitis is not well defined. Improvement rarely occurs, but stabilization is reported in a few cases. Aside from more intensive treatment of GVHD, including corticosteroids and inhaled and oral bronchodilators, one should seek out and treat specific airways infection. Immune globulin therapy might be useful in selected cases. Chronic aspiration can be considered in the differential diagnosis if the GVHD is accompanied by severe esophageal dysfunction.

G. Long-Term Changes in Lung Function

Springmeyer et al. (1983) studied lung function in selected patients from a large group that had received allogeneic BMT over a 3-year period. Seventy-nine were reevaluated at 1 year, 23 at 2 years, and 10 and 14 at 3 and 4 years posttransplant, respectively. TLC was mildly (65–80%) or moderately (50–65%) reduced at 1 year in 28% of the patients, but those who were studied at later times showed only mild reductions in 13% of the cases. Few patients (about 4%) had a FEV_1/FVC of $< 60\%$ at 1 or 2 years, but this proportion increased sharply to 13% at 3 and 4 years (three and five patients, respectively). The authors were not persuaded that the presence of GVHD was associated with reduced FEV_1/FVC, although they recognized that others had described severe, late-onset COPD in a few patients, all with chronic GVHD.

Another study from Seattle (Clark et al., 1987) examined changes in pulmonary function about 1 year after transplant. A total of 281 of 506 survivors of 941 transplant patients aged 18 years or older were available for study. Of these 281 patients, 261 had received allogeneic BMT from a sibling and 14 from a parent or child. Among 185 patients with chronic GVHD, there was an excessive number (20) with $FEV_1/FVC < 55\%$. Values ranged down to 30%. Only 1 of 96 patients without GVHD had a FEV_1/FVC as low as 55%. The analysis of change of FEV_1/FVC (pretransplant versus 1 year posttransplant) also showed that 13% of 143 patients with GVHD had a decrease in FEV_1/FVC ratio as large as 20%.

Patients who had received prolonged methotrexate treatment in the postgraft period also appeared to be at risk for excessive decline in FEV_1/FVC. It was suggested speculatively that methotrexate might induce class II MHC antigen expression on lung cell membrances, making these cells vulnerable to attack by the GVH reaction (Clark et al., 1987).

A prospective study of 44 chronic myelogenous leukemia patients who received allogeneic BMT was reported by Sutedja et al. (1987). Thirty-four survivors were followed at 3-monthly intervals. Modest decreases in pulmonary CO-diffusing capacity were observed but there appeared to be some recovery at 24 months. Abnormalities in VC were paralleled by those in FEV_1 and were mild. The changes were most marked at 6 months and were greater in those patients who had developed acute GVHD. Only one patient developed a severe decrease in FEV_1/FVC.

Overall, it appears that mild restrictive impairment is not uncommon as a long-term sequel to BMT. Multiple causative factors can be invoked. Moderate to severe obstructive disease, on the other hand, is limited to chronic GVHD patients and may have serious consequences. Obstructive bronchiolitis contributes importantly to this syndrome.

VIII. Lymphomas

A. Hodgkin's Disease

When the pulmonologist approaches a patient with known or suspected Hodgkin's disease, three general issues should be considered. First, although Hodgkin's disease is a lymphoid neoplasm, the disease can manifest itself outside the lymphoreticular system. Second, all patients with Hodgkin's disease should be regarded as immunosuppressed. Moreoever, this immunosuppression is not restricted to cell-mediated immunity; functional abnormalities of T cells and macrophages as well as lymphopenia contribute to a generalized disturbance of host defenses. Finally, patients are treated with radiation therapy, chemotherapy, or both modalities, which have known pulmonary toxicities (Gross, 1977; Cooper et al., 1986; Rosiello and Merrill, 1990).

Pulmonary abnormalities may therefore be due to tissue infiltration by Hodgkin's disease, or infection, or a result of therapy. A number of chest x-ray findings have been reported as due to Hodgkin's disease alone. These include solitary masses, lobar infiltration with or without cavitation (Scully et al., 1989), and pleural effusion (Ludmerer and Kissane, 1988). These abnormalities usually occur in conjunction with disease at other sites, particularly hilar and mediastinal node enlargement, although rarely the lungs may be the only site of disease (Prakash, 1989). For any of these pulmonary abnormalities, there are no findings on physical examination or on the x-ray pathognomonic of Hodgkin's disease. Diagnosis requires histological confirmation. The least invasive procedure is BAL, which may show Reed-Sternberg cells, but this is infre quently positive. A second option is transbronchial biopsy, which is also not likely to lead to a diagnosis owing to small amounts of tissue obtained (Peters et al., 1988). In many instances, open lung biopsy is required (McCabe et al., 1989).

The spectrum of pulmonary infectious pathogens in Hodgkin's disease is large. Bacterial, fungal, viral, mycobacterial, and other opportunistic pathogens have been found (Notter et al., 1980), a diversity that prohibits construction of an algorithm for empirical therapy. Extensive examination and culturing of sputum and bronchial washings should be done before initiation of therapy and should consider all categories of pathogens.

Two types of pulmonary toxicity are related to radiation therapy. The first is radiation pneumonitis, which has been defined pathologically and clinically. Pathologically, there are early and late changes in the lungs (Gross, 1977; 1981; Rosiello and Merrill, 1990). Early, 4–12 weeks, after completion of radiation therapy, engorgement of small vessels, intimal proliferation, desquamation of epithelial cells, and fibrin deposits are seen. Later, beyond 6 months, pulmonary fibrosis appears. Clinically, a syndrome of dry cough and dyspnea begins several months after radiation. The chest x-ray shows a shaggy appearance at the borders of the mediastinum as well as a streaky infiltrate at the mediastinal-lung border. The distribution conforms to the radiation ports. Pulmonary function tests show a decrease in vital capacity.

The value of treatment is debatable because most patients have resolution of symptoms during the next 2–4 months. If treatment is given, it consists of corticosteroids, begun at 40 mg of prednisone daily, which is slowly tapered over several months. Occasionally, whether or not the patient receives treatment, the syndrome does not resolve and the patient progresses to severe dyspnea, hypoxemia, and death. In these instances, a large dose of radiation was given to an extensive portion of the lungs.

The second toxicity in radiated patients is the development of lung cancer. In a 17-year follow-up study of 1507 Hodgkin's disease patients treated at Stanford University Medical Center, 14 developed lung cancer. All 14 had a smoking history and had been treated with chest radiation therapy (Tucker et al., 1988). A similar incidence was found in another report of patients followed over a 12-year period (List et al., 1985). In this series, small-cell lung cancer was the most common histological type. Almost all patients had received radiation therapy, but a smoking history was reported in only half the lung cancer patients.

Three commonly used chemotherapeutic agents in Hodgkin's disease cause pulmonary damage. Bleomycin, part of the ABVD regimen (adriamycin, bleomycin, vinblastine, DTIC), results in pulmonary fibrosis (Jules-Elysee and White, 1990; Chandler, 1990). This reaction appears to be idiosyncratic in that it has been reported after a few treatments with bleomycin. Even careful monitoring of asymptomatic patients with serial chest x-rays or pulmonary function tests has not been shown to prevent or mitigate this complication (Bell et al., 1985). The reaction may resolve spontaneously or can be fatal. Some patients have responded to corticosteroid administration, although these reports are anecdotal (Bell et al., 1985). Adriamycin, also a component of ABVD, may cause pulmonary toxicity in patients previously treated with radiation (Twohig and Matthay, 1990), because of Adriamycin's ability to enhance the effects of radiation. The end result is tissue damage in areas of prior radiation, and can occur even when Adriamycin is given months to years after radiotherapy. In a few patients treated with procarbazine, part of the MOPP regimen (nitrogen mustard, vincristine, procarbazine, prednisone), infiltrates have been seen on chest x-ray. These are generally diffuse interstitial infiltrates and the patients exhibit peripheral eosinophilia. The syndrome resolves with discontinuation of the drug (Ecker et al., 1978).

B. Non-Hodgkin's Lymphoma

There are many similarities between non-Hodgkin's lymphoma and Hodgkin's disease. These include extranodal disease and disease-induced immunosuppression. In addition, many of the chemotherapeutic drugs used in the treatment of Hodgkin's disease are also used to treat patients with non-Hodgkin's lymphoma. Because of these similarities, the pulmonologist can approach the patient with known or suspected non-Hodgkin's lymphoma in much the same way as discussed previously for Hodgkin's disease patients.

A substantial literature exists describing pulmonary parenchymal involvement due to non-Hodgkin's lymphoma. Patterns on chest x-ray include solitary or multiple nodules, diffuse infiltration, cavitating mass, and pleural effusion (Moormeier et al., 1990); Ludmerer and Kissane, 1988; Scully et al., 1989). Most of these findings occur in the presence of nodal enlargement, although primary lung involvement has been reported. Diagnosis is most often made by open lung biopsy (McCabe et al., 1989). An alternative method is to obtain multiple transbronchoscopic biopsies with a goal of providing enough material for surface marker studies. Finding only B- or T-cell antigens in the absence of epithelial markers may allow a diagnosis of lymphoma (Ludmerer and Kissane, 1988).

The spectrum of pulmonary infection superimposed on non-Hodgkin's lymphoma is as varied as that reported with Hodgkin's disease. This is due to the use of aggressive chemotherapy coupled with immunosuppression from the disease itself. Therapy should be based on examination of sputum and bronchial washings. There is a role for empirical antimicrobial therapy if the patient is granulocytopenic secondary to chemotherapy (<500/μL). In this case antibiotics covering common gram-positive and gram-negative organisms, including *Pseudomonas* species, should be started. Particular attention should be paid to the patient with hemoptysis, as this may be an indication of fungal pneumonia. A retrospective study of patients with hematological malignancy and hemoptysis reported six fatalities from hemoptysis. All these patients had fungal pneumonia (Panos et al., 1988).

Treatment-related pulmonary toxicity is largely due to chemotherapy because this modality plays a much greater role than radiation in the treatment of non-Hodgkin's lymphoma. Agents used in non-Hodgkin's lymphoma that may cause pulmonary toxicity are bleomycin, cyclophosphamide, and cytosine arabinoside. Cyclophosphamide administration may lead to pulmonary fibrosis months to years after the drug is stopped. Patients present with dyspnea and cough and their chest x-rays show diffuse infiltrates. There is no known treatment and patients usually die. Fortunately, this is an uncommon complication of cyclophosphamide use (Cooper et al., 1986). Noncardiogenic pulmonary edema has been reported in patients receiving cytosine arabinoside (Haupt et al., 1981) and was observed either during drug administration or within 1 month of its cessation. Most patients died of this complication, although a few survived with mechanical ventilation and careful management of fluid status. At autopsy, a highly proteinaceous fluid was seen in the intraalveolar and interstitial spaces. The cause of this complication is not known, but it does not appear related to the amount of cytosine arabinoside given.

IX. Multiple Myeloma

Classical myeloma is a relatively common hematological malignancy among middle-aged adults. The malignant cells are derived from B lymphocytes, which proliferate and differentiate into autonomous clones of immunoglobulin (Ig)-producing, plasma-cell-like forms. IgG or IgA myelomas are most common; IgD and IgE myelomas are rare. IgM is confined to Waldenström's macroglobulinema (see below).

Myeloma first develops in the microenvironment of the bone marrow. It often erodes bone and causes the appearance of typical "punched-out" osteolytic lesions without reactive changes. Marrow-based tumor may extend locally into other tissues, including the chest wall and pleura. Less commonly, myeloma deposits grow in extramedullary locations, including lung parenchyma and airways.

Myeloma is accompanied by severely impaired humoral immunity because of suppression of normal polyclonal Ig synthesis. Pulmonary infection with encapsulated bacteria, often *Strep. pneumoniae*, is a classical manifestation, but other organisms are also commonly found. Additional suppression of host defenses by corticosteroid and cytotoxic therapy may also contribute to infection by a variety of organisms.

In some patients myeloma causes significant remote pathology because of the secretion into the circulation by the tumor of large quantities of monoclonal Ig. Monoclonal Ig light chains may also be produced. These "M" proteins are potentially amyloidogenic and are associated with diffuse pulmonary parenchymal deposition of amyloid, respiratory muscle amyloidosis, amyloidosis of the tongue, and cardiac amyloidosis. These manifestations are discussed in the section on amyloidosis. Myeloma also commonly causes hypercalcemia due to bone resorption and impaired renal function and may therefore cause metastatic calcification in the lung parenchyma.

Table 4 lists the pulmonary and chest wall manifestations associated directly or indirectly with myeloma.

The most extensive review of thoracic and pulmonary abnormalities in myeloma remains that of Kintzer et al. (1978) based on 958 cases of myeloma seen at the Mayo Clinic. Rib lesions were the initial finding in 15% of the patients and were found in a total of 268 (38%). The bone lesions were most often solitary. A few cases of severe kyphosis secondary to vertebral involvement were complicated by respiratory failure.

Intrathoracic plasmacytomas (113 patients) were generally of intramedullary origin related to rib lesions. The masses are smooth and radiologically homogeneous. They are accessible to percutaneous biopsy.

Only 11 patients with myeloma had extramedullary plasmacytomas affecting the respiratory tract. These lesions usually involved the lung parenchyma, but symptomatic paratracheal or laryngeal lesions also occurred (Kintzer et al., 1978). They may exhibit extensive calcification (Morinaga et al., 1987). Herskovic et al. (1965) reported a 7% incidence of intrathoracic plasmacytoma among 303 patients with myeloma. Roikjaer and Thomsen (1986) described two pulmonary plasmacytomas, of different immunological types that occurred at a 5-year interval in an elderly woman and were treated effectively with resectional surgery. Plasmacytoma should be differentiated morphologically from plasma cell granuloma, inflammatory pseudotumor, and pseudolymphoma (Bahadori and Liebow, 1973) by immunocytochemical demonstration of monoclonality of surface Ig.

Extramedullary plasmacytoma may occur in the absence of myeloma in the marrow. Wiltshaw (1976) reviewed 257 cases of isolated extramedullary plasmacytoma and found that the tumor exhibited an extraordinary affinity for supralaryngeal airways. Lower airways and lung were involved in only 13 cases in his report.

Ten percent of the Mayo Clinic myeloma patients (Kintzer et al., 1978) developed pulmonary infiltrates. Three-quarters of these were due to infection

Table 4 Myeloma and the Respiratory System

- I. Bone
  - A. Ribs
    1. Single or multiple "punched-out" osteolytic lesions
    2. Pathological fractures
    3. Diffuse osteoporosis
  - B. Vertebrae
- II. Chest wall
  - A. Extension of rib lesion to form an extrapleural mass
  - B. Pleural effusion
    1. Malignant (exudative, sanguineous, usually left sided, and associated with IgA myeloma)
    2. Benign (transudative, associated with amyloid cardiomyopathy)
  - C. Amyloidosis of respiratory muscles with restrictive impairment, weakness, respiratory failure
- III. Parenchyma
  - A. Pneumonia
    1. Encapsulated bacteria
    2. Other organisms
  - B. Myelomatous invasion (rare)
    1. Extramedullary plasmacytoma (mass)
    2. Infiltrative disease
  - C. Diffuse alveolar disease
    1. Septal amyloidosis
    2. Metastatic calcification
- IV. Airways
  - A. Intrapulmonary (rare cases of submucosal infiltration in IgA myeloma that may cause obstruction and atelectasis)
  - B. Supralaryngeal extramedullary plamacytoma
  - C. Amyloidosis of tongue
- V. Vascular
  - A. Amyloidosis
  - B. Thromboembolism

and were lobar or segmental. The remaining quarter had more diffuse infiltrates. Some of these were due to infection, but a few represented myelomatous parenchymal invasion, suggesting enhanced malignant potential of the neoplastic cells (Garewal and Durie, 1982). An unusual case of IgA myeloma with right-lung atelectasis secondary to extensive, bronchoscopically demonstrated submucosal plasma cell invasion appeared to respond temporarily to corticosteroids and cyclophosphamide (Gilchrist et al., 1988). Diagnosis of malignant plasma cells in sputum or bronchial washings is difficult using ordinary cytological techniques (Riazmontazer and Bedayat, 1989) and has rarely been described (Geisinger et al., 1986).

Pleural involvement by malignant plasma cells is notably left sided and usually follows spread from chest wall lesions in advanced myeloma (Kintzer et al., 1978; Airoldi et al., 1986). However, pleural effusion has also been described as a presenting finding (Estrov et al., 1983; Chee and Chea, 1984; Witt et al., 1986). About 80% of cases of myelomatous pleural effusion involve IgA myeloma (Airoldi et al., 1986). The exudative effusions are sanguineous and a cytological diagnosis can generally be established (Gondos et al., 1976; Scullin and Cohen, 1979; Geisinger et al., 1986). Intrapleural chemotherapy may be helpful (Iannitto et al., 1988).

Pleural effusion in myeloma is more commonly secondary to cardiac disease, especially myocardial amyloidosis (Kintzer et al., 1978), than to direct extension of the tumor. Pulmonary embolism must also be considered, although it is not particularly common (Pasqualetti et al., 1989).

Diffuse metastatic alveolar septal calcification has been reported in hypercalcemic myeloma patients. The calcification may develop initially in the upper zones, probably because of the higher V_A/Q ratios with consequent hypocapnia and akalosis in these regions. Local hypoperfusion secondary to embolism can cause localization of metastatic calcification to the affected area for similar reasons. The diffuse pulmonary infiltrates may progress and cause death from respiratory failure, despite control of serum calcium (Paladini et al., 1986; Morassi et al., 1985).

Scintigraphy with 99m Tc-labeled bone-seeking agents is a sensitive technique for detecting metastatic lung calcification. It is more sensitive than chest x-ray (Morassi et al., 1985) and may detect abnormality in the absence of pulmonary symptoms. Scintigraphy may also be useful in distinguishing metastatic calcification in hypercalcemic myeloma patients from other infiltrative processes such as diffuse amyloidosis, infection, or myelomatous infiltration.

X. Waldenström's Macroglobulinemia

The malignant clone of B lymphocytes produces monoclonal IgM in patients with this disease. As in myeloma, anemia, epistaxis, and other evidence of coagulopathy are common. Despite marrow involvement, osteolytic lesions and bone pain are not a feature, but invasion of the liver, spleen, and lymph nodes occurs as the disease progresses.

Pulmonary manifestations include bacterial pneumonia, infiltrative parenchymal disease, mediastinal adenopathy, malignant pleural effusion, and focal airways involvement (Winterbauer et al., 1974). If amyloidosis occurs, it is more likely to be associated with areas of malignant plasma cell tissue invasion rather than to be a remote manifestation as in myeloma.

A special feature, attributable to the large quantities of circulating IgM, is the hyperviscosity syndrome, which particularly affects the cerebral and retinal circulations. Plasmapheresis is effective therapy unless hemorrhage has supervened. Pulmonary abnormalities are attributable to increased plasma volume with pulmonary vascular congestion or even edema (Bloch and Maki, 1973).

XI. Amyloidosis

Amyloid is an acellular deposit of homogeneous material with distinctive tinctorial properties. Various unrelated peptides are capable of forming amyloid deposits. Prominent among such peptides are Ig light chains and serum amyloid A protein. Amyloidogenic polypeptides form antiparallel arrays of molecules in the β-pleated sheet conformation. This fibrillar structure confers on amyloid its characteristic green birefringence in polarized light when stained with Congo red. In the presence of calcium, the amyloid fibrils bind a normal serum α_1-glycoprotein of hepatic origin that confers periodic acid-Schiff positivity (Glenner, 1980).

In the great majority of patients with clinically significant cardiorespiratory amyloidosis, the fibrils are probably of Ig-light-chain origin. However, certain cases of metastatic carcinoma in the lung have shown amyloid in association with tumor cells (Cordier et al., 1986). In these cases, the amyloid is probably formed from a polypeptide locally produced by the tumor (calcitonin in the case of medullary carcinoma of the thyroid). Patients with chronic inflammatory disease may develop systemic amyloidosis related to serum amyloid protein A, but neither clincally significant nor radiologically apparent deposits of amyloid A are found in the respiratory tract (Celli et al., 1978; Rubinow et al., 1978).

A. Systemic Amyloidosis

Amyloidosis may involve the lower respiratory tract as part of a more generalized process. Other areas of involvement include the gastrointestinal tract (particularly esophagus and rectum), the tongue, peripheral and autonomic nerves, skeletal muscles, heart, and kidney. Lung involvement is usually of the diffuse alveolar septal variety and may lead to progressive dyspnea with hypoxemia, restrictive impairment, and respiratory failure. The amyloidosis may be idiopathic or associated with multiple myeloma (Stone and Frenkel, 1975; Kyle and Greipp, 1983; Alexanian et al., 1984; Topilow et al., 1986; Morgan et al., 1987). A case of pulmonary hypertension with diffuse pulmonary vascular infiltration but mild alveolar septal involvement has been described in a patient with myeloma (Shiue and McNally, 1988).

Massive infiltration of the tongue can obstruct the oral airway and may cause obstructive sleep apnea, which can be treated with nasal continuous positive airway pressure (Lesser et al., 1988). Amyloid infiltration of the respiratory muscles may result in pump failure (Streeten et al., 1986; Santiago et al., 1987). Myocardial amyloidosis can cause restrictive myocardiopathy, conduction abnormalities, and congestive heart failure with transudative pleural effusion (Smith et al., 1979).

B. Localized Lower Respiratory Tract Amyloidosis

The principal types of idiopathic amyloidosis confined to the airways, lung, and intrathoracic lymph nodes were categorized by Thompson and Citron (1983) on the basis of a review including 126 such patients. Most cases either diffusely involved the tracheobronchial submucosa (57 cases) or were confined to the parenchyma as one or more discrete nodules (55 cases). Isolated, single tumor-like tracheal or bronchial masses of amyloid were found in 10 cases. Diffuse, interstitial (alveolar septal) amyloid was found in only four cases. A basically similar distribution of localized, lower respiratory tract amyloid was reported by Hui et al. (1986) in a series of 48 cases. The series of Cordier et al. (1986) reported a higher proportion of interstitial parenchymal amyloid. However, they included a number of cases associated with neoplasm.

Diffuse tracheobronchial submucosal amyloidosis narrows the airways and causes chronic wheezing, dyspnea, cough, hemoptysis, atelectasis, and chronic infection. Endoscopy reveals multiple areas of ridging and stenosis. Endobronchial biopsy and suitable histological examination of the tissue confirms the diagnosis. In two patients, immunocytochemical analysis revealed a disproportionate number of lambda-light-chain-bearing plasma cells in proximity to the amyloid (Hui et al., 1986). Treatment by repeated transbronchoscopic piecemeal removal of submucosal plaques may provoke severe hemoptysis. Laser surgery may provide an effective and safer alternative.

Nodular parenchymal amyloidosis is usually asymptomatic (although hemoptysis may occur) and is detected on a chest radiograph. One or more nodules, either unilateral or bilateral, ranging up to 15 cm in diameter are present. Immunocytochemical analysis of mononuclear cells in proximity to the nodules showed a polyclonal pattern in several cases. Although plasma cells and giant cells were relatively numerous in relation to these nodules, the polyclonality implies that the cellular infiltrate is reactive rather than causal in the amyloid generating process (Hui et al., 1986). Nodules may grow slowly and may cavitate or become calcified. Treatment is generally unnecessary although single nodules are commonly resected to rule out carcinoma. A pulmonary A-V fistula within a large amyloid nodule has been described, probably due to vascular wall involvement (Kamei et al., 1989). Two cases of Sjögren's syndrome in which multiple pulmonary bullae were associated with multinodular parenchymal amyloid have been published (Kobayashi et al., 1988; Kornfeld et al., 1989).

Diffuse amyloidosis involves the alveolar septa and causes a picture of diffuse infiltration that can slowly progress to cause restrictive impairment, hypoxemia, and respiratory insufficiency. The diagnosis is generally not apparent but can be established by transbronchial biopsy (Klein et al., 1985) or even percutaneous needle aspiration biopsy (Scott and Scott, 1985). Nevertheless, hemorrhage is always a risk in biopsying amyloid in internal organs (Yood et al., 1983), and spontaneous bleeding in tracheobronchial amyloidosis has been discussed above. A case of spontaneous hemoptysis with medial dissection of medium-sized pulmonary arteries involved with amyloid has been reported (Road et al., 1985). Strange et al. (1987) described a patient with extensive diffuse parenchymal amyloidosis who died of severe hemorrhage and air embolism immediately following a transbronchial biopsy.

C. Miscellaneous

Amyloid rarely causes hilar and mediastinal adenopathy that may be massive and undergo calcification (Thompson et al., 1983). Amyloid pleural involvement with effusion has been described (Graham and Ahmad, 1987; Knapp et al., 1988) but is rare.

XII. Summary

In this chapter we have discussed hematological diseases that affect the pulmonary microcirculation (sickle cell disease, hyperleukocytosis), briefly indicated approaches to dealing with coagulopathies in the patient requiring invasive procedures, and discussed malignant B- and T-cell disorders (Hodgkin's disease, non-Hodgkin's lymphoma, multiple myeloma, and Waldenström's macroglobulinemia). Although they may be associated with myeloma, the pulmonary manifestation of amyloidosis are considered separately. Finally, we have given particular emphasis to the manifold pulmonary problems associated with bone marrow transplantation, an increasingly utilized treatment for a large number of oncological and hematological diseases.

References

Airoldi, M., Fantasia, R., Giorgetti, A., and Stefanetti, C. (1986). Pleural involvement in multiple myeloma. *Haematologica* **71**:56–59.

Albelda, S. M., Talbot, G. M., Gerson, S. L., Miller, W. T., and Cassileth, P. A. (1985). Pulmonary cavitation and massive hemoptysis in invasive pulmonary aspergillosis. Influence of bone marrow recovery in patients with acute leukemia. *Am. Rev. Respir. Dis.* **131**:115–120.

Alexanian, R., Fraschini, G., and Smith, L. (1984). Amyloidosis in multiple myeloma or without apparent cause. *Arch. Intern. Med.* **144**:2158–2160.

Appelbaum, F. R., Meyers, J. D., Fefer, A., Flournoy, N., Cheever, M. A., Greenberg, P. D., Hackman, R., and Thomas, E. D. (1982). Nonbacterial nonfungal pneumonia following marrow transplantation in 100 identical twins. *Transplantation* **33**:265–268.

Bahadori, M., and Liebow, A. A. (1973). Plasma cell granuloma of the lung. *Cancer* **31**:191–208.

Bakris, G. L., Sauter, E. R., Hussey, J. L., Fisher, J. W., Gaber, A. O., and Winsett, R. (1990). Effects of theophylline on erythropoietin production in normal subjects and in patients with erythrocytosis after renal transplantation. *N. Eng. J. Med.* **323**:86–90.

Bell, M. R., Meredith, D. J., and Gill, P. G. (1985). Role of carbon monoxide diffusing capacity in the early detection of major bleomycin-induced pulmonary toxicity. *Aust. NZ J. Med.* **15**:235.

Beschorner, W. E., Hutchins, G. M., Burns, W. H., Saral R., Tutschka, P. J. and Santos, G. W. (1980). Cytomegalovirus pneumonia in bone marrow transplant recipients: military and diffuse patterns. *Am. Rev. Respir. Dis.* **122**:107–114.

Bishop, J. M., Donald, K. W., and Wade, O. L. (1955) Circulatory dynamics at rest and on exercise in the hyperkinetic states. *Clin. Sci.* **14**:329–360.

Bloch, K. J., and Maki, D. G. (1973). Hyperviscosity syndromes associated with immunoglobulin abnormalities. *Semin. Hematol.* **10**:113–124.

Bortin, M. M., and Rimm, A. A. (1986). Increasing utilization of bone marrow transplantation. *Transplantation* **42**:229–234.

Bromberg, P. A. (1974). Pulmonary aspects of sickle cell disease. *Arch. Intern. Med.* **133**:652–657.

Bromberg, P. A., and Jensen, W. N. (1967). Arterial oxygen unsaturation in sickle cell disease. *Am. Rev. Respir. Dis.* **96**:400–407.

Bromberg, P. A., and Ross, D. W. (1988). The lung in hematologic disease. In *Textbook of Respiratory Medicine*, Chapter 90. Edited by J. F. Murray and J. A. Nadel. Saunders, Philadelphia, pp. 1906–1920.

Buckner, C. D., Meyers, J. D., Springmeyer, S. C., Sullivan, K. M., Hackman,R. C., Flournoy, N., Clift, R., Storb, R., Witherspoon, R. P.,

Petersen, F. B., and Thomas, E. D. (1984). Pulmonary complications of marrow transplantation: review of the Seattle experience. *Exp. Hematol.* **12**:1–5.

Bunin, N. J., Kunkel, K., and Callihan, T. R. (1987). Cytoreductive procedures in the early management in cases of leukemia and hyperleukocytosis in children. *Med. Pediatr. Oncol.* **15**:232–235.

Callaghan, T. A., and Fitzsimons, E. J. (1989). Atypical presentation of the hyperleucocytic syndrome: acute myeloid leukaemia with iliac artery occlusion. *Clin. Lab. Haematol.* **11**:147–151.

Celli, B. R., Rubinow, A., Cohen, A. S., and Brody, J. S. (1978). Patterns of pulmonary involvement in systemic amyloidosis. *Chest* **74**:543–547.

Chan, C. K., Hyland, R. H., Hutcheon, M. A., Minden, M. D., Alexander, M. A., Kossakowske, A. E., Urbanski, S. J., Fyles, G. M., Fraser, I. M., Surtis, J. E., and Messner, H. A. (1987). Small-airways disease in recipients of allogeneic bone marrow transplants. *Medicine* **66**:327–340.

Chan, C. K., Hyland, R. H., and Hutcheon, M. A. (1990). Pulmonary complications following bone marrow transplantation. *Clin. Chest Med.* **11**:323–332.

Chandler, D. B. (1990). Possible mechanisms of bleomycin-induced fibrosis. *Clin. Chest Med.* **11**:21–30.

Chao, N. J., Duncan, S. R., Long, G. D., Horning, S. J., and Blume, K. G. (1991). Corticosteroid therapy for diffuse alveolar hemorrhage in autologous bone marrow transplant recipients. *Ann. Intern. Med.* **114**:145–146.

Charache, S., Scott, J., and Charache, P. (1979). "Acute chest syndrome" in adults with sickle cell anemia. *Arch. Intern. Med.* **139**:67–69.

Chee, Y. C., and Chea, E. (1984). IgA myeloma with primary pleural involvement. *Eur. J. Respir. Dis.* **65**:136–138.

Clark, J. G., Schwartz, D. A., Flournoy, N., Sullivan, K. M., Crawford, S. W. and Thomas, E. D. (1987). Risk factors for airflow obstruction in recipients of bone marrow transplants. *Ann. Intern. Med.* **107**:648–656.

Collins, F. S., and Orringer, E. P. (1982). Pulmonary hypertension and cor pulmonale in the sickle hemoglobinopathies. *Am. J. Med.* **73**:814–821.

Consensus Development Conference (1987). Platelet transfusion therapy. *JAMA* **257**:1777–1780.

Cooper, J. A. D., White, D. A., and Matthay, R. A. (1986). Drug-induced pulmonary disease. Part I: Cytotoxic drugs. *Am. Rev. Respir. Dis.* **133**:321–340.

Cordier, J. F., Loire, R., and Brune, J. (1986). Amyloidosis of the lower respiratory tract. *Chest* **90**:827–831.

Cordonnier, C., Bernaudin, J-F., Bierling, P., Huet, Y., and Vernant, J-P. (1986). Pulmonary complications occurring after allogeneic bone marrow transplantation: a study of 130 consecutive transplanted patients. *Cancer* **58**:1047–1054.

Cordonnier, C., Escudier, E., Nicolas, J-C, Fleury, J., Deforges, L., Ingrand, D., Bricout, F., and Bernaudin, J-F. (1987). Evaluation of three assays on alveolar lavage fluid in the diagnosis of cytomegalovirus pneumonitis after bone marrow transplantation. *J. Infect. Dis.* **155**:495–500.

Crawford, S. W., Raleigh, A. B., Hackman, R. C., Gleaves, C. A., Meyers, J. D., and Clark, J. G. (1988). Rapid detection of cytomegalovirus pulmonary infection by bronchoalveolar lavage and centrifugation culture. *Ann. Intern. Med.* **108**:180–185.

Creutzig, U., Ritter, J., Budde, M., Sutor, A., Schellong, G., and the German BFM Study Group (1987). Early deaths due to hemorrhage and leukostasis in childhood acute myelogenous leukemia. *Cancer* **60**:3071–3079.

Davies, S. C., Luce, P. J., Win, A. A., Riordan, J. F., and Brozovic, M. (1984). Acute chest syndrome in sickle-cell disease. *Lancet* **1**:36–38.

Davies, S. C., Stebbens, V. A., Samuels, M. P., and Southall, D. P. (1989). Upper airways obstruction and cerebrovascular accident in children with sickle cell anaemia. *Lancet* **121**:283–284.

De Ceulaer, K., McMullen, K. W., Maude, G. H., Keatinge, R., and Serjeant, G. R. (1985). Pneumonia in young children with homozygous sickle cell disease: risk and clinical features. *Eur. J. Pediatr.* **144**:255–258.

Denning, D. W., and Stevens, D. A. (1990). Antifungal and surgical treatment of invasive aspergillosis: review of 2,121 published cases. *Rev. Infect. Dis.* **12**:1147–1201.

Dickout, W. J., Chan, C. K., Hyland, R. H., Hutcheon, M. A., Fraser, I. M., Morgan, C. D., Curtis, J. E., Messner, H. A. (1987). Prevention of acute pulmonary edema after bone marrow transplantation. *Chest* **92**:303–309.

DiMarco, A. T. (1988). Carbon monoxide poisoning presenting as polycythemia. *N. Eng. J. Med.* **318**:874.

Drew, W. L., Finley, T. N., and Golde, D. W. (1977). Diagnostic lavage and occult pulmonary hemorrhage in thrombocytopenic immunocompromised patients. *Am. Rev. Respir. Dis.* **116**:215–221.

Ecker, M. D., Jay, B., and Keohane, M. F. (1978). Procarbazine lung. *Am. J. Roentgenol.* **131**:527–528.

Editorial (1987). Pseudopolycythaemia. *Lancet* **121**:603–604.

Editorial (1989). Polycythaemia due to hypoxaemia: advantage or disadvantage? *Lancet* **121**:20–22.

Edwards, J. R., and Matthay, K. K. (1989). Hematologic disorders affecting the lungs. *Clin. Chest Med.* **10**:723–746.

Emmanuel, D., Cunningham, I., Jules-Elysee, K., Brochstein, J. A., Kerman, N. A., Laver, J., Stover, D., White, D. A., Fels, A., Polsky, B.,

Castro-Malaspina, H., Peppard, J. R., Bartus, P., Hammerling, U., and O'Reilly, R. J. (1988). Cytomegalovirus pneumonia after bone marrow transplantation treated with the combination of ganciclovir and high-dose intravenous immune globulin. *Ann. Intern. Med.* **109**:777–782.

Englund, J. A., Sullivan, C. J., Jordan, M. C., Dehner, L. P., Vercellotti, G. M. and Balfour, H. H. Jr. (1988). Respiratory syncytial virus infection in immunocompromised adults. *Ann. Intern. Med.* **108**:203–208.

Estrov, Z., Berrebi, A., Hazani, E., and Resnitzky, P. (1983). Pleural effusion and ascites as presenting signs of IgA myeloma. *Haematologica (Pavia)* **68**:104–109.

Galgiani, J. N. (1990). Fluconazole, a new antifungal agent. *Ann. Intern. Med.* **113**:177–179.

Garewal, M. and Durie, B. G. M. (1982). Aggressive phase of multiple myeloma with pulmonary plasma cell infiltrates. *JAMA* **248**:1875–1876.

Gaston, M. H., Verter, J. I., Woods, G., Pegelow, C., Kelleher, J., Presbury, G., Zarkowsky, H., Vichinsky, E., Iyer, R., Lobel, J. S., Diamond, S., Holbrook, C. T., Gill, F. M., Ritchey, K., and Faletta, J. M. (1986). Prophylaxis with oral penicillin in children with sickle cell anemia. *N. Eng. J. Med.* **314**:1593–1599.

Geisinger, K. R., Buss, D. H., Kawamoto, E. H., and Ahl, E. T. (1986). Multiple myeloma: the diagnostic role and prognostic significance of exfoliative cytology. *Acta Cytol.* **30**:334–340.

Gilchrist, D., Chan, C. K., LaRoye, G. J., Messner, H. A., and Curtis, J. E. (1988). Bronchial mucosal infiltration and unilateral lung collapse: an unusual complication of multiple myeloma. *Am. J. Med.* **85**:740–741.

Glenner, G. G. (1980). Amyloid deposits and amyloidosis: the β-fibrilloses. *N. Eng. J. Med.* **302**:1283–1292, 1333–1343.

Gondos, B., Miller, T. F., and King, E. B. (1976). Cytologic diagnosis of multiple myeloma and macroglobulinemia in effusions. *Ann. Clin. Lab. Sci.* **8**:11–16.

Graham, D. R., and Ahmad D. (1987). Clinical aspects of pulmonary amyloidosis. *Chest.* **92**:576–577.

Gross, N. (1977). Pulmonary effects of radiation therapy. *Ann. Intern. Med.* **86**:81–92.

Gross, N. (1981). The pathogenesis of radiation-induced lung damage. *Lung.* **159**:115–125.

Grundy, J. E., Shanley, J. D., and Griffiths, P. D. (1987). Is cytomegalovirus interstitial pneumonitis in transplant recipients an immunopathological condition? *Lancet.* **2**:996–999.

Hammond, T. G., and Mosesson, M. W. (1989). Fatal small-bowel necrosis and pulmonary hypertension in sickle cell disease. *Arch. Intern. Med.* **149**:447–448.

Hardy, R. E., Cummings, C., Thomas, F., and Harrison, D. (1986). Cryptococcal pneumonia in a patient with sickle cell disease. *Chest*. **89**:892–894.

Hasleton, P. S., Orr, K., Webster, A., and Lawson, R. A. M. (1989). Evolution of acute chest syndrome in sickle cell trait: an ultrastructural and light microscopic study. *Thorax* **44**:1057–1058.

Haupt, H. M., Hutchins, G. M., and Moore, G. W. (1981). Ara-C lung: noncardiogenic pulmonary edema complicating cytosine arabinoside therapy of leukemia. *Am. J. Med.* **70**:256–261.

Haupt, H. M., Moore, G. W., Bauer, T. W., and Hutchins, G. M. (1982). The lung in sickle cell disease. *Chest* **81**:332–337.

Herskovic, T., Andersen, H. A., and Bayrd, E. D. (1965). Intrathoracic plamacytomas. Presentation of 21 cases and review of literature. *Dis Chest* **47**:1–6.

Hertz, M. I., Englund, J. A., Snover, D., Bitterman, P. B. and McGlave, P. B. (1989). Respiratory syncytial virus-induced acute lung injury in adult patients with bone marrow transplants: a clinical approach and review of the literature. *Medicine* **68**:269–281.

Holland, H. K., Wingard, J. R., Beschorner, W. E., Saral, R., and Santos, G. W. (1988). Bronchiolitis obliterans in bone marrow transplantation and its relationship to chronic graft-v-host disease and low serum IgG. *Blood* **72**:621–627.

Holtz, H., Bielory, L., Freund, N., and Lasker, N. (1990) Clinical decision making. *New Jersey Med.* **87**:305–309.

Hug, V., Keating, M., McCredie, K., Hester, J., Bodey, G. P., and Freireich, E. J. (1983). Clinical course and response to treatment of patients with acute myelogenous leukemia presenting with a high leukocyte count. *Cancer* **52**:773–779.

Hui, A. N., Koss, M. N., Hochholzer, L., and Wehunt, W. D. (1986). Amyloidosis presenting in the lower respiratory tract. *Arch. Pathol. Lab. Med.* **110**:212–218.

Iannitto, E., Scaglione, R., Musso, M., Abbadess, W. and Licata, G. (1988). Intrapleural adriamycin in treatment of myelomatous pleural effusion: a case report. *Haematologica* **73**:325–327.

Jiwa, N. M., Van Gemert, G. W., Raap, A. K., Van De. Rijke, F. M., Mulder, A., Lens, P. F., Salimans, M. M. M., Zwaan, F. E., Van Dorp, W., and Van der Ploeg, M. (1989). Rapid detection of human cytomegalovirus DNA in peripheral blood leukocytes of viremic transplant recipients by the polymerase chain reaction. *Transplantation* **48**:72–76.

Jules-Elysee, K., and White, D. A. (1990). Bleomycin-induced pulmonary toxicity. *Clin. Chest Med.* **11**:1–20.

Kamei, K., Kusumoto, K., and Suzuki, T. (1989). Pulmonary amyloidosis with pulmonary arteriovenous fistula. *Chest* **96**:1435–1436.

Kintzer, J. S. Jr., Rosenow, E. C., and Kyle, R. A. (1978). Thoracic and pulmonary abnormalities in multiple myeloma: a review of 958 cases. *Arch. Intern. Med.* **138**:727–730.

Kirkpatrick, M. B., Haynes, Jr. J., and Bass, Jr. J. B. (1991). Results of bronchoscopically obtained lower airway cultures from adult sickle cell disease patients with the acute chest syndrome. *Am. J. Med.* **90**:206–210.

Klein, L. R., Dise, C. A., Ferro, T. J., and Hansen-Flaschen, J. H. (1985). Diagnosis of pulmonary amyloidosis by transbronchial biopsy. *Am. Rev. Respir. Dis.* **132**:191–194.

Knapp, M. J., Roggli, V. L., Kim, J., Moore, J. O., and Shelburne, J. D. (1988). Pleural amyloidosis. *Arch. Pathol. Lab. Med.* **112**:57–60.

Kobayashi, H., Kitamura S., and Tsunoda, N. (1988). Sjögren's syndrome with multiple bullae and pulmonary nodular amyloidosis. *Chest* **94**:438–440.

Kollef, M. H., McCormack, M. T., Caras, W. E., Reddy, V. V. B., and Bacon, D. (1990). The fat overload syndrome: successful treatment with plasma exchange. *Ann. Intern. Med.* **112**:545–546.

Kornfeld, S., Molina, P., Canfield, W., and Gonzalez, J. G. (1989). Clinical-pathologic conferences: subcutaneous masses and adenopathy in a 77-year-old man with Sjögren's syndrome and amyloidosis. *Am. J. Med.* **86**:585–590.

Koshy, M., Burd, L., Wallace, D., Moawad, A., and Baron, J. (1988). Prophylactic red-cell transfusions in pregnant patients with sickle cell disease. *N. Engl. J. Med.* **319**:1447–1452.

Krowka, M. J., Rosenow, E. C. III, and Hoagland, H. C. (1985). Pulmonary complications of bone marrow transplantation. *Chest* **87**:237–246.

Kyle, R., and Greipp, P. (1983). Amyloidosis (AL): clinical and laboratory features in 229 cases. *Mayo. Clin. Proc.* **58**:665–683.

Labi, M., Haponik, E. F., Welsh, R. A., and Summer, W. R. (1989). Alveolar cell carcinoma complicating sickle cell anemia: a chance occurrence? *Am J. Hematol.* **32**:222–225.

Lazarus, H. (1990). Granulocyte transfusions: have we learned anything? (editorial). *J. Lab. Clin. Med.* **115**:271–272.

Lesser, B. A., Leeper, K. V. Jr., and Conway, W. (1988). Obstructive sleep apnea in amyloidosis treated with nasal continuous positive airway pressure. *Arch. Intern. Med.* **148**:2285–2287.

Lind, S. E. (1991). The bleeding time does not predict surgical bleeding. *Blood* **77**:2547–2552.

List, A. F., Doll, D. C., and Greco, F. A. (1985). Lung cancer in Hodgkin's disease: association with previous radiotherapy. *J. Clin. Oncol.* **3**:215.

Ludmerer, K. M., and Kissane, J. M. (1988). A 77 year-old man with a pleural effusion. *Am. J. Med.* **84**:941–948.

Lum, L. G. (1987). The kinetics of immune reconstitution after human marrow transplantation. *Blood* **69**:369–380.

Maddern, B. R., Reed, H. T., Ohene-Frempong, K., and Beckerman, R. C. (1989). Obstructive sleep apnea syndrome in sickle cell disease. *Ann. Otol. Rhinol. Laryngol.* **98**:174–178.

Maurer, H. S., Steinherz, P. G., Gaynon, P. S., Finklestein, J. Z., Sather, H. N., Reaman, G. H., Bleyer, W. A., and Hammond, G. D. (1988). The effect of initial management of hyperleukocytosis on early complications and outcome of children with acute lymphoblastic leukemia. *J. Clin. Oncol.* **6**:1425–1432.

McCabe, R. E., Brooks, R. G., Catterall, J. R., and Remington, J. S. (1989). Open lung biopsy in patients with non-Hodgkin's lymphoma and pulmonary infiltrates. *Chest* **96**:319–324.

McKee, L. C., and Collins, R. D. (1974). Intravascular leukocyte thrombi and aggregates as a cause of morbidity and mortality in leukemia. *Medicine* **53**:463–478.

Meyers, J. D. (1985). Infection in recipients of bone marrow transplants. *Curr. Clin. Top. Infect. Dis.* **6**:261–292.

Meyers, J. D., Reed, E. C., Shepp, D. H., Thornquist, M., Dandliker, P. S., Vicary, C. A., Flournoy, N., Kirk, L. E., Kersey, J. H., Thomas, E. D., and Balfour, H. H., Jr. (1988). Acyclovir for prevention of cytomegalovirus infection and disease after allogeneic marrow transplantation. *N. Engl. J. Med.* **318**:70–75.

Milburn, H. J., Prentice, H. G., and Du Bois, R. M. (1987). Role of bronchoalveolar lavage in the evaluation of interstitial pneumonitis in recipients of bone marrow transplants. *Thorax* **42**:766–772.

Miller, G. J., Serjeant, G. R., Sivaprogasam, S., Petch, M. C. (1973). Cardiopulmonary responses and gas exchange during exercise in adults with homozygous sickle cell disease (sickle-cell anemia). *Clin. Sci.* **44**:113–128.

Milne, N., Light, R. W., and Chetty, K. G. (1990). Exercise-induced changes in left ventricular function after phlebotomy in patients with polycythemic COPD. *J. Thorac. Imaging* **5**:68–72.

Milner, P. F. (1974). Oxygen transport in sickle cell anemia. *Arch. Intern. Med.* **133**:565–572.

Moormeier, J. A., Williams, S. F., and Golomb, H. M. (1990). The staging of non-Hodgkin's lymphomas. *Semin. Oncol.* **17**:43–50.

Morassi, P., Paladini, G., Mazzanti, G., Cataldo, R., Cantalupi, D., and Versari, A. (1985). Bone scintigraphy in the diagnosis of pulmonary calcification in multiple myeloma. *Eur. J. Nucl. Med.* **11**:327–329.

Morgan, J. E., Rodriguez, F. H., deShazo, R. D., and Banks, D. E. (1987). Pulmonary immunologic features of alveolar septal amyloidosis associated with multiple myeloma. *Chest* **94**:704–708.

Morinaga, S., Watanabe, H., Gemma, A., Mukai, K., Nakajima, T., Shimosato, Y., Goya, T., and Shinoda, T. (1987). Plasmacytoma of the lung associated with nodular deposits of immunoglobulin. *Am. J. Surg. Pathol.* **11**:989–995.

Morrow, J. D. (1991). Fluconazole: a new triazole antifungal agent. *Am. J. Med. Sci.* **302**:129–132.

Murtaza, L. N., Stroud, C. E., Davis, L. R., and Cooper, D. J. (1981). Admissions to hospital of children with sickle-cell anaemia: a study in south London. *Br. Med. J.* **282**:1048–1051.

Nagler, A., Brenner, B., Zuckerman, E., Hazani, A., and Israel, O. (1988). Acute respiratory failure in hyperleukocytotic acute myeloid leukemia: the role of perfusion lung scintigraphy. *Am. J. Hematol.* **17**:65–66.

Newball, H. A., and Brahim, S. A. (1977). Chronic obstructive airway disease in patients with Sjögren's syndrome. *Am. Rev. Respir. Dis.* **115**: 295–304.

Notter, D. T., Grossman, P. L., Rosenberg, S. A., and Remington, J. S. (1980). Infections in patients with Hodgkin's disease: a clinical study of 300 consecutive adult patients. *Rev. Infect. Dis.* **2**:761–800.

Oppenheimer, E. H., and Esterly, J. R. (1971). Pulmonary changes in sickle cell disease. *Am. Rev. Respir. Dis.* **103**:858–859.

Paladini, G., Morassi, P., Melato, M., and Falconieri, G. (1986). Massive pulmonary calcification in multiple myeloma. Report of a case. *Haematologica* **71**:313–316.

Panos, R. J., Barr, L. F., Walsh, T. J., and Silverman, H. J. (1988). Factors associated with fatal hemoptysis in cancer patients. *Chest* **94**:1008–1013.

Pasqualetti, P., Casale, R., and Colantonio, D. (1989). Pulmonary thromboembolism in multiple myeloma. *Haematologica* **74**:625–626.

Pecego, R., Hill, R., Appelbaum, F. R., Amos, D., Buckner, C. D., Fefer, A., and Thomas, E. D. (1986). Interstitial pneumonitis following autologous bone marrow transplantation. *Transplantation* **42**:515–517.

Petch, M. C., and Serjeant, G. R. (1970). Clinical features of pulmonary lesions in sickle-cell anaemia. *Br. Med. J.* **3**:31.

Peters, S. G., Meadows, J. A., and Gracey, D. R. (1988). Outcome of respiratory failure in hematologic malignancy. *Chest* **94**:99–102.

Pianosi, P., D'Souza, S. J. A., Esseltine, D. W., Charge, T. D., and Coates, A. L. (1991). Ventilation and gas exchange during exercise in sickle cell anemia. *Am. Rev. Respir. Dis.* **143**:226–230.

Poncz, M., Kane, E., and Gill, F. M. (1985). Acute chest syndrome in sickle cell disease: etiology and clinical correlates. *J. Pediatr.* **107**:861–866.

Powars, D., Weidman, J. A., Odom-Maryon, T., Niland, J. C., and Johnson, C. (1988). Sickle cell chronic lung disease: prior morbidity and the risk of pulmonary failure. *Medicine* **67**:66–76.

Prakash, U. B. S. (1989). Hematologic diseases. In *Textbook of Pulmonary Diseases*, 4th ed. Edited by G. L. Baum and E. Wolinsky. Little Brown, Boston, pp. 1291–1323.

Ralph, D. D., Springmeyer, S. C., Sullivan, K. M., Hackman, R. C., Storb, R., and Thomas, E. D. (1984). Rapidly progressive air-flow obstruction in marrow transplant recipients: possible association between obliterative bronchiolitis and chronic graft-versus-host disease. *Am. Rev. Respir. Dis.* **129**:641–644.

Reed, E. C., Bowden, D. A., Dandliker, P. S., Lilleby, K. E., and Meyers, J. D. (1988). Treatment of cytomegalovirus pneumonia with gangciclovir and intravenous cytomegalovirus immune globulin in patients with bone marrow transplants. *Ann. Intern. Med.* **109**:783–788.

Riazmontazer, N., and Bedayat, G. (1989). Cytology of plasma cell myeloma in bronchial washing. *Acta Cytol.* **33**:519–522.

Road, J. D., Jacques, J., and Sparling, J. R. (1985). Diffuse alveolar septal amyloidosis presenting with recurrent hemoptysis and medial dissection of pulmonary arteries. *Am. Rev. Respir. Dis.* **132**:1368–1370.

Robbins, R. A., Linder, J., Stahl, M. G., Thompson, A. B. III, Haire, W., Kessinger, A., Armitage, J. O., Arneson, M., Woods, G., Vaughan, W. P., and Rennard, S. I. (1989). Diffuse alveolar hemorrhage in autologous bone marrow transplant recipients. *Am. J. Med.* **87**:511–518.

Roikjaer, O., and Thomsen, J. K. (1986). Plasmacytoma of the lung. A case report describing two tumors of different immunoglobulin type in a single patient. *Cancer* **58**:2671–2674.

Rosiello, R. A., and Merrill, W. W. (1990). Radiation-induced lung injury. *Clin. Chest Med.* **11**:1–20.

Rubinow, A., Celli, B. R., Cohen, A. S., Rigden, B. G., and Brody, J. S. (1978). Localized amyloidosis of the lower respiratory tract. *Am. Rev. Respir. Dis.* **118**:603–611.

Santiago, R. M., Scharnhorst, D., Ratkin, G., and Crouch, E. C. (1987). Respiratory muscle weakness and ventilatory failure in AL amyloidosis with muscular pseudohypertrophy. *Am. J. Med.* **83**:175–178.

Scott, P. P., and Scott, W. W. (1985). Isolated nodular pulmonary amyloidosis: diagnosis by percutaneous needle aspiration biopsy. *South Med. J.* **78**: 467–471.

Scullin, D. C., Jr., and Cohen, H. J. (1979). Myelomatous pleural effusion: clinical course and immunologic chracterization of the pleural fluid cells. *Am. J. Hematol.* **6**:267–273.

Scully, R. E., Mark, E. J., McNeely, W. F., and McNeely, B. U. (1989). Case records of the Massachusetts General Hospital. *N. Eng. J. Med.* **321**: 102–110.

Shapiro, M. P., and Hayes, J. A. (1984). Fat embolism in sickle cell disease. *Arch. Intern. Med.* **144**:181–182.

Shiue, S. T., and McNally, D. P. (1988). Pulmonary hypertension from prominent vascular involvement in diffuse amyloidosis. *Arch. Intern. Med.* **148**:687–689.

Smith, C. B. (1989). Cytomegalovirus pneumonia: state of the art. *Chest* 95(suppl):182S–187S.

Smith, R. R., Hutchins, G. M., Moore, G. W., Humphrey, R. L. (1979). Type and distribution of pulmonary parenchymal and vascular amyloid: correlation with cardiac amyloidosis. *Am. J. Med.* **66**:96–104.

Snyder, A. B., Barone, J. G., DiGiacomo, C., and Barone, J. E. (1990). Postoperative pulmonary leukostasis. *Crit. Care Med.* **18**:116–117.

Snydman, D. R. (1990). Cytomegalovirus immunoglobulins in the prevention and treatment of cytomegalovirus disease. *Rev. Infect. Dis.* **12**:839–848.

Spector, S. A. (1990). Diagnosis of cytomegalovirus infection. *Semin. Hematol.* **27**:11–16.

Springmeyer, S. C., Flournoy, N., Sullivan, K. M., Storb, R., and Thomas, E. D. (1983). Pulmonary function changes in long-term survivors of allogeneic marrow transplantation. In *Recent Advances in Bone Marrow Transplantation*. Alan R. Liss, New York, pp. 343–353.

Sproule, B. J., Mitchell, J. H., and Miller, W. F. (1960). Cardiopulmonary responses to heavy exercise in patients with anemia. *J. Clin. Invest.* **39**:378–388.

Stone, M. J., and Frenkel, E. P. (1975). The clinical spectrum of light chain myeloma. *Am. J. Med.* **58**:601–618.

Stover, D. E., Zaman, M. B., Hajdu, S. I., Lange, M., Gold, J., and Armstrong, D. (1984). Bronchoalveolar lavage in the diagnosis of diffuse pulmonary infiltrates in the immunosuppressed host. *Ann. Intern. Med.* **101**:1–7.

Strange, C., Heffner, J. E., Collins, B. S., Brown, F. M., and Sahn, S. A. (1987). Pulmonary hemorrhage and air embolism complicating transbronchial biopsy in pulmonary amyloidosis. *Chest* **92**:367–369.

Strauss, A., and LaCandia, S. (1989). Sickle cell disease and cocaine abuse—a deadly mixture? *South. Med. J.* **82**:1455–1456.

Streeten, E. A., de la Monte, S. M., and Kennedy, T. P. (1986). Amyloid infiltration of the diaphragm as a cause of respiratory failure. *Chest* **89**:760–762.

Sullivan, K. M. (1987). Immunoglobulin therapy in bone marrow transplantation. *Am. J. Med.* **83**:34–45.

Sutedja, T. G., Apperley, J. F., Hughes, J. M. B., Aber, V. R., Kennedy, H. G., Nunn, P., Jones, L., Hopper, L., and Goldman, J. M. (1987). Pulmonary function after bone marrow transplantation for chronic myeloid leukaemia. *Thorax* **43**:163–169.

Theodore, J., Starns, V. A., and Lewiston, N. J. (1990). Obliterative bronchiolitis. *Clin. Chest Med.* **11**:309–321.

Thompson, P. J., and Citron, K. M. (1983). Amyloid and the lower respiratory tract. *Thorax* **38**:84–87.

Thompson, P. J., Jewkes, J., Corwin, B., and Citron, K. M. (1983). Primary bronchopulmonary amyloid tumor with massive hilar adenopathy. *Thorax* **38**:153–154.

Topilow, A. A., Gopal, I., and Rock, P. (1986). Systemic amyloidosis with pulmonary involvement in IgD myeloma. *N.J. Med.* **83**:739–742.

Tucker, M. A., Coleman, C. N., Cox, R. S., Varghese, A., and Rosenberg, S. A. (1988). Risk of second cancers after treatment for Hodgkin's disease. *N. Eng. J. Med.* **318**:76–81.

Twohig, K. J., and Matthay, R. A. (1990). Pulmonary effects of cytotoxic agents other than bleomycin. *Clin. Chest Med.* **11**:31–54.

Urbanski, S. J., Kossakowska. A. E., Durtis, J., Chan, C. K., Hutcheon, M. A., Hyland, R. H., Messner, H., Minden, M., and Sculier, J. P. (1987). Idiopathic small airways pathology in patients with graft-versus-host disease following allogeneic bone marrow transplantation. *Am. J. Surg. Pathol.* **11**:965–971.

van Buchem, M. A., Wondergem, J. H., Kool, L. J. S., te Velde, J., Kluin, P. M., Bode, P. J., and Busscher, D. L. T. (1987). Pulmonary leukostasis: radiologic pathologic study. *Radiology* **165**:739–741.

Weiland, D., Ferguson, R. M., Peterson, P. K., Snover, D. C., Simmons, R. L., and Najarian, J. S. (1983). Aspergillosis in 25 renal transplant patients. Epidemiology, clinical presentation, diagnosis and management. *Ann. Surg.* **198**:622–629.

Wiltshaw, E. (1976). The natural history of extramedullary plasmacytoma and its relation to solitary myeloma of bone and myelomatosis. *Medicine (Baltimore)* **55**:217–238.

Wingard, J. R., Mellits, E. D., Sostrin, M. B., Chen, D. Y., Burns, W. H., Santos, G. W., Vriesendorp, H. M. Beschorner, W. E., and Saral, R., (1988). Interstitial pneumonitis after allogeneic bone marrow transplantation: nine-year experience at a single institution. *Medicine (Baltimore)* **67**:175–186.

Wingard, J. R., Piantadosi, S., Burns, W. H., Zahurak, M. L., Santos, G. W., and Saral, R. (1990). Cytomegalovirus infections in bone marrow transplant recipients given intensive cytoreductive therapy. *Rev. Infect. Dis.* **12**:793–804.

Winston, D. J., Ho, W. G., and Champlin, R. E. (1990). Cytomegalovirus infections after allogeneic bone marrow transplantation. *Rev. Infect. Dis.* **12**:776–792.

Winterbauer, R. H., Riggins, R. C. Griesman, F. A., and Bauermeister, D. E. (1974). Pleuropulmonary manifestations of Waldenström's macroglobulinemia. *Chest* **66**:368–375.

Witherspoon, R. P., Lum, L. G., and Storb, R. (1984). Immunologic reconstitution after human marrow grafting. *Semin. Hematol.* **21**:2–10.

Witt, D. H., Zalusky, R., Castella, A., and Mercer, W. D. (1986). Light chain myeloma with meningeal and pleural involvement. *Am. J. Med.* **80**:1213–1216.

Yood, R. A., Skinner, M., Rubinow, A., Talarico, L. and Cohen, A. S. (1983). Bleeding manifestations in 100 patients with amyloidosis. *JAMA* **249**:1322–1324.

Zaia, J. A., Kovacs, A., and Forman, S. J. (1987). Human cytomegalovirus-associated pneumonitis: pathogenesis, prevention and treatment. *Transplant. Proc.* **19**:125–131.

Zinkham, W. H., and Winslow, R. M. (1989). Unstable hemoglobins: influence of environment on phenotypic expression of a genetic disorder. *Medicine (Baltimore)* **68**:309–319.

6

Endocrine and Metabolic Disease

MICHAEL A. MATTHAY

University of California, San Francisco
San Francisco, California

I. Introduction

The purpose of this chapter is to consider the clinically important manifestations of endocrine disorders on the respiratory system. Some of the effects of endocrine dysfunction are direct in their influence on pulmonary function, whereas other effects are more indirect. In patients with diabetes mellitus, for example, there is a higher risk of both acute and chronic pulmonary infections that may lead to acute respiratory failure. In some patients with severe hypothyroidism, however, mechanical lung function may be mildly abnormal, but in others, acute hypercapnic respiratory failure may develop because of a decrease in central ventilatory drive.

This chapter will also discuss the relatively new concept that the lung itself is an endocrine organ. The basis of this approach derives from a rapidly growing body of knowledge about biogenic amines, neuropeptides, and various other hormones that are produced in the lungs under both normal and abnormal conditions and that have both local and systemic effects. This area has emerged recently as a field of major interest to both scientists and some clinical investigators.

II. Diabetes Mellitus

The most common endocrine disorder in clinical medicine is diabetes mellitus. The most important overall effect of diabetes mellitus on the respiratory system is an increased incidence of both acute and chronic pulmonary infections. Large surveys of mortality in patients with diabetes mellitus before 1924 revealed that 19% of deaths in diabetic patients were due to infections, most of which were pulmonary (Marble, 1985). In a classic review of diabetes mellitus and tuberculosis, it was stated, "In the latter half of the 19th century the diabetic patient appeared doomed to die of pulmonary tuberculosis if he succeeded in escaping diabetic coma" (Root, 1934a). After the introduction of insulin and antimicrobial therapy, the death rate from infection in patients with diabetes mellitus declined. Nevertheless, approximately 10% of diabetic patients still die from infections, the majority of which are acute or chronic pulmonary infections (Marble, 1985).

Studies of diabetic patients with bacterial pneumonia have documented the frequent occurrence of *Staphylococcus aureus* and gram-negative pneumonias. In one study of *Escherichia coli* pneumonia, diabetes mellitus was present in 69% of patients (Tillotson and Lerner, 1967). Also, Winterbauer and colleagues (1969) reported that diabetes mellitus was a major cause of recurrent pneumonia in a study of 158 patients. Pneumococcal pneumonia occurs with higher frequency in patients with diabetes mellitus, and the mortality from bacteremic pneumococcal pneumonia is also higher in diabetic patients than in the general population. However, there is still controversy regarding the use of pneumococcal vaccine for diabetics. Because it has been shown that the vaccine results in a reasonable antibody response, some have recommended that patients with long-standing diabetes complicated by cardiac, peripheral vascular, or chronic renal disease be given the vaccine (Marble, 1985).

The pathophysiological basis for the increased susceptibility to acute and chronic infection in patients with diabetes mellitus has been explored in a number of studies. The usual clinical explanations for increased susceptibility are dehydration, malnutrition, impaired neutrophil function, vascular insufficiency, and chronic renal disease. The phagocytic function of neutrophils has been shown to be defective in some patients with diabetes, especially in the presence of acidosis and hyperglycemia (Bagdale et al., 1972). One study demonstrated that these abnormalities were reversible with insulin treatment, suggesting that normal metabolism of glucose was necessary to provide energy for phagocytes and killing of microorganisms (Bagdale et al., 1974). Some studies of neutrophil chemotaxis from diabetic patients have demonstrated impaired chemotactic function of neutrophils in both adult- and juvenile-onset diabetes, but this has not been a consistent finding (Marble, 1985).

There is also an increased susceptibility in diabetic patients to chronic pulmonary infection. For example, in 1952, results from the Philadelphia Survey indicated that chest radiographs of 3106 diabetics demonstrated an 8.4% incidence of tuberculosis versus a 4.3% incidence in 71,767 control patients (Boncot et al., 1952). Overall, diabetics are more susceptible to the reactivation of pulmonary tuberculosis (Edsall et al., 1970).

The increased risk of diabetics to develop pulmonary tuberculosis is well established in both older studies (Root, 1934b) and more recent studies (Burke et al., 1979), but the reason for this increased risk has not been established. Some studies have noted an association clinically with hyperglycemia and the number of episodes of ketosis and the development of pulmonary tuberculosis (Turner-Warwick, 1957). Also, an interesting series of 20 patients with tuberculosis and diabetes mellitus reported that four patients had the disease confined to the lower lobes and another patient to the right lower lobe (Weaver, 1974). Conceivably, this unusual type of involvement might represent progression of the initial (primary), lower lung region inoculum because of failure of host defense mechanisms.

In addition, diabetics have a higher susceptibility to a variety of fungal infections. For instance, it is well known that diabetics have a particular propensity for developing rhinocerebral mucormycosis, but it is less well known that they have an increased risk for developing pulmonary mucormycosis. A localized form of pulmonary mucormycosis with involvement of the major airways and a propensity for life-threatening hemoptysis has been reported in a number of patients with diabetes (Donohue, 1983; Bigby et al., 1986). Figure 1 is a chest radiograph of a patient with diabetic ketoacidosis who developed hemoptysis from pulmonary mucormycosis with a paratracheal abscess. The cellular basis for the higher risk of chronic fungal and mycobacterial infection may be a defect in monocyte chemotactic responses as well as a decrease in monocyte phagocytic activity (Hill et al., 1983).

It has also been well documented that patients with acute diabetic ketoacidosis have a greater incidence of pulmonary infections as well as an increased risk of urinary tract and skin infection (Marble, 1985). In addition, a few recent clinical reports have noted the development of the adult respiratory distress syndrome as a complication of diabetic ketoacidosis in the absence of the usual associated causes (i.e., sepsis, aspiration, or acute pancreatitis) (Russel et al., 1981; Powner et al., 1975). One of these reports was particularly well documented, with measurements of a normal pulmonary artery wedge pressure in association with a high protein concentration in the edema fluid in the absence of pulmonary infection (Fig. 2). The mechanism for increased permeability pulmonary edema is unknown in diabetic patients with ketoacidosis, although it has been reported that diabetics have a higher baseline permeability of the systemic capillaries (Alpert et al., 1972).

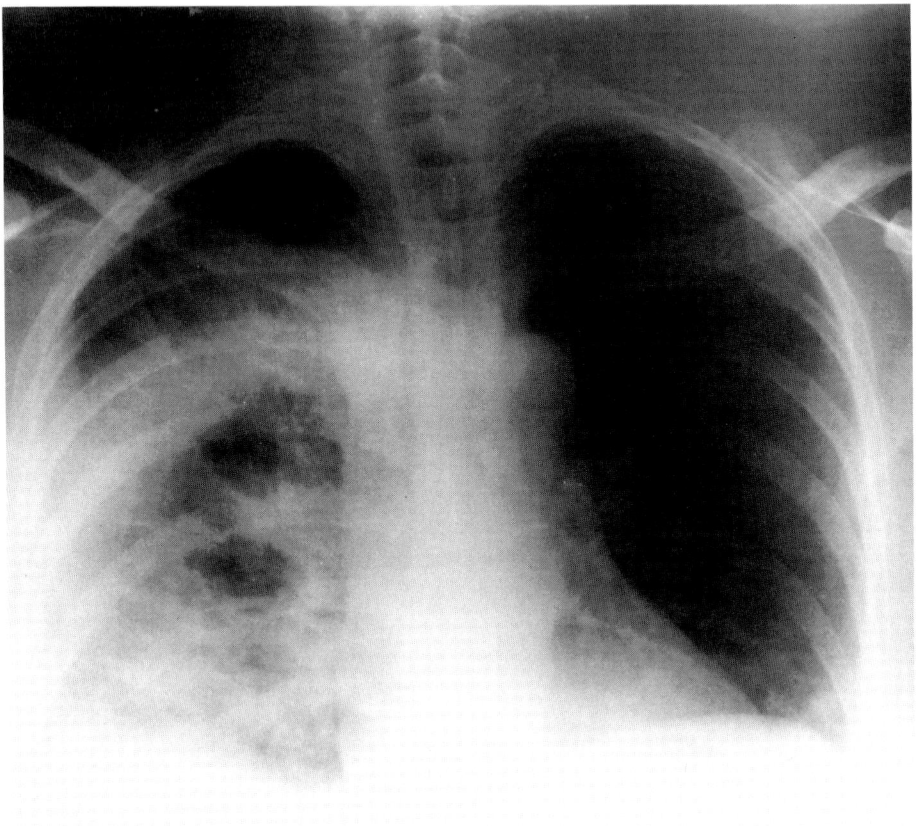

Figure 1 Anteroposterior chest radiograph of a 59-year-old diabetic woman who died with gross hemoptysis shortly after this chest radiograph was taken. There are diffuse infiltrates throughout the right lung field, with two cavities appearing in the right middle lung field. Postmortem studies revealed pulmonary mucormycosis with a right paratracheal mycormycosis abscess. This is a good example of an opportunistic infection that occurs more frequently in patients with diabetes mellitus than a normal host. [Reprinted with permission of the American College of Chest Physicians, from Bigby, et al. (1986).]

Other manifestations of diabetes mellitus in the respiratory system depend on the development of specific complications of diabetes. For example, ischemic heart disease is common in diabetics, and it may lead to the development of acute or chronic cardiogenic pulmonary edema with respiratory insufficiency from congestive heart failure, either from coronary artery disease or from diabetic cardiomyopathy (Kannel et al., 1974; Hamby et al., 1974). Diabetics who

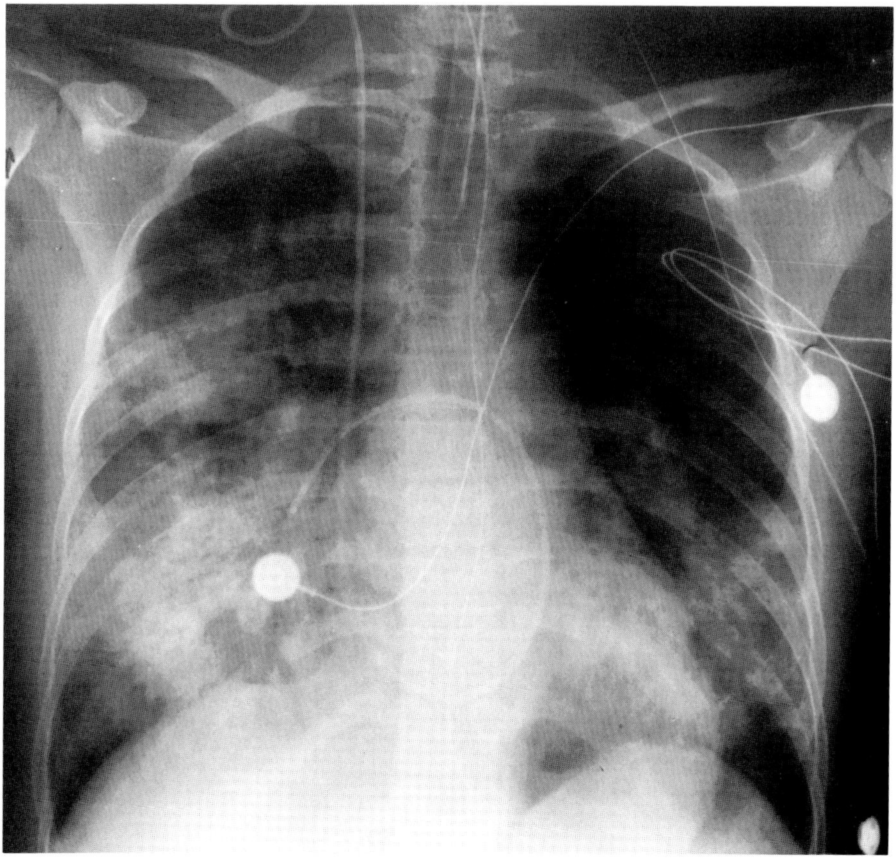

Figure 2 Anteroposterior chest radiograph of 40-year-old woman who developed fulminant pulmonary edema in association with diabetic ketoacidosis. The pulmonary edema fluid albumin concentration was 95% of the plasma albumin concentration. Pulmonary artery wedge pressure was 11 mmHg. The usual clinical causes of adult respiratory distress syndrome, such as sepsis, gastric aspiration, and acute pancreatitus, were excluded by the clinical workup as well as postmortem examination (patient died within 24 hr of onset of pulmonary edema). [Reprinted with permission of the *Western Journal of Medicine*, from Russel et al. (1981).]

develop chronic renal failure may develop the nephrotic syndrome, which in turn may result in the development of large, transudative pleural effusions.

Recently, a well-designed study of pulmonary function in 40 nonsmoking, insulin-dependent diabetics indicated that 60% of the patients had either a mild reduction in the elastic recoil of the lung or a reduction in pulmonary diffusing capacity. These abnormalities were correlated with the duration of diabetes mellitus, but not with other organ involvement. There were no abnormalities of lung volume, air flow, or gas distribution (Sandler et al., 1987). In addition, there is some evidence that basal airway tone controlled by vagal nerve activity can be altered by autonomic diabetic neuropathy (Douglas, 1979). Diabetic neuropathy can also affect the autonomic nervous system and may reduce the ventilatory response to hypoxia (Soler, 1982).

III. Thyroid Disorders

A variety of respiratory abnormalities may occur in patients with hypothyroidism and hyperthyroidism. The effect on the respiratory system may be mediated by changes in central respiratory drive or by the development of either pleural effusions or muscle weakness. A number of texts discuss in detail the physiology of thyroid hormone excess or deficiency and the endocrine manifestations of these abnormalities. This section will consider the respiratory disturbances that may develop in patients with thyroid disease.

A. Hypothyroidism

The classic study of pulmonary function in patients with hypothyroidism was reported in 1960 (Wilson and Bedell, 1960). The investigators in that study demonstrated that patients with myxedema without obesity had normal lung volumes and normal alveolar ventilation. In contrast, patients with myxedema and obesity had moderate reductions of inspiratory capacity, expiratory reserve volume, vital capacity, residual volume, and total lung capacity. In addition, patients with both myxedema and obesity had evidence of alveolar hypoventilation and moderate oxygen desaturation (Table 1). These investigators did not study the mechanism of hypoventilation, but it was believed to be due to a combination of respiratory muscle weakness and decreased central ventilatory drive (Ingbar and Woebar, 1974).

Table 1 Pulmonary Function Tests in Four Patients with Myxedema and Obesity Before and After Treatment

	Vital capacity (% predicted)	Total lung capacity (% predicted)	Arterial O_2 saturation (%)	$Paco_2$ (mmHg)
Before treatment	68 ± 17	64 ± 13	80 ± 4	61 ± 15
After treatment	95 ± 20	82 ± 20	92 ± 4	40 ± 5

In a subsequent study, ventilatory drive to both hypoxia (Figure 3) and hypercapnia (Figure 4) in myxedema patients was found to be depressed (Zwillich et al., 1975). All abnormalities of pulmonary function and ventilatory drive returned to normal when patients were treated with appropriate thyroid hormone replacement.

Clinically there is an important association between severe myxedema and acute respiratory failure (Buchanan et al., 1967). Previously unsuspected hypothyroidism is one of the causes for failure to wean from mechanical ventilation in patients who have required mechanical ventilation for medical or surgical problems. Clinically significant myxedema that is sufficient to cause respiratory failure is usually correlated with a marked decrease in deep tendon reflexes (Ingbar and Woebar, 1974). There is also a clinically important association between myxedema and obstructive sleep apnea (Orr et al., 1981). In one study of three patients with obesity and myxedema, obstructive sleep apnea was documented to result in severe arterial oxygen desaturation. The obstructive sleep apnea

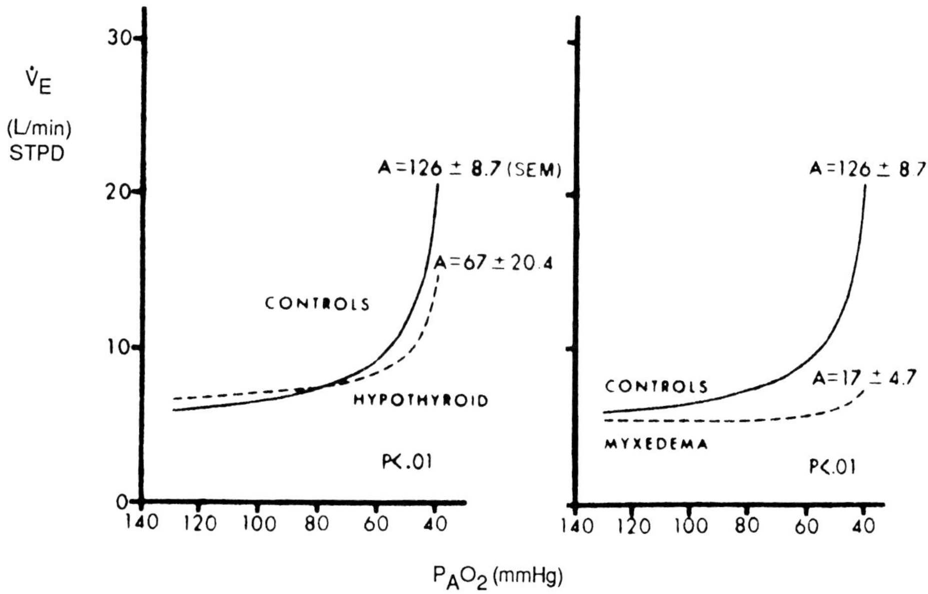

Figure 3 Ventilatory responses to hypoxia shown as the relation between alveolar oxygen tension (Pao_2) and minute ventilation (V̇Ê), standard temperature and dry pressure (STDP). In the hypothyroid group, hypoxic ventilatory drive was moderately depressed, whereas in the groups with myxedema, hypoxic ventilatory drive was markedly depressed. [Reprinted with permission of the *New England Journal of Medicine*, from Zwillich et al. (1975).]

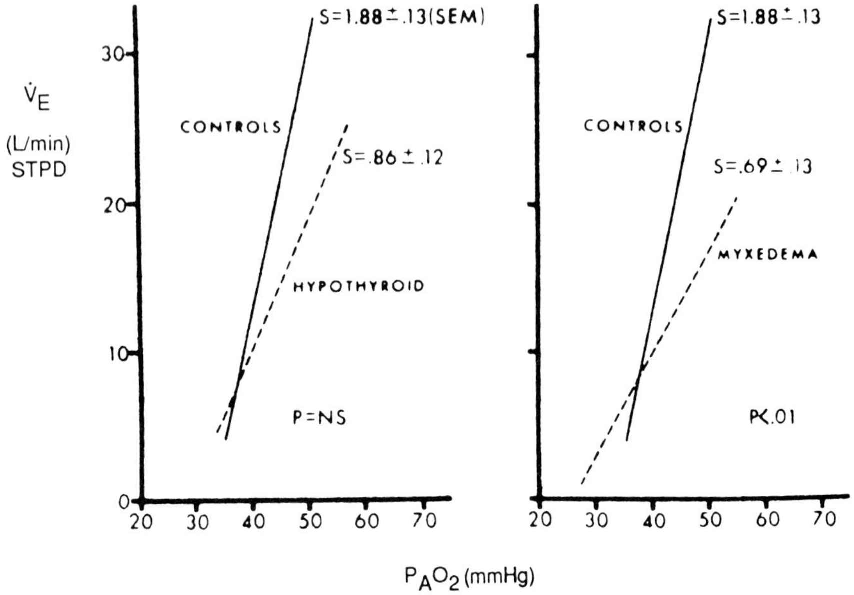

Figure 4 Ventilatory responses to hypercapnia are shown as the relation between alveolar carbon dioxide tension ($Paco_2$) and minute ventilation ($\dot{V}E$). Hypercapnic ventilatory drive was depressed in the hypothyroid group, but was even more strikingly depressed in the group with myxedema. [Reprinted with permission of the *New England Journal of Medicine*, from Zwillich et al. (1975).]

resolved with thyroid hormone replacement, although the patients remained obese. The cause of the upper airway obstruction may relate to deposition of mucopolysaccharides and protein extravasation in the face, tongue, and pharyngeal structures, which may predispose to upper airway obstruction during rapid eye movement sleep (Parving et al., 1979).

Patients with myxedema often have evidence of pericardial and pleural effusions (Fig. 5). The reported protein concentration of the pericardial effusions has ranged from 2.2 to 7.6 g/dl (Schneierson and Katz, 1958; Smolar et al., 1976). The mechanism for the development of pleural effusions is uncertain, although it may be related to abnormalities of transcapillary filtration of liquid and protein. Patients with hypothyroidism may also have a substernal goiter that can present as an anterior mediastinal mass (Paré and Fraser, 1983) and, rarely, can cause superior venal caval obstruction (Mahajan et al., 1975).

In several in vitro and animal studies, thyroid hormone has been shown to accelerate fetal lung maturation by increasing the size of type II pneumocytes and increasing surfactant production (Morishige et al., 1982; Redding et al.,

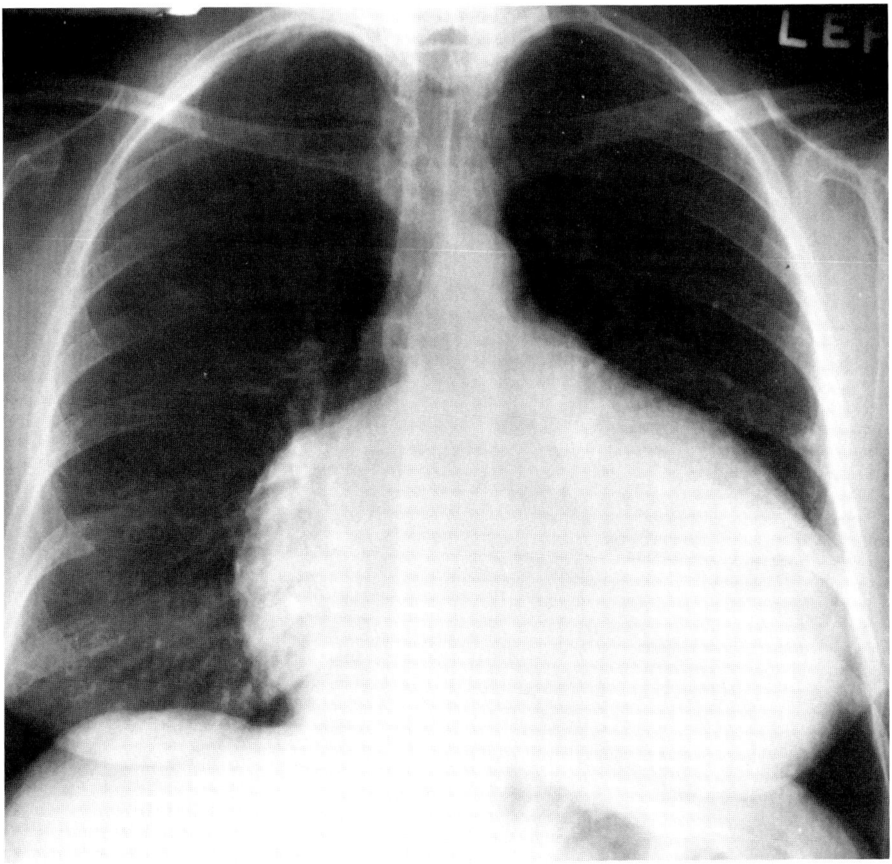

Figure 5 Posteroanterior chest radiograph of a 55-year-old woman with severe myxedema and a large cardiac silhouette. Echocardiogram demonstrated a large pericardial effusion. In addition, a small left pleural effusion was noted on the echocardiogram. [Courtesy of W. B. Saunders Co., from Murray and Nadel, (1988).]

1972). Mashiach and co-workers (1978) demonstrated in a nonrandomized study of pregnant women that the intra-amniotic administration of thyroxine decreased the incidence of infant respiratory distress syndrome of fetuses at high risk for developing the syndrome.

B. Hyperthyroidism

Over 50 years ago, investigators studying pulmonary function in hyperthyroid patients found a high incidence of dyspnea and a decrease in vital capacity in most patients with thyrotoxicosis (Peabody and Wentworth, 1917; Femor, 1924). Subsequently, Stein and colleagues (1961) reported a comprehensive study of pulmonary function in 13 hyperthyroid patients. The vital capacity was reduced in only three patients, and other lung volume measurements were normal in all patients. The mean vital capacity did increase, however, in seven patients who were restudied after treatment for hyperthyroidism. There was a significant increase in minute ventilation in the hyperthyroid patients during exercise (26.1 ± 5.7 L/min/m^2), which was more than twice the minute ventilation of exercising, euthyroid control patients (12.5 ± 3.8 L/min/m^2) at comparable levels of exercise. At rest, mean oxygen consumption was higher in hyperthyroid patients than in euthyroid control patients, but during exercise at the same workload, oxygen consumption values were not significantly different in the two groups.

The presence of dyspnea in hyperthyroid patients probably is not related to abnormalities of lung volume or mechanics of breathing, but rather to the increase in central ventilatory drive (Massey et al., 1967). The results of one

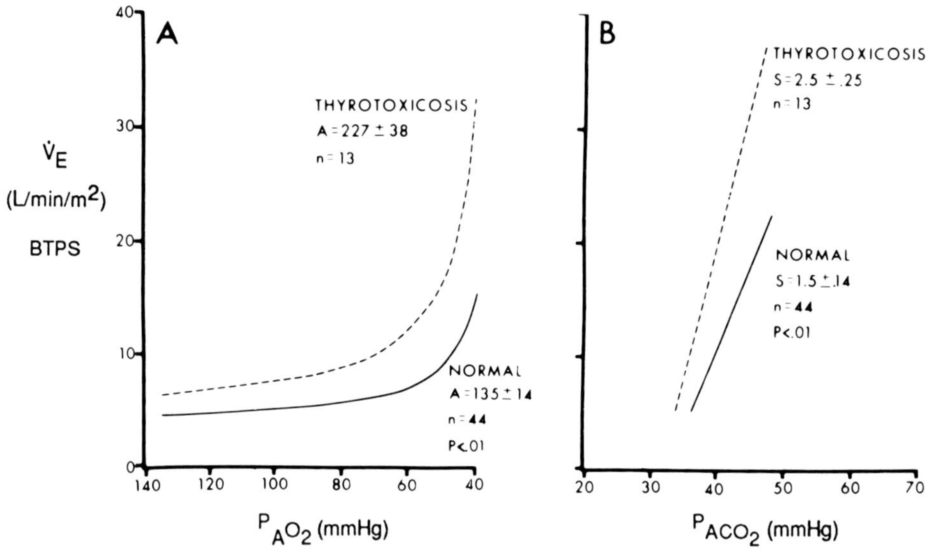

Figure 6 Mean ventilatory responses to hypoxia, (A) and hypercapnia (B) are shown for 13 patients with thyrotoxicosis compared with 44 normal subjects. Note that the hypoxic ventilatory response was steeper in the patients with thyrotoxicosis and that ventilation ($\dot{V}_E$) at a Pa_{O_2} = 40 mmHg was twofold greater. The hypercapnic response was also significantly increased in the thyrotoxicosis patients compared with the normal subjects. Beta blockade with high doses of propranolol did not alter these increased ventilatory responses, whereas definitive treatment of the hyperthyroid state with surgery or ^{131}I resulted in normalization of ventilatory drives to both hypoxia and hypercapnia. [Reprinted with permission of the Endocrine Society, from Zwillich et al. (1978).

study demonstrated that there was a marked increase in both hypoxic and hypercapnic ventilatory drives in patients with thyrotoxicosis compared with healthy control subjects (Fig. 6) (Zwillich et al., 1978). Although treatment with beta-sympathomimetic blockade diminished many of the signs and symptoms of thyrotoxicosis, there was no evidence that the increases in metabolic rate, resting ventilation, or ventilatory responses to hypoxia or hypercapnia could be reversed by this form of therapy. On the other hand, specific treatment of the hyperthyroid state resulted in normalization of both the hypoxic and hypercapnic ventilatory drives.

No large studies link reactive airway disease to thyrotoxicosis, although there has been an anecdotal report of resolution of intractable asthma after treatment of thyrotoxicosis in five patients (Settipane et al., 1972). Patients with severe thyrotoxicosis may develop high-output cardiac failure and even cardiogenic pulmonary edema (Fig. 7), although the hyperkinetic state in hyperthyroidism does not usually lead to congestive heart failure unless there is underlying cardiac or coronary artery disease (Braunwald, 1980).

IV. Parathyroid Disease

In general, patients with hyperparathyroidism or hypoparathyroidism do not have major abnormalities referable to the respiratory system. However, patients with hyperparathyroidism do occasionally have significant neuromuscular weakness, which may manifest as mild restrictive lung disease. In addition, the chest radiograph will often show some of the classic findings of hyperparathyroidism, with severe osteopenia and osteitis fibrosa cystica at the ends of the clavicle or in the scapula (Paré and Fraser, 1983). Soft tissue calcification may also be evident on chest or shoulder films (Fig. 8). Occasionally, a parathyroid adenoma will be located within the thorax and will be visible on the chest radiograph as a mediastinal mass (Fig. 9).

Patients with hypoparathyroidism may have hypocalcemia sufficient to result in generalized muscle weakness and mild restrictive respiratory disease as well. Following thyroid or parathyroid surgery, localized edema may cause postoperative upper airway obstruction. Postoperative hypocalcemia from removal of parathyroid glands and inadequate postoperative supplementation may lead to laryngeal spasm (Sabiston, 1986).

V. Pituitary, Adrenal, and Reproductive System Disorders

In general, patients with hypothalamic, pituitary, adrenal, or ovarian diseases do not have major respiratory manifestations. The exceptions to this generalization include, of course, patients who have recently had pituitary surgery and may

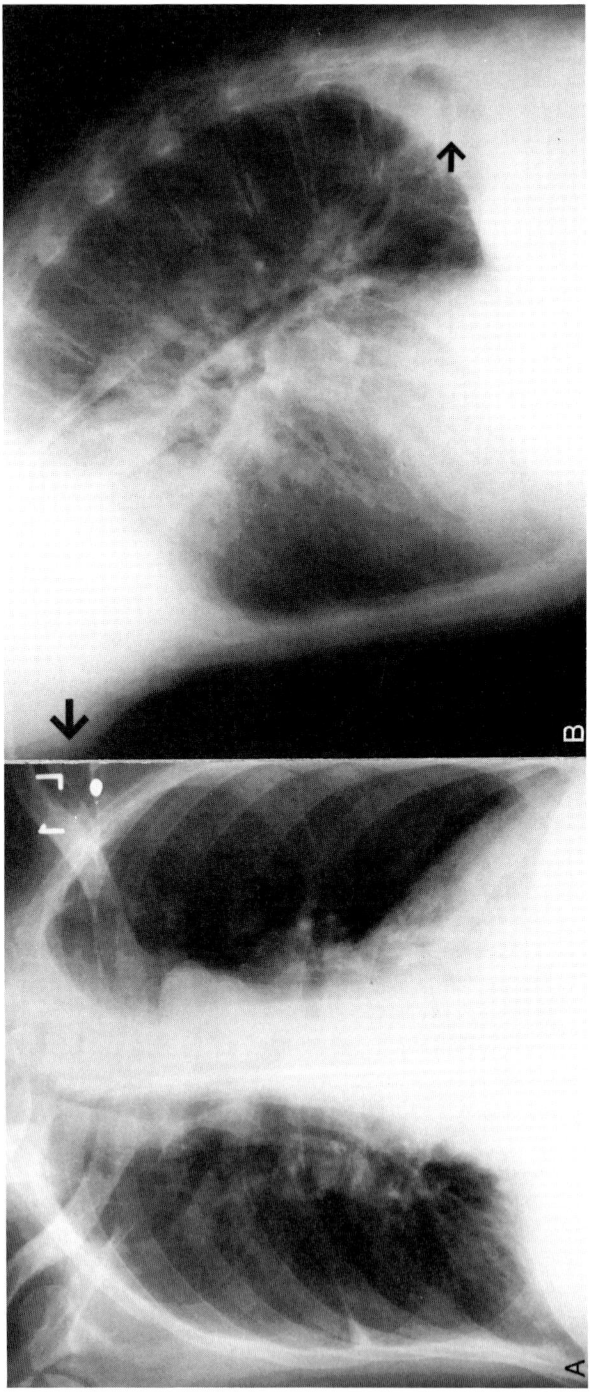

Figure 7

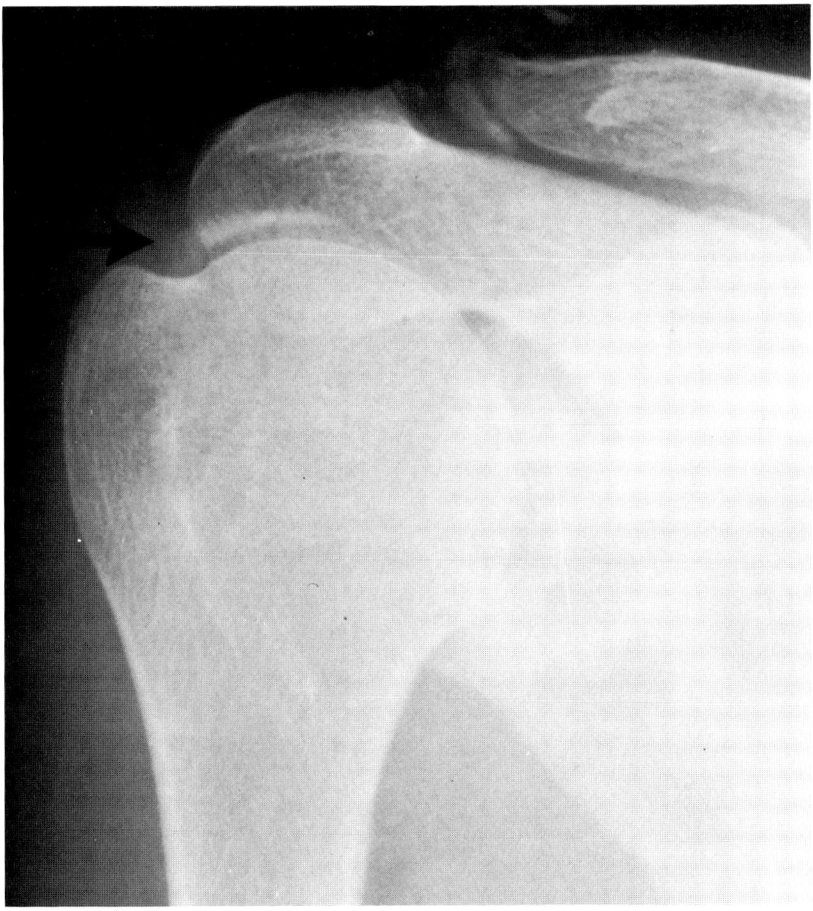

Figure 8 Right shoulder and scapula film of a patient with primary hyperparathyroidism showing soft tissue calcification (arrow) of the acromioclavicular joint and the articular cartilage and cystic changes in the scapula. These are classic radiographic signs of primary hyperparathyroidism. [Courtesy of W. B. Saunders Co., from Murray and Nadel (1988).]

Figure 7 Chest radiographs of a 65-year-old woman with thyrotoxicosis and a goiter who developed atrial fibrillation and congestive heart failure. (A) Posteroanterior chest radiograph reveals bilateral pleural effusions, interstitial pulmonary edema, and an increased density in the lower neck and superior mediastinum. (B) Lateral chest film shows a prominent neck mass (*upper left arrow*) and posterior tracking of pleural effusions (*lower right arrow*). Patient did have underlying ischemic heart disease. [Courtesy of W. B. Saunders Co., from Murray and Nadel (1988).]

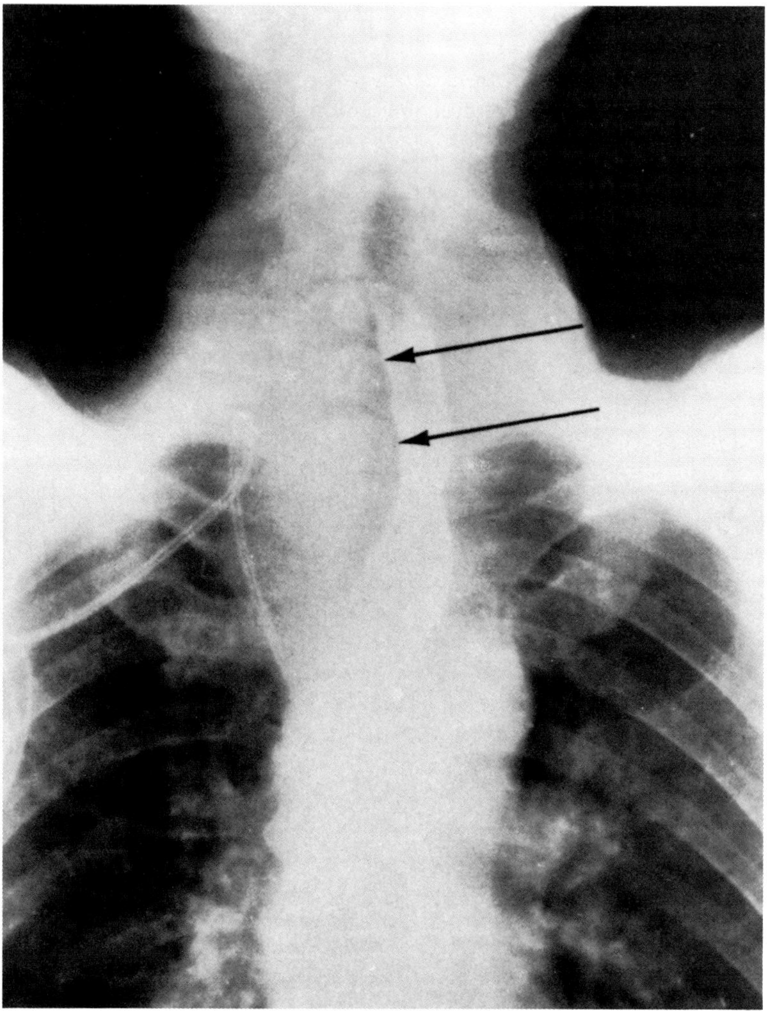

Figure 9 Posteroanterior chest radiograph of a patient during a barium swallow demonstrating an anterior mediastinal mass that displaced the esophagus to the left (*arrows*). The lesion turned out to be a 24-g parathyroid tumor of the left inferior gland that had migrated into the posterior-superior mediastinum. [Courtesy of Grune & Stratton, from Paloyan et al. (1973).]

have a decreased mental status with a greater tendency for gastric aspiration and acute respiratory failure. Patients with Cushing's syndrome may be predisposed to some opportunistic infections because of their excessive endogenous glucocorticoids. Also, impressive widening of the mediastinum may occur with mediastinal lipomatosis in Cushing's syndrome (Fig. 10).

In addition, patients with acromegaly may present with an increase in lung size, a narrowing of the airways, and pulmonary venous hypertension (Evans et al., 1977; Harrison et al., 1978; Kitahara, 1971). In a classic study of six acromegalic men, pulmonary function testing demonstrated increased lung volumes without evidence of airflow obstruction or air trapping (Brody et al.,

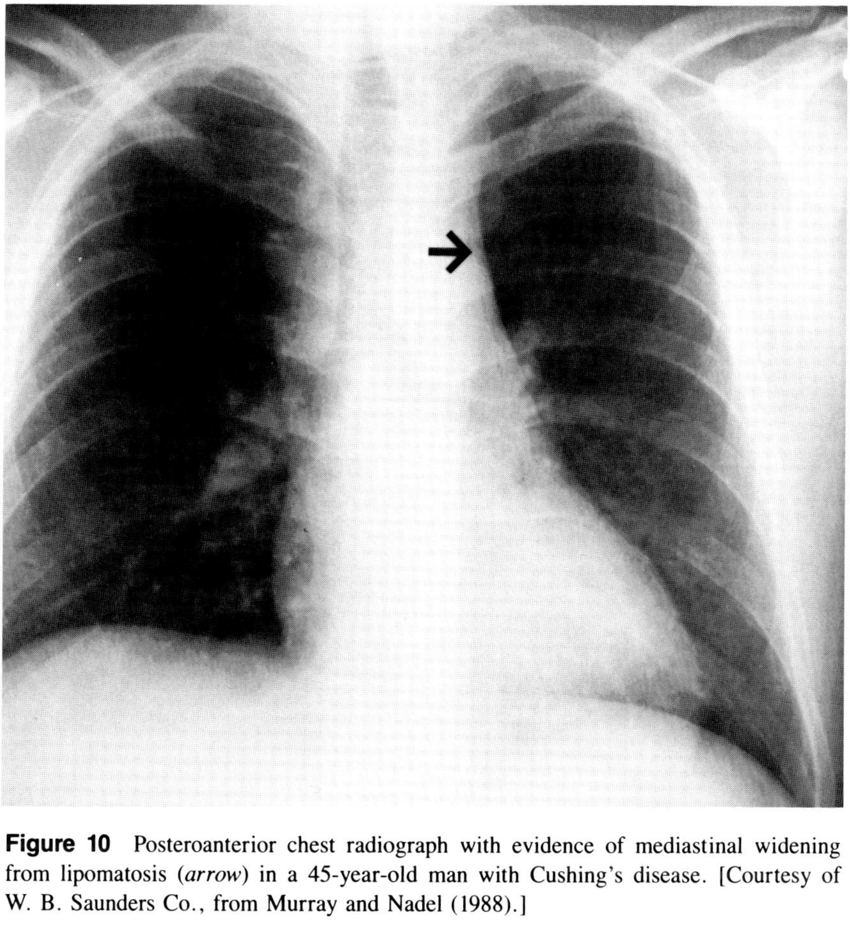

Figure 10 Posteroanterior chest radiograph with evidence of mediastinal widening from lipomatosis (*arrow*) in a 45-year-old man with Cushing's disease. [Courtesy of W. B. Saunders Co., from Murray and Nadel (1988).]

1970). The diffusing capacity was normal, suggesting that the lung enlargement resulted from an increase in the size rather than in the number of alveoli.

Interestingly, lung volumes were normal in four acromegalic women, suggesting that sex hormones may modify the effect of growth hormones on the lung. Also, an increase in the frequency of sleep apnea has been reported in patients with excessive growth hormone secretion and can be either obstructive or central in origin (Cadieux et al., 1982; Mezon et al., 1980; Milman et al., 1983). Recently, sleep apnea associated with acromegaly has been reported to improve rapidly after short-term treatment with the somatostatin analog SMS 201-995 (Chanson et al., 1986).

In patients with a pheochromocytoma, the primary tumor may be located within the thorax. In the chest, these tumors are thought to arise from para-aortic paraganglion cells associated with the sympathetic chain (the islands of Zuckerhandl). They are highly vascular and therefore can usually be visualized by an aortic angiogram (Sabiston et al., 1983). Metastatic adrenal medullary pheochromocytoma can be excluded by demonstrating normal adrenal glands on computed-tomography scan before making a diagnosis of primary intrathoracic pheochromocytoma.

The Meigs-Salmon syndrome (pleural effusions, ascites, and ovarian tumors) was originally described in association with ovarian fibromas (Salmon, 1934). The syndrome is now known to be associated with a wide variety of primary pelvic neoplasms, including fibroma, thecoma, granulosa cell tumors, Brenner tumors, cystadenoma, adenocarcinoma, and even extraovarian pelvic tumors such as fibromyoma of the uterus (Paré and Fraser, 1983). The ascites appears to result from secretion of large amounts of fluid by the tumors (Meigs, 1954). Pleural effusions may be massive; they are most frequently on the right side, but may be on the left side or bilateral (Fig. 11). The pleural fluid is usually a transudate, but occasionally contains blood. The pleural effusions probably result from ascitic fluid passing through pores in the diaphragm into the pleural space (Light, 1983). Removal of the pelvic tumor is usually followed by disappearance of both hydrothorax and the ascites (Paré and Fraser, 1983).

On rare occasions, endometrial tissue can deposit on the pleural spaces. During menstruation, this problem can lead to pneumothorax (catamenial pneumothorax), usually on the right side (Shearin et al., 1974). Further discussion of the pulmonary manifestations of endometriosis and other gynecological conditions is presented in Chapter 11.

VI. Abnormalities of Mineral Metabolism

A number of other disorders with associated abnormalities of mineral metabolism may manifest with respiratory system involvement. Renal osteodystrophy

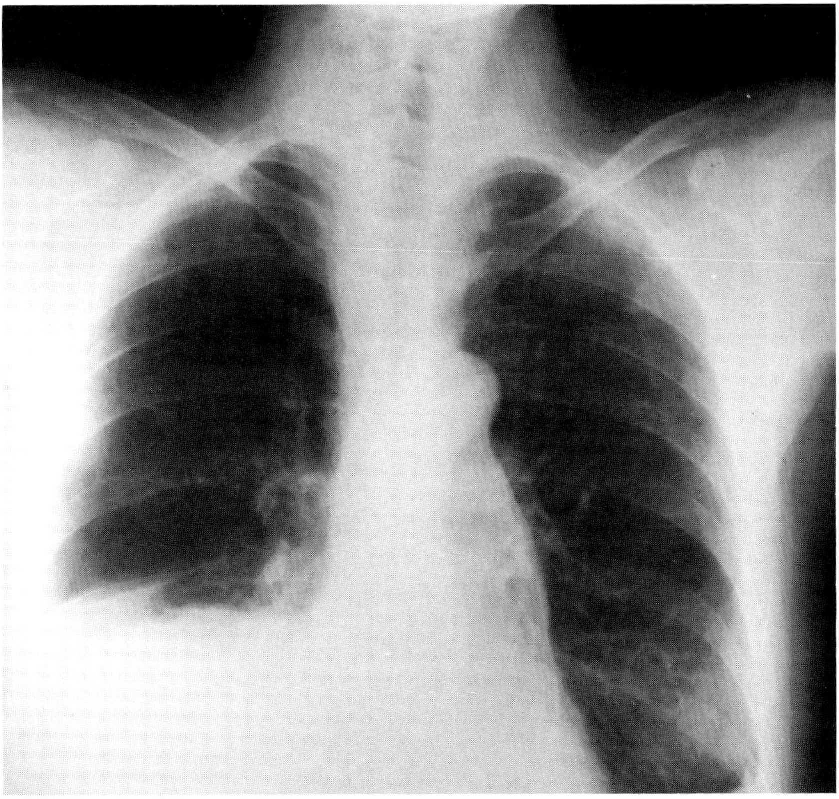

Figure 11 Posteroanterior chest radiograph of 29-year-old woman with Meigs-Salmon syndrome manifested by ascites and bilateral pleural effusions. Note that the left pleural effusion is less than the right because 1000 ml of pleural fluid has recently been removed. [Courtesy of W. B. Saunders Co., from Murray and Nadel (1988).]

can lead to extraskeletal calcifications within the lungs, which, at times, may cause restrictive lung disease (Conger et al., 1975). Rickets and osteomalacia can cause thoracic malformation that, when severe, may lead to a restrictive pulmonary disease, as discussed in Chapter 7, "Neuromuscular and Skeletal Disease," and possibly to an increased risk of infection.

Paget's disease can affect the respiratory system in several ways. In severe cases, the increased vascularity of the involved bones may to high cardiac output failure with resulting pulmonary edema (Deuxchaines and Krane, 1964). On rare occasions, the process can involve the bone at the base of the skull, a site at which subsequent bone expansion can compress the neighboring respiratory center in the brainstem and impair respiratory control (Schmidek, 1977). Finally, vertebral fractures are often present in patients with Paget's disease. These fractures may cause kyphosis, which, as described in Chapter 7, can lead to restrictive lung disease (Bergofsy, 1979).

The hypophosphatemia often associated with disorders of mineral metabolism may lead to muscular weakness and result in respiratory insufficiency (Newman et al., 1977). A more common manifestation of hypophosphatemia is difficulty of weaning of patients already being mechanically ventilated for other indications (Aubier et al., 1985). Furthermore, chronic hypophosphatemia can cause a decrease in 2,3-diphosphoglycerate, which increases the affinity of oxygen to hemoglobin, thereby decreasing the delivery of oxygen to the tissues.

VII. The Lung as an Endocrine Organ

The lung is a very active metabolic organ that degrades, transforms, and activates many circulating substances that derive from extrapulmonary sources and traverse the pulmonary circulation (Table 2). For example, bradykinin, angiotensin I, norepinephrine, 5-hydroxytryptamine, and several of the prostaglandins are all subjected to degradation and metabolism in the lung. In addition, a new area of interest has emerged regarding chemical messenger substances that are synthesized and released within the lung in both health and disease (Becker and Gazdar, 1984).

A. Neuropeptides

Several neuropeptides that have been localized by immunochemical studies to neurons within the central nervous system have also been localized to neurons within the lungs. Some of the peptides that have been identified within pulmonary nerves include substance P, vasoactive intestinal peptide (VIP), and somatostatin. In addition, a number of hormonal substances are known or are strongly suspected to be synthesized in normal lungs and may have important roles in both health and pathological states. Most of these substances are polypeptides, but a few are arachidonic acid metabolites and others are biogenic amines. Table 2 lists some of the potentially most important chemical messengers that may have effects within the lungs. Despite the remarkable metabolic diversity of these substances, with few exceptions, their roles in maintaining homeostasis of the body and of the lungs are poorly understood.

B. Pulmonary Calcitonin

Calcitonin is a 32-amino-acid polypeptide, which is normally produced by the C cells of the thyroid gland, but which is also present in the lungs. In general,

Table 2 Pharmacological and/or Physiological Effects of Biogenic Amines, Hormones, and Arachidonic Acid Metabolites Found in the Lung

ACTH	Promotes fetal lung maturation
Angiotensin II	Pulmonary vasoconstriction
Bradykinin	Pulmonary vasodilation or contraction Causes bronchoconstriction, perhaps by prostaglandin release Competitively inhibits enzyme conversion of angiotensin I to angiotensin II
Calcitonin	Increases endothelial prostacyclin synthesis Centrally, can increase tidal volume
Substance P	Releases histamine from mast cells Stimulates synthesis and release of tracheobronchial mucus
Prostaglandin E2	Pulmonary vasodilator Inhibits platelet aggregation Maintains patency of ductus arteriosus in fetus
Prostaglandin F2x	Pulmonary vasoconstriction and bronchoconstriction
Thromboxane A2	Promotes platelet aggregation and causes pulmonary vasoconstriction and bronchoconstriction
Leukotrienes	Pulmonary bronchoconstriction and vasoconstriction or vasodilation May increase capillary permeability Increase mucus release

calcitonin is believed to have a major role in calcium metabolism by decreasing bone resorption through an inhibition of osteoclastic activity (Chambers, 1982). Although the concentration of calcitonin in the thyroid gland exceeds that in the lungs, if the total weight of the two organs is considered, then the total calcitonin content in pulmonary endocrine cells is greater than in the total thyroid gland in humans (Becker and Gazdar, 1984). Within respiratory tract tissue, calcitonin has been extracted from the trachea, bronchi, and both lungs, with the highest concentrations usually noted in the right middle and upper lobes. However, it is not known whether pulmonary calcitonin production and release contributes to normal calcium metabolism.

Evidence of increased serum and urine levels of calcitonin has been found in nonneoplastic pulmonary diseases (Becker et al., 1981). In one study of 50 patients with chronic obstructive pulmonary disease (COPD), 18 patients with tuberculosis, and 22 patients with acute pneumonia, serum or urine calcitonin

Table 3 Percentage of Patients with Acute and Chronic Pulmonary Disease Whose Serum and/or Urine Calcitonin Levels Were Elevated

Condition	No. of patients	Serum levels	Urine levels
COPD	50	15%	47%
Tuberculosis	18	25%	31%
Pneumonia	22	37%	45%
Total	90	24%	44%

levels exceeded the upper limits of normal in approximately 50% of the patients (Table 3). There was no correlation, however, between blood gas abnormalities and the levels of calcitonin in the patients with COPD. Serum and urine calcitonin levels have been reported to be elevated in the majority of smoking patients (Becker and Gazdar, 1984). It has also been demonstrated that urinary levels of calcitonin are higher in current cigarette smokers than in previous cigarette smokers and nonsmokers. Interestingly, the urine calcitonin level of previous smokers was strongly correlated with the number of pack-years of smoking (Becker and Gazdar, 1984).

Thus, serum and urine calcitonin concentrations may be indices of disease activity in some acute and chronic lung diseases. Perhaps the higher level of calcitonin in acute pneumonia is due to acute hypersecretion or necrosis of pulmonary endocrine cells. In COPD, the high calcitonin level may be related to pulmonary endocrine cell hyperplasia. The increased levels of calcitonin in the urine of cigarette smokers may be related to changes in the bronchial epithelium.

VIII. Summary

The discussion in this chapter has considered the pulmonary manifestations of various endocrine diseases, chiefly diabetes mellitus and thyroid disorders. In addition, attention has been directed toward the role of the lungs themselves as an endocrine organ. The lungs seem to have substantial endocrine activity that involves the metabolism, storage, and release of many different hormones. However, the precise contribution of the lungs to endocrine homeostasis and how this role is affected by pulmonary diseases are unknown and await further study.

Acknowledgments

I appreciate the assistance of Carol Baumeister in preparation of this manuscript. The work was supported in part by NIH Pulmonary Vascular SCOR Grant HL19155.

References

Alpert, J. S., Cocman, J.. D., Balodimos, N. C., et al. (1972). Capillary permeability and blood flow in skeletal muscle of patients with diabetes mellitus. *N. Engl. J. Med.* **286**:454–460.

Aubier, M., Murciano, D., Lecocguic, Y., Viires, N., Jacquens, Y., Squara, P., and Pariente, R. (1985). Effect of hypophosphatemia on diaphragmatic contractility in patients with acute respiratory failure. *N. Engl. J. Med.* **313**:420–424.

Bagdale, J. N., Nielson, K. L., and Bulger, R. J. (1972). Reversible abnormalities of phagocytic function in poorly controlled diabetic patients. *Am. J. Med.* **263**:451–456.

Bagdale, J. N., Root, R. K., and Bulger, R. J. (1974). Impaired leukocyte function in poorly controlled diabetic patients. *Diabetes* **23**:9–16.

Becker, K. L., and Gazdar, A. F. (1984). *The Endocrine Lung*. Saunders, Philadelphia, 1984.

Becker, K. L., Nash, D., Silva, O. L., Snider, R. H., and Moore, C. F. (1981). Increased serum and urinary calcitonin in patients with pulmonary disease. *Chest* **79**:211–216.

Bergofsky, E. H. (1979). Respiratory failure in disorders of the thoracic cage. *Am. Rev. Respir. Dis.* **1219**:643–678.

Bigby, T., Serota, M., Tierney, L. M., and Matthay, M. A. (1986). The clinical spectrum of pulmonary mucormycosis. *Chest* **89**:435–439.

Boncot, K. P., Cooper, P., Dillon, E. S., et al. (1952). Tuberculosis among diabetics. *Am. Rev. Tuberc.* **65**:(suppl.):1–30.

Braunwald, E. (1980). Thyrotoxic heart disease. In *Heart Disease*. Edited by E. Braunwald. Saunders, Philadelphia.

Brody, J. S., Fisher, A. B., Gocmen, A., and DuBois, A. B. (1970). Acromegalic pneumonomegaly: lung growth in the adult. *J. Clin. Invest.* **49**:1051–1060.

Buchanan, K. D., McKiddie, M. T., and Reid, J. M. (1967). Respiratory acidosis in hypothermic myxedema coma. *Postgrad. Med. J.* **43**:114–130.

Burke, R. M., Schwartz, L. P., and Snider, D. F., Jr. (1979). The Ottawa county project: a report of a tuberculosis screening project in a small mining community. *Am. J. Public Health* **69**:340–347.

Cadieux, R. J., Kales, A., and Santen, R. J., et al. (1982). Endoscopic findings in sleep apnea associated with acromegaly. *J. Clin. Endocrinol. Metab.* **55**:18–22.

Chambers, T. J. (1982). Osteoblasts release osteoclasts from calcitonin-induced quiescence. *J. Cell. Sci.* **57**:247–260.

Chanson, P., Timsit, J., Benoit O., et al. (1986). Rapid improvement in sleep apnea of acromegaly after short-term treatment with somastatin analogue. SMS 201–995. *Lancet* **1**:1270–1271.

Conger, J. D., Hammond, W. S., and Alfrey, A. C. (1975). Pulmonary calcification in chronic dialysis patients. *Ann. Intern. Med.* **83**:330–360.

Deuxchaines, C. N., and Krane, S. M. (1964). Paget's disease of the bone: clinical and metabolic observations. *Medicine* **43**:233–266.

Donohue, J. F. (1983). Endobronchial mucormycosis. *Chest* **83**:585–586.

Edsall, J., Collins, J. G., and Gray, J. A. (1970). The reactivation of tuberculosis in New York in 1967. *Am. Rev. Respir. Dis.* **102**:725–736.

Evans, C. C., Hipkin, L. J., and Murray, G. M. (1977). Pulmonary function in acromegaly. *Thorax* **32**:322–327.

Hamby, R. I., Zoneraich, S., and Sherman, L. (1974). Diabetic cardiomyopathy. *JAMA* **229**:1749–1754.

Harrison, B. D. W., Millhouse, K. A., Harrington, M., et al. (1978). Lung function in acromegaly. *Q. J. Med.* **47**:517–532.

Hill, H. R., Augustine, N. H., Rollison, M. C., and Santos, J. I. (1983). Defective monocyte chemotactic responses in diabeties mellitus. *J. Clin. Immunol.* **3**:70–77.

Ingbar, S. H., and Woebar, K. A. (1974). The thyroid gland. In *Williams' Textbook of Endocrinology*, 7th ed. Edited by J. B. Wilson and D. W. Foster. Saunders, Philadelphia, pp. 95–232.

Kannel, W. B., Hjortlan, M., and Castelli, W. P. (1974). Role of diabeties in congestive heart failure. *Am. J. Cardiol.* **34**:29–34.

Kitahara, L. M. (1971). Airway difficulties associated with anaesthesia in acromegaly. *Br. J. Anaesth.* **43**:1187–1190.

Lemon, W. S., and Moersch, H. J. (1924). Basal metabolism and vital capacity. *Arch. Intern. Med.* **33**:130–135.

Light, R. W. (1983). *Pleural Diseases*. Lee & Febiger, Philadelphia, pp. 177–186.

Mahajam, V., Strimlan, V., and Van Ordstrand, H. S. (1975). Benign superior vena cava syndrome. *Chest* **68**:32–35.

Marble, A. (1985). Joslin's diabetes mellitus. Lea & Feibiger, Philadelphia.

Mashiach, S. G., Barkai, Sack, J., et al. (1978). Enhancement of fetal lung maturity by intra-amniotic administration of thyroid hormone. *Am. J. Obstet. Gynecol.* **130**:289–193.

Massey, P. G., Bechlake, M. R., McKenyie, J. M., and Bates, D. V. (1967). Circulatory and ventilatory response to exercise in thyrotoxicosis. *N. Engl. J. Med.* **276**:1104–1112.

Meigs, J. V. (1954). Fibroma of the ovary associated with ascites and hydrothorax—Meig's syndrome. *Am. J. Obstet. Gynecol.* **67**:962–987.

Mezon, B. J., West, P., Maclean, J. P., et al. (1980). Sleep apnea in acromegaly. *Am. J. Med.* **69**:615–617.

Milman, R. P., Bevilacqua, J., and Peterson, D. D. (1983). Central sleep apnea in hypothyroidism. *Am. Rev. Respir. Dis.* **127**:504–507.

Morishige, W. K., Joun, N. S., and Guernsey, D. L. (1982). Thyroidal influence on postnatal lung development in the rat. *Endocrinology* **110**:444–451.

Murray, J. F., and Nadel, J. A., eds. (1988). *Textbook of Respiratory Medicine*. Saunders, Philadelphia.

Newman, J. H., Neff, T. A., and Ziporin, P. (1977). Acute respiratory failure associated with hypophosphatemia. *N. Engl. J. Med.* **296**:1101–1103.

Orr, W. C., Males, J. L., and Imes, N. K. (1981). Myxedema and obstructive sleep apnea. *Am. J. Med.* **70**:1060–1066.

Paloyan, E., Lawrence, A., and Straus, F. (1973). *Hyperparathyroidism*. Grune & Stratton, New York.

Paré, J. A. P., and Fraser, R. (1983). *Synopsis of Diseases of the Chest*. Saunders, Philadelphia.

Parving, H. H., Hansen, J. M., Nielsen, S. L., Rossing, N., Mumck, O., and Lessen, N. A. Mechanisms of edema formation in myxedema—increased protein extravasation and relative slow lymphatic drainage. *N. Engl. J. Med.* **301**:460–465.

Peabody, F. W., and Wentworth, J. (1917). Clinical studies of the respiration. IV. The vital capacity of the lungs and its relation to dyspnea. *Arch. Intern. Med.* **20**:443–448.

Powner, D., Snyder, J. V., and Grenwich, A. (1975). Altered pulmonary capillary permeability recovering from diabetic ketoacidosis. *Chest* **68**: 253–256.

Redding, R. A., Douglas, W. H. J., and Stein, M. (1972). Thyroid hormone influence upon lung surfactant metabolism. *Science* **175**:994.

Root, H. F. (1934a). The association of diabetes and tuberculosis. *N. Engl. J. Med.* **210**:1–13.

Root, H. F. (1934b). The association of diabetes and tuberculosis: epidemiology, pathology, treatment, and progression. *N. Engl. J. Med.* **201**:1–15.

Russel, J., Follansbee, S., and Matthay, M. A. (1981). Adult respiratory distress syndrome complicating diabetes ketoacidosis. *West. J. Med.* **135**:148–150.

Sabiston, D. C., Jr. (1986). *Textbook of Surgery: The Biological Basis of Modern Surgical Practice*, 13th ed. Saunders, Philadelphia.

Sabiston, D. C., Jr., and Oldham, H. N., Jr. (1983). The mediastinum. In *Gibbon's Surgery of the Chest*, 4th ed. Edited by D. C. Sabiston, Jr., and F. C. Spencer. Saunders, Philadelphia.

Salmon, U. J. (1934). Benign pulvic tumors associated with ascites and pleural effusion. *J. Mt. Sinai Hosp.* **1**:169–179.

Sandler, M. A., Bunn, and Stewart, R. (1987). Cross-section study of pulmonary function in patients with insulin-dependent diabetes mellitus. *Am. Rev. Respir. Dis.* **135**:223–229.

Schmidek, H. H. (1977). Neurologic and neurosurgical sequilae of Paget's disease of bone. *Clin. Orthop.* **127**:70–77.

Schneierson, S. J., and Katz, M. (1958). Solitary pleural effusions due to myxedema. *JAMA* **168**:1003–1005.

Settipane, G. A., Schoenfeld, E., and Hamolsky, M. V. (1972). Asthma and hyperthyroidism. *J. Allergy Clin. Immunol.* **49**:348–355.

Shearin, R. P. N., Hepper, N. G. G., and Payne, W. S. (1974). Recurrent spontaneous pneumothorax concurrent with menses. *Mayo Clin. Proc.* **49**:98–101.

Smolar, E. N., Rubin, J. E., Avranides, A., and Carter, A. C. (1976). Hypothyroidism. Cardiac tamponade and review of the literature. *Am. J. Med. Sci.* **272**:345–352.

Stein, M., Kimball, P., and Johnson, R. L. (1961). Pulmonary function in hyperthyroidism. *J. Clin. Invest.* **40**:348–363.

Tillotson, J. R., and Lerner, A. M. (1967). Characteristics of pneumonia caused by *Escherichia coli*. *N. Engl. J. Med.* **277**:115–120.

Turner-Warwick, M. (1957). Pulmonary tuberculosis and diabetes mellitus. *Q. J. Med.* **26**:31–42.

Weaver, R. A. (1974). Unusual radiolographic presentation of pulmonary tuberculosis presentation of pulmonary tuberculosis in diabetic patients. *Am. Rev. Respir. Dis.* **109**:162–163.

Wilson, W. R., and Bedell, G. N. (1960). Pulmonary abnormalities in myxedema. *J. Clin. Invest.* **39**:42–55.

Winterbauer, R. H., Bedon, G. A., and Ball, W. C., Jr. (1969). Recurrent pneumonia: predisposing illness and clinical pattern of 158 patients. *Ann. Intern. Med.* **70**:689–695.

Zwillich, C. W., Pierson, D. J., Hofeldt, F. D., Lufkin, E. G., and Weil, J. V. (1975). Ventilatory control in myxedema and hypothyroidism. *N. Engl. J. Med.* **292**:662–666.

Zwillich, C. W., Matthay, M. A., Potts, D. E., Adler, R., Hofeldt, F., and Weil, J. V. (1978). Thyrotoxicosis: comparison of effects of thyroid ablation and beta-adrenergic ventilatory control. *J. Clin. Endocrinol. Metab.* **46**:491–500.

7

Neuromuscular and Skeletal Disease

DUDLEY F. ROCHESTER and LARRY J. FINDLEY

University of Virginia Health Sciences Center
Charlottesville, Virginia

I. Introduction

A. Effects of Neuromuscular and Skeletal Diseases on the Respiratory System

The principal effect of neuromuscular and skeletal diseases on the respiratory system is restriction of breathing. Neuromuscular diseases restrict breathing by weakening or paralyzing the respiratory muscles responsible for the act of breathing. In contrast, skeletal and some nonskeletal disorders, such as obesity, alter the structure of the thorax and thereby limit its excursion.

Features in common to all these disorders are limitation of the capacity to breathe, impaired gas exchange, and ventilatory failure. The lungs and airways are intrinsically normal, but become secondarily affected by the limited respiratory excursion. Additional complications include inability to cough or swallow effectively, compromise of pulmonary defense mechanisms, atelectasis, and pneumonia. Ultimately, patients with more severe forms of neuromuscular and skeletal diseases develop ventilatory failure.

Morbid obesity is included here because it too leads to hypoxia and ventilatory failure. In the obesity-hypoventilation syndrome, restriction of chest wall motion is usually not as severe as in advanced neuromuscular or skeletal disease, cough is better preserved, and problems of aspiration, atelectasis, and pneumonia are less prominent. However, the obesity-hypoventilation syndrome is compounded by obstructive sleep apnea and all its complications.

B. Scope of This Chapter

The section on *neuromuscular diseases* is concerned with conditions that cause weakness or paralysis of the various muscle groups involved in the act of breathing. The muscles of interest are those which collectively comprise the air pump, including respiratory muscle groups in the neck, rib cage, and abdomen. To a lesser extent, this section is also concerned with the muscles responsible for maintaining the patency of the upper airway during breathing. However, neuromuscular diseases that primarily and predominantly affect the control of breathing rather than the muscular act of breathing and disorders such as the obstructive sleep apnea syndrome or other forms of upper airway obstruction are beyond the scope of this chapter.

The first part of the section on *skeletal disorders of the chest wall* is concerned with skeletal diseases such as kyphoscoliosis, ankylosing spondylitis, sternal deformities, thoracoplasty, and flail chest. The second part covers *obesity and the obesity-hypoventilation syndrome*. Obesity is included in this section because of its profound effects on the mechanical properties of the chest wall, and because it is a leading cause of ventilatory failure.

The *respiratory complications of neuromuscular and skeletal disorders* are summarized in a separate section, because most of the complications occur in skeletal as well as neuromuscular diseases. This section is organized into three parts. The first covers mechanical factors that broach pulmonary defense mechanisms and lead to atelectasis and pneumonia. The second part is concerned with the control of breathing in neuromuscular and skeletal diseases, and the third reviews the pathogenesis of ventilatory failure.

The last section is concerned with treatment of *ventilatory failure* in neuromuscular and skeletal diseases. The major topics are the various modalities available for therapy, including new techniques and reapplications of old techniques. Specific treatments of the underlying neurological disease, skeletal deformity, or obesity are beyond the scope of this chapter, but are mentioned briefly in the appropriate sections.

This chapter focuses on newer developments in the pathophysiology, clinical presentation, and management of the respiratory effects of neuromuscular and skeletal disorders that restrict breathing. Space limitations preclude comprehensive coverage of the older literature. The reader is referred to selected older original articles (Bergofsky et al., 1959; Black and Hyatt, 1971; Newsom-Davis et al., 1976; Ferris et al., 1952a; Inkley et al., 1974; Stone and Keltz, 1963) and several reviews (Aldrich and Aldrich, 1986; Bergofsky, 1979;

De Troyer and Pride, 1985; Gibson, 1989; Kaminski and Young, 1985; Bennett and Bleck, 1988; Kelly and Luce, 1991; Rochester and Enson, 1974; Rochester and Findley, 1988) for more detailed documentation of earlier work.

II. Neuromuscular Diseases

A. General Considerations

The Respiratory Muscles

Innervation

The muscles responsible for maintaining the patency of the upper airway and for the act of breathing are striated skeletal muscles under neural control. All the upper airway muscles derive their innervation from cranial nerves (V, VII, IX, X, XI, and XII). The upper motor neurons involved in automatic breathing lie in the brainstem, whereas upper motor neurons involved in voluntary control of ventilatory acts lie in the motor cortex. Axons from the brainstem descend ipsilaterally in the ventrolateral aspect of the spinal cord. Axons from the motor cortex descend in the internal capsule, decussate in the brainstem, and descend contralaterally in the lateral columns of the spinal cord. Because the automatic and voluntary respiratory upper motor neurons follow different pathways, it is possible for voluntary respiration to be paralyzed while automatic breathing is maintained, and vice versa (Kuperman et al., 1971; Newsom-Davis, 1974; Rizvi et al., 1974).

The upper motor neurons synapse with respiratory lower motor neurons in the anterior horns of the spinal cord. The lower motor neurons cluster together in pools, such as the phrenic motor neuron pool in the cervical portion of the cord. Axons from respiratory lower motor neurons emerge from the spinal cord via the ventral roots and come together as efferent fibers in respiratory nerves. Finally, these fibers make contact with respiratory muscles at the neuromuscular junction, which is usually located midway along the length of the muscle fiber.

Neuromuscular diseases can affect breathing at every level of the chain, from the upper motor neuron to the muscle cell. Most neuromuscular disorders affect the respiratory system by causing muscle weakness or paralysis. Some neuromuscular diseases that commonly involve the respiratory system are classified according to their neurological location in Table 1.

Muscle Groups and Interactions

For the air pump muscles to perform their task efficiently, the upper airway must remain patent during inspiration and expiration. During quiet breathing, this is mainly the task of muscles that adduct the vocal cords. At higher levels of ventilatory effort many other muscle groups may come into play, including muscles that dilate the nose, the soft palate, the lips, the pharynx, and the larynx.

Table 1 Anatomical Classification of Neuromuscular Diseases that Affect Respiratory Muscle Function

Anatomic location	Disease
Brainstem	Trauma Tumor
Spinal cord	Anterior horn cell diseases Tetanus
Motor nerve	Trauma Neuropathy
Neuromuscular junction	Myasthenia gravis Eaton-Lambert syndrome Organophosphate poisoning
Muscle	Dystrophy Myopathy Myotonia

Pharyngeal muscles include the tongue (genioglossus) in the upper pharynx and a number of strap muscles attached to the hyoid bone in the lower pharynx. Because some of the latter attach to the mandible, even the masseter muscle of the jaw may be considered an accessory upper airway muscle (Hollowell and Suratt, 1989).

The muscles that comprise the air pump are divided into inspiratory and expiratory groups. The designations refer to the primary function of the particular muscle or muscle group, but owing to interactions among inspiratory and expiratory muscles, the expiratory muscles may at times serve to facilitate inspiration. The principal inspiratory muscles are the diaphragm, the parasternal intercostal muscles, and the scalene muscles in the neck. Additional inspiratory support is provided by the sternocleidomastoid and lateral intercostal muscles. The principal expiratory muscles are the internal and external oblique muscles of the abdomen and the transversus abdominis. Additional expiratory support is provided by the internal intercostal, transversus thoracis, and rectus abdominis muscles. The principal muscles of both the upper airway and the air pump, and their innervation, are summarized in Table 2.

During quiet breathing in the supine position, inspiration is accomplished almost exclusively by the diaphragm, and expiration is passive. Shifting to a seated or standing position immediately recruits the inspiratory scalene and parasternal intercostal muscles and the abdominal expiratory muscles. Whenever a higher level of ventilatory effort is needed, there is increased activation of muscles already recruited, and additional muscle groups are recruited as

Table 2 Innervation of the Respiratory Muscles

Muscle group	Muscle	Nerve	Level
Upper airway	Pharyngeal	IX	Medulla
	Tongue	XII	Medulla
	Laryngeal	X	Medulla
Inspiratory	Diaphragm	Phrenic	C_{3-5}
	Scalenes		C_{4-8}
	Sternocleidomastoid	XI	C_{1-2}
	Parasternals	Intercostal	T_{1-7}
	External intercostal	Intercostal	T_{1-12}
Expiratory	Internal intercostal	Intercostal	T_{1-12}
	Transversus thoracis	Intercostal	T_{1-12}
	Abdominal obliques	Lumbar	T_7–L_1
	Transversus abdominis	Lumbar	T_7–L_1
	Rectus abdominis	Lumbar	T_7–L_1

needed. Recruitment of respiratory muscles also occurs when a major primary muscle such as the diaphragm is paralyzed.

Classification

The clinical and physiological manifestations of respiratory involvement in neuromuscular disease vary with the type of disease, its location, and its severity. Thus neuromuscular diseases are often classified according to type and site of involvement (Table 1) or according to the innervation of the various groups of respiratory muscles (Table 2). Although we appreciate the value of these classifications, particularly in establishing the correct diagnosis, we also like to classify neuromuscular diseases in a way that integrates anatomical, clinical, and functional aspects of their impact on the respiratory system (Table 3). This arrangement is based on whether the presentation is focal or diffuse, and whether the functional deficit stems from respiratory muscle weakness or paralysis.

B. Dysfunction Limited to the Diaphragm

Unilateral Paresis or Paralysis

Paralysis or weakness of hemidiaphragm is relatively common. This condition is sometimes referred to as eventration of the diaphragm, but inasmuch as most or all cases are caused by partial or complete denervation, it is preferable to call it paresis or paralysis.

Table 3 Functional Classification of Neuromuscular Diseases, According to the Type of Ventilatory Deficit

Diseases limited to the diaphragm
Unilateral paralysis
Bilateral paralysis
Postoperative dysfunction
Spinal cord injury
High cervical
Mid- to low cervical
Thoracic
Other forms of localized paralysis
Hemiplegia
Poliomyelitis
Diffuse neuromuscular diseases
Acute onset
Acute inflammatory polyneuropathy
Myasthenia gravis, Lambert-Eaton syndrome
Poisoning (botulinism, organophosphate)
Gradual onset
Amyotrophic lateral sclerosis
Muscular dystrophy
Myopathy (congenital, acquired)

Etiology

There is often no obvious cause for unilateral paralysis of the diaphragm (Piehler et al., 1982). When the cause is apparent, it is almost always related to trauma or to an adjacent lesion. Examples of the latter include cervical osteoarthritis, pleurisy or pneumonia, and aneurysm or tumor (Lisboa et al., 1986; Mellem et al., 1987; Hillman and Finucane, 1988; Graham et al., 1990). However, in a series of 142 patients, intrathoracic malignant neoplasms were responsible for diaphragmatic paralysis in less than 5% of cases (Piehler et al., 1982). Sporadic cases have been reported to be the result of carbon monoxide poisoning (Joiner et al., 1990), spinal cord injury, poliomyelitis, and muscular dystrophy.

Numerous traumatic causes of unilateral phrenic nerve injury have been summarized elsewhere (Rochester and Findley, 1988). They include birth injury, spinal manipulation, and central or jugular venous catheterization. Thoracotomy and pneumonectomy do not affect the phrenic nerves (De Troyer and Vanderhoeft, 1982), but the left phrenic nerve is subject to injury during repair of esophageal hiatus hernia (Arborelius et al., 1975).

Currently the leading cause of unilateral diaphragmatic paralysis is open heart surgery (Estenne et al., 1985; Large et al., 1985; Wheeler et al., 1985; Wilcox et al., 1988a). Indeed, injury to one phrenic nerve may occur in 10–20% of patients undergoing open heart surgery. Left lower lobe atelectasis is also quite common after open heart surgery, but it cannot be attributed to phrenic nerve injury in most cases (Wilcox et al., 1988a).

This type of phrenic nerve injury has usually been attributed to cold cardioplegia (Benjamin et al., 1982) or to stretching the nerve (Wilcox et al., 1990a). The cold-injury hypothesis is supported by reports indicating that use of a cardiac insulation pad markedly reduced the incidence of diaphragmatic paralysis (Wheeler et al., 1985; Laub et al., 1991). Abd et al. (1989) proposed a third interesting hypothesis, i.e., that using the internal mammary arteries for coronary artery bypass compromises the blood supply of the phrenic nerves. At present, the evidence for this mechanism is circumstantial.

Clinical Features

Piehler et al. (1982) retrospectively studied 142 patients with unilateral diaphragmatic paralysis. There was no particular age distribution, with cases occurring from infancy to old age. In this series, men were affected twice as often as women. Approximately 60% of cases were on the left, and 40% on the right side. Others have found a relatively equal distribution of paralysis between the sexes and the side of involvement (Hillman and Finucane, 1988).

Over half the patients had no respiratory symptoms initially, and a quarter had exertional dyspnea. About 5% had either chest wall pain, cough, or a combination of dyspnea, chest pain, and cough (Piehler et al., 1982). Some patients have more severe exertional dyspnea (Graham et at., 1990) and may experience dyspnea at rest if they lie with the paralyzed side down (Arborelius et at., 1975). As espected, the symptoms to unilateral diaphragmatic paralysis are worse in patients who have coexistent lung disease (Wright et al., 1985; Lisboa et al., 1986).

Physical examination reveals that the excursions of the chest and abdomen are diminished on the affected side. This sign is best elicited by having the patient inspire slowly and deeply, in the supine or semirecumbent position. The abdomen should protrude with inspiration on the normal side, and its outward excursion is minimal or absent on the paralyzed side. There is dullness to percussion, and breath sounds are diminished to absent, over the involved hemidiaphragm. Occasionally one may hear crackles over the compressed portion of the lung.

Diagnosis

The usual clue to the diagnosis of unilateral diaphragmatic paralysis is an elevated hemidiaphragm on the chest roentgenogram. It must be kept in mind that this is a nonspecific finding, because unilateral pulmonary diseases (atelectasis, embolism, edema) also elevate the hemidiaphragm. Subpulmonic pleural effusions, trauma with diaphragmatic rupture, and agenesis of the hemidiaphragm (Tzelepis et al., 1988) can mimic the chest radiographic appearance of the paralyzed diaphragm. Therefore, it is desirable to have additional ways to assess the functional status of the diaphragm and the phrenic nerve.

The traditional test is to fluoroscope the patient and observe the motion of the diaphragm while the patient sniffs (sniff test). In a positive test, the normal side of the diaphragm moves downward (caudad) and the paralyzed side moves upward (craniad). The false positive rate for the sniff test is normal subjects is as high as 6% (Alexander, 1966), and a better test may be to examine diaphragmatic excursion during a slow, deep inspiration made in the semirecumbent or supine position (Paré and Fraser, 1983). Ultrasound imaging from the subcostal position can be used instead of fluoroscopy (Balaji et al., 1990).

Another approach to diagnosis is to observe the electrical and mechanical consequences of phrenic nerve stimulation. A single shock, delivered by a percutaneous electrode overlying the cervical portion of either phrenic nerve, should produce a twitch contraction of the ipsilateral hemidiaphragm. The mechanical twitch response can be detected fluoroscopically or by ultrasound (McCauley and Labib, 1984), and the electrical response can be detected as a compound action potential recorded from electrodes placed on the anterolateral chest wall in the 8th or 9th intercostal space (Mier et al., 1987). The time from delivery of the single shock to the onset of the compound action potential is referred to as a "latency," because it includes the time required for the electrical impulse to traverse the tissues of the neck and chest wall, as well as the phrenic nerve conduction time. The normal value of phrenic latency in adults is about 7.0 msec (Estenne et al., 1985; Mier et al., 1987).

In the presence of phrenic nerve disease, the latency may be prolonged (Mier et al., 1987), but often the nerve does not respond at all to stimulation (McCauley and Labib, 1984). The phrenic nerve stimulation test is probably more reliable when combined with fluoroscopic assessment of diaphragmatic twitch (McCauley and Labib, 1984). The reliablility of the phrenic latency test is unclear. The phrenic nerve contains thousands of nerve fibers, many of them afferent in nature. There are no data to define how many fibers have to be injured or how serious the injury must be in order to prolong the phrenic latency or to define the threshold at which the nerve becomes unresponsive to stimulation.

Physiological Abnormalities

Unilateral diaphragmatic paralysis alone has only a small effect on pulmonary function (Rochester and Findley, 1988). It generally reduces vital capacity (VC) and forced vital capacity (FVC), total lung capacity (TLC), and maximal voluntary ventilation (MVV) by 15–25%, whereas the effects on functional residual capacity (FRC) and residual volume (RV) are small and variable. In the absence of underlying obstructive lung disease, the forced expiratory volume in 1 sec (FEV_1) is reduced by 20–40%, whereas the ratio FEV_1/FVC is normal. Not surprisingly, pulmonary function is substantially worse when unilateral diaphragmatic paralysis develops in the presence of underlying lung disease (Lisboa et al., 1986).

Regional function of the lung is mildly to moderately abnormal. Both ventilation and perfusion tend to be less on the involved side, especially adjacent to the paralysis. Assuming the supine position causes regional lung function to become worse, and arterial Po_2 falls. Venous admixture is usually less than 10% of the cardiac output, and diffusing capacity is normal.

Patients with uncomplicated paralysis of one hemidiaphragm developed maximal inspiratory pressures that were about 80% predicted, whereas patients with unilateral diaphragmatic paralysis and coexisting lung disease developed only 35% of the predicted inspiratory pressure (Lisboa et at., 1986). The VC in these two groups was 74% and 52%, respectively. Even unilateral paralysis can diminish the inspiratory component of abdominal pressure. This shifts the ratio of the inspiratory abdominal to inspiratory pleural pressure swing ($\Delta Pab/\Delta Ppl$) from its normally negative value toward zero, or even to a positive value (Hillman and Finucane, 1988).

Treatment

Most patients with isolated unilateral paralysis of the diaphragm do not need treatment, although they should be encouraged to stay as physically active as they can be without undue distress. Surgical intervention is indicated for some categories of patients. Infants and children tolerate unilateral diaphragmatic paralysis poorly, being subject to atelectasis, pneumonia, and ventilatory failure (Shoemaker et al., 1981; Moorthy et al., 1985), and have responded well to plication of the diaphragm (Shoemaker et al., 1981); in one case where plication failed, surgical reconstruction was accomplished using Marlex mesh (Bowen et al., 1982). Adults suffering from dyspnea consequent to diaphragmatic paralysis also benefitted from plication, with improvement in pulmonary function and blood gas composition, as well as a significant reduction in dyspnea (Wright et al., 1985; Graham et al., 1990).

Bilateral Paralysis

Etiology

Bilateral diaphragmatic paralysis is often caused by the same processes that cause unilateral paralysis, including surgery on the heart, thorax, or cervical spine (Abd et al., 1989; Chandler et al., 1984; Kreitzer et al., 1978a; Mier-Jedrzejowicz et al., 1988b) and trauma. Unlike unilateral paralysis, bilateral severe weakness or paralysis frequently occurs in nontraumatic neuromuscular disorders, including multiple sclerosis (Aisen et al., 1990) and motor neuron diseases (Newsom-Davis et al., 1976; Haas et al., 1981). Diaphragmatic weakness also complicates muscular dystrophy and myopathy (Newsom-Davis, 1976; Skatrud et al., 1980; Mier-Jedrzejowicz et al., 1988b). In two patients, diaphragmatic myopathy (polymyositis, amyloidosis) was the only manifestation of myopathy (Schiavi et al., 1984; Streeten et al., 1986). Bilateral diaphragmatic paralysis that occurred in the fifth decade in homozygous twin brothers was considered to be of genetic origin, but no specific nerve or muscle disease could be identified (Molho et al., 1987).

It seems likely that many of the unexplained cases of unilateral and bilateral diaphragmatic paralysis are due to neuropathy. Several cases have been reported in which diaphragmatic paralysis was associated with the neuropathy of myxedema (Hamly et al., 1975), carbon monoxide or amiodarone toxicity (Joiner et al., 1990; Miller et al., 1988), and paraneoplastic syndrome (Thomas et al., 1984). Phrenic neuropathy has also been reported in association with neuralgic amyotrophy or brachial neuritis (Graham et al., 1985; Gregory et al., 1990) and hereditary neuropathies (Newsom-Davis, 1967; Chan et al., 1987; Dyer and Callahan, 1987; Laroche et al., 1988b; Gilchrist et al., 1989; Hardie et al., 1990). In one series, 40 of 200 patients with Charcot-Marie-Tooth disease had respiratory symptoms, and 15 of these had significant respiratory muscle dysfunction (Nathanson et al., 1989).

Phrenic neuropathy can also occur in peripheral neuropathy of unknown cause (Newsom-Davis, 1967; Goldstein et al., 1974), and it would not be surprising to find it as a complication of diabetic or alcoholic neuropathy. It is of particular interest that polyneuropathy is relatively common in critically ill patients, and that it often involves the phrenic nerves functionally (Witt et al., 1991) and pathologically (Zochodne et al., 1987).

Clinical Features

Unlike unilateral paralysis, bilateral paralysis of the diaphragm almost always causes severe morbidity and profound abnormalities of pulmonary function in adults. Many patients develop ventilatory failure, which is frequently complicated by right ventricular failure, atelectasis, and pneumonia. However, if there is isolated diaphragmatic weakness and the remaining respiratory muscles are strong, respiratory failure does not occur, even during sleep (Laroche et al., 1988b). Early in the disease, dyspnea is present at rest and is severely aggravated by exercise or by assuming the supine position (Mier-Jedrzejowicz et al., 1988b). Patients may become acutely hypercapnic at night and experience early-morning headache. Other symptoms may include anxiety, insomnia, excessive daytime somnolence, and even more severe neurological manifestations such as confusion and motor impairment. Both resting and exertional dyspnea may abate somewhat as the other inspiratory muscles become better adapted.

Physical examination generally reveals mild tachypnea, with the respiratory rate 20–25 breaths per minute (Newsom-Davis et al., 1976). The inspiratory contraction of the scalene and sternocleidomastoid muscles is usually augmented. Percussion of the chest reveals dullness over the lower lung fields with limited to absent excursion of the diaphragm, and auscultation reveals diminished to absent breath sounds at the lung bases bilaterally. None of these signs are specific, and they can be mimicked by bialteral pleural effusions.

The most important physical sign is paradoxical inward movement of the abdomen during inspiration (Abd et al., 1989; Newsom-Davis et al., 1976; Chandler et al., 1984; Mier-Jedrzejowicz et al., 1988b). This sign is best elicited with the patient in the supine or semirecumbent position. When the patient inspires slowly and as deeply as possible, the chest will clearly move outward. However, the abdomen will be drawn inward with inspiration, which is just the opposite of its normal excursion. In order for abdominal paradox to occur consistently, the diaphragm must be extremely weak (Mier-Jedrzejowicz et al., 1988b).

Diagnosis

The chest roentgenogram often shows elevation of both hemidiaphragms, but not infrequently the chest roentgenogram has been considered to be normal (Alexander, 1966; Abd et al., 1989; Chandler et al., 1984; Laroche et al., 1988b; Mier-Jedrzejowicz et al., 1988b). The respiratory excursion of the diaphragm is usually absent, but may be present (Spiteri et al., 1985). The sniff test is helpful if it detects paradoxical motion of the diaphragm, but it is often misleading (Newsom-Davis, et al., 1976; Chandler et al., 1984).

As an alternative to the sniff test, one may examine the excursion of the diaphragm between full expiration and full inspiration (Paré and Fraser, 1983). The standing patient initially inspires fully from FRC to TLC. During this maneuver, the chest expands, but the abdomen is drawn inward as the severely weakened or paralyzed diaphragm is sucked upward (craniad) by negative pleural pressure. During passive expiration back to FRC, the abdomen protrudes as the diaphragm descends. During the active phase of expiration from FRC to RV, the abdominal muscles contract, constrict the abdomen, and push the paralyzed diaphragm upward. When the patient relaxes, the diaphragm descends, the abdomen moves outward, and the patient passively inspires back to FRC. Diaphragmatic and abdominal excursions in the last part of the cycle, passive inspiration from RV back to FRC, resemble those of normal inspiration, but these are purely passive motions.

When the diagnosis cannot be made with certainty from physical roentgenographic examination, it is helpful to stimulate the phrenic nerves (McCauley and Labib, 1984; Mier et al., 1987)., With this technique, one can determine whether the phrenic nerve latency is normal or prolonged, and whether the diaphragm responds to the stimulation. In the absence of any electrical or mechanical response, one might still want to try stimulating the nerve directly using needle electrodes, rather than using the percutaneous stimulation technique.

The definitive diagnosis of significant diaphragmatic weakness or paralysis can only be made by measuring the pressure swing across the diaphragm during inspiratory efforts (Mier-Jedrzejowicz et al., 1988b). This pressure swing, referred to as the transdiaphragmatic pressure (Pdi), equals the difference between abdominal (gastric) and pleural (esophageal) pressure. Normally, Pdi at the end of an inspiration to TLC is greater than 25 cm H_2O (Newsom-Davis et al., 1976; De Troyer and Estenne, 1981). When the normal subject makes a maximal inspiratory effort against a closed airway (Mueller maneuver), Pdi is usually greater than 90 cm H_2O, but may be as low as 18 cm H_2O (De Troyer and Estenne, 1981). The Pdi can also be measured during vigorous sniffs, and this technique yields somewhat higher and more reproducible values (Mier-Jedrzejowicz et al., 1988b; Rochester, 1988).

In the presence of complete paralysis of the diaphragm, the active inspiratory component of Pdi is zero, whether it is measured after inspiration to TLC or during the Mueller maneuver. However, it should be pointed out that the paralyzed diaphragm can sustain an end-expiratory passive pressure, that is, pressure resulting from stretch of the flaccid diaphragm. Diseases that weaken but do not paralyze the diaphragm reduce maximal inspiratory pressure measured at the mouth (PI_{max}), as well as Pdi measured during Mueller maneuvers or vigorous sniffs (Abd et al., 1989; Mier-Jedrzejowicz et al., 1988b). Indeed, all these pressures are affected to the same extent. Because of the wide range of values in normal subjects (De Troyer and Estenne, 1981), diaphragmatic weakness can be considered to be severe when Pdi measured by any technique lies between 0 and 20 cm H_2O (Gibson, 1989; Mier-Jedrzejowicz et al., 1988b).

One consequence of severe diaphragmatic weakness and inability to generate any active Pdi is that the abdominal pressure component of the inspiratory transdiaphragmatic pressure swing is sharply reduced or absent. One way of expressing this is a fall in the numerical value of the ratio $\Delta Pga/\Delta Pdi$ from its normal value of approximately 0.2–0.4 to 0 or even negative values (Maeda et al., 1988). Alternatively, the numerical value of the ratio $\Delta Pab/\Delta Pbl$ ($\Delta Pga/\Delta Pes$) changes from negative to positive (Hillman and Finucane, 1988). The ratio is normally negative, with a numerical value of -0.5 to -1.0, because during inspiration there is a positive abdominal (gastric) pressure and a nearly equal negative pleural (esophageal) pressure. When the diaphragm is paralyzed, the inspiratory pleural pressure remains negative, but the inspiratory abdominal pressure also becomes negative as the diaphragm is sucked up into the chest. This finding can be of diagnostic value, especially in patients who are unable to make reproducible maximal efforts.

Differential Diagnosis

When bilateral diaphragmatic paralysis causes ventilatory failure, it is often mistaken for alveolar hypoventilation secondary to brainstem or high spinal cord disease. Patients with central alveolar hypoventilation generally have normal respiratory muscle strength, lung volumes, and maximal voluntary ventilation. Thus these patients can voluntarily hyperventilate to normalize the Pa_{CO_2} for a short time, but so can some patients with neuromuscular disease. The ventilatory response to CO_2 inhalation is virtually absent in central alveolar hypoventilation, but it is often impaired in neuromuscular disease as well (see Section IV.C, "Pathogenesis of CO_2 Retention"). To confirm a diagnosis of phrenic nerve or diaphragmatic dysfunction, one should look for paradoxical inward motion of the abdomen, test for phrenic nerve dysfunction by electrical stimulation, and verify that diaphragmatic motion and transdiaphragmatic pressure are markedly reduced.

Physiological Abnormalities

The paradoxical inward inspiratory movement of the abdomen can be detected using magnetometers (Kreitzer et al., 1978a) or the respiratory inductance plethysmograph. Paradoxical motion is present in both sitting and supine positions when weakness is severe, but only in the supine posture in moderate weakness, and there is no paradoxical motion when weakness is mild to moderate (Mier-Jedrzejowicz et al., 1988b; Laroche et al., 1988b).

Pulmonary function tests show a far more severe restrictive pattern than is characteristic of unilateral diaphragmatic paralysis. Typically, the VC and TLC are approximately 50% and 60% predicted, respectively, and the FRC is also reduced in most patients (Abd et al., 1989; Chandler et al., 1984; Laroche et al., 1988b; Mier-Jedrzejowicz et al., 1988b; Newsom-Davis et al., 1976). The RV is affected to a variable degree, ranging from reduced by 50% to increased by 50%, but on average the RV is normal (Laroche et al., 1988a; Mier-Jedrzejowicz et al., 1988b). The FEV_1 is reduced in proportion to the VC (Mier-Jedrzejowicz et al., 1988b), so the ratio FEV_1/FVC is normal (Laroche et al., 1988b).

Patients with severe weakness or paralysis of both hemidiaphragms tolerate the supine posture and immersion in water very poorly. In the supine position, the weight of the abdominal contents presses on the paralyzed diaphragm and forces it into the chest. This causes dyspnea and limits the inspiratory excursion. Thus, the supine VC is more than 25% lower than the upright VC in patients with severe weakness or paralysis (Allen et al., 1985; Mier-Jedrzejowicz et al., 1988b; Molho et al., 1987). When upright patients are immersed in water to the level of the abdomen, the inspiratory effect of abdominal relaxation is negated, and the paralyzed diaphragm is no longer pulled downward by the weight of the abdominal viscera (McCool and Mead, 1989). Again, inspiratory excursion is limited and patients become dyspneic.

Table 4 Respiratory Muscle and Pulmonary Function Test Results in Unilateral and Bilateral Paralysis of the Diaphragm[a]

Variable	Unilateral	Bilateral
PI_{max} (cm H_20)	−70	−20
RV	100	55
FRC	100	60
TLC	85	55
VC	75	45
FEV_1	70	50

[a]Values expressed as percentage of predicted normal, unless otherwise specified.

Hypoxemia with a modest elevation of the alveolar-arterial oxygen tension difference (A-a)Po_2 is the most consistent finding on arterial blood gas analysis (Laroche et al., 1988b; Loh et al., 1979). The (A-a)Po_2 is higher in supine and decubitus positions, reflecting a poorer matching of ventilation to perfusion than when upright (Loh et al., 19790. Isolated diaphragmatic paralysis reduces the diffusing capacity, probably owing to poor inspiratory effort, because the transfer coefficient for CO is normal or increased (Laroche et al., 1988b).

The $Paco_2$ may be normal during the daytime (Laroche et al., 1988b; Loh et al., 1979), but is is often elevated (Goldstein et al., 1974; Kreitzer et al., 1978a; Loh et al., 1979; Molho et al., 1987; Skatrud et al., 1980). Laroche et al. (1988b) concluded that daytime CO_2 retention does not occur in isolated diaphragmatic paralysis or severe weakness, as long as the other respiratory muscles and the lungs are normal. Hypoventilation may worsen in the supine position or during sleep (Newsom-Davis et al., 1976, Skatrud et al., 1980). The acute rise in $Paco_2$ overnight accounts for the morning headache.

Treatment

Treatment of bilateral diaphragmatic paralysis is supportive. Some kind of mechanical ventilation is often necessary, especially early in the course of the disease. Abd et al. (1989) found the rocking bed to be particularly valuable for patients whose isolated diaphragmatic paralysis resulted from open heart surgery. Others have used a negative-pressure body ventilator (Kreitzer et al., 1978a). Recovery of phrenic nerve and diaphragmatic function may take 2–19 months after trauma or open heart surgery (Merav et al., 1983; Abd et al., 1989; Wilcox et al., 1990b). Patients with brachial neuritis (neuralgic amyotrophy) may recover partial function of the diaphragm after 2–3 years (Graham et al., 1985).

Even when the phrenic nerve and diaphragm do not recover, patients often improve with regard to overall functional status. This appears to reflect a training effect on the other inspiratory muscles, so they are better able to compensate for the loss of diaphragmatic function. Two of our patients, who were physically fit prior to their phrenic paralysis, recovered their ability to walk in 1–2 months, well in advance of any change in diaphragmatic function. However, their ability to tolerate the supine position remained poor until they had regained some active inspiratory diaphragmatic excursion.

Postoperative Diaphragmatic Dysfunction

Abdominal Surgery

Upper abdominal surgery is followed by a limitation of diaphragmatic motion (Ford et al., 1983; Simonneau et al., 1983). The tidal volume is markedly reduced and is accomplished by expansion of the rib cage instead of the combined rib cage and abdomen (Chuter et al., 1990). Studies in animals show that this phenomenon does not result from general anesthesia alone, nor does it follow lower abdominal surgery (Road et al., 1984). Dureuil et al. (1986) showed that in dogs subjected to upper abdominal surgery, diaphragmatic dysfunction was apparent during spontaneous breathing, but the Pdi response to electrical stimulation of the phrenic nerves was normal. Thus, it appears that the phrenic nerve and diaphragm are normal, but the diaphragmatic contraction is inhibited reflexly, perhaps by stimuli arising from inflammation of the peritoneum or stimulation of the gallbladder (Ford et al., 1983).

Thoracic Surgery

Thoracotomy does not usually affect phrenic nerve function (De Troyer and Vanderhoeft, 1982), but it does cause diaphragmatic dysfunction during spontaneous breathing (Maeda et al., 1988). This, like the dysfunction after upper abdominal surgery, is manifest by a significant reduction in the abdominal pressure component of the transdiaphragmatic pressure swing and reduction in voluntary Pdi_{max}. The inspiratory Pdi during quiet breathing was unchanged, indicating that there was greater activation of rib cage and neck inspiratory muscles to compensate for the impairment in diaphragmatic function.

Clinical Significance

The magnitude of postoperative diaphragmatic dysfunction is maximal immediately after surgery, and diaphragmatic function returns to normal within 7–10 days (Ford et al., 1983; Simonneau et al., 1983; Maeda et al., 1988). It is thought that the postoperative limitation of diaphragmatic motion contributes significantly to lower lobe atelectasis as well as the reduction in tidal volume (Chuter et al., 1990, 1991). Neither relief of postoperative pain (Simonneau et al., 1983) nor incentive spirometry (Chuter et al., 1990) alleviated the problem, but voluntarily adopting a diaphragmatic pattern of breathing improved diaphragmatic motion and abdominal excursion (Chuter et al., 1990). It remains to be seen whether diaphragmatic breating training will reduce postoperative complications. Thoracotomy reduces maximal cough pressures (Byrd and Burns, 1975), and postthoracotomy diaphragmatic dysfunction was associated with overt ventilatory failure and the need for mechanical ventilation, in patients whose work of breathing was already elevated preoperatively (Maeda et al., 1988).

C. Spinal Cord Injury

General Considerations

Most spinal cord injuries result from trauma consequent to motor vehicle, industrial, or sports accidents. Nontraumatic causes include tumors, vascular malformations, transverse myelitis, syringomyelia, and epidural abscesses. Regardless of the cause, the outcome is similar whether the paralysis is abrupt or gradual in onset.

Spinal cord injury is a devastating event that is often attended by serious medical complications, which include loss of bowel, bladder, and sexual function, decubitus ulcers, infections of skin, urinary tract, and lungs, poor nutrition, and wasting of the nonparalyzed muscles. Some of these problems, especially muscle wasting and weakness, have significant impact on the respiratory system. The other important issue with regard to respiratory function is the level of the injury.

High Cervical Lesions

Clinical Features

Injuries above the C3 level almost completely paralyze the respiratory muscles. Some innervation of the sternocleidomastoid and trapezius muscles is derived from the C1–2 levels, but innervation of the scalene, phrenic, intercostal, and abdominal motor neuron pools is totally interrupted. Disruption of reticulospinal pathways in the ventral aspect of the high cervical spinal cord produces a syndrome that resembles central alveolar hypoventilation (Kuperman et al., 1971; Rizvi et al., 1974), whereas lesions limited to the lateral columns disrupt voluntary ventilation without impinging on automatic control of breathing (Newsom-Davis, 1974). Trauma almost always interrupts both automatic and voluntary pathways. A recent case report describes an adult patient in whom the clinical presentation of type I Arnold-Chiari malformation began with pneumonia, which was followed by ventilatory failure and late-onset quadriplegia (Tsao et al., 1991).

Patients with high cervical lesions can scarcely breathe or talk, and they cannot cough. The patients are dyspneic and have difficulty with secretions. Physical examination may reveal apnea or prominent contraction of the sternocleidomastoid and trapezius muscles. These muscles tend to become hypertrophied in time. Breath sounds are faint, and rhonchi are frequently heard. The respiratory excursion of the diaphragm is lost, but the diaphragm does descend when the patient is brought to the sitting position. The abdominal muscles as well as the limb and other truncal muscles are flaccid.

Such pulmonary function data as are available show that the spontaneous tidal volume is extremely small, ranging from 60 to 500 ml (James et al., 1977; Nochomovity et al., 1984; Bach and Alba, 1990c), and the expiratory reserve volume (ERV) is essentially zero because the patients have no expiratory function at all. Thus RV equals FRC and FRC is usually reduced, probably due to atelectasis. Measurements of maximal inspiratory and expiratory pressures at the mouth in one patient showed that PI_{max} was −20 cm H_2O and PE_{max} was +70 cm H_2O (James et al., 1977). In this patient, the expiratory pressure came from glossopharyngeal muscles, not expiratory muscles. Glossopharyngeal breathing is a tehnique in which the patient gulps air and learns to force it into the lungs. After 10–20 gulps, the patient can inflate the lungs enough to produce a VC of a liter or more (Montero et al., 1967; James et al., 1977). This maneuver is not useful for tidal breathing, but does help restore speech and limited cough.

Patients with high spinal cord injury have been shown by electromyographic measurements to recruit as inspiratory muscles not only the sternocleidomastoid, which is known to be an accessory inspiratory muscle, but also the trapezius, platysma, myelohyoid, and sternohyoid muscles, which are not usually employed in breathing (De Troyer et al., 1986). When the neck muscles contract, the sternum is pulled cranially and the anteroposterior diameter of the upper rib cage increases, but the diameters of the lower rib cage and abdomen decrease (Danon et al., 1979; De Troyer et al., 1986). The negative inspiratory pressure produced by contraction of the neck inspiratory muscles is small, being −16 cm H_2O in one patient at FRC and falling off progressively as lung volume was increased above FRC (Danon et al., 1979).

Treatment

Patients with high spinal cord injury require some form of artificial ventilation. Because they are unable to cough and clear secretions effectively, virtually all these patients undergo tracheostomy, in part to allow pulmonary toilet, and in part to provide access for mechanical ventilation. Although volume-cycled ventilators are most often used in the acute phase, by the time the condition has become chronic, one may use portable volume ventilators, mouth pressure ventilators, or negative-pressure body ventilators (see Section V). If the spinal cord injury is high enough to spare the phrenic motoneuron pool, then electrophrenic respiration may be employed.

Mid- to Lower Cervical Lesions

Clinical Features

Patients with lesions at levels C3–C8 are quadriplegic, but have variable degrees of respiratory impairment. The nerves to the conventional expiratory muscles lie below C8, so expiratory function and cough are severely compromised. However, some expiratory function is assumed by the clavicular head of the pectoralis major muscles (De Troyer et al., 1986; Estenne and De Troyer, 1990). One would expect that inspiratory function would be worse in patients with lesions at the C3–C5 levels, because they would involve the phrenic motor neuron pool. In fact, although the vital capacity is somewhat smaller in patients with C4 lesions than in patients with C5–C7 lesions, there is considerable overlap in this and in inspiratory muscle strength (Gross et al., 1980; Ledsome and Sharp, 1981).

Physiological Abnormalities

Typical values for respiratory muscle and pulmonary function, based on data from many laboratories, are summarized in Table 4. As with other forms of neuromuscular disease, the deficit is restrictive in nature, with normal expiratory flow rates after correction for the loss in VC. The reduction in VC results in part from a reduction in inspiratory capacity (IC) and in part from a reduction in expiratory reserve volume (ERV). The relative loss of ERV is much greater than that in IC, because expiratory muscles are affected out of proportion to inspiratory muscles. As a corollary of the fall in ERV, the RV is increased. It should be noted that this is not the result of airway obstruction. The patients simply cannot exhale, and their FRC is normal.

Pulmonary resistance is usually normal, and lung compliance is reduced in quadriplegia (Stone and Keltz, 1963; Bergofsky, 1964; De Troyer et al., 1986), but compliance corrected for the reduction in lung volume is normal (De Troyer and Heilporn, 1980). Lung compliance is better in patients who, despite a cervical cord injury, retain some function of the parasternal intercostal muscles (De Troyer and Heilporn, 1980). Chest wall and rib cage compliance are reduced by 30% and 45%, respectively, whereas the compliance of the abdomen is almost 3 times normal (Estenne and De Troyer, 1986). The work and oxygen cost of breathing are moderately elevated (Silver 1963; Stone and Keltz, 1963). Some of the increased work is done by the diaphragm in displacement of the abdominal viscera (Bergofsky, 1964), but extra work is also done when diaphragmatic inspiration deforms the upper rib cage (Mortola and Sant'Ambrogio, 1978; Estenne and De Troyer, 1985; Urmey et al., 1986).

Posture has a significant impact on pulmonary function in quadriplegic patients. In the supine position, their VC and PI_{max} increase, whereas FRC and RV decrease (Hultgren et al., 1980). The increase in VC when supine results from the decrease in RV rather than any increase in TLC (Estenne and De Troyer, 1987). These volume changes come about from the effects of posture on the abdominal viscera and diaphragm position. When the patient is sitting, the weight of the abdominal contents pulls the diaphragm down, and the flaccid abdominal wall offers little resistance. In contrast, when the patient is supine, the abdominal contents push the diaphragm up into the chest, and it is this effect that causes the RV to fall and the VC to rise.

Pulmonary function after cervical spinal cord injury improves over time. Relatively rapid improvement in vital capacity occurs early on, so the VC doubles in the first 3 months (Ledsome and Sharp, 1981). The VC, IC, and TLC continue to improve during the first year, after which only the VC exhibits a small additional improvement (Haas et al., 1985). Lung compliance falls in the first month after injury to approximately 45% of normal and then increases during the next 12 months to 65% of normal (Scanlon et al., 1989). As lung compliance improves, rib cage distortion lessens.

Ventilatory Failure

Most patients with mid- to lower cervical spinal cord injury are not dependent on mechanical ventilation, although some with lesions that destroy the phrenic motor neurons are partially ventilator dependent. The $\mathrm{Paco_2}$ is either normal or mildly elevated when patients are awake (Stone and Keltz, 1963; Bergofsky, 1964; Gross et al., 1980). These patients are usually mildly hypoxemic, with an increase in the $\mathrm{(A\text{-}a)PO_2}$ (Ledsome and Sharp, 1981). Pulmonary physiological testing reveals a normal ratio of dead space to tidal volume (VD/VT) and carbon monoxide diffusion capacity (DLCO), and a nearly normal regional distribution of ventilation (Stone and Keltz, 1963; Bergofsky, 1964). Thus, the hypoxemia probably results from abnormally low ventilation-perfusion ratios in collapsed or partially collapsed areas of lung, primarily in the lower lobes (Bake et al., 1972b).

Wicks and Menter (1986) reported that 76 of 134 patients (57%) who were initially ventilator-dependent could be weaned from mechanical ventilation during the first hospitalization. Weaning success was associated with a lower cervical level of injury, a higher initial VC, and greater improvement in VC during the hospitalizaiton. The survival rates for patients who remained ventilator-dependent at the time of discharge from hospital were 90% at 1 year, 56% at 3 years, and 33% at 5 years.

Thoracic Lesions

Paraplegia at the thoracic level has much less effect on the respiratory system than injuries in the cervical region of the spinal cord. The principal problem is impaired capacity to cough effectively. Midthoracic lesions cause as much expiratory muscle weakness as cervical lesions, whereas lower thoracic and upper lumbar injuries cause less severe expiratory weakness (Arora et al., 1978). The FRC and $\mathrm{FEV_1/FVC}$ are the same in thoracic and cervical cord injury, but with thoracic lesions the RV and ERV are normal because expiratory muscle strength is better preserved (Table 4).

Table 5 Maximal Inspiratory and Expiratory Pressures and Pulmonary Function Test Results in Patients with Quadriplegia, Showing the Difference Between Mid- to Lower Cervical and Thoracic Levels of Injury[a]

Variable	C_{4-7} level	T_{3-12} level
PI_{max} (cm H_20)	65	80
PE_{max} (cm H_20)	40	100
MVV	50	60
VC	50	70
FEV_1/VC	85	80
IC	70	—
ERV	20	65
RV	140	90
FRC	85	85
TLC	70	80

[a]Values expressed as percentage of predicted normal, unless otherwise specified

Patients with midthoracic spinal cord injury use their scalene and parasternal intercostal muscles as well as their diaphragms, when breathing quietly in the seated posture (De Troyer and Estenne, 1990). The abdominal muscle paralysis increases the compliance and the inspiratory outward excursion of the abdomen, relative to normal. These patients depart from the relaxed configuration of the respiratory system during quiet breathing, which means that they expend extra energy in deforming the chest wall, instead of inflating the lungs.

D. Other Focal Paralyses of the Respiratory Muscles

Hemiplegia

Hemiplegia is most often the result of cerebrovascular disease (stroke), but it often occurs with trauma as well. Paralysis in hemiplegia results from damage to upper motor neurons, somewhere between the cortex and the spinal cord. Lower motor neurons are spared, but they are subject to stimulation by sensorimotor reflex arcs at the spinal level. Thus, hemiplegia initially is characterized by flaccid paralysis, but later by spastic paralysis.

The respiratory muscles are driven by two anatomically and functionally discrete upper motor neuronal pathways. The corticospinal tracts, which lie in the pyramidal system and descend in the lateral columns of the spinal cord, mediate voluntary respiratory motions such as breath holding and performance of pulmonary function tests. The reticulospinal pathways, which arise in the "medullary respiratory center" and descend in ventral columns of the spinal cord, are responsible for the automatic control of breathing. Patients with hemiplegia sustain damage to the corticospinal tracts, but the reticulospinal pathways are spared unless the medulla is directly involved by the lesion (infarction, tumor, trauma, etc.). Diaphragmatic motion as assessed fluoroscopically and movements of the chest measured with calipers are slightly impaired on the affected side (Fluck, 1966; Korcyzn et al., 1969). Differences between the affected and nonaffected side are more apparent during deep breathing than they are at rest. Neither of these tests is of diagnostic value.

Santamaria and Ruiz (1988) retrospectively evaluated supine chest films of 62 consecutive patients with acute stroke and 92 control patients with acute ischemic heart disease. Half the patients had right-sided paralysis, and half had left-sided paralysis. Hemiplegia was considered to be severe in 55% of patients, and large lesions (>40 ml) were found in 45%. The difference between the heights of the right and left hemidiaphragms was 7 ± 14 mm (right side higher) in the controls, less than that in patients with right-sided neurological lesions (left hemiplegia), and much greater than control in patients with left-sided neurological lesions (right side paralyzed). Differences in hemidiaphragm height were greater when the hemiplegia was more severe, when the volume of the neurological lesions exceeded 40 ml, and when the lesions involved the genu of the internal capsule and/or the near anterolateral area.

De Troyer et al. (1981) measured the electrical activity (electromyogram, EMG) of the diaphragm and parasternal intercostal muscles of hemiplegic patients. On the paralyzed side, parasternal activity was lower in 19 of 20 patients, whereas diaphragmatic activity was lower in 15 of 20 patients. There were no apparent differences between patients whose diaphragms were equally active on both sides and those who exhibited less activity on the paralyzed side. It was concluded that upper motor neuron innervation of the respiratory muscles was significantly mediated by decussating fibers (De Troyer et al., 1981).

Poliomyelitis

The poliomyelitis virus attacks motoneurons in the medulla (bulbar polio) and anterior horns of the spinal cord. The resulting muscle paralysis may involve any striated skeletal muscle, including those responsible for speech and swallowing, the respiratory muscles, and muscles of the trunk and limbs. Muscle weakness and paralysis are most severe in the early, febrile stage of the disease, and partial recovery is common during convalescence. Significant respiratory paresis occurred in 15% of patients studied after a 1953 epidemic (Linderholm and Werneman, 1956). The distribution and severity of respiratory muscle involvement are quite variable, such that some patients exhibit more expiratory than inspiratory weakness, others have more inspiratory weakness, and still others have approximately equal loss of strength in both respiratory muscle groups.

The reduction in vital capacity is not wholly due to respiratory muscle weakness (De Troyer et al., 1980). The compliance ofthe respiratory system is reduced to between 40% and 70% of its normal value (Brody et al., 1964; Ferris et al., 1952a), with a relatively greater reduction in the compliance of the lung than of the chest wall (Ferris et al., 1952a). By and large, the VC in polio is lower in relation to the degree of respiratory muscle weakness than in other forms of neuromuscular disease (De Troyer et al., 1980); this may reflect improved respiratory therapy between the 1950s and the 1970s.

The result of two series (Ferris et al., 1952a; Brody et al., 1964) show the relationship between ventilatory capacity, pulmonary function, and respiratory muscle strength (Table 6). Three groups of patients are presented: group 1 comprises patients who were dependent on mechanical ventilation >12 hr/day, group 2 comprises patients who were dependent on mechanical ventilation <12 hr/day, and patients in group 3 had never required mechancial ventilatory assistance. In group 1, respiratory muscle strength is less than one-quarter of normal, VC is even lower, and MVV is only 2–3 times the resting ventilation. In group 2, respiratory muscle strength, VC, and MVV are all about one-third of normal, whereas in group 3 these indices of ventilatory function are approximately at half their normal values. Analysis of data from convalescing patients (Ferriset al., 1955) shows that ventilatory endurance time, i.e., the time a patient can breathe spontaneously without mechanical ventilator support, was related to VC by the formula: endurance time (hr) = 0.54 VC (% predicted) −3.2 ($r = 0.75$, $p < 0.001$). The pathogenesis of ventilatory failure in neuromuscular disease, and its treatment, are discussed in detail in subsequent sections of this chapter.

Table 6 Maximal Respiratory Pressures and Spirometric Data in Patients with Poliomyelitis[a]

Variable	Group 1	Group 2	Group 3
PI_{max}	25	35	45
PE_{max}	25	40	55
MVV	20	35	75
VC	15	35	55
IC	10	25	45
ERV	0	5	25

[a]Values are expressed as percentage of predicted normal.
Group 1 = dependent on mechanical ventilation > 12 hr/day; Group 2 = dependent on mechanical ventilation < 12 hr/day; Group 3 = not dependent on mechanical ventilatory support.

Patients with poliomyelitis, as well as those with other forms of neuromuscular disease, may exhibit a number of abnormalities in the control of breathing, including poor ventilatory responses to inhalation of CO_2 and sleep-related breathing disorders (Linderholm and Werneman, 1956; Plum and Swanson, 1958; Solliday et al., 1974; Hill et al., 1983; Steljes et al., 1990). Plum and Swanson (1958) found that the impaired ventilatory response to CO_2 inhalation was more related to respiratory muscle paralysis than to bulbar polio.

Although poliomyelitis is unlikely to recur in epidemic form in developed countries, sporadic cases may occur, especially in patients who, for whatever reason, fail to receive vaccination. Therefore, physicians must be alert to the possibility of polio when they encounter febrile patients with myalgias and weakness. In addition, it is now recognized that there is a ''postpolio syndrome'' characterized by new or accelerating weakness decades after the original illness (Fischer, 1985; Cashman et al., 1987; Steljes et al., 1990). The patients who are most likely to be dyspneic and predisposed to develop ventilatory failure are characterized by lower VC and maximal respiratory pressures, especially a low PE_{max} (Dean et al., 1991).

E. Diffuse Neuromuscular Disease

The diseases considered in this section are unrelated as to etiology, but have two features in common: the involvement of the respiratory muscles is diffuse, and it is relatively symmetrical with regard to inspiratory and expiratory muscle groups. It is clinically important to distinguish between the disorders that are likely to have an acute onset (acute inflammatory polyneuropathy, myasthenia gravis, botulism, organophosphate poisoning, or aminoglycoside anitbiotic toxicity) and those that occur gradually, even insidiously (amyotrophic lateral sclerosis, muscular dystrophies, and myopathies). The clincial characeristics of the underlying neurological dysfunction have been described elsewhere (Kaminski and Young, 1985; De Troyer and Pride, 1985; Aldrich and Aldrich, 1986; Bennett and Bleck, 1988), so the focus of this chapter is on the respiratory system manifestations of the neuromuscular disease.

Diseases with Acute Onset

Acute Inflammatory Polyneuropathy

Acute inflammatory polyneuropathy (Landry-Guillain-Barré-Stohl syndrome) is a prototypical model of acute respiratory muscle weakness. Owing to the ascending nature of the paralysis, the chest wall and abdominal muscles are affected prior to involvement of laryngeal and pharyngeal muscles, so the disease affords an opportunity to see ventilatory insufficiency and failure from respiratory muscle weakness in pure form. Complications characteristic of botulism or organophosphate poisioning are absent, as are secondary features of prolonged neuromuscular disease.

The clinical presentation is characterized by progressive weakness, dyspnea, and difficulty with coughing (Rochester and Findley, 1988). As the disease progresses, patients also experience dysphagia and difficulty with speech. On physical examination early in the course, one can easily demonstrate weakness of limb and truncal muscles, but examination of the respiratory system in the earlier stages reveals only tachypnea. Later manifestations may include use of the neck (accessory) inspiratory muscles, failing voice, and loss of the gag reflex.

The results of arterial blood gas analysis in acute inflammatory polyneuropathy are characteristic of diffuse respiratory muscle weakness of any cause (Braun, et al., 1983). Typically, the Pa_{O_2} is somewhat low, the $(A\text{-}a)P_{O_2}$ is increased, and the Pa_{CO_2} is low in patients who are able o breathe spontaneously. Ventilatory failure with hypercapnia develops only after the VC has fallen below one-third of normal. Patients with progressive dyspnea and tachypnea are at high risk of developing ventilatory failure abruptly, with rapid progression to respiratory arrest. Therefore, all patients with even minor respiratory symptoms should be closely followed, by having their VC and maximal respiratory pressures (PI_{max}, PE_{max}) measured at frequent intervals. Moreover, they should receive mechanical ventilatory support prior to overt respiratory arrest.

At the Mayo Clinic, 25% of patients with acute inflammatory polyneuropathy required admission to an intensive care unit, and 13 of 79 patients had to be ventilated mechanically (Gracey et al., 1982). Mechanical ventilation lasted 10–104 days (mean 58 days), and the process of weaning took 7–93 days (mean 37 days). Because most patients afflicted with acute inflammatory polyneuropathy have a prolonged course, early tracheostomy should be given serious consideration. Weaning from mechanical ventilation was associated with increases in transdiaphragmatic pressure per breath (Pdi) and maximum transdiaphragmatic pressure (Pdi_{max}), PI_{max}, and tidal volume (VT); improvement in Pdi_{max} was the best predictor of recovery (Borel et al., 1991).

Myasthenia Gravis

Myasthenia gravis is an immunological disease of the neuromuscular junction (motor end-plate). The pathogenesis of the disease is binding of IgG autoantibodies to acetylcholine receptors on the muscle cells. This prevents acetylcholine, which is released from the terminal portion of the motoneuron, from exciting the muscle cell to initiate contraction. In mild disease, receptor blockade is incomplete and weakness is mild, but in advanced disease weakness is profound. It is characteristic of myasthenia gravis that weakness is aggravated by repeated contraction.

Respiratory muscle involvement is common, but there is little or no correlation between the degree of respiratory muscle weakness and the grade of myasthenia, the strength of the quadriceps muscle, or the severity of dyspnea (Mier-Jedrzejowica et al., 1988a). Maximal inspiratory and expiratory pressures were approximately half of normal, but diaphragmatic contractile responses to bilateral phrenic nerve stimulation were normal in 14 of 17 patients. Peripheral nerve function is normal, as manifest by normal phrenic nerve conduction times (Mier-Jedrzejowicz et al., 1988a).

The diagnosis of myasthenia gravis can be difficult, and it behooves the physician to consider this possibility in all cases of unexplained muscle weakness or ventilatory failure. Among the clinical manifestations, dysphagia, diplopia, ptosis, and aggravation of weakness by activity are helpful indicators (Dushay et al., 1990; Mier et al., 1990b). The diagnosis is highly likely when one can demonstrate a significant improvement, such as loss of diplopia or ptosis, improved pulmonary function, or increased strength of any muscle group, following intravenous injection of 2–10 mg of edrophonium hydrochloride (Tensilon). Indeed, pulmonary function, ventilatory capacity, and maximal respiratory pressures improved by approximately 30% in 15 of 17 patients after injection of Tensilon, and the two failures had had severe, long-standing myasthenia gravis (Mier-Jedrzejowicz et al., 1988a). When the Tensilon test fails, one may still obtain a response from an anticholinesterase such as neostigmine, and the diagnosis of myasthenia gravis can be confirmed by deomonstrating the presence of antistriated muscle and acetylcholine receptor antibodies (Dushay et al., 1990).

Two recent case reports remind us that myasthenia gravis can present as isolated ventilatory failure (Dushay et al., 1990; Mier et al., 1990b). In both cases, processes other than myasthenia gravis (obesity-hypoventilation syndrome with obstructive sleep apnea, surgical removal of part of the diaphragm) were initially considered to have been responsible for the patient's condition. It is important to recognize that patients with myasthenia gravis can have severe respiratory muscle weakness, even when involvement of the peripheral muscles is mild (Mier-Jedrzejowicz et al., 1988a).

Treatment of myasthenia gravis is directed at removing the IgG autoantibodies by plasmapheresis (Gracey et al., 1984b; Dau, 1985) and enhancing the concentration of acetylcholine at the motor end-plate by using anticholinesterase drugs such as prostigmine, physostigmine, pyridostigmine (Mestinon), or neostigmine (Radwan et al., 1988). Corticosteroid therapy has been variably successful. The degree of improvement in respiratory muscle strength and ventilatory capacity after treatment with neostigmine is 20–30%, i.e., about the same as after diagnostic injection of Tensilon.

Management of myasthenia gravis is beset with problems, and those which are most likely to precipitate prolonged ventilatory failure are myasthenic crisis, cholinergic crisis, and surgery, especially thymectomy (Gracey et al., 1983). Factors that predispose to the need for postoperative ventilator support are bulbar involvement (Gracey et al., 1984a) and expiratory muscle weakness (Younger et al., 1984).

Lambert-Eaton Syndrome

The Lambert-Eaton syndrome is another autoimmune disorder of the neuromuscular transmission; approximately half of those afflicted have small-cell carcinoma of the lung (O'Neill et al., 1988). In this syndrome, IgG antibodies to presynaptic calcium channels lead to their down-regulation, which in turn impairs the release of acetylcholine from cholinergic nerve terminals (McEvoy et al., 1989; Laroche et al., 1989). The weakness mainly affects proximal truncal muscles, and in contradistinction to myasthenia gravis, muscle strength in the Lambert-Eaton syndrome improves with sustained contraction. Other features are hyporeflexia and autonomic dysfunction.

Inspiratory muscle, specifically diaphragmatic, involvement may be prominent, and PI_{max} improves with repeated PI_{max} testing (Wilcox et al., 1988b). Although not common, ventilatory failure has been reported (Gracey and Southorn, 1987). Coexistent pulmonary disease and use of muscle relaxants may contribute to the pathogenesis of ventilatory failure, but need not. Laroche et al. (1989) studied six patients and found that all of them had mild to moderate weakness of the diaphragm. In addition, four patients had expiratory and leg muscle weakness, and two were in ventilatory failure.

In addition to appropriate supportive therapy, treatment should be directed at the associated small-cell carcinoma, when present, and at enhancing the release of acetylcholine with 3, 4-diaminopyridine (McEvoy et al., 1989; Laroche et al., 1989). Plasmapheresis has been used, but if it has an effect, it is substantially delayed, as compared to the response in myasthenia gravis (Gracey and Southorn, 1987).

Botulism

Botulism also causes acute respiratory muscle paralysis by poisoning the neuromuscular junction. Botulism characteristically produces symptoms of visual impairment, dry mouth, slurred speech, dysphagia, nausea, vomiting and diarrhea, weakness, dizziness, and dyspnea. Physical signs include ptosis, paralysis of extraocular muscles, dysarthria, tachypnea, and extreme muscle weakness. The manifestations of type A and type B botulism are similar, but patients with type B botulism develop symptoms more slowly, come to medical attention later, and are less likely to require mechanical ventilation (St. Louis et al., 1988). Patients with type B botulism are often misdiagnosed as having myasthenia gravis, stroke, or psychiatric disorder. In recent outbreaks the foods responsible were vegetable roots or tubers that had been cooked and coated with oil, thereby providing an anaerobic environment (St. Louis et al., 1988).

Pulmonary complications and ventilatory failure are characteristic of botulism (Schmidt-Nowara et al., 1983), and the patients who have the most severe symptoms and signs are most likely to need mechanical ventilation. Both respiratory and upper airway muscle involvement are commonly present, and respiratory muscle weakness is manifest early in the course (Wilcox et al., 1990a). Most recovery of function occurs in the first 12 weeks, but it may take a year for full recovery to occur.

As is true for all forms of respiratory muscle weakness, VC and maximal respiratory pressures should be measured frequently, and one should not wait for the appearance of hypercapnia to institute mechanical ventilation in a patient whose respiratory muscles are failing rapidly. Treatment is mainly supportive and is frequently prolonged. Mortality has been reduced to about 5%, but residual symptoms of dyspnea and fatigue are common long after recovery from ventilatory failure.

Antimicrobial Drugs

Aminoglycoside and polymyxin antibiotics can produce a clinical picture very similar to botulism (Lindesmith et al., 1968). The risk is greatest in patients with renal failure, but recognition of the problem, avoidance of some antibiotics such as sodium colistimethate, and careful attention to dosage schedules have combined to make this syndrome virtually unheard of at present. Anticholinesterase therapy can reverse the effects of aminoglycosides, but not those of polymyxin or sodium colistimethate.

Organophosphorus Poisoning

Quarternary organophosphate and carbonate compounds are used as agricultural insecticides (parathion, malathion, carbaryl) or as nerve gases. They cause muscle paralysis by inhibiting acetylcholinesterase, thus leading to excessive concentrations of acetylcholine at the neuromuscular junction and other cholinergic synaptic sites. Edrophonium and drugs like neostigmine are therapeutic members of the quarternary class of drugs; their excessive use accounts for the cholinergic crisis of myasthenia gravis.

Symptoms of acute organophosphate intoxication reflect both muscarnic and nicotinic effects. The former include sweating, salivation, nausea, vomiting, abdominal cramps, bradycardia, and hypotension. Nicotinic effects include muscle fasciculation, weakness, and paralysis. Central nervous system manifestations of organophosphate toxicity include ataxia, loss of reflexes, confusion, convulsions, and coma. Neurotoxic effects may be rapid in onset or delayed for 2–3 weeks. Senanayake and Karalliedde (1987) described 10 patients in whom paralysis of proximal limb, neck, and respiratory muscles occurred 24–96 hr after poisoning and lasted 2–3 weeks.

The principal respiratory manifestations are laryngospasm, excessive tracheobronchial secretions, bronchoconstriction, respiratory muscle weakness, and central depression of ventilation. Mechanical ventilatory support may be needed urgently (Senanayake and Karalliedde, 1987). Treatment is directed at reversing the muscarinic effects with atropine and the nicotinic effects of the neuromuscular junction paralysis with pralidoxime (Protopam). Both drugs should be given intravenously, as soon as possible. Prophylactic use of oral pyridostigmine, 30 mg every 8 hr, for 1–7 days produced minimal side effects (Keeler et al., 1991).

Diseases with Gradual Onset

The diffuse neuromuscular diseases with a subacute or chronic course that affect the respiratory muscles fall into three major groups: amyotrophic lateral sclerosis, a disease of unknown etiology that attacks motoneurons in the anterior horns of the spinal cord (Kreitzer et al, 1978b; Kaminski and Young, 1985), several types of muscular dystrophy (Fallat et al., 1979; Jammes et al., 1985), and diverse myopathies (Black and Hyatt, 1971; Braun et al., 1983; Aldrich and Aldrich, 1986). Virtually all varieties of myopathy involve the respiratory muscles. They may be congenital disorders of muscle metabolism (Braun et al., 1983; Margolis and Hill, 1986) or acquired myopathies related to nutritional status (Arora and Rochester, 1982), endocrinopathy (Silverstein et al., 1983; Laroche et al., 1988a;, Mier et al., 1989), infection, or inflammation (Morgan et al., 1982; Ivey et al., 1991). Myopathy is also a prominent component of autoimmune diseases such as systemic lupus erythematosus and scleroderma (Gibson et al., 1977a; Chausow et al., 19874; Thompson et al., 1985).

The clinical course varies according to the nature of the underlying disease. The distribution of muscle involvement may be predominantly proximal, as in myopathies, distal, or both distal and proximal. Patients may experience muscle cramps, and muscle fasciculations or atrophy is sometimes present on physical examination. Patients usually are aware of limb muscle weakness before they have respiratory symptoms, but there are notable exceptions to this general rule. The average life expectancy of patients with amyotrophic lateral sclerosis is 3–4 years after the onset of symptoms. It is somewhat longer in muscular dystrophies, and these patients usually die of respiratory failure.

Most of the congenital myopathies seen in adults have a slowly progressive course, whereas the varieties seen in infants tend to be rapidly fatal. The course of acquired myopathies is widely variable, according to the type of myopathy and the extent of comorbidity. Some reverse spontaneously (Morgan et al. 1982). Inflammatory or autoimmune myopathies frequently respond to anti-inflammatory or immunosuppressive therapy, and myopathies caused by malnutrition or thyroid dysfunction stabilize or improve with appropriate corrective treatment (Laroche et al., 1988a; Mier et al., 1989). Myopathies attributable to alcohol or corticosteroid therapy often improve when the offending agent is discontinued.

Clinical Features

The distribution of weakness among the inspiratory and expiratory muscles is usually symmetrical (Black and Hyatt, 1971; Arora and Rochester, 1982; Braun et al., 1983), but sometimes expiratory weakness exceeds inspiratory weakness (Kreitzer et al., 1978b; Demedts et al., 1982). Vincken et al. (1987) analyzed the relationship between respiratory muscle weakness and other aspects of the disease in 30 patients with polyneuropathy, myasthenia gravis, motor neuron disease, or myopathy. Maximal respiratory pressures were about 67% of normal, but there was no correlation between respiratory and general muscle strength. Expiratory muscle strength varied according to the type of disease, but duration of disease and nutritional status did not influence respiratory muscle strength. It is important to keep in mind that the respiratory muscles may be far weaker than the limb muscles, and that diaphragmatic dysfunction may exceed that of the other respiratory muscles (Newsom-Davis et al., 1976; Skatrud et al., 1980; Chausow et al., 1984; Mier-Jedrzejowicz et al., 1988a).

The principal respiratory symptoms are fatigue and dyspnea on exertion. As weakness becomes more severe, patients may be dyspneic at rest and have difficulty in coughing, speaking, and swallowing. The symptoms of disturbed sleep, morning headache, and daytime somnolence are characteristic of acute nocturnal respiratory failure, and patients with long-standing nocturnal respiratory failure or chronic ventilatory failure often develop symptoms of heart failure. Physical examination of the respiratory system may be normal or may reveal only tachypnea. In more advanced disease, physical signs of poor diaphragmatic movement, sternocleidomastoid atrophy, atelectasis, and impaired gag reflex may be present.

Diagnosis

The diagnostic workup of patients suspected of having neuromuscular disease should include careful evaluation of the neuromuscular system. General guidelines are briefly mentioned below; details specific to different disorders are covered in several reviews (Kaminski and Young, 1985; Aldrich and Aldrich, 1986; Bennett and Bleck, 1988). One should note, on physical examination, the pattern of muscle weakness, the presence or absence of findings consistent with upper motor neuron disease, and the presence or absence of fasciculations that indicate lower motor neuron disease. In addition, electrophysiological techniques to study nerve conduction, motor end-plate potentials, and muscle electrical activity are useful in differentiating between denervation, motor end-plate disease, dystrophies, and myopathies. Muscle biopsy and serum levels of muscle enzymes such as creatine kinase and aldolase are also of value. Galloway et al. (1991) took advantage of elective tracheostomy to biopsy the sternohyoid muscle. Frequently it is necessary to assess the response to intravenous Tensilon, to rule out myasthenia gravis.

Physiological Abnormalities

Routine pulmonary function tests such as spirometry are the first step in the objective evaluation of the respiratory system in neuromuscular disease. Objective assessment is critical, because it has been demonstrated that 50% reductions of VC and MVV could not be detected on routine clinical examination (Fallat et al., 1979). The characteristic finding in neuromuscular disease is a restrictive pattern; i.e., the FVC is small but there is no obstructive component. The reduction in VC is out of proportion to what would be expected from muscle weakness alone (De Troyer et al., 1980; Braun et al., 1983), probably because of decreased distensibility of the lungs from microtelectasis coupled with a decrease in the outward recoil of the chest wall (De Troyer et al., 1980).

Measurement of lung volumes reveals that RV is increased in most patients with respiratory muscle weakness, TLC is usually but not always reduced, and FRC is also normal or low (Kreitzer et al., 1978b; Demedts et al., 1982; Braun et al., 1983). Thus both subdivisions of VC, the inspiratory capacity (IC) and the expiratory reserve volume (ERV), are also reduced. The diffusing capacity is normal in neuromuscular disease, provided it is corrected for the reduction in TLC (Demedts et al., 1982).

The peak expiratory and inspiratory flow rates are reduced more or less in proportion to the reduction of VC, the FEV_1/FVC ratio is normal, and the MVV is almost always low (Black and Hyatt, 1971; Jammes et al., 1985; Braun et al., 1983). Airway resistance is slightly increased, but specific airway conductance is either normal or higher than normal (Riley et al., 1977; Demedts et al., 1982). Thus, the slight increase in airway resistance can be attributed to reduction in lung volume, and the reductions in forced inspiratory and expiratory flow rates result from respiratory muscle weakness rather than from any airway disease.

The only sure way to determine the distribution and severity of respiratory muscle weakness is to measure maximal inspiratory and expiratory pressures (Black and Hyatt, 1971; Braun et al., 1983; Vincken et al., 1987). This is a simple, noninvasive procedure, but when patients are unable to perform the test properly, respiratory muscle strength will be underestimated. If one suspects that is the case, it is necessary to place a balloon catheter in the esophagus to measure pleural pressure swings during inspiratory and expiratory efforts. Maneuvers such as inspiring to TLC, sniffing, and coughing are easier for some patients to do because they are more natural than the Muller and expiratory maneuvers required to obtain maximal pressures, and they yield reliable results (Rochester, 1988). These tests provide a global evaluation of respiratory muscle strength, but more specific information can be obtained by selectively assessing diaphragmatic strength using the sniff test and/or bilateral stimulation of the phrenic nerves (Mier-Jedrezejowicz et al., 1988b).

All the pulmonary function tests worsen as neuromuscular disease progresses. Early in the course of neuromuscular diseases, the spirometric tests, especially VC and FVC, may remain normal although PI_{max} and PE_{max} are as low as half normal (Black and Hyatt, 1971; Braun et al., 1983; Jammes et al., 1985). However, as respiratory muscle strength falls from 50% to 20% of predicted, VC falls progressively to one-quarter normal. Other tests of pulmonary function are linearly correlated with respiratory muscle function. For example, RV (% predicted) is significantly and inversely related to PE_{max} (% predicted), and MVV (% predicted) correlates well with respiratory muscle strength (the mean of PI_{max} and PE_{max}, % predicted) (Braun et al., 1983).

Neuromuscular disease is frequently accompanied by coexisting obstructive or interstitial lung disease (Black and Hyatt, 1971; Gibson et al., 1977b; Braun et al., 1983; Chausow et al., 1984; Thompson et al., 1985). One would think that this would affect pulmonary function out of proportion to the degree of respiratory muscle weakness, but this was found to be true only for the MVV (Braun et al.,1983). Thus, MVV and RV are more likely to be abnormal early in the course of neuromuscular disease than is the VC, and MVV for any degree of respiratory muscle weakness will be lower in patients with coexistent lung disease.

The respiratory complictations of diffuse neuromuscular disease and their managemen are by and large similar to those of bilateral diaphragmatic paralysis and spinal cord injury. Moreover, the respiratory complications and management of ventilatory failure consequent to skeletal disorders and obesity are also nearly identical (see Section III). For these reasons, the complications are discussed in Section IV, and treatment of respiratory complications and ventilatory failure is covered in Section V of this chapter.

III. Skeletal Disorders and Obesity

A. Deformities of the Chest Wall

This section deals with the related group of respiratory disorders that originate from diseases of the chest wall. Because respiratory muscles act on the chest wall, it is not surprising that the neuromuscular diseases that affect respiratory muscle function have features in common with diseases of the chest wall (Bergofsky, 1985). Obesity is included in this section because of its profound effects on the mechanical properties of the chest wall, breathing during sleep, and gas exchange.

Kyphoscoliosis

Etiology

Kyphoscoliosis is an excessive curvature of the spine. The increased spinal curvature may be posterior (kyphosis) or lateral (scoliosis). This disorder is caused by defects in the vertebrae, the vertebral connective tissue, or the neuromuscular system supporting the spinal column (Table 7). Various disease processes associated with severe kyphoscoliosis include neuromuscular disease (muscular dystrophy), vertebral disease (osteomalacia), and connective tissue disorders (Marfan's syndrome). Idiopathic disease accounts for approximately 80% of cases of kyphoscoliosis (James, 1976). Hereditary factors probably play a role in idiopathic kyphoscoliosis, although the exact mode of genetic transmission is not clear (Litwin, 1978).

Clinical Features

Although slight deviation in spinal curvature may occur in as many as 10% of otherwise healthy people, severe kyphoscoliosis accounts for less than 1% of chronic ventilatory failure in adults. Kyphoscoliosis must be of a severe degree to cause ventilatory failure in adults with otherwise normal lungs. Bergofsky et al., (1959) demonstrated that ventilatory failure is most marked in those patients with the most severe degree of spinal deformity. In addition, this study showed that the lateral and posterior deformities of the spine are additive in producing ventilatory failure; in other words, a combination of moderate kyphosis and scoliosis is equivalent to a severe degree of either one alone. Bergofsky and associates (1959) suggested that in the absence of kyphosis greater than 20°, a scoliosis of less than 100° fails to cause ventilatory failure. The correlation

Table 7 Etiologies of Kyphoscoliosis

Idiopathic	
Neuromuscular disease	Muscular dystrophy
	Poliomyelitis
	Cerebral palsy
	Friedreich's ataxia
Vertebral disease	Osteoporosis
	Osteomalacia
	Vitamin D–resistant rickets
	Tuberculous spondylitis
	Neurofibromatosis
Connective tissue disease	Marfan's syndrome
	Ehlers-Danlos syndrome
	Morquio's Syndrome
Thoracic cage abnormalities	Empyema
	Thoracoplasty

between degrees of skeletal deformity and the clinical status is sufficient to suggest that adults with greater than 100° of scoliosis are likely to develop symptoms of ventilatory failure.

The clinical presentation in patients with kyphoscoliosis varies according to the patient's age and degree of spinal deformity (Bergofsky et al., 1959; Kafer, 1976; Libby et al., 1982; Lisboa et al., 1985). Patients younger than 35 years, even though they may have severe degrees of kyphoscoliosis, may be asymptomatic. However, middle-aged patients with severe degrees of kyphoscoliosis tend to develop dyspnea, decreased exercise tolerance, and repeated acute respiratory infections, and often go on to develop frank ventilatory failure with cor pulmonale.

Physical examination often reveals little besides the marked thoracic cage abnormalities in younger, asymptomatic patients, whereas patients with cardiorespiratory failure will have findings such as cyanosis, distended neck veins, edema, and hepatomegaly. Chest radiographs often show no obvious abnormality, except the marked spinal deformity. Cardiac size and subtle pulmonary infiltrates are often difficult to recognize in the radiographs of the more severely deformed patients.

Physiological Abnormalities

Adolescents with mild idiopathic scoliosis have a mild restrictive pattern, with VC less than 80% of predicted (Smyth et al., 1984). The VC correlated with maximal respiratory pressures (PI_{max}, PE_{max}) but not with the degree of thoracic curvature. As a consequence of the reduction in lung volume, both static and dynamic lung compliances are reduced, but the low lung capacity has been attributed to defective mechanical coupling between the inspiratory muscles and the chest wall (Jones et al., 1981; Cooper et al., 1984). Lung volumes, including TLC and VC, are uniformly decreased in patients with scoliosis greater than 90° (Table 8). Both TLC and VC are diminshed roughly in proportion to the severity of spinal deformity (Weber et al., 1975; Weinstein et al., 1981). The FEV_1 and forced midexpiratory flow rate (FEF_{25-75}) are decreased only in proportion to the decreased VC, unless the patient has superimposed obstructive lung disease (Caro and DuBois, 1961).

Compliance of the chest wall and lung and the pulmonary diffusing capacity are markedly reduced in adults with kyphoscoliosis (Caro and DuBois, 1961; Sinha and Bergofsky, 1972; Weber et al., 1975; Kafer, 1975; Jones et al., 1981). In contrast, chest wall compliance is normal in children, even in those with severe spinal deformity (Caro and DuBois, 1961; Jones et al., 1981). The reduction in lung volumes and ventilatory performance results from both mechanical distortion of the chest and impaired respiratory muscle function.

In younger patients with a mean scoliosis angle of approximately 50%, both PI_{max} and PE_{max} are mildly decreased, to 70% and 80% of control,

Table 8 Pulmonary Function Test Results in Kyphoscoliosis (KS), Ankylosing Spondylitis (AS), Obesity (OB), and the Obesity-Hypoventilation Syndrome (OHS)[a]

Variable	KS	AS	OB	OHS
FVC	50	75	80	60
FEV_1/FVC	80	85	80	85
FRC	75	125	85	60
MVV	40	85	80	55
PI_{max}	70	—	100	70

[a]All values expressed as percentage of predicted normal.

respectively (Caro and DuBois, 1961; Jones et al., 1981; Cooper et al., 1984; Smyth et al., 1984). However, in older patients with a somewhat greater scoliosis, PI_{max} was about half normal in eucapnic patients, and one-quarter normal in hypercapnic patients (Lisboa et al., 1985). the reduction in PE_{max} is partly due to the decrease in TLC (Rochester, 1988). However, the decline in PE_{max} and PI_{max} may also arise from mechanical disadvantages due to abnormal respiratory muscle lengths, shapes, and insertions in the markedly distorted thoracic cage.

The capacity of patients with mild to moderate kyphoscoliosis for physical exercise is reduced, to 60–85% of normal depending on the severity of the scoliosis (Shneerson, 1978; Kesten et al., 1991). Maximal oxygen consumption was linearly correlated with FVC, FEV_1, and MVV (Shneerson, 1978). During exercise, VT increased linearly with VE, and although the absolute VT is smaller than normal, the VT_{max}/VC ratio was approximately 0.5 which is normal. Kesten et al. (1991) found that the dyspnea index, defined as VE_{max}/MVV was 69%, also normal, and that the anaerobic threshold was 57% of maximal oxygen consumption. These patients, whose Cobb angle was between 25° and 70°, had low-normal hypoxic and hypercapnic ventilatory responses. Thus, it was concluded that the impairment of exercise performance in moderate scoliosis is probably due to physical deconditioning, rather than to either mechanical limitation to breathing or impaired chemoreceptor sensitivity (Kesten et al., 1991).

Hypoxemia without hypercapnia is characteristic of moderate to severe kyphoscoliosis. Radionuclide ventilation-perfusion studies demonstrate that mismatch tends to occur in patients with scoliosis greater than 65° (Bake et al., 1972a; Shannon et al., 1971). One uncontrolled study showed that patients with severe kyphoscoliosis have reduced oxyhemoglobin saturation during sleep, the greatest reduction occurring during rapid eye movement (REM) sleep (Mazon et al., 1980).

Patients with acute or chronic ventilatory failure have hypercapnia, severe hypoxemia, and an increased (A-a)Po_2 (Bergofsky et al., 1959; Kafer, 1976; Libby et al., 1982). The severity of hypercapnia does not correlate well with the degree of thoracic deformity, but, instead, with the patients age and inspiratory muscle strength (Lisboa et al., 1985). Although respiratory muscle weakness may contribute to ventilatory failure, the converse may also be true. In one series, PI_{max} was low in all patients with kyphoscoliosis, but PI_{max} was lowest in the hypercapnic patients (Lisboa et al., 1985). Moreover, PI_{max} correlated much better with Pco_2 and Po_2 than with the degree of spinal curvature. Patients with kyphoscoliosis have a fairly good prognosis after the onset of acute ventilatory failure, despite the severity of their restrictive deficit (VC 30% predicted, FEV_1 23% predicted), probably because the VC and FEV_1 decline relatively slowly thereafter (Libby et al., 1982).

Pathological Abnormalities

The spinal deformity in kyphoscoliosis leads to small lung volumes and a decreased pulmonary vascular bed (Naeye, 1961). Pathological studies have shown the lungs to be between 30% and 65% of normal size in patients with kyphoscoliosis with ventilatory failure. In addition to the loss of lung volume and pulmonary vascular bed, the deformed chest cage undergoes unknown structural changes as the patient ages, causing the chest wall to become even less compliant (Jones et al., 1981). As the patient ages, the stiff chest wall increases the work of breathing and leads to hypoventilationn (Bergofsky et al., 1959), and respiratory muscle weakness leads to a decrease in the tidal volume (Kafer, 1976; Lisboa et al., 1985).

With progression of ventilation-perfusion mismatch and hypoventilation, pulmonary hypertension consequent to hypoxic pulmonary vasoconstriction ensues. This is aggravated by the decreased pulmonary vascular bed and any superimposed intrinsic lung disease (Naeye, 1961). Pathological studies of the lungs in patients with severe kyphoscoliosis show that as many as one-third with kyphoscoliosis have additional lung diseases such as emphysema and bronchiectasis. The remaining two-thirds of patients usually show atelectasis as the only parenchymal lung pathology.

Treatment

Patients with only mild degrees of spinal deformity do not require special treatment to prevent vetilatory failure. A styudy of 219 patients with untreated idiopathic scoliosis demonstrated that significant reduction in pulmonary function occurs only in patients with thoracic scoliosis curves of greater than 100° (Jones et al., 1981). Patients with lesser degrees of thoracic scoliosis are not significantly different from a control population with regard to symptoms and pulmonary function tests results.

Although surgical correction of thoracic cage deformity may be helpful in children and adolescents, such surgical procedures have not been demonstrated to significantly improve the pulmonary function in adults with severe kyphoscoliosis. Surgical therapy for severe kyphoscoliosis has been shown to decrease the severity of thoracic deformity in young children and adolescents. Some investigators have reported slight improvement in pulmonary function testing after surgical placement of a Harrington rod in adolescents (Cooper et al., 1984). Others failed to confirm these findings (Shannon et al., 1971; Swank et al., 1981). A study of 222 patients over the age of 20 years documented that spinal fusion and Harrington rod placement do not significantly improve the FVC, FEV_1, or resting arterial Po_2 (Swank et al., 1981). This study also showed that Harrington rod placement and spinal fusion have a complication rate of greater than 50%. A study in 13 young patients with kyphoscoliosis undergoing spinal fusion demonstrated significant deterioration of their total respiratory system mechanics (Baydur et al., 1990b).

The medical therapy for the adult with kyphoscoliosis is both preventive and supportive. Immunization, adequate hydration, prompt care for respiratory infection, avoidance of sedatives, and carefully monitored supplemental O_2 are the mainstays of therapy. One study showed that 5 min of intermittent positive-pressure breathing produced a marked improvement in the lung mechanics and resting arterial Pco_2 in six patients with severe kyphoscoliosis and chronic ventilatory failure (Sinha and Bergofsky, 1972). The $Paco_2$ fell by approximately 12 mmHg and the work of breathing fell by half. These effects lasted up to 3 h after the treatment. The intermittent positive-pressure breathing probably decreases microatelectasis and increases lung compliance. The improved lung compliance, in turn, probably decreases the work of breathing and improves ventilation-perfusion matching in the lung. Thus, intermittent positive-pressure breathing may have a clinical benefit in patients with severe kyphoscoliosis and chronic ventilatory failure. Finally, the results of several studies of adult patients with severe kyphoscoliosis in chronic ventilatory failure suggest that chronic nocturnal mechanical ventilation is safe and effective therapy in such patients (Garay et al., 1981b; Hoeppner et al., 1984; Fulkerson et al., 1984).

Ankylosing Spondylitis

Etiology

Ankylosing spondylitis is a rheumatic disorder of unknown etiology, which causes fibrosis and ossification of ligamentous structures of the spine and rib cage. The close association of this disease with the HLA-B27 histocompatibility antigen and the increased familial prevalence suggest a strong genetic susceptibility to ligamentous and joint capsule ossification. Approximately 20% of Caucasians with HLA-B27 will manifest some feature of ankylosing spondylitis. In addition, 95% of Caucasions with primary ankylosing spondylitis have the HLA-B27 type.

Ankylosing spondylitis is a systemic disorder whose diagnosis is made using clinical criteria (Calin, 1985). The clinical criteria for diagnosis include: (1) chronic low back pain with limitation of spinal motion; (2) radiographic evidence of bilatera sacroiliitis; and (3) limitation of chest wall expansion (less than 2.5 cm measured at the level of the 4th intercostal space). This disease is a common one in that approximately 1% of Caucasians may have both the HLA-B27 type and one or more of the clinical criteria for ankylosing spondylitis. This disease is systemic in that iritis, cardiac disease (aortic insufficiency and heart block), and peripheral arthritis may be involved in as many as 10–20% of patients with long-term ankylosing spondylitis. The pulmonary complications of ankylosing spondylitis are discussed in Chapter 8.

Clinical Features

The clinical presentation of the majority of patients with ankylosing spondylitis is one of back pain. Few of these patients have predominant complaints of pulmonary disease, although some may experience mild exercise intolerance. Less than 1% of these patients develop the classic bamboo spine. Ventilatory failure is uncommon unless the patient has underlying lung disease or diaphragmatic dysfunction.

Although the motion of the rib cage may be severely restricted, patients usually display only small restrictive ventilatory dificit on pulmonary function testing (Gacad and Hamosh, 1973; Grimby et al., 1974). Descent of the diaphragm is unimpaired, which partially accounts for the fact that the restrictive deficit is mild (Table 8). There is a decrease in vital capacity and total lung capacity that is proportional to the radiographic severity of spinal ankylosis. Because the thoracic cage is often restricted in an inspiratory position, both functional residual capacity and residual volume are increased above the predicted levels. The diffusing capacity and lung compliance are normal. The Pao_2 may be slightly decreased with a widened alveolar-arterial difference; this is due to increased venous admixture and ventilation-perfusion mismatching. Some exercise limitation may also be present in patients with ankylosing spondylitis (Elliot et al., 1985).

Treatment

The medical therapy for adult patients with ankylosing spondylitis is both preventive and supportive. Patients with ankylosing spondylitis should not smoke tobacco. These patients should be managed by a clinician skillful in the treatment of rheumatic disease. Baseline chest films and spirometry are clearly indicated. Referral to a pulmonologist is indicated for abnormal chest films, deteriorating lung volumes, hypoxemia, hypercapnea, or symptoms of pulmonary disease.

Thoracoplasty

The use of thoracoplasty as a form of collapse therapy for cavitary pumonary tuberculosis ceased when effective chemotherapy was introduced. However, many patients who were subjected to thoracoplasty are still alive and are experiencing significant respiratory insufficiency and failure. Phillips et al. (1987) traced 171 patients who had been operated on between 1951 and 1953 and found over half to be alive in 1985. Of the 65 deaths, 19 were attributed to cardiorespiratory failure, and eight of the survivors had developed respiratory failure. Significant risk factors included preoperative cavitary disease, a previous articil pneumothorax on the opposite side, older age at operation, and male sex.

The pulmonary functional impairment is predominantly restrictive, but has an obstructive component (Bredin, 1989). Fifteen patients who had survived for 30 years had, on average, 50%reductions in VC and MVV, a 60% reduction in $FEV_1$and a 40% reduction in TLC. The FRC was 70%, and RV 90% of predicted; RV/TLC was 50% and FEV_1/FVC was 60%. The single breath diffusing capacity was 65% of predicted, but when corrected for lung volume, the diffusing capacity was normal. There was no correlation with the extent of the thoracoplasty (number of ribs removed or the number of surgical stages), and part of the pulmonary functional deficit in these patients was thought to have been caused by cigarette smoking and/or the extent of lung destruction by tuberculosis. Two of these patients developed ventilatory failure.

Flail Chest

The term "flail chest" denotes a condition in which the chest deforms markedly with quiet breathing, consequent to multiple rib fractures (Todd and Shamji, 1985). It is the result of blunt trauma, incurred as a result of falls from high places, automobile accidents, and airplane crashes. Patients with flail chest frequently have severe associated injuries such as fractures of long bones or vertebrae, head trauma, rupture of the aortic arch or other arteries, and laceration of the liver or spleen. Other pulmonary complications, which occur in about 60% of patients, include pulmonary contusion and hemothorax or pneumothorax (Landercasper et al., 1984). Not surprisingly, the mortality rate is high and long-term disability is relatively common; in one series, chest tightness, pain, or dyspnea and mild spirometric abnormalities were present in over half of 32 patients, and only 12 had returned to full-time work (Landercasper et al., 1984).

Mechanical ventilation as a "pneumatic splint" has been a mainstary of therapy since its introduction in 1956, but this did not reduce mortality. For example, the mortality rate for 543 patients treated with tracheostomy and continuous mechanical ventilation was 31% (Shackleford et al., 1976). Three reports compared the effects of continuous mechanical ventilation with a volume-cycled ventilator in 65 patients with either intermittent mandatory ventilation (IMV) and positive end-expiratory pressure (PEEP) in 16 patients (Cullen et al., 1975) or no mechanical ventilation in 21 patients (Trinkle et al., 1975; Shackleford et al., 1976). The mortality rate averaged 18% for the continuous mechanical ventilation group, 6% for the IMV—PEEP group, and 0% for the nonventilated group. The corresponding complication rates were 73%, 38%, and 28%, respectively; i.e., the rate of complications related to treatment was significantly lower when there was either no mechanical ventilation or ventilation with IMV and PEEP instead of continuous mechanical ventilation. Part of the problem is that mechanical ventilation increases rather than decreases the distortion of the chest wall (Tzelepis et al., 1989).

Despite these results, the issue of whether or not the distortion of the chest is important remains controversial. It is clear that the underlying lung contusion is a major part of the flail chest syndrome, and the more serious complications include pneumonia, adult respiratory distress syndrome, pleural effusions, and tracheal injury consequent to long-term intubation and tracheostome. The essential components of treatment include pain control, incentive spirometry, mechanical ventilation with PEEP for severe hypoxemia, and adjustment of ventilatroy settings to minimize or avoid negative swings in pleural pressure. Surgical fixation of the rib cage may be indicated in some patients (Thomas et al., 1978).

Other Deformities

Pectus Excavatum

The sternum may be abnormally depressed (pectus excavatum) or abnormally protuberant (pectus carinatum). Pectus excavatum is probably due to a congenital defect in the connective tissue surrounding the sternum. Pectus excavatum is frequently associated with congenital connective tissue disorders, including Marfan's syndrome. Pectus carinatum is of unknown etiology and is associated with congenital heart disease (atrial septal defect and ventricular septal defect). In addition, pectus carinatum has been associated with severe childhood asthma and rickets.

The majority of patients with congenital deformities of the sternum are free of pulmonary symptoms. These patients generally show no significant abnormalities on pulmonary function testing although some patients do have a mildly decreased vital capacity (Castile et al., 1982; Mead et al., 1985). Exercise testing is also generally normal, although a minority of patients show a small decrease in their exercise tolerance. Since congenital deformities of the sternum rarely produce cardiorespiratory debility, surgical therapy is usually reserved as a correction of the cosmetic deformity in these patients. One potential complication of the extensive surgery required to correct sternal deformities is a small decrease in both FEV_1 and FVC (Derveaux et al., 1988, 1989).

Achondroplasia

Achondroplasia is a skeletal dysplasia characterized by shortening of the proximal limbs, a large head, and narrowing of the spinal canal. Respiratory complications, including recurrent pulmonary infiltrates, sleep apnea, chronic hypoxemia, cor pulmonale, and sudden death, occur in about 10% of children with achondroplasia (Stokes et al., 1988). For the most part these problems are related to the abnormalities of ventilatory control. Chest wall deformities also occur, including pectus excavatum, thoracic kyphosis, and lumbar lordosis (Stokes et al., 1990). The VC is approximately 70% of that predicted for normally proportioned subjects and is thought to be reduced out of proportion to the patients' size (Stokes et al., 1988, 1990).

B. Obesity

Uncomplicated Obesity

Obesity is a common and potentially serious medical problem. Obesity is an excess of adipose tissue; this excess tissue is often expressed by the relationship of body weight to an "ideal body weight" normalized for height and sex. In general, body weights of greater than 110–120% of ideal weight are said to represent obesity. This condition is common in that approximately one-third of adults in the United States weight more than 120% of their ideal body weight. Even moderate degrees of obesity may endanger health; the Framingham study shows a body weight of greater than 120% ideal body weight is associated with increased health risks. Other studies show that the risks of atherosclerotic cardiovascular disease, diabetes mellitus, and degenerative joint disease are increased in obese patients.

The precise degree of obesity associated with respiratory compromise is unclear. However, most of the respiratory studies in obese patients define obesity as being 150–200% of ideal body weight. Another estimate of overweight is the body mass index, which is the ratio of body weight (kg) to height (m) squared. The upper limit of normal is 28 kg/m^2, and morbidly obese patients generally exceed 40 kg/m^2 (Kelly et al., 1988). It is important to recognize that for a given degree of overweight, the hypercapnic obese subjects, i.e., those with the obesity-hypoventilation syndrome (OHS), are as different physiologically from eucapnic obese subjects (OB) as the eucapnic obese subjects are from normal subjects (Zwillich et al., 1975).

Respiratory Mechanics

The effects of simple obesity uncomplicated by upper or lower airway deisease were revealed in a study of 43 healthy, young, nonsmoking obese subjects whose body weight exceeded 160% of ideal (Ray et al., 1983). The VC, FRC, TLC, and MVV were within the normal range by standard predictive equations in all but the most obese subjects. Only those subjects whose weight/height ratio (kg/cm) was greater than unity had lung volumes below the predicted normal value. Similar results were obtained by Kelly et al. (1988), who studied 45 patients whose average age was 38 years, and whose weight was 180% of ideal. Airway resistance as measured by the ratio of FEV_1/FVC is not increased in obese patients without underlying lung disease (Zwillich et al., 1975; Leech et al., 1987).

Obesity may have profound effects on the compliance of the respiratory system and the work of breathing (Sharp et al., 1964). The compliance of the chest wall is relatively normal in simple obesity (Suratt et al., 1984), even though one would expect that the increased weight pressing on the thoracic cage and abdomen of markedly obese subjects would make the chest wall stiff and noncompliant (Zwillich et al., 1975). In fact, the weight does present an added load, but it is of the threshold type, that is, a weight that has to be lifted to inspire (Suratt et al., 1984). Chest wall compliance falls when obese subjects change from the sitting to the supine position (Morgan and Zwillich, 1978). Compliance of the lung is also decreased in obesity, in part due to the increased pulmonary blood volume (Rochester and Enson, 1974), and in part to increased closure of dependant airways (Zwillich et al., 1975). Given the stiffer lungs and, at times, chest walls, it is not surprising that mechanical work and oxygen cost of breathing are increased (Rochester and Enson, 1974; Zwillich et al., 1975; Morgan and Zwillich, 1978).

Obesity produces a restrictive ventilatory deficit that becomes clearly evident as patients become increasingly obese (Table 8). The compression of lung tissue by the excess fat on the thoracic cage and in the abdomen decrease FRC, ERV, and TLC in patients with severe obesity (Zwillich et al., 1975; Morgan and Zwillich, 1978; Leech et al., 1987; Chan et al., 1989). In addition, both VC and MVV are decreased in obese subjects, in proportion to their body weight and chest wall compliance (Zwillich et al., 1975; Morgan and Zwillich, 1978; Lopata and Onal, 1982). Both impaired respiratory muscle function and a noncompliant respiratory system appear to play a role in the decreases in VC and MVV (Rochester and Enson, 1974; Zwillich et al., 1975; Lopata and Onal, 1982).

Gas Exchange

Severely obese subjects are hypoxemic with a widened A-aPO_2 difference (Rochester and Enson, 1974; Zwillich et al., 1975; Morgan and Zwillich, 1978). Ventilation and perfusion are mismatched, because the well-perfused lung bases are underventilated due to airway closure and alveolar collapse (Garay et al., 1981a; Jones et al., 1985; Hurewitz et al., 1985). The majority of patients with severe obesity are eucapnic, even though obesity produces a greater demand on the ventilatory system to maintain a normal $PaCO_2$. Obese subjects have a larger carbon dioxide production than nonobese subjects (Rapoport et al., 1986; Leech et al.,

1987) and must expend an increased amount of work to excrete CO_2 owing to the increased stiffness of the respiratory system.

Respiratory Muscle Function

Eucapnic obese patients have normal respiratory muscle strength, as evidenced by normal maximal respiratory pressures. However, the energy required to breathe is increased (Rochester and Enson, 1974), and obese patients manifest an increased diaphragmatic electrical activity (EMG) compared to normal subjects, both at rest and with CO_2-stimulated hypercapnia (Lourenco, 1969; Millman, 1986). This suggests that respiratory muscle efficiency is decreased owing to mechanical disadvantage.

Respiratory Effects of Weight Loss

Several reports describe pulmonary function and arterial blood gases before and after weight loss, induced by small-bowel bypass or gastric surgery (Jacobsen et al., 1974; Thomas et al., 1989; Sugerman et al., 1986) or by very-low-calorie diets (Farebrother et al., 1974). In general, these studies show that in massively obese subjects, weight loss of 10–50 kg increases vital capacity, ERV, and MVV and has little or no effect on airway resistance (FEV_1/FVC). Weight loss of 40–50 kg may also increase Pa_{O_2} in eucapnic obese patients (Chan et al., 1989), but not always (Farebrother et al., 1974).

Obesity-Hypoventilation Syndrome

Definition and Etiology

The obesity-hypoventilation syndrome (OHS) is characterized by the clinical triad of obesity, daytime hypoventilation, and excessive somnolence (Morgan and Zwillich, 1978). It appears that most patients with OHS also have obstructive sleep apnea (Block et al., 1979; Harman et al., 1981). OHS is an uncommon condition that has been extensively studied by investigators interested in the control of breathing and disordered breathing during sleep. Most studies on the etiology of OHS have focused on the problem of hypoventilation and have demonstrated that hypoventilation is not simply due to extreme obesity, but probably results from an imbalance between ventilatory drive and ventilatory load (Rochester and Enson, 1974; Zwillich et al., 1975; Garay et al., 1981b; Lopata and Onal, 1982; Jones et al., 1985; Chan et al., 1989).

The decrease in ventilatory drive may be either inherited or acquired as a result of sleep deprivation, excessive alcohol intake, or use of other sedatives. The increased ventilatory loads inhibiting ventilation and gas exchange in these patients include: *obesity* with its increased work of breathing and interference with the mechanical efficiency of ventilation (Rochester and Enson, 1974); *heart failure* (Rochester and Enson, 1974); *diffuse airway obstruction* (Bradley et al., 1986; Krieger et al., 1989); and the recurrent apneas and blood gas derangements of *obstructive sleep apnea* (Jones et al., 1985; Rapoport et al., 1986).

Recent studies suggest that there may be several subgroups of patients with OHS, based on their predominant clinical features. Some patients have diffuse airway obstruction (Bradley et al., 1986; Krieger et al., 1989), whereas other patients have little clinical or physiological evidence of obstruction (Rochester and Enson, 1974; Jones et al., 1985; Chan et al., 1989). Some patients with OHS have little or no obstructive sleep apnea, but the majority of the patients do have this complication (Tassinari et al., 1972; Millman, 1986). There are also differences in the response to treatment. Some obese patients with obstructive sleep apnea improve their daytime ventilation after successful treatment of the sleep apnea with tracheostomy or nasal continuous positive airway pressure (CPAP), whereas in others the daytime hypercapnia persists despite successful treatment of the apnea (Rapoport et al., 1986). Thus, the etiology of OHS may well differ among these subgroups.

Clinical Features

OHS is significantly correlated with the presence of recurrent apneas and hypoxemia during sleep in men and postmenopausal women (Block et al., 1979; Harman et al., 1981). The findings on history and physical examination define this syndrome. Patients are severely hypersomnolent and fall asleep at the most inappropriate times; they may fall asleep while eating, while standing, or while being interviewed by their physician. Although snoring is not a universal finding, these patients are often legendary snorers with a long history of loud and disruptive snoring. On physical examination, the patients are obese, often weighing more than 50% above their predicted weights. They may have a ruddy complexion and/or cyanosis due to hypoxemia and secondary erythrocytosis. They often have a short, thick neck, an enlarged uvula, and a small oropharynx. Examination of the chest may disclose crackles or wheezes, and one may be able to demonstrate hepatomegaly, peripheral edema, and other findings of right ventricular heart failure.

Chest radiographs show an enlarged heart and small lung fields with pulmonary congestion. Electrocardiograms often demonstrate right atrial and ventricular enlargement. Arterial blood gases show hypoxemia and hypercapnia, with a widened (A-a)PO_2 difference. However, these patients can voluntarily hyperventilate and normalize their $PaCO_2$. Approximately one-half of these patients have erythrocytosis. Spirometry demonstrates lowered VC, FEV_1, and MVV. Some patients also have evidence of superimposed airway obstruction, i.e., FEV_1/FVC of less than 75%. The deficits in VC and MVV are far worse in OHS than in simple obesity, in part because in OHS, the compliance of the lungs and chest wall are so low (Rochester and Enson, 1974).

Respiratory muscle weakness and mechanical disadvantage contribute to poor performance on the pulmonary function tests, and almost certainly to ventilatory failure as well. Patients with OHS have moderate decreases in inspiratory muscle strength (Rochester and Arora, 1980; Kelly et al., 1988), and this persists after treatment (Sampson and Grassino, 1983). In severely obese subjects the diaphragm may be overstretched, at least in the supine position (Sharp et al., 1986), which places the muscle at a mechanical disadvantage, and which therefore contributes to the decreased inspiratory strength and ventilatory efficiency observed in obese patients. In addition, the oxygen cost and mechanical work of breathing are especially high in OHS.

Diagnosis

The clinical evaluation of patients with OHS should focus on any conditions that could contribute to persistent daytime hypoventilation, i.e., hypothyroidism, severe sleep apnea, or respiratory muscle weakness. In addition, one must consider other sources of ventilatory impairment, such as left ventricular heart failure and diffuse airway disease. Each patient should have a careful history and complete physical examination, thyroid function tests, arterial blood gases, spirometry, and measurement of maximal mouth inspiratory and expiratory pressures. Tests of ventilatory control show a diminished response to both hypercapnia an hypoxemia. All patients with OHS should also have a full-night sleep study; these usually demonstrate moderate to severe obstructive sleep apnea with prolonged apneic periods accompanied by profound arterial oxymemoglobin desaturation. However, one may also find severe hypopnea or central apnea.

Prognosis

There are no reports describing the results of long-term follow-up of large numbers of patients with OHS. However, the studies that are available suggest that these patients have a high risk of in-hospital morbidity and mortality from their disorder. Miller and Granada (1974) followed 10 patients for 5 years and found that 70% died; three patients died due to hypercapnic respiratory failure, three died of pulmonary embolism, and one died of acute renal failure. MacGregor et al. (1970) followed 22 patients with OHS and also found a high mortality rate, with 7 of the 22 patients dying within a 10 year period and the surviving patients having many complications from their disease. They concluded that serious complications are frequent in this group of patients and that sudden unexpected death is common.

Treatment

Patients with OHS have a life-threatening disorder that may be reversible with appropriate treatment. An aggressive approach to evaluation and treatment is necessary to avoid the complications of acute ventilatory decompensation and sudden death. The principles of therapy are to *reduce the ventilatory load* and to *increase ventilatory drive*.

Ventilatory drive can be enhanced by progesterone, and treatment with progesterone and analogs has improved daytime ventilation and oxygenation in some patients with sleep apnea (Sutton et al., 1975; Kimura et al., 1989). The use of these agents is limited by concerns about the occurrence of male sexual impotency and a possible increase in the risk of cardiovascular or thromboembolic disease. The potential risk of thromboembolic desease is of particular concern, because obesity and inactivity are also significant risk factors for deep-vein thrombosis and pulmonary embolism. Sedatives and other ventilatory depressants should also be avoided. Nocturnal and daytime oxygen supplementation must be used with caution to avoid ventilatory depression and worsening hypercapnia.

The most important step in decreasing ventilatory load is to lose weight. Weight loss decreases the work of breathing, increases vital capacity, and increases ventilatory drive in patients with OHS (Rochester and Enson, 1974). Moreover, reduction of body weight of 20–40 kg has normalized $Paco_2$ in patients with OHS (Rochester and Enson, 1974; Sugerman et al., 1986). In addition, weight loss in both massively and moderately obese patients is associated with an improvement in apneas and hypoxemia during sleep (Harman et al., 1982; Smith et al., 1985; Suratt et al., 1987). Unfortunately, it is very difficult for patients with OHS to maintain a permanent weight loss. It may require long-term in-hospital treatment or surgical therapy to realize this goal. Treating obstructive airways disease and left heart failure will also diminish ventilatory load and improve ventilation.

Treating sleep apnea with either tracheostomy or nasal continuous positive airway pressure improves daytime ventilation and normalizes daytime $Paco_2$ in approximately half of patients with OHS and obstructive sleep apnea who are so treated (Rapoport et al., 1986). Preventing the recurrent apneas and blood gas derangements of obstructive sleep apnea may decrease ventilatory load as well as improve daytime ventilatory drive. However, the exact mechanism responsible for the improvement in daytime ventilation remains unclear (Findley, 1987). Recent reports show successful treatment of central alveolar hypoventilation during sleep with intermittent positive-pressure ventilation through a nasal mask (Ellis et al., 1987; Guillenimault et al., 1989; Bach and Alba, 1990a). Although these subjects were nonobese, these studies suggest a role for nasal ventilation in treating the obesity-hypoventilation syndrome. Positive-pressure ventilation by nose mask and other means is covered in more detail in Section V.

IV. Complications of Neuromuscular and Skeletal Diseases

A. Mechanical Factors That Compromise Pulmonary Defenses

Predisposing Factors

Both the muscles responsible for maintaining the caliber of the upper airways and those responsible for pharyngeal function and swallowing are often involved in various diffuse neuromuscular diseases. A break in the integrity of the swallowing mechanism allows spillage of oropharyngeal contents into the trachea and subsequent aspiration into the lungs. Aspiration is especially likely to cause pneumonia in patients with neuromuscular disease because they cannot cough effectively. In addition, the restriction of chest wall motion characteristic of neuromuscular and skeletal diseases also predisposes to the development of atelectasis and pneumonia.

Atelectasis and pneumonia are the principal respiratory complications of spinal cord injury. Mansel and Norman (1990) recommend frequent position changes, deep breaths, assisted coughs, chest percussion, bronchoscopy as indicated, and bronchodilators. Aspiration, atelectasis, and pneumonia are also well-recognized complications in patients with other forms of severe respiratory muscle weakness and ventilatory failure who require prolonged mechanical ventilation (Gracey et al., 1982; Schmidt-Nowara and Altman, 1984).

Respiratory System Compliance

The vital capacity in neuromuscular disease is almost always substantially lower than can be explained by muscle weakness alone (De Troyer et al., 1980). That is because the compliance of the respiratory system is considerably reduced in neuromuscular diseases (Ferris et al., 1952b; Gibson et al., 1977b; De Troyer et al., 1980). Much of the reduction in respiratory system compliance can be attributed to large reductions in lung compliance, although the reason for this is not readily apparent. Leading hypotheses are, first, that there is "microatelectasis," second, that surfactant activity is decreased by the long-standing limitation to lung inflation, and third, that the fibrous skeleton of the lung is remodeled. Positive-pressure breathing to inflate the lungs two to three times the patient's inspiratory capacity had no effect on lung compliance or volumes in neuromuscular diseases (De Troyer and Deisser, 1981; McCool et al., 1986).

The other cause of decreased respiratory system compliance is increased stiffness of the chest wall (Ferris et al., 1952b; Estenne et al., 1983; Estenne and De Troyer, 1986). Typically, the compliance of the chest wall is about two-thirds of normal. For the most part, the reduction in chest wall compliance results from a sharp reduction in the compliance of the rib cage, with relatively little change in abdominal compliance (Estenne and De Troyer, 1986). The mechanism of the rib cage stiffness in not known, but could reflect changes in rib articulations with the spine, in ligaments, or in muscles.

Respiratory system compliance is also abnormally low in skeletal disorders. Again, the deficit is partly in the lungs and partly in the chest wall (Sinha and Bergofsky, 1972; Kafer, 1975; Jones et al., 1981; Cooper et al., 1984). However, unlike the situation in neuromuscular disease, positive-pressure breathing and lung inflation improved lung compliance in patients with kyphoscoliosis by 70%, and the improvement lasted for 3 hr (Sinha and Bergofsky, 1972). After prolonged intermittent positive-pressure hyperinflation, the improvement in VC persisted for 9 months (Simonds et al., 1989). Lung compliance is normal in uncomplicated ankylosing spondylitis (Gacad and Hamosh, 1973), and chest wall excursion is diminished because of the impaired rib motion (Grimby et al., 1974).

Cough Mechanics

In order for cough to be effective, there must be an initial deep inspiration followed by adduction of the vocal cords. With the cords adducted, the abdominal muscles contract against the diaphragm to generate a large head of expiratory pressure (Van Lunteren et al., 1988). With sudden opening of the vocal cords, there is immediate dynamic compression of the vocal cord into a slit so that the explosive outrush of air achieves a very high velocity and kinetic energy (Knudson et al., 1974). Studies of curarized normal volunteers suggest that the loss of dynamic tracheal compression is a more important consequence of expiratory muscle weakness than loss of expiratory volume (Arora and Gal, 1981). Thus, it can be seen that cough depends on the adequacy of three sets of muscles: those that govern the integrity of the upper airway and those that regulate the strength of inspiration and expiration.

Szeinberg et al. (1988) evaluated cough capacity in 22 adolescents with muscular dystrophy and found that only 10 patients were able to generate the transients of peak flow that reflect dynamic compression of the airways. Patients who could not develop these flow transients had lower values of PEFR, FVC, and PE_{max}, and PE_{max} was the best predictor of the ability to produce flow transients. In effect, flow transients were present when PE_{max} exceeded 60 cm H_2O, and absent when PE_{max} was less than 45 cm H_2O. Patients with high thoracic and low to midcervical spinal cord injury lose motor innervation to abdominal and thoracic expiratory muscles and have a very limited cough capacity (Siebens et al., 1964). Estenne and De Troyer (1990) have shown that the clavicular portion of the pectoralis major muscle plays a major role in coughing in tetraplegic patients, and they suggest that training the pectoralis muscle might result in more effective cough. To overcome the inefficiency that results from protrusion of the abdomen, abdominal compression would also be needed.

Mucociliary Clearance

Mucus production is abnormal and tracheal bronchial clearance is impaired in some patients with neuromuscular diseases. About 20% of patients with acute quadriplegia produce an excessive volume of tenacious sputum, rich in glycoprotein (Bhaskar et al., 1991). As this syndrome has a sudden onset and spontaneous recovery, it is thought to represent an abnormality of autonomic nervous system control. In a group of patients who had severe bilateral weakness of the diaphragm, mucociliary clearance from the trachea and bronchi was markedly depressed (Mier et al., 1990a). Although the initial topographic distribution of radioactive aerosol was similar in patients and normal controls, the extent of clearance after 6 hr was only half the normal value in the patients with neuromuscular diseases. It is not yet clear to what extent the limitation in clearance is due to compromise of mucociliary function, as opposed to being a consequence of the severe mechanical restriction of lung inflation.

B. Pulmonary Embolism

Deep venous thrombosis is said to be present in almost all patients with spinal cord injury (Myllynen et al., 1985). Therefore, routine heparin prophylaxis is recommended (Merli et al., 1988). Pulmonary embolism is relatively uncommon, but a syndrome closely simulating acute pulmonary embolism in quadriplegic patients can result from acute mucus plugging (Dee et al., 1984). In other forms of neuromuscular disease, fatal pulmonary embolism has been quite common in the past, occurring in up to 20% of patients with acute inflammatory polyneuropathy (Raman et al., 1971). The two deaths attributed to pulmonary embolism by Gracey et al. (1982) occurred in patients who did not receive prophylactic therapy.

Pulmonary hypertension due to small-vessel disease has been described in polymyositis and dermatomyositis and may be relatively common (see also Chapter 8, "Rheumatological Diseases"). In one series, 7 of 11 patients with polymyositis had echo/Doppler evidence of pulmonary hypertension, even though maximal respiratory pressures were normal. Pulmonary function was within normal limits in five patients and minimally restrictive in two others (Hebert et al., 1990).

C. Pathogenesis of CO_2 Retention

Control of Breathing

Decreased Neural Drive

It has been well documented that a few patients with neuromuscular disease exhibit impaired ventilatory control while awake, which is manifest by impaired ventilatory responses to hypercapnia, hypoxia, or both (Solliday et al., 1974; Bellamy et al., 1975; Riley et al., 1977; Carroll et al., 1977; Wilson et al., 1987). The impaired ventilatory control cannot readily be ascribed to muscle weakness per se, since the patients described in these reports had minimal to mild weakness. The diagnoses of these patients included poliomyelitis (Solliday et al., 1974), myotonic dystrophy (Carroll et al., 1977), and congenital myopathies (Bellamy et al., 1975; Riley et al., 1977; Weng et al., 1985; Wilson et al., 1987). It should be emphasized that these cases occur sporadically and infrequently, and that the principal cause of ventilatory failure in the great majority of patients with neuromuscular disease is muscle weakness, not an abnormally low neural drive to breathe.

Reduction in ventilatory drive may also contribute to the pathogenesis of OHS. Specifically, patients with OHS have markedly decreased hypoxic ventilatory responses to hypoxia or to hypoxia and hypercapnia (Lourenco, 1969; Kronenberg et al., 1977; Zwillich et al., 1975; Lopata and Onal, 1982; Bradley et al., 1986). Of interest, the depressed hypercapnic response could be restored toward normal by a ketogenic diet (Fried et al., 1976). The responses of mouth occlusion pressure ($P_{0.1}$) and diaphragmatic electrical activity to hypercapnic stimuli are also reduced (Lourenco, 1969; Lopata and Onal, 1982). Notwithstanding these observations, it seems likely that obstructive sleep apnea plays a far larger role in the pathogenesis of OHS than does the reduction of ventilatory drive (Block et al., 1979; Harman et al., 1981; Lopata and Onal, 1982).

Abnormal Breathing During Sleep

In many patients with neuromuscular disease the abnormality of ventilatory control manifests itself primarily during sleep (Skatrud et al., 1980; Carre et al., [1988; Smith et al., 1988a, 1989; Steljes et al., 1990). These patients exhibit profound hypopnea and hypoxemia, especially during REM sleep. The same phenomena occur in patients with OHS (Jones et al., 1985; Rapoport et al., 1986) and kyphoscoliosis (Sawicka and Branthwaite, 1987). These patients do not have obstructive sleep apnea. Instead, their minute ventilation falls, especially in REM sleep, because the tidal volume (VT) is too small; This phenomenon reflects the reduction in the activity of limb, postural, and respiratory muscles that is characteristic of REM sleep (Johnson and Remmers, 1984; Millman et al., 1988).

Increased Ventilatory Drive

Neural drive to breathe is increased—not decreased—in most patients with muscle weakness, neuromuscular disease, skeletal disease, and obesity. Neural drive cannot be measured directly, but can be inferred from mouth occulsion pressure ($P_{0.1}$). An experiment that involved administration of *d*-tubocurarine, to normal subjects showed that the $P_{0.1}$ reflects ventilatory drive, despite severe muscle weakness. With increasing doses of *d*-tubocurarine, the $P_{0.1}$ increased exponentially as PI_{max} decreased, so that when PI_{max} had fallen to 23% of its baseline value, the $P_{0.1}$ measured at a $Paco_2$ of 45 mmHg was 2.2 times its baseline value (Holle et al.,1984). In other words, the $P_{0.1}$ test is nearly impervious to severe muscle weakness.

Patients with neuromuscular disease have a similar increase in $P_{0.1}$. This is true for diffuse neuromuscular diseases where PI_{max} was approximately half normal (Begin et al., 1982; Baydur, 1991). Another indicator of ventilatory drive is the mean inspiratory flow rate, which is the tidal volume (VT) divided by the duration of inspiration (Ti). In contrast to $P_{0.1}$, VT/Ti is normal in neuromuscular disease (Begin et al., 1982; Baydur 1991). Indeed, in normal subjects breathing CO_2, the $P_{0.1}$ increases faster than VT/Ti, thus giving rise to the concept of the "effective impedance" of the respiratory system. Effective impedance, expressed as $P_{0.1}$/(VT/Ti), is approximately twice normal in patients with neuromuscular disease (Begin et al., 1982; Baydur, 1991). Values for $P_{0.1}$, VT/Ti, and effective impedance in neuromuscular disease, eucapnic obesity, and normal subjects are summarized in Table 9.

Patients with kyphoscoliosis have either normal or slightly low ventilatory responses to CO_2 inhalation (Bergofsky, 1979), and the magnitude of the response is proportional to the degree of mechanical limitation and lung volume restriction (Kafer, 1975). Eucapnic obese patients generally have increased hypoxic and hypercapnic ventilatory drives (Lourenco, 1969; Lopata and Onal, 1982; Leech et al., 1987; Krieger et al., 1989), and these responses return toward normal after weight loss (Chapman, Himal and Rebuck, 1990). In simple obesity and former OHS patients, $P_{0.1}$ is approximately twice normal (Sampson and Grassino, 1983). Unlike neuromuscular disease, VT/Ti is elevated in the eucapnic obese subjects (Sampson and Grassino, 1983; Burki and Baker, 1984). In addition, the effective impedance, $P_{0.1}$/(VT/Ti), is higher than normal.

Pattern of Breathing

Values that characterize the pattern of breathing, respiratory rate (RR), tidal volume, (VT), and fractional duration of inspiration (Ti/Ttot), in patients with neuromuscular disease and eucapnic obesity and in normal subjects are summarized in Table 9. The data in the table have been calculated from mean values from four reports (Begin et al., 1982; Sampson and Grassino, 1983; Burki and Baker, 1984; Baydur, 1991). It can be seen that the respiratory rate is higher, and the tidal volume smaller, in patients with neuromuscular disease. In two

Table 9 Values that Characterize the Pattern of Breathing and the Drive to Breathe in Neuromuscular Disease (NMD), Eucapnic Morbid Obesity (OB), and Normal Subjects (NLS)

Variable	NMD	OBE	NLS
RR (br/min)	24	16	14
VT (ml)	400	730	570
Ti/Ttot	0.43	0.38	0.44
VT/Ti (l/sec)	0.35	0.50	0.36
$P_{0.1}$ (cm H_20)	1.7	2.0	0.9
$P_{0.1}$/(VT/Ti)	4.9	4.0	2.6

well-studied patients, the pattern of breathing was analyzed in terms of regional ventilation (Easton et al., 1983) or rib cage and abdominal components (Grimman and Whitelaw, 1983). Both patients exhibited new patterns of respiratory muscle contraction, consistent with the patterns adopted by normal subjects who are confronted by increased ventilatory loads.

The eucapnic obese patients have a near-normal pattern of breathing (Sampson and Grassino, 1983; Burki and Baker, 1984). Evidently this requires an increased neural drive, to overcome the added ventilatory load. Tidal volume is also normal in ankylosing spondylitis (Grimby et al., 1974), but in kyphoscoliosis VT is reduced to the same extent that it is in neuromuscular diseases, i.e., approximately 70% of normal.

Hypercapnic patients have significantly smaller tidal volumes and higher respiratory rates than their eucapnic counterparts (Table 10). The hypercapnic patients with kyphoscoliosis have slightly, but not significantly, larger scoliosis angles, and they are older than the eucapnic kyphoscoliosis patients (Kafer, 1976). The hypercapnic obese patients (OHS) do not weigh significantly more than the eucapnic obese subjects (Kaufman et al., 1959). In both groups of hypercapnic patients, the RR is approximately 33% greater, and the VT is 33% smaller, than in the eucapnic counterparts. Comparable data are not available for neuromuscular disease, but the VT is smaller during acute ventilatory failure. In acute inflammatory polyneuropathy and myasthenia gravis, the VT recovers during recovery from ventilatory failure and weaning from mechanical ventilation (Borel et al., 1991). Moreover, during trials of weaning from mechanical ventilation, failure to wean was significantly correlated with the magnitude of decrement in VT during the trial.

Table 10 Physiological Variables in Eucapnic and Hypercapnic Patients with Kyphoscoliosis (KS) or Obesity (OB-OHS)

Group	Variable	Eucapnic	Hypercapnic
KS	$Paco_2$ (mmHg)	39	52
	Scoliosis angle (°)	79	99
	RR (br/min)	17	22
	VT (ml)	420	300
	PI_{max} (cm H_20)	53	27
OB-OHS	$Paco_2$ (mmHg)	39	56
	Body weight (% ideal)	179	196
	RR (br/min)	18	23
	VT (ml)	500	330
	PI_{max} (cm H_20)	90	65

Inspiratory Effort

In neuromuscular diseases, the pressure required to inspire during quiet breathing (P_{breath}) is about 40% higher than normal (Borel et al., 1991), probably owing to the modest reductions in the compliance of the lungs and chest wall (Section IV.A.). Values of P_{breath} are not available for patients with kyphoscoliosis, but extrapolating from VT, lung resistance, and dynamic elastance of the repiratory system (Kafer, 1975, 1976; Baydur et alk., 1990a), it can be estimated that P_{breath} would be approximately twice normal in this disorder. In eucapnic obese patients, P_{breath} is also about twice normal (Sampson and Grassino, 1983), and it is probably either the same or slightly higher in OHS, considering the available data on respiratory system compliance and the oxygen cost of breathing (Rochester and Arora, 1980).

The magnitude of P_{breath} depends not only on respiratory system resistance and compliance, but also on the size of the breath. Because patients with neuromuscular disease, kyphoscoliosis, and OHS have smaller than normal tidal volumes (Tables 9, 10), their P_{breath} is about 40% lower than it would be if the size of the VT were normal. However, the absolute magnitude of P_{breath} is not nearly as important as its relative magnitude, which is expressed as the ratio of P_{breath} to PI_{max}. Normally, during quiet breathing P_{breath} is -5 cm H_2O, PI_{max} is -100 cm H_2O, and P_{breath}/PI_{max} is 0.05. Since PI_{max} is reduced in neuromuscular disease, kyphoscoliosis, and OHS (Tables 9, 10), P_{breath}/PI_{max} is typically two to five times normal, or even higher.

Muscle Fatigue

When P_{breath}/PI_{max} exceeds 0.3–0.4, the inspiratory muscles are subject to becoming fatigued. That does not happen unless the fatiguing pattern of breathing is sustained for several hours or more. Equally important, when P_{breath}/PI_{max} is so high, the patient perceives this as respiratory distress (Killian and Jones, 1988). It seems highly likely that the response to an increase in P_{breath}/PI_{max} to this magnitude is to reduce the size of VT, so as to minimize the sense of respiratory effort. This conclusion is supported by experiments in patients and animals subjected to inspiratory loads (Oliven et al., 1985; Adams et al., 1988), as well as by analysis of the reasons for success versus failure in trials of weaning from mechanical ventilation (Jabour et al., 1991). The reduction in VT helps to avoid inspiratory muscle fatigue, but the small tidal volume may be too small for gas exchange, expecially when dead space is increased by rapid, shallow breathing (Jabour et al., 1991).

To summarize, it is unlikely that overt *respiratory muscle fatigue* is the proximate cause of ventilatory failure. However, *respiratory muscle weakness* is a critical element in the pathogenesis of ventilatory failure, because of its effect on PI_{max}, P_{breath}, P_{breath}/PI_{max} and the sense of respiratory effort. The reductions in compliance of the lungs and chest wall, combined with any increase in airway resistance that may be present, serve to increase P_{breath}. Although the ventilatory drive, expressed as the $P_{0.1}$, remains elevated, the pattern of breathing changes in response to the elevation of P_{breath}/PI_{max}. The VT falls, which minimizes dyspnea. Because there is a compensatory increase in RR, VE is unchanged. However, because rapid shallow breathing increases dead space, the small VT is inadequate for gas exchange, and hypercapnia ensues.

V. Treatment of Ventilatory Failure

A. Body Respirators

Negative Pressure Ventilators

The first widely used mechanical ventilatory was the Drinker respirator, also known as the "iron lung" or the "tank ventilator" (Rochester and Martin, 1985). It is quiet, powerful, and works well in neuromuscular and skeletal disorders. However, owing to its weight and bulk, it is awkward to use at home. It also requires sufficient floor space to permit the inner stretcher platform to be pulled out of the outer cylinder. Putting a patient with significant generalized muscle weakness into a tank ventilator requires at least two assistants. Considerable skill is required to bring the patient's head through the end-plate, and to adjust the neck seal to minimize leakage of air. It is also important to adjust the levels of the head and body supports for optimal comfort. Complications include claustrophobia, discomfort consequent to the enforced supine position, and inadvertent aerophagia.

Two other types of negative-pressure body ventilators have been developed to overcome some of the disadvantages of the iron lung. One is the "cuirass" ventilator, which consists of a rigid shell applied to the anterior aspect of the chest and abdomen. The shell is sealed to the body by a foam rubber ring, and negative pressure is cyclically generated within the shell by an electric-motor-driven pump. The body wrap ventilator consists of a back plate and a chest cage, surrounded by a poncho-like plastic garment that can be made airtight. An electrically driven pump cyclically reduces the pressure inside the body wrap to below atmospheric, just as with the cuirass respirator.

Despite their disadvantages, negative-pressure ventilators have been used successfully for patients with a variety of neuromuscular diseases (Riley et al., 1977; Loh et al., 1979; Marino and Braun, 1982; Curran and Colbert, 1989; Mohr and Hill, 1990). In addition to relieving symptoms of polycythemia and right ventricular failure, nocturnal negative-pressure ventilation has been found to lower the $Paco_2$ by 10 mmHg or more and to increase Pao_2 to a comparable degree in patients who are able to breathe spontaneously during the day. Nocturnal mechanical ventilation was also associated with improved respiratory muscle strength and endurance (Braun and Marino, 1982; Celli et al., 1987;

Kinnear et al., 1988a). As expected, overall ventilatory and limb muscle function ultimately fails in progressive diseases such as muscular dystrophy. Nonetheless, use of negative-pressure body ventilators increased survivorship by 6 years (Curran and Colbert, 1989).

A major drawback to the use of negative-pressure ventilators is nocturnal desaturation due to obstructive sleep apnea. This can be managed using a tricyclic drug or nasal continuous positive airway pressure (Goldstein et al., 1987). In one series, significant sleep desaturation occurred in 22 of 37 patients with neuromuscular diseases and was alleviated by switching to noninvasive positive-pressure ventilation (Bach and Penek, 1991).

The cuirass and body wrap respirators have also been of great benefit to patients with kyphoscoliosis, or with chest wall deformity secondary to thoracoplasty. Sometimes it is necessary to custom-fit the cuirass to the body contours of the particular patient (Wiers et al., 1977; Fulkerson et al., 1984). Chronic nocturnal ventilation at home relieved dyspnea, pulmonary hypertension, and right ventricular failure and improved blood gas composition (Wiers, et al., 1977; Garay et al., 1981b; Sawicka et al., 1983; Fulkerson, et al., 1984; Kinnear et al., 1988b). Some patients have been followed for up to 10 years, mainly at home. One of the main benefits of negative-pressure ventilation in chest wall disease is that it markedly reduces the need for hospitalization (Wiers et al., 1977; Garay et al., 1981b; Sawicka et al., 1983). Similar results have been obtained using nocturnal ventilation via tracheostomy (Hoeppner et al., 1984). One patient was maintained with a tracheostomy and a portable ventilator for 27 years (Woolf, 1990).

Rocking Bed

For selected patients, the rocking bed is an attractive alternative to negative-pressure ventilators. This device consists of a conventional hospital bed mounted on a frame that enables it to go through an excursion of 30° feet down to 15° head down, up to 20 cycles/min. Ventilation is effected by the alternating headward and footward motion of the diaphragm, driven by the force of gravity acting on the abdominal contents. Abd et al., (1989) found the rocking bed to be particularly valuable for patients whose isolated diaphragmatic paralysis resulted from open heart surgery. The patients rapidly learned how to use the bed, and they tolerated it much better than other forms of body ventilation. The rocking bed was also useful in improving sleep architecture in quadriplegic patients (Iber, et al., 1989).

B. Noninvasive Positive-Pressure Ventilation

Nasal Intermittent Positive-Pressure Ventilation

Intermittent positive-pressure ventilation via a nasal mask is noninvasive, convenient, and relatively inexpensive. Some devices function in almost the same fashion as the far more expensive pressure support ventilators. Nasal intermittent positive-pressure ventilation (NIPPV) at night has been used successfully to treat patients with both neuromuscular disease (Ellis et al., 1987; Heckmatt et al., 1990; Bach and Alba, 1990a; Baydur et al., 1990a; Gay et al., 1991) and kyphoscoliosis (Carroll and Branthwaite, 1988; Bach and Alba, 1991a; Carrey et al., 1990; Goldstein et al., 1991). Daytime blood gas composition and ventilatory endurance are improved to approximately the same extent that occurs with negative-pressure ventilation.

Nasal ventilation may obviate the need for tracheostomy (Bach and Alba, 1990a). Nasal ventilation with positive pressure may prevent upper airway obstruction and oxyhemoglobin desaturation during sleep (Heckmatt et al., 1990), and it overcomes the upper airway obstructive phenomena seen with negative-pressure ventilators (Goldstein et al., 1987; Bach and Penek, 1991).

The complications of nose mask ventilation are mainly leaks and pressure symptoms such as irritation and ulceration, especially on the bridge of the nose. Special circuits that do not contact the nasal bridge may be used (Gay et al., 1991). Some patients tolerate nose mask ventilation poorly for psychological or other reasons, but overall acceptance seems to be around 80% (Gay et al., 1991).

Other Positive-Pressure Modalities

Mouth Intermittent Positive-Pressure Ventilation

Bach and Alba (1990c) reported their extensive experience with mouth intermittent positive-pressure ventilation (MIPPV) in quadriplegic patients with high spinal cord injury. Of 80 patients who were originally ventilator-dependent, 25 remained so. Of these, 23 were able to convert from IPPV via tracheostomy to MIPPV or to negative-pressure ventilators. Four of these patients were weaned completely, three died, and the others use MIPPV or negative-pressure ventilation from 1 to 16 hr daily. Curran and Colbert (1989) also administer MIPPV, using a Sippy mouthpiece. One would think that the leakage problem would defeat this regimen, but patients learn to take air from the mouthpiece without significant leakage.

Tracheostomy Intermittent Positive-Pressure Ventilation

In most cases of severe ventilator dependency, patients with neuromuscular or skeletal diseases have a tracheostomy. Although other forms of ventilator support such as NIPPV or MIPPV have eliminated the need for IPPV via tracheostomy (TIPPV) in many patients, some still need it. Here too, recent advances have simplified care. Bach and Alba (1990b) showed that tracheostomy ventilation may be accomplished with the cuff deflated, or even with cuffless tubes, in over 90% of totally ventilator-dependent patients. The criteria for switching to TIPPV without cuff seal are adequate ability to swallow and adequate compliance of the respiratory system.

Abdominal Positive-Pressure Ventilation

Bach and Alba (1991) have also reported their experience with abdominal positive-pressure ventilators. These devices consist of a corset under which is an air bladder. The air bladder is filled and emptied by an external pump. Filling the bladder compresses the abdomen and forces the patient to exhale. The subsequent inspiration is accomplished by passive recoil from RV to FRC. This modality was most useful for daytime support. Minute ventilation and end-tidal Pco_2 were maintained normal, and SaO_2 was generally 95% or better, with the minimum SaO_2being 86%.

Abdominal positive-pressure ventilation works best in patients with neuromuscular disease without coexisting pulmonary disease. The compliance of the respiratory system must not be too low, and the patient must be able to sit at 30° to 75°. Patients with skeletal deformity are for the most part unable to use an abdominal positive-pressure device. For the right patient, the abdominal positive-pressure mode can be used for many years, and up to 24 hr daily. One advantage of abdominal positive pressure, MIPPV, and NIPPV for patients who are nearly totally ventilator-dependent is that they can get rid of the tracheostomy tube. This in turn enables them to learn glossopharyngeal breathing (Bach and Alba, 1991).

C. Electrophrenic Respiration

High spinal cord injury is one of the few indications for electrophrenic respiration. Because the phrenic motor neurons lie at levels C3, C4, and C5 in humans, these motoneurons are largely intact when the level of injury is above C3. Thus the phrenic nerves are intact and capable of responding to electrical stimulation. Technical details have been summarized by Glenn et al. (1980). The phrenic nerves are stimulated in the neck, usually percutaneously. However, if there is no response to percutaneous stimulation, it may be necessary to expose the nerves to test their response.

Once the viability of the nerve has been established, the phrenic pacemaker is surgically implanted. It is easier to place it in the neck, but the diaphragm is more fully activated when the pacemaker is located in the thorax. It is customary to implant a pacemaker over each phrenic nerve, so they may be used in alternating fashion. After implantation, the pacemaker is activated by an external programmable power supply A typical stimulation regimen would be 10–15 impulses/sec, for 1.3 sec, 12 times a minute. The current per impulse is increased until the stimulated tidal volume is maximal. If a bipolar waveform is used and higher stimulation frequencies are avoided, there is little damage to either the nerve or the muscle (Glenn et al., 1980); Ciesielski et al., 1983).

When electrophrenic respiration is initiated long after the original injury had occurred, the diaphragm is severely atrophied and will fatigue rapidly when stimulated (Glenn et al., 1980; Nochomovitz et al., 1984). Therefore, it is necessary to begin by stimulating the phrenic nerves for only a few minutes at a time, every hour for 4–6 hr. Each day the duration and number of periods of stimulation can be increased, until the tidal volume remains constant for at least half an hour. Thereafter, the schedule is advanced to 30 min of pacing alternating with 30 min of rest, for several hours at a time. The ultimate goal is to achieve 6–12 hr of continuous pacing, which allows the patient to be free of the mechanical ventilator.

Although tidal volumes and transdiaphragmatic pressures are about 50% higher when both hemidiaphragms contract, it is not always necessary or desirable to stimluate both phrenic nerves together. Some patients do better when one hemidiaphragm is stimulated for 6 hr, then switching to the other. Overall, the process of restoring diaphragmatic contractility through electrical stimulation of the phrenic nerves is a form of muscular training. It has to start gently in order to avoid fatigue and damage to the muscle, and even after the muscle has regained contractility, care must be taken not to overstimulate or fatigue either the nerve or the muscle.

The pattern of breathing with electrophrenic respiration is quite different from spontaneous breathing. Inspiration lasts for only 25% of the breath, ,and the patient is caused to breathe slowly and deeply. Electrophrenic respiration causes outward excursions of the lower rib cage and abdomen, but the upper rib cage is pulled inward (Danon et al., 1979; Mead et al., 1984). Diaphragmatic pacing is more effective when the patients are supine, because the abdominal viscera push the diaphragm farther up into the chest during expiration, thus enabling it to sweep a large volume displacement when it is stimulated. Sitting up causes the end-expiratory position of the diaphragm to descend, so the inspiratory volume displacement is reduced (Danon et al., 1979; Mead et al., 1984). An abdominal binder offsets this problem (Mead et al., 1984). Continuous positive airway pressure (CPAP) was shown to reduce the tidal volume generated by electrophrenic respiration, as well as reducing respiratory system compliance and diaphragm length, in one well-studied patient (Harpin et al., 1986).

Vanderlinden et al. (1988) reported on the use of electrophrenic respiration in 24 patients, eight of whom had C1, C2-level spinal cord injury. Pacing was successful in all patients with high spinal cord injury and in most patients with neurogenic apnea or central alveolar hypoventilation. However, the diapragm could not be paced in two patients, and pacing did not help in one patient with myopathy and two patients with COPD. Fodstad (1989) reported his experience with 35 patients, aged 2–69 years. Diagnoses included central alveolar hypoventilation (''Ondine's curse''), and brainstem and high spinal cord lesions. After a follow-up period of 2 months to 10 years, 15 patients were weaned completely, and eight used phrenic pacing during the day and mechanical ventilation at night.

The complications of electrophrenic respiration are nerve damage (Glenn et al., 1980), infection (McMichan et al., 1979), upper airway obstruction (Scharf et al., 1978), and failure of the radio receiver or other implanted components (Vanderlinden et al., 1988; Weese-Meyer et al., 1989). As with negative-pressure ventilation, upper airway obstruction during electrophrenic respiration results from failure to activate the muscles that open the vocal cords. Tracheostomy circumvents this problem. Weese-Mayer et al. (1989) reported that the implanted pacer components fail on average in 56 months, and overall failures could be attributed to receiver failure, broken wires or insulation, infection necessitating implant removal, and nerve damage. The phrenic nerves can be stimulated noninvasively, using magnetic coils, but this technique is still experimental.

D. Respiratory Muscle Training

Inspiratory Resistive Training

The inspiratory muscles can be trained by having patients inspire through a device that imposes an added inspiratory load. The load may be of the threshold or the resistive type. A threshold load must be overcome in order to initiate inspiration, and it is independent of the inspiratory flow rate. A resistive load is present throughout inspiration, and it is very sensitive to the inspiratory flow rate. For optimal results, one should control the pattern of breathing through the inspiratory load with either technique.

Inspiratory muscle weakness in quadriplegia usually results from undernutrition and infection, and when these factors are controlled, the muscles can respond well to training regimens. Inspiratory resistive training, used 30 min day, 6 days a week, for 8, 12, and 16 weeks, improved inspiratory muscle strength and endurance of quadriplegic patients (Gross et al., 1980). Their initial PI_{max} was 62 cm H_2O, about half normal. It increased by 25% at 8 weeks and 35% at 12 weeks, and thereafter remained at 85 cm H_2O. These patients were able to tolerate higher resistive loads without electromyographic signs of inspiratory muscle fatigue after training.

Inspiratory resistive training may also be of value in weaning patients with quadriplegia or kyphoscoliosis from mechanical ventilation and otherwise improving their ventilatory endurance and exercise capacity (Hornstein et al., 1987; Lerman and Weiss 1987). In one patient with a high spinal cord injury, repetitive stimulation of the phrenic nerves was used to enhance diaphragmatic strength and endurance (Nochomovitz et al., 1984). Transdiaphragmatic pressure increased by 75% from the third to the sixteenth week of training, and endurance increased ninefold.

Training has also been tried in progressive muscle diseases, with mixed results. Two reports describe approximately doubling inspiratory muscle strength (Martin et al., 1983) or endurance (DiMarco et al., 1985) in an adult with acid maltase deficiency and in adults and children with muscular dystrophy. However, others report no increase in PI_{max}, PE_{max}, or VC and little or no change in endurance (Martin et al., 1986; Smith et al., 1988b).

Cough Training

Another use for respiratory muscle training is to improve cough. To this end, two techniques have been employed in patients with cervical spinal cord injuries. *Glossopharyngeal breathing* involves gulping air with the mouth and using oral and pharyngeal muscles to force the air into the trachea. Patients learn to add 500–1000 ml of air to their vital capacity in 10–20 gulps, which is enough to help them cough effectively (Montero et al., 1967; Mazza et al., 1984). Glossopharyngeal breathing also enables some patients to have time off the ventilator (Bach and Alba, 1991)

A newer approach involves *training the clavicular portion of the pectoralis major muscle*, which has been shown to have an expiratory action (De Troyer et al., 1986a). Isometric exercises were performed by six quadriplegic patients, while another six who received routine pulmonary rehabilitation served as controls (Estenne et al., 1989). Training consisted of 10 isometric contractions at 80% of maximal voluntary strength, held for 6 sec, with 6 sec rest. This routine was repeated once daily, 5 days/week, for 6 weeks. In the trained patients, muscle strength increased by 55%, and expiratory reserve volume increased by 47%. The FRC did not change, and RV decreased by 14%. Such responses should help quadriplegic patients cough bettcr, but that point remains to be tested.

VI. Summary

The physiological characteristics of ventilatory impairment in neuromuscular and skeletal disorders are similar. Both produce a restrictive pattern on pulmonary function testing, which is characterized by reductions in vital capacity (VC) and total lung capacity (TLC). The respiratory rate is higher than normal, and the tidal volume tends to be smaller than normal, especially in more advanced disease. The compliance of the respiratory system is lower than normal, due in part to the direct effects of neuromuscular and skeletal diseases on the chest wall and in part to secondary effects of these disorders on the lungs. In addition, there may be a considerable degree of ventilation-perfusion (V/Q) imbalance, mainly in the dependent lung regions, which have a very low ratio of ventilation to perfusion.

The functional consequences of neuromuscular and skeletal disease are a reduced capacity for physical exercise and activities of daily living and the possible onset of ventilatory failure. Restriction of the ventilatory capacity is often as important as the peripheral effects of neuromuscular or skeletal disease in limiting the patient's functional class. In neuromuscular diseases, the primary deficit is respiratory muscle weakness or paralysis, and the work of breathing is normal. In skeletal diseases, the respiratory muscles are normal, but the skeletal disorder restricts thoracic motion and increases the work of breathing. However, owing to secondary consequences of both types of disorder, respiratory muscle weakness becomes prominent in advanced skeletal disease, and respiratory system compliance falls in neuromuscular diseases.

The pathogenesis of ventilatory failure in both neuromuscular and skeletal disorders involves either respiratory muscle weakness or an increase in the work of breathing, or combinations of both. These abnormalities impair CO_2 elimination mainly through their effect on the pattern of breathing. As ventilatory reserve dwindles, the balance between the work of breathing and the capacity of the respiratory muscles to cope with the ventilatory load becomes progressively unfavorable. When the tidal volume (VT) falls below a critical level, alveolar ventilation becomes inadequate and the partial pressure of carbon dioxide in arterial blood ($Paco_2$) rises. Minute ventilation does not accurately reflect the effect of the reducation in VT, because of the increase in the respiratory rate.

A similar sequence of events occurs in OHS, but there are several important differences. First, OHS is associated with upper airway obstruction during sleep. Patients with neuromuscular disease develop upper airway obstruction with negative-pressure ventilation or electrophrenic respiration, but do not usually have it spontaneously. Second, patients with OHS probably have inadequate ventilatory drive, in the sense that mouth occlusion pressure ($P_{0.1}$) is normal when it should be increased, as in simple obesity.

Complications are similar among all three groups of patients, but patients with diffuse neuromuscular diseases are most apt to have aspiration pneumonia, because their laryngeal and pharyngeal muscles are abnormal. All three groups of patients are at relatively high risk to develop deep venous thrombosis and pulmonary embolism, but the major complication is ventilatory failure.

Management of ventilatory failure is much the same for patients with neuromuscular and skeletal diseases. More and more attention is being given to noninvasive techniques for delivering positive-pressure ventilation, including nose masks, mouth tubes, noncuffed tracheostomy tubes, and abdominal pressure belts. Negative-pressure ventilation is being supplanted by the noninvasive positive-pressure regimens, because the latter are less cumbersome and they also prevent upper airway obstruction. Nonetheless, negative-pressure ventilation has been the mainstay of therapy for patients with kyphoscoliosis. The rocking bed has been revived, especially for patients with isolated diaphragmatic paralysis. These patients do not seem to have a problem with upper airway obstruction while using the rocking bed, but potentially could. Patients with OHS need nasal CPAP, but generally do not need NIPPV.

There is a broader awareness that patients with neuromuscular and skeletal diseases have limited ventilatory endurance. When the patient's own ventilatory endurance is exceeded, additional support by intermittent noninvasive ventilation is indicated, usually at night, but whenever it is convenient. Such regimens can be implemented in nursing homes and at home and do not require intensive-care units. Hospitals are developing intermediate-care units to facilitate initiation of partial ventilator support, and to arrange for appropriate discharge planning. Patients who obtain such ventilator support do very well out of the hospital, even when their underlying disease is slowly progressive.

References

Abd, A. G., Braun, N. M. T., Baskin, M. I., O'Sullivan, M. M., and Alkaitis, D. A. (1989) Diaphragmatic dysfunction after open heart surgery: treatment with a rocking bed. *Ann. Intern. Med.* **111**:881–886.

Adams, J. M., Farkas, G. A., and Rochester, D. F. (1988). Vagal afferents, diaphragm fatigue and inspiratory resistance in the anesthetized dog. *J. Appl. Physiol.* **64**:2279–2286.

Aisen, M., Arlt, G., and Foster, S. (1990). Diaphragm paralysis without bulbar or limb paralysis in multiple sclerosis. *Chest* **98**:499–501.

Aldrich, T. K., and Aldrich, M. S. (1986). Primary muscle diseases: respiratory mechanisms and complications. In *Pulmonary Aspects of Neurologic Disease*. Edited by S. L. Kanholz. SP Scientific and Medical Books, New York.

Alexander, C. (1966). Diaphragm movements and the diagnosis of diaphragmatic paralysis. *Clin. Radiol.* **17**:79–83.

Allen, S. M., Hunt, B., and Green, M. (1985). Fall in vital capacity with posture. *Br. J. Dis. Chest* **79**:267–271.

Arborelius, M. J., Lilja, B., and Senyk, J., (1975). Regional and total lung function studies in patients with hemidiaphragmatic paralysis. *Respiration* **32**:253–264.

Arora, N. S., and Gal, T. J. (1981). Cough dynamics during progressive expiratory muscle weakness in healthy curarized subjects. *J. Appl. Physiol.* **51**:494–498.

Arora, N. S., and Rochester, D. F. (1982). Respiratory muscle strength and maximal voluntary ventilation in undernourished patients. *Am. Rev. Respir. Dis.* **126**:5–8.

Arora, N. S., Suratt, P. M., and Rochester, D. F. (1978). Respiratory muscle and ventilatory function in spinal cord injury. *Clin. Res.* **26**:443A.

Bach, J. R., and Alba, A. S. (1990a). Management of chronic alveolar hypoventilation by nasal ventilation. *Chest* **97**:52–57.

Bach, J. R., and Alba, A. S. (1990b). Tracheostomy ventilation. A study of efficacy with deflated cuffs and cuffless tubes. *Chest* **97**:679–683.

Bach, J. R., and Alba, A. S. (1990c). Noninvasive options for ventilatory support of the traumatic high level quadriplegic patient. *Chest* **98**:613–619.

Bach, J. R., and Alba, A. S. (1991). Intermittent abdominal pressure ventilator in a regimen of noninvasive ventilatory support. *Chest* **99**:630–636.

Bach, J. R., and Penek, J. (1991). Obstructive sleep apnea complicating negative-pressure ventilatory support in patients with chronic paralytic/restrictive ventilatory dysfunction. *Chest* **99**:1386–1393.

Bake, B., Bjure, J., Kasalichy, J., and Nachemson, A. (1972a). Regional pulmonary ventilation and perfusion distribution in patients with untreated idiopathic scoliosis. *Thorax* **27**:703–712.

Bake, B., Fugl-Meyer, A. R., and Grimby, G. (1972b). Breathing patterns and regional ventilation distribution in tetraplegic patients and in normal subjects. *Clin. Sci.* **42**:117–128.

Balaji, S., Kunovsky, P., and Sullivan, I. (1990). Ultrasound in the diagnosis of diaphragmatic paralysis after operation for congenital heart disease. *Br. Heart. J.* **64**:20–22.

Baydur, A. (1991). Respiratory muscle strength and control of ventilation in patients with neuromuscular disease. *Chest* **99**:330–338.

Baydur, A., Gilgoff, I., Prentice, W., Carlson, M., and Fischer, D. A. (1990a). Decline in respiratory function and experience with long-term assisted ventilation in advanced Duchenne's muscular dystrophy. *Chest* **97**: 884–889.

Baydur, A., Swank, S. M., Stiles, C. M., and Sassoon, C. S. H. (1990b). Respiratory mechanics in anesthetized young patients with kyphoscoliosis: immediate and delayed effects of corrective spinal surgery. *Chest* **97**:1157–1164.

Begin, R., Bureau, M. A., Lupien, L., Bernier, J-P., and Lumieux, B. (1982). The mechanical factors. Pathogenesis of respiratory insufficiency in myotonic dystrophy. *Am. Rev. Respir. Dis.* **125**:312–318.

Bellamy, D., Davis, J. M. N., Hickey, B. P., Benatar, S. R., and Clark, T. J. H. (1975). A case of primary alveolar hypoventilation associated with mild proximal myopathy. *Am. Rev. Respir. Dis.* **112**:867–873.

Benjamin, J. J., Cascade, P. N., Rubenfire, M., Wajszczuk, W., and Kerin, N. Z. (1982). Left lower lobe atelectasis and consolidation following cardiac surgery: the effect of tropical cooling on the phrenic nerve. *Radiology* **142**:11–14.

Bennett, D. A., and Bleck, T. P. (1988). Diagnosis and treatment of neuromuscular causes of acute respiratory failure. *Clin. Neuropharmacol.* **11**: 303–347.

Bergofsky, E. H. (1979). Respiratory failure in disorders of the thoracic cage. *Am. Rev. Respir. Dis.* **119**:643–669.

Bergofsky, E. H. (1964). Mechanism for respiratory insufficiency after cervical cord injury. *Ann. Intern. Med.* **61**:435–447.

Bergofsky, E. H. (1985). Thoracic deformities. In *The Thorax (Part B)*. Edited by C. Roussos and P. T. Macklem. Marcel Dekker, New York, chapter 32, pp. 941–978.

Bergofsky, E., Turino, G., and Fishman, A. (1959). Cardiorespiratory failure in kyphoscoliosis. *Medicine* **38**:263–317.

Bhaskar, K. R., Brown, R., O'Sullivan, D. D., Melia, S., Duggan, M., Reid, L., and the Respiratory Therapists. (1991). Bronchial mucus hypersecretion in acute quadriplegia. Macromolecular yields and glycoconjugate composition. *Am. Rev. Respir. Dis.* **143**:640–648.

Black, L. F., and Hyatt, R. E. (1971). Maximal static respiratory pressures in generalized neuromuscular disease. *Am. Rev. Respir. Dis.* **103**:641–650.

Block, A., Boysen, P., Wynne, J., and Hunt, L. (1979). Sleep apnea, hypopnea, and oxygen desaturation in normal subjects. *N. Engl. J. Med.* **300**: 513–517.

Borel, C. O., Tilford, C., Nichols, D. G., Hanley, D. F., and Traytsman, R. J. (1991). Diaphragmatic performance during recovery from acute ventilatory failure in Guillain-Barré syndrome and myasthenia gravis. *Chest* **99**:444–451.

Bowen, T. E., Zajtchuk, R., and Albus, R. A. (1982). Diaphragmatic paralysis managed by diaphragmatic replacement. *Ann. Thorac. Surg.* **33**:184–188.

Bradley, D., Rutherford, R., Lue, F., et al. (1986). Role of diffuse airway obstruction in the hypercapnia of obstructive sleep apnea. *Am. Rev. Respir. Dis.* **134**:920–924.

Braun, N. M. T., Arora, N. S., and Rochester, D. F. (1983). Respiratory muscle and pulmonary function in polymyositis and other proximal myopathies. *Thorax* **38**:616–623.

Bredin, C. P. (1989). Pulmonary function in long-term survivors of thoracoplasty. *Chest* **95**:18–20.

Brody, A. W., O'Halloran, P. S., Connolly, J. J., Jr., Wander, H. J., and Schwertley, F. W. (1964). Ventilatory mechanics and strength in subjects paralyzed after poliomyelitis. *Chest* **46**:263–275.

Burki, N., and Baker, R. (1984). Ventilatory regulation in eucapnic morbid obesity. *Am. Rev. Respir. Dis.***129**:538–543.

Byrd, R. B., and Burns, J. R. (1975). Cough dynamics in the post-thoracotomy state. *Chest* **67**:654–657.

Calin, A. (1985). Ankylosing spondylitis. *Clin. Rheum. Dis.* **11**:41–60.

Caro, C. G., and DuBois, A. B. (1961). Pulmonary function in kyphoscoliosis. *Thorax* **16**:282–290.

Carre, P. C., Didier, A. P., Tiberge, Y. M., Arbus, L. J., and Leophonte, P. J. (1988). Amyotrophic lateral sclerosis presenting with sleep hypopnea syndrome. *Chest* **93**:1309–1312.

Carrey, Z., Gottfried, S. G., and Levy, R. D. (1990). Ventilatory muscle support in respiratory failure with nasal positive pressure ventilation. *Chest* **97**:150–158.

Carroll, J. E., Zwillich, C. W., and Weil, J. V. (1977). Ventilatory response in myotonic dystrophy. *Neurology* **27**:1125–1128.

Carroll, N., and Branthwaite, M. A. (1988). Control of nocturnal hypoventilation by nasal intermittent positive pressure ventilation. *Thorax* **43**: 349–353.

Cashman, N. R., Maselli, R., Wollman, R. L., Roos, R., Simon, R., and Antel, J. P. (1987). Late denervation in patients with antecendent paralytic poliomyelitis. *N. Engl. J. Med.* **317**:7–12.

Castile, R., Staats, B., and Westbrook, P. (1982). Symptomatic pectus deformities of the chest. *Am. Rev. Respir. Dis.* **126**:564–568.

Celli, B. R., Rassulo, J., and Corral, R. (1987). Ventilatory muscle dysfunction in patients with bilateral idiopathic diaphragmatic paralysis: reversal by intermittent external negative pressure ventilation. *Am. Rev. Respir. Dis.* **136**:1276–1278.

Chan, C. K., Mohsenin, V., Loke, J., Virgulto, J., Sipski, L., and Ferranti, R. (1987). Diaphragmatic dysfunction in siblings with hereditary motor and sensory neuropathy (Charcot-Marie-Tooth disease). *Chest* **91**:567–570.

Chan, S., Grunstein, R., Bye, P., Woolcock, A., and Sullivan, C. (1989). Obstructive sleep apnea with severe chronic airflow limitation. *Am. Rev. Respir. Dis.* **140**:1274–1278.

Chandler, K. W., Rozas, C. J., Kory, R. C., and Goldman, A. L. (1984). Bilateral diaphragmatic paralysis complicating local cardiac hypothermia during open heart surgery. *Am. J. Med.* **77**:243–249.

Chapman, K. R., Himal, H. S., and Rebuck, A. S. (1990). Ventilatory responses to hypercapnia and hypoxia in patients with eucapnic morbid obesity before and after weight loss. *Clin. Sci.* **78**:541–545.

Chausow, A. M., Kane, T., Levinson, D., and Szidon, J. P. (1984). Bilateral diaphragmatic paralysis complicating local cardiac hypothermia during open heart surgery. *Am. J. Med.* **77**:243–249.

Chuter, T. A. M., Weissman, C., Mathews, D. M., and Starker, P. M. (1990). Diaphragmatic breathing maneuvers and movement of the diaphragm after cholecystectomy. *Chest* **97**:1110–1114.

Chuter, T. A. M., Weissman, C., and Starker, P. M. (1991). Respiratory patterns after cholecystectomy. Effects of posture and CO_2 stimulation. *Chest* **100**:23–27.

Ciesielski, T. E., Fukuda, Y., Glenn, W. W. L., Gorfien, J., Jeffery, K., and Hogan, J. F. (1983). Response of the diaphragm muscle to electrical stimulation of the phrenic nerve. *J. Neurosurg.* **58**:92–100.

Cooper, D. M., Rojas, J., Mellins, R. B., Keim, H. A., and Mansell, A. L. (1984). Respiratory mechanics in adolescents with idiopathic scoliosis. *Am. Rev. Respir. Dis.* **130**:16–22.

Cullen, P., Modell, J. H., Kirby, R. R., Klein, E. F., Jr., and Long, W. (1975). Treatment of flail chest. Use of intermittent mandatory ventilation and positive end-expiratory pressure. *Arch. Surg.* **110**:1099–1103.

Curran, F. J., and Colbert, A. P. (1989). Ventilator management in Duchenne muscular dystrophy and postpoliomyelitis syndrome: twelve years' experience. *Arch. Phys. Med. Rehab.* **70**:180–185.

Danon, J., Druz, W. S., Goldberg, N. B., and Sharp, J. T. (1979). Function of the isolated paced diaphragm and the cervical accessory muscles in C1 quadriplegics. *Am. Rev. Respir. Dis.* **119**:909–919.

Dau, P. (1985). Respiratory failure in myasthenia gravis. *Chest* **85**:712–722.

Dean, E., Ross, J., Road, J. D., Courtenay, L., and Madill, K. J. (1991). Pulmonary function in individuals with a history of poliomyelitis. *Chest* **100**:118-23.

Dee, P. M., Suratt, P. M., Bray, S. T., and Rose, C. E., Jr. (1984). Mucous plugging simulating pulmonary embolism in patients with quadriplegia. *Chest* **85**:363–366.

Demedts, M., Beckers, J., Rochette, F., and Bulcke, J. (1982). Pulmonary function in moderate neuromuscular disease without respiratory complaints. *Eur. J. Respir. Dis.* **63**:62–72.

Derveaux, L., Ivanoff, I., Rochette, F., and Demedts, M. (1988). Mechanism of pulmonary function changes after surgical correction for funnel chest. *Eur. Respir. J.* **1**:823–825.

Derveaux, L., Clarysse, I., Ivanoff, I., and Demedts, M. (1989). Preoperative and postoperative abnormalities in chest x-ray indices and in lung function in pectus deformities. *Chest* **95**:850–856.

De Troyer, A., and Deisser, P. (1981). The effects of intermittent positive pressure breathing on patients with respiratory muscle weakness. *Am. Rev. Respir. Dis.* **124**:132–137.

De Troyer, A., and Estenne, M. (1981). Limitations of transdiaphragmatic pressure in detecting diaphragm weakness. *Thorax* **36**:169–174.

De Troyer, A., and Estenne, M. (1990). Chest wall motion in paraplegic subjects. *Am. Rev. Respir. Dis.* **141**:332–336.

De Troyer, A., and Heilporn, A., (1980). Respiratory mechanics in quadriplegia. The respiratory function of the intercostal muscles. *Am. Rev. Respir. Dis.* **122**:591–600.

De Troyer, A., and Pride, N. B. (1985). The respiratory system in neuromuscular disorders. *In The Thorax (Lung Biology in Health and Disease*. Marcel Dekker, New York, Edited by C. Roussos and P. T. Macklem. pp. 1089–1121.

De Troyer, A., and Vanderhoeft, P. (1982). Phrenic nerve function after pneumonectomy. *Chest* **81**:212–214.

De Troyer, A., Borenstein, S., and Cordier, R. (1980). Analysis of lung volume restriction in patients with respiratory muscle weakness. *Thorax* **35**: 603–610.

De Troyer, A., De Beyl, D. Z., and Thirion, M. (1981). Function of the respiratory muscles in acute hemiplegia. *Am. Rev. Respir. Dis.* **123**: 631–632.

De Troyer, A., Estenne, M., and Heilporn, A., (1986). Mechanism of active expiration in tetraplegic sugjects. *N. Engl. J. Med.* **314**:740–744.

De Troyer, A., Estenne, M., and Vincken, W. (1985b). Rib cage motion and muscle use in high tetraplegics. *Am. Rev. Respir. Dis.* **133**:1115–1119.

DiMarco, A. F., Kelling, J. S., DiMarco, M. S., Jacobs, I., Shields, R., and Altose, M. D. (1985). The effects of inspiratory resistive training on respiratory muscle function in patients with muscular dystrophy. *Muscle Nerve* **8**:284–290.

Dureuil, B., Viires, N., Cantineau, J-P., Aubier, M., and Desmonts, J-M. (1986). Diaphragmatic contractility after upper abdominal surgery. *J. Appl. Physiol.* **61**:1775–1780.

Dushay, K. M., Zibrak, J. D., and Jensen, W. A. (1990). Myasthenia gravis presenting as isolated respiratory failure. *Chest* **97**:232–234.

Dyer, E. L., and Callahan, A. S. (1987). Charcot-Marie-Tooth disease and respiratory failure. *Chest* **92**:957.

Easton, P. A., Fleetham, J. A., De La Rocha, A., and Anthonisen, N. R. (1983). Respiratory function after paralysis of the right hemidiaphragm. *Am. Rev. Respir. Dis.* **27**:125–128.

Elliott, C., Hill, T., Adams, T., Crapo, R., Nietrzeba, R., and Gardner, R., (1985). Exercise performance of subjects with ankylosing spondylitis and limited chest expansion. *Bull. Eur. Physiopathol. Respir.* **21**:363–368.

Ellis, E. R., Bye, P. T. P., Bruderer, J. W., and Sullivan, C. E. (1987). Treatment of respiratory failure during sleep in patients with neuromuscular disease: positive-pressure ventilation through a nose mask. *Am. Rev. Respir. Dis.* **135**:148–152.

Estenne, M., and De Troyer, A. (1985). Relationship between respiratory muscle electromyogram and rib cage motion in tetraplegia. *Am. Rev. Respir. Dis.* **132**:53–59.

Estenne, M., and De Troyer, A., (1986). The effects of tetraplegia on chest wall statics. *Am. Rev. Respir. Dis.* **134**:121–124.

Estenne, M., and De Troyer, A. (1987). Mechanism of the postural dependence of vital capacity in tetraplegic subjects. *Am. Rev. Respir. Dis.* **135**:367–371.

Estenne, M., and De Troyer, A., (1990). Cough in tetraplegic subjects. An active process. *Ann. Intern. Med.* **112**:22–28.

Estenne, M., Heilporn, A., Delhez, L., Yernault, J-C., and De Troyer, A. (1983). Chest wall stiffness in patients with chronic respiratory muscle weakness. *Am. Rev. Respir. Dis.* **128**:1002–1007.

Estenne, M. Yernalt, J. C., De Smet, J. M., and De Troyer, A., (1985). Phrenic and diaphragm function oafter coronary artery bypass grafting. *Thorax* **40**:293–299.

Estenne, M., Knopp, C., Vanvaerenbergh, J., Heilporn, A., and De Troyer, A., (1989). The effect of pectoralis muscle training in tetraplegic subjects. *Am. Rev. Respir. Dis.* **139**:1218–1222.

Fallat, R. J., Jewitt, B., Bass, M., Kamm, B., Norris, F. H., Jr. (1979). Spirometry in amyothrophic lateral sclerosis. *Arch. Neurol.* **36**:74–80.

Farebrother, M., McHardy, G., and Munro, J. (1974). Relation between pulmonary gas exchange and closing volume before and after substantial weight loss in obese subjects. *Br. Med. J.* **3**:391–393.

Ferris, B. G., Jr., Whittenberger, J. L., and Affeldt, J. E. (1952a). Pulmonary function in convalescent poliomyelitic patients. I. Pulmonary subdivisions and maximum breathing capacity. *N. Engl. J. Med.* **246**:919–923.

Ferris, B. G., Jr., Mead, J., Whittenberger, J. L., and Saxton, G. A., Jr. (1952b). Pulmonary function in convalescent poliomyelitis patients. III. Compliance of the lungs and thorax. *N. Engl. J. Med.* **247**:390–393.

Ferris, B. G., Jr, Warren, A., and Beals, C. A. (1955). The vital capacity as a measure of the spontaneous breathing ability in poliomyelitis. *N. Engl. J. Med.* **252**:618–621.

Findley, L. (1987). The close but mysterious ties between obstructive sleep apnea and the obesity-hypoventilation syndrome. *Chest* **92**:772–773.

Fischer, D. A. (1985). Poliomyelitis: late pulmonary complications and management. In *Late Effects of Poliomyelitis*. Edited by L. S. Halstead and D. O. Wiechers. Symposium Foundation, Miami, pp. 185–192.

Fluck, D. C. (1966). Chest movements in hemiplegia. *Clin. Sci.* **31**:383–388.

Fodstad, H. (1989). Pacing of the diaphragm to control breathing in patients with paralysis of central nervous system origin. *Stereotact. Funct. Neurosurg.* **53**:209–222.

Ford, G. T., Whitelaw, W. A., Rosenal, T. W., Cruse, P. J. and Guenter, C. A. (1983). Diaphragm function after upper abdominal surgery in humans. *Am. Rev. Respir. Dis.* **127**:431–436.

Fried, P. I., McClean, P. A., Zamel, N., Murray, F. T., and Marliss, E. B. (1976). Effect of ketosis on respiratory sensitivity to carbon dioxide in obesity. *N.* Engl. *J. Med.* **294**:1081–1086.

Fulkerson, W. J., Wilkins, J. K., Esbenshade, A. M., Eskind, J. B., and Newman, J. H. (1984). Life threatening hypoventilation in kyphoscoliosis: successful treatment with a molded body brace-ventilator. *Am. Rev. Respir. Dis.* **129**:185–187.

Gacad, G., and Hamosh, P. (1973). The lung in ankylosing spondylitis. *Am. Rev. Respir. Dis.* **107**:286–289.

Galloway, G., Fedok, F. G., Wiegand, D. A., and Towfighi, J. (1991). Sternohyoid muscle biopsy. A diagnostic technique in respiratory failure of neuromuscular origin. *Chest* **100**:540–543.

Garay, S. M., Rapoport, D., Sorkin, B., Epstein, H., Feinberg, I., and Goldring, R. M. (1981a). Regulation of ventilation in the obstructive sleep apnea syndrome. *Am. Rev. Respir. Dis.* **124**:451–457.

Garay, S. M., Turino, G. M., and Goldring, R. M. (1981b). Sustained reversal of chronic hypercapnia in patients with alveolar hypoventilation syndromes. *Am. J. Med.* **70**:269–274.

Gay, P. C., Patel, Am M., Viggiono, R. W., and R. D. Hubmayr. (1991). Nocturnal nasal ventilation for treatment of patients with hypercapnic respiratory failure. *Mayo Clin. Proc.* **66**:695–703.

Gibson, G. J. (1989). Diaphragmatic paresis: pathophysiology, clinical features and investigation. *Thorax* **44**:960–970.

Gibson, G. J., Edmonds, J. P., and Hughes, G. R. V. (1977a). Diaphragm function and lung involvement in systemic lupus erythematosus. *Am. J. Med.* **63**:926–932.

Gibson, G. J., Pride, N. B., Davis, J. N., and Loh, L. C. (1977b). Pulmonary mechanics in patients with respiratory muscle weakness. *Am. Rev. Respir. Dis.* **115**:389–395.

Gilchrist, D., Chan, C. K., and Deck, J. H. N. (1989). Phrenic involvement in Charcot-Marie-Tooth disease. *Chest* **96**:1197–1199.

Glenn, W. W. L., Hogan, J. F., and Phelps, M. L. (1980). Ventilatory support of the quadriplegic patient with respiratory paralysis by diaphragm pacing. *Surg. Clin. North Am.* **60**:1055–1078.

Goldstein, R. L., Hyde, R. W., Lapham, L. W., Gazioglu, K., and dePapp, Z. G. (1974). Peripheral neuropathy presenting with respiratory insufficiency as the primary complaint. *Am. J. Med.* **56**:443–449.

Goldstein, R. S., Molotiu, N. Skrastins, R., Long, S., De Rosie, J., Contreras, M., Popkin, J., Rutherford, R., and Phillipson, E. A. (1987). Reversal of sleep-induced hypoventilation and chronic respiratory failure by nocturnal negative pressure ventilation in patients with restrictive ventilatory impairment. *Am. Rev. Respir. Dis.* **135**:1049–1055.

Goldstein, R. S., DeRosie, J. A., Avendano, M. A. and Dolmage, T. E. (1991). Influence of noninvasive positive pressure ventilation on inspiratory muscles. *Chest* **99**:408–415.

Gracey, D. R., and Southorn, P. A. (1987). Respiratory failure in Lambert-Eaton myasthenic syndrome. *Chest* **91**:716–718.

Gracey, D. R., McMichan, J. C., Divertie, M. B., and Howard, F. M., Jr. (1982). Respiratory failure in Guillain-Barré syndrome. *Mayo Clin. Proc.* **57**:742–746.

Gracey, D. R., Divertie, M. B., and Howard, F. M., Jr. (1983). Mechanical ventilation for respiratory failure in myasthenia gravis. *Mayo Clin. Proc.* **58**:597–602.

Gracey, D. R., Divertie, M. B., Howard, F. M., Jr., and Payne, W. S. (1984a). Postoperative respiratory care after transsternal thymectomy in myasthenia gravis. *Chest* **86**:67–71.

Gracey, D. R., Howard, F. M., Jr., and Divertie, M. B. (1984b). Plasmapheresis in the treatment of ventilator-dependent myasthenia gravis patients. *Chest* **85**:739–743.

Graham, A. N., Martin, P. D., and Haas, L. F. (1985). Neuralgic amyothrophy with bilateral diaphragmatic palsy. *Thorax* **49**:635–636.

Graham, D. R., Kaplan, D., Evans, C. C., Hind, C. R. K., and Donnelly, R. J. (1990). Diaphragmatic plication for unilateral diaphragmatic paralysis: a 10-year experience. *Ann. Thorac. Surg.* **49**:248–252.

Gregory, R. P., Loh, L., and Newsom-Davis, J. (1990). Recurrent isolated alternating phrenic nerve palsies: a variant of brachial neuritis? *Thorax* **45**:420–421.

Grimby, G., Fugl-Meyer, A. R., and Blomstrand, A. (1974). Partitioning of the contributions of rib cage and abdomen to ventilation in ankylosing spondylitis. *Thorax* **29**:179–184.

Grinman, S., and Whitelaw, W. A. (1983). Pattern of breathing in a case of generalized respiratory muscle weakness. *Chest* **84**:770–772.

Gross, D., Ladd, H. W., Riley, E. J., Macklem, P. T., and Grassino, A. (1980). The effect of training on strength and endurance of the diaphragm in quadriplegia. *Am. J. Med.* **68**:27–35.

Guilleminault, C., Stoohs, R., Schneider, H., Posdszus, T., Peter, J., and Wichert, P. (1989). Central alveolar hypoventilation and sleep: treatment by intermittant positive pressure ventilation through nasal mask in an adult. *Chest* **96**:1210–1212.

Haas, F., Axen, K., Pineda, H., Gancino, D., and Haas, A., (1985). Temporal pulmonary function changes in cervical cord injury. *Arch. Phys. Med. Rehab.* **66**:139–144.

Haas, H., Johnson, L. R., Gill, T. H., and Armentrout, T. S. (1981). Diaphragm paralysis and ventilatory failure in proximal spinal muscular atrophy. *Am. Rev. Respir. Dis.* **123**:465–467.

Hamly, F. H., Timms, R. M., Minh, V. D., and Moser, K. M. (1975). Bilateral, phrenic paralysis in myxedema. *Am. Rev. Respir. Dis.* **111**:911–912.

Hardie, R., Harding, A. E., Hirsch, N., Gelder, C., Macrae, A. D., and Thomas, P. K. (1990). Diaphragmatic weakness in hereditary motor and sensory neuropathy. *J. Neurol. Neurosurg. Psychiatry* **53**:348–350.

Harman, E., Wynne, J., Block, A., and Malloy-Fisher, L. (1981). Sleep-disordered breathing and oxygen desaturation in obese patients. *Chest* **79**:256–260.

Harman, E., Wynne, J., and Block, A. (1982). The effect of weight loss on sleep-disordered breathing and oxygen desaturation in morbidly obese men. *Chest* **82**:291–294.

Harpin, R. P., Gignac, S. P., Epstein, S. W., Gallacher, W. N., and Vanderlinden, R. G. (1986). Diaphragm pacing and continuous positive airway pressure. *Am. Rev. Respir. Dis.* **134**:1321–1323.

Hebert, C. A., Byrnes, T. J., Baethge, B. A., Wolf, R. E., and Kinasewitz, G. T. (1990). Exercise limitation in patients with polymyositis. *Chest* **98**:352–357.

Heckmatt, J., Loh, L. and Dubowitz, V. (1990). Night-time nasal ventilation in neuromuscular disease. *Lancet* **335**:579–582.

Hill, A. R., Robbins, A. W., Messing, R., and Arora, N. S. (1983). Sleep apnea syndrome after poliomyelitis. *Am. Rev. Respir. Dis.* **127**:129–131.

Hillman, D. R., and Finucane, K. E. (1988). Respiratory pressure partitioning during quiet inspiration in unilateral and bilateral diaphragmatic weakness. *Am. Rev. Respir. Dis.* **137**:1401–1405.

Hoeppner, V. H., Crockcroft, D. W., Dosman, J. A., and Cotton, D. J. (1984). Nighttime ventilation improves respiratory failure in secondary kyphoscoliosis. *Am. Rev. Respir. Dis.* **129**:240–243.

Holle, R. H. O., Schoene, R. B., and Pavlin, E. J. (1984). Effect of respiratory muscle weakness on Po.1 induced by partial curarization. *J. Appl. Physiol.* **57**(4):1150–1157.

Hollowell, D. E., and Suratt, P. M. (1989). Activation of masseter muscles with inspiratory resistance loading. *J. Appl. Physiol.* **671**:270–275.

Hornstein, S., Inman, S., and Ledsome, J. R. Jr. (1987). Ventilatory muscle training in kyphoscoliosis. *Spine* **12**:859–863.

Hultgren, A.-C., Fugl-Meyer, A. R., Jonasson, E., Bake, B. (1980). Ventilatory dysfunction and respiratory rehabilitation in post-traumatic quadriplegia *Eur. J. Respir. Dis.* **61**:347–356.

Hurewitz, A., Susskind, H., and Harold, W. (1985). Obesity alters regional ventilation in lateral decubitus position. *J. Appl. Physiol.* **59**:774–783.

Iber, C., Davies, S. F., and Mahowald, M. W. (1989). Nocturnal rocking bed therapy: improvement in sleep fragmentation in patients with respiratory muscle weakness. *Sleep* **12**:405–412.

Inkley, S. R., Oldenburg, F. C., and Vignos, P. J., Jr. (1974). Pulmonary function in Duchenne muscular dystrophy related to stage of disease. *Am. J. Med.* **56**:297–306.

Ivey, M., Eichenborn, M. S., Glasberg, M. R., and Hyzy, R. C. (1991). Hypercapnic respiratory failure due to L-tryptophan-induced eosinophilic polymyositis. *Chest* **99**:756–757.

Jabour, E. R., Rabil, D. M., Truwit, J. D., and Rochester, D. F. (1991). Evaluation of a new weaning index, based on ventilatory endurance and the efficiency of gas exchange. *Am. Rev. Respir. Dis.* **144**:531–537.

Jacobsen, E., Dano, P., and Skovsted, P. (1974). Respiratory function before and after weight loss following intestinal shunt operation for obesity. *Scand. J. Respir. Dis.* **55**:332–339.

James, J. (1976). *Scoliosis*. Churchill-Livingstone, Edinburgh, pp. 1–12, 147–185.

James, W. S., III, Minh, V., Minteer, M. A., and Moser, K. M. (1977). Cervical accessory respiratory muscle function in a patient with a high cervical cord lesion. *Chest* **71**:59–64.

Jammes, Y., Pouget, J., Grimaud, C., and Serratrice, G. (1985). Pulmonary function and electromyographic study of respiraatory muscles in myotonic dystrophy. *Muscle Nerve* **8**:586–594.

Johnson, M. W., and Remmers, J. E. (1984). Accessory muscle activity during sleep in chronic obstructive pulmonary disease. *J. Appl. Physiol.* **57**(4):1011–1017.

Joiner, T. A., Sumner, J. R., and Catchings, T. T. (1990). Unilateral diaphragmatic paralysis secondary to carbon monoxide poisoning. *Chest* **97**: 498–499.

Jones, J., Wilhoit, S., Findley, L., and Suratt, P. (1985) Oxyhemoglobin saturation during sleep in subjects with and without the obesity-hypoventilation syndrome. *Chest* **88**:9–15.

Jones, R. S., Kennedy, J. D., Hasham, F., Owen, R., and Taylor, J. F. (1981). Mechanical inefficiency of the thoracic cage in scoliosis. *Thorax* **36**: 456–461.

Kafer, E. R. (1975). Idiopathic scoliosis: mechanical properties of the respiratory system and the ventilatory response to carbon dioxide. *J. Clin. Invest.* **55**:1153–1163.

Kafer, E. R. (1976). Idiopathic scoliosis-gas exchange and the age dependence of arterial blood gases. *J. Clin. Invest.* **58**:825–833.

Kaminski, M. J., and Young, R. R. (1985). Neuromuscular and neurologic disorders affecting respiration. *The Thorax* (*Part B*), Edited by C. Roussos and P. T. Macklem. Marcel Dekker, New York, Chapter 35, pp. 1023–1087.

Kaufman, B. J., Ferguson, M. H., and Cherniack, R. M. (1959). Hypoventilation in obesity. *J. Clin. Invest.* **38**:500–507.

Keeler, J. R., Hurst, C. G., and Dunn, M. A. (1991). Pyridostigmine used as a nerve agent pretreatment under wartime conditions. *JAMA* **266**: 693–695.

Kelly, B. J., and Luce, J. M. (1991). The diagnosis and management of neuromuscular diseases causing respiratory failure. *Chest* **99**:1485–1494.

Kelly, T. M., Jensen, R. L., Elliott, C. G., and Crapo, R. O. (1988). Maximum respiratory pressures in morbidly obese subjects. *Respiration* **54**:73–77.

Kesten, S., Garfinkel, S. K., Wright, T., and Rebuck, A. S. (1991). Impaired exercise capacity in adults with moderate scoliosis. *Chest* **99**:663–666.

Killian, K. J., and Jones, N. L. (1988). Respiratory muscles and dyspnea. *Clin. Chest Med.* **9**:237–248.

Kimura, H., Tatsumi, K., Kunitomo, F., Okita, S., Tojima, H., Kouchiyama S., Masuyama, S., Shinozaki, T., Honda, Y., and Kuryama, T., (1989). Progesterone therapy for sleep apnea syndrome evaluated by occulusion pressure responses to exogenous loading. *Am. Rev. Respir. Dis.* **139**: 1198–1206.

Kinnear, W., Hockley, S., Harvery, J., and Shneerson, J., (1988a). The effects of one year of nocturnal cuirass-assisted ventilation in chest wall disease. *Eur. Respir. J.* **1**:204–208.

Kinnear, W., Petch, M., Taylor, G., and Shneerson, J. (1988b). Assisted ventilation using cuirass respirators. *Eur. Respir. J.* **1**:198–203.

Knudson, R. J., Mead, J., and Knudson, D. E. (1974). Contribution of airway collapse to supramaximal expiratory flows. *J. Appl. Physiol.* **36**(6): 653–667.

Korcyzn, A. D., Leibowitz, U., and Bruderman, I. (1969). Involvement of the diaphragm in hemiplegia. *Neurology* **19**:97–100.

Kreitzer, S. M., Feldman, N. T., Saunders, N. A., and Ingram, R. H., Jr. (1978a). Bilateral diaphragmatic paralysis with hypercapnic respiratory failure. *Am. J. Med.* **65**:89–95.

Kreitzer, S. M., Saunders, N. A., Tyler, H. R., Ingram, R. H., Jr. (1978b). Respiratory muscle function in amyotrophic lateral sclerosis. *Am. Rev. Respir. Dis.* **117**:437–447.

Krieger, J., Sforza, E., Apprill, M., Lampert, E., Weitzenblum, E., and Ratomaharo, J. (1989). Pulmonary hypertension, hypoxemia, and hypercapnia in obstructive sleep apnea patients. *Chest* **96**:729–737.

Kronenberg, R. S., Drage, C. W., and Stevenson, J. E. (1977). Acute respiratory failure and obesity with normal ventilatory response to carbon dioxide and absent hypoxic ventilatory drive. *Am. J. Med.* **62**:772–776.

Kuperman, A. S., Krieger, A. J., and Rosonoff, H. L. (1971). Respiratory function after cervical cordotomy. *Chest* **59**:128–132.

Landercasper, J., Cogbill, T. H., and Lindesmith, L. A. (1984). Long-term disability after flail chest injury. *Trauma* **24**:410–414.

Large, S. R., Heywood, L. J., Flower, C. D., Cory-Pearch, R., Wallwork, J., and English, T. A. H. (1985). Incidence and aetiology of a raised hemidiaphragm after cardiopulmonary bypass. *Thorax* **40**:444–447.

Laroche, C. M., Cairns, T., Moxham, J., and Green, M. (1988a). Hypothyroidism presenting with respiratory muscle weakness. *Am. Rev. Respir. Dis.* **138**:472–474.

Laroche, C. M., Carroll, N., Moxham, J., and Green, M. (1988b). Clinical significance of severe isolated diaphragm weakness. *Am. Rev. Respir. Dis.* **138**:862–866.

Laroche, C. M., Mier, A. K., Spiro, S. G., Newsom-Davis, J., Moxham, J., and Green, M. (1989). Respiratory muscle weakness in the Lambert-Eaton syndrome. *Thorax* **44**:913–918.

Laub, G. W., Muralidharan, S., Chen, C., Perritt, A., Adkins, M., Pollock, S., Bailey, B., and McGrath, L. B. (1991). Phrenic nerve injury. A prospective study. *Chest* **100**:376–379.

Ledsome, J. R., and Sharp, J. M. (1981). Pulmonary function in acute cervical cord injury. *Am. Rev. Respir. Dis.* **124**:41–44.

Leech, J., Onal, E., Baer, P., and Lopata, M. (1987). Determinants of hypercapnia in occlusive sleep apnea syndrome. *Chest* **92**:807–813.

Lerman, R. M., and Weiss, M. S. (1987). Progressive resistive exercise in weaning high quadriplegics from the ventilator. *Paraplegia* **25**:130–135.

Libby, D. M., Briscoe, W. A., Boyce, B., and Smith, J. P. (1982). Acute respiratory failure in scoliosis or kyphosis. *Am. J. Med.* **73**:532–538.

Linderholm, H., and Werneman, H. (1956). On respiratory regulation in poliomyelitis convalescents. *Acta Med. Scand.* **154**(suppl 316):135–157.

Lindesmith, L. A., Baines, R. D., Jr., Bigelow, D. B., and Petty, T. L. (1968). Reversible respiratory paralysis associated with polymixin therapy. *Ann. Intern. Med.* **68**:318–327.

Lisboa, C., Moreno, R., Fava, M., Ferretti, R., and Cruz, E. (1985). Inspiratory muscle function in patients with severe kyphoscoliosis. *Am. Rev. Respir. Dis.* **132**:48–52.

Lisboa, C., Pare, P. D., Pertuze, J., et al. (1986). Inspiratory muscle function in unilateral diaphragmatic paralysis. *Am. Rev. Respir. Dis.* **134**:488–492.

Litwin, S. D. (1978). *Genetic Determinants of Pulmonary Disease*. Marcel Dekker, New York, pp. 182–188.

Loh, L., Hughes, J. M. B., and Davis, J. N. (1979). Gas exchange problems in bilateral diaphragm paralysis. *Bull. Eur. Physiopathol.* **15**:137–141.

Lopata, M., and Onal, E. (1982). Mass loading, sleep apnea, and the pathogenesis of obesity hypoventilation. *Am. Rev. Respir. Dis.* **126**:640–645.

Lourenco, R., (1969). Diaphragm activity in obesity. *J. Clin. Invest.* **48**:1609–1614.

MacGregor, M. I., Block, A. J., and Ball, W. C., Jr. (1970). Serious complications and sudden death in the Pickwickian syndrome. *Johns Hopkins Med. J.*. **126**:279–304.

Maeda, H., Nakahaara, K., Ohno, K., Kido, T., Ikeda, M., and Kawashima, Y. (1988). Diaphragm function after pulmonary resection. Relationship to postoperative respiratory failure. *Am. Rev. Respir. Dis.* **137**:678–681.

Mansel, J. K., and J. R. Norman. (1990). Respiratory complications and management of spinal cord injuries. *Chest* **97**:1446–1452.

Margolis, M. L., and Hill, A. R. (1986). Acid maltase deficiency in an adult. Evidence for improvement in respiratory function with high-protein dietary therapy. *Am. Rev. Respir. Dis.* **134**:328–331.

Marino, W., and Braun, N. M. T. (1982). Reversal of the clinical sequelae of respiratory muscle fatigue by intermittent mechanical ventilation. *Am. Rev. Respir. Dis.* **125**(Part 2):85.

Martin, A. J., Stern, L., Yeates, J., Lepp, D., and Little J. (1986). Respiratory muscle training in Duchenne muscular dystrophy. *Dev. Med. Child Neurol.* **28**:314–318.

Martin, R. J., Sufit, R. L., Ringel, S. P., Hudgel, D. W., and Hill, P. L. (1983). Respiratory improvement by muscle training in adult-onset acid maltase deficiency. *Muscle Nerve* **6**:201–203.

Mazza, F. G., DiMarco, A. F., Altose, M. D., and Strohl, K. P. (1984). The flow-volume loop during glossopharyngeal breathing. *Chest* **85**: 638–640.

McCauley, R. G. K., and Labib, K. B. (1984). Diaphragmatic paralysis evaluated by phrenic nerve stimulation during fluoroscopy or real-time ultrasound. *Radiology* **153**:33–36.

McCool, F. D., and Mead, J., (1989). Dyspnea on immersion: mechanisms in patients with bilateral diaphragm paralysis. *Am. Rev. Respir. Dis.* **139**:275–276/

McCool, F. D., Mayewski, R. F., Shayne, D. S., Gibson, C. J., Griggs, R. C., and Hyde, R. W. (1986). Intermittent positive pressure breathing in patients with respiratory muscle weakness. Alterations in total respiratory system compliance. *Chest* **90**:546–552.

McEvoy, K. M., Windebank, A. J., Daube, J. R., and Low, P. A. (1989). e,4-Diaminopyridine in the treatment of Lambert-Eaton syndrome. *N. Engl. J. Med.* **321**:1567–1571.

McMichan, J. C., Piepgras, D. G., Gracey, D. R., Marsh, H. M., and Sittipong, R. (1979). Electrophrenic respiration. *Mayo Clin. Proc.* **54**: 662–668.

Mead, J., Banzett, R. B., Lehr, J., Loring, S. H., and O'Cain, C. F. (1984). Effect of posture on upper and lower rib cage motion and tidal volume during diaphragm pacing. *Am. Rev. Respir. Dis.* **130**:320–321.

Mead, J., Sly, P., Lesouef, P., Hibbert, M., and Phelan, P. (1985). Rib cage mobility in pectus excavatum. *Am. Rev. Respir. Dis.* **130**:1223–1228.

Mellem, H., Johansen, B., Nakstad, P., Russell, D., and Seim, H. (1987). Unilateral phrenic nerve paralysis caused by osteoarthritis of the cervical spine. *Eur. J. Respir. Dis.* **71**:56–58.

Merav, A. D., Attai, L. A., and Condit, D. D. (1983). Successful reepair of a transected phrenic nerve with restoration of diaphragmatic function. *Chest* **84**:642–644.

Merli, G. J., Herbison, G. J., Ditunno, J. F., Weitz, H. H., Henzes, J. H, Park, C. H., and Jaweed, M. M. (1988). Deep vein thrombosis: prophylaxis in acute spinal cord injured patients. *Arch. Phys. Med. Rehabil.* **69**: 661–664.

Mezon, B., West, P., Israels, J., and Kryger, M. (1980). Sleep breathing abnormalities in kyphoscoliosis. *Am. Rev. Respir. Dis.* **122**:617–621.

Mier, A., Brophy, C., Moxham, J., and Green, M. (1987). Phrenic nerve stimulation in normal subjects and in patients with diaphragmatic weakness. *Thorax* **42**:885–888.

Mier, A., Brophy, C., Wass, J. A. H., Besser, G. M., and Green, M. (1989). Reversible respiratory muscle weakness in hyperthyroidism. *Am. Rev. Respir. Dis.* **139**:529–533.

Mier, A., Laroche, C., Agnew, J. E., Vora, H., Clarke, S. W., Green, M., and Pavia, D. (1990a). Tracheobronchial clearance in patients with bilateral diaphragmatic weakness. *Am. Rev. Respir. Dis.* **142**:545–548.

Mier, A., Laroche, C., and Green, M. (1990b). Unsuspected myasthenia gravis presenting as respiratory failure. *Thorax* **45**:422–423.

Mier-Jedrzejowicz, A. K., Brophy, C., and Green, M. (1988a). Respiratory muscle function in myasthenia gravis. *Am. Rev. Respir. Dis.* **138**:867–873.

Mier-Jedrzejowicz, A., Brophy, C., Moxham, J., and Green, M. (1988b). Assessment of diaphragm weadkness. *Am. Rev. Respir. Dis.* **137**:877–883.

Miller, A., and Granada, M. (1974). In-hospital mortality in the Pickwickian syndrome. *Am. J. Med.* **56**:144–150.

Miller, B., Skupin, A., Rubenfire, M., and Bigman, O. (1988). Respiratory failure produced by severe procainamide intoxication in a patient with preexisting peripheral neuropathy caused by amiodarone. *Chest* **94**:663–664.

Millman, R. P. (1986). Did the fat boy snore? *Chest* **89**:621–622.

Millman, R. P., Knight, H., Kline, L. R., Shore, E. T., Chung, D-C., and Pack A. I. (1988). Changes in compartmental ventilation in association with eye movements during REM sleep. *J. Appl. Physiol.* **65**(3):1196–1202.

Mohr, C. H., and Hill, N. S. (1990). Long-term follow-up of nocturnal ventilatory assistance in patients with respiratory failure due to Duchenne-type muscular dystrophy. *Chest* **97**:91–96

Molho, M., Katz, I., Schwartz, E., Shemesh, Y., Sadeh, M., and Wolf, E. (1987). Familial bilateral paralysis of diaphragm. *Chest* **91**:464–467.

Montero, J. C., Feldman, D. J., and Montero, D. (1967). Effects of glossopharyngeal breathing on respiratory function after cervical cord transection. *Arch. Phys. Med. Rehab. il.* **48**:650–653.

Moorthy, S. S., Markand, O. N., Mahomed, Y., and Brown, J. W. (1985). Electrophysiologic evaluation of phrenic nerves in severe respiratory insufficiency requiring mechanical ventilation. *Chest* **88**:211–214.

Morgan, E., and Zwillich, C., (1978). The obesity-hypoventilation syndrome. *West. J. Med.* **129**:387–393.

Morgan, E. J., Altmeyer, R., Khakoo, R., and Lapp, N. L. (1982). Pulmonary function in infectious mononucleosis. *Chest* **81**:699–700.

Mortola, J. P., and Sant'Ambrogio, G. (1978). Motion of the rib cage and the abdomen in tetraplegic patients. *Clin. Sci. Mol. Med.* **54**:25–32.

Myllynen, P., Kammonen, M., Rokkanen, P., Bostman, O., Lalla, M., and Lassonen, E. (1985). Deep venous thrombosis and pulmonary embolism in patients with acute spinal cord injury: a comparison with nonparalyzed patients immobilized due to spinal fractures. *Trauma* **25**:541–543.

Naeye, R. (1961). Kyphoscoliosis and cor pulmonale. *Am. J. Pathol.* **38**: 561–571.

Nathanson, B. N., Yu, D-G., and Chan, C. K. (1989). Respiratory muscle weakness in Charcot-Marie-Tooth disease. *Arch. Intern. Med.* **149**: 1389–1391.

Newsom-Davis, J. (1967). Phrenic nerve conduction in man. *J. Neurol. Neurosurg. Psychiatry* **30**:420–426.

Newsom-Davis, J., (1974). Autonomous breathing. *Arch. Neurol.* **30**:480–483.

Newsom-Davis, J., Goldman, M., Loh, L., and Casson, M. (1976). Diaphragm function and alveolar hypoventilation. *O. J. Med.* **177**:87–100.

Nochomovitz, M. L., Hopkins, M., Brodkey, J., Montenegro, H., Mortimer, J. T., and Cherniack, N.S. (1984). Conditioning of the diaphragm with phrenic nerve stimulation after prolonged disuse. *Am. Rev. Respir. Dis.* **130**:685–688.

Oliven, A., Kelsen, S. G., Deal, E. C., Jr., and Cherniack, N. S. (1985). Respiratory pressure sensation. Relationship to changes in breathing pattern and PC02 during acute increase in airway resistance in patients with chronic obstructive pulmonary disease. *Am. Rev. Respir. Dis.* **132**: 1214–1218.

O'Neill, J. H., Murray, N. M. F., and Newson-Davis, J. N. (1988). The Lambert-Eaton myasthenic syndrome. *Brain* **111**:577–596.

Paré, J. A. P., and Fraser, R. G. (1983). *Synopsis of Diseases of the Chest.* Saunders, Philadelphia, pp. 737–740.

Phillips, M. S., Kinnear, W. J. M., and Shneerson, J. M. (1987). Late sequelae of pulmonary tuberculosis treated by thoracoplasty. *Thorax* **42**:445–451.

Piehler, J. M., Pairolero, P. C., Gracey, D. R., and Bernatz, P. E. (1982). Unexplained diaphragmatic paralysis: a harbinger of malignant disease? *J. Thorac. Cardiovasc. Surg* **84**:861–864.

Plum, F., and Swanson, A. G. (1958). Abnormalities in central regulation of respiration in acute and convalescent poliomyelitis. *Arch. Neurol. Psychiatry* **80**:267–285.

Radwan, L., Strugaluska, M., and Koziorowski, A., (1988). Changes in respiratory muscle function after neostigmine injection in patients with mysthenia gravis. *Eur. Respir. J.* **1**:119–121.

Raman, K., Blake, J. A., and Harris, T. M. (1971). Pulmonary embolism in Landry-Guillain-Barre-Strohl syndrome. *Chest* **60**:555–557.

Rapoport, D., Garay, S., Epstein., and Goldring, R. (1986). Hypercapnia in the obstructive sleep apnea syndrome. *Chest* **89**:627–635.

Ray, C. S., Sue, D. Y., Bray, G., Hansen, J. E., and Wasserman, K. (1983). Effects of obesity on respiratory function. *Am. Rev. Respir. Dis.* **128**: 501–506.

Riley, D. J., Santiago, T. V., Daniele, R. P., Schall, B., and Edelman, N. H. (1977). Blunted respiratory drive in congenital myopathy. *Am. J. Med.* **63**:459–466. 131:A331.

Rizvi, S. S., Ishikawa, S., Faling, L. J., Schlessinger, L., Satia, J., and Seckel, B. (1974). Defect in automatic respiration in a case of multiple sclerosis. *Am. J. Med.*.**56**:433–436.

Road, J. D., Burgess, K. R., Whitelaw, W. A., and Ford, G. T. (1984). Diaphragm function and respiratory response after upper abdominal surgery in dogs. *J. Appl. Physiol. Respir. Environ. Exercise. Physiol.* **57**: 576–582.

Rochester, D. F. (1988). Tests of respiratory muscle function. *Clin. Chest Med.* **9**:249–261.

Rochester, D. F., and Arora, N. J. (1980). Respiratory failure from obesity. In *Medical Complications of Obesity*. Edited by M. Mancini, B. Lewis, and F. Contaldo. Academic Press, New York, pp. 183–190.

Rochester, D., and Enson, Y. (1974). Current concepts in the pathogensis of the obesity-hypoventilation syndrome. *Am. J. Med.* **57**:402–420.

Rochester, D. F., and Findley, L. J. (1988). The lungs and neuromuscular and chest wall diseases. In *Textbook of Respiratory Medicine*. Edited by J. T. Murray and J. A. Nadel. Philadelphia, Saunders, Chapter 93, pp. 1942–1971.

Rochester, D. F., and Martin, L. L. (1985). Respiratory muscle rest. In *The Thorax (Part B)*. Edited by C. Roussos and P. T. Macklem. Marcel Dekker, New York, Chapter 43, pp. 1303–1328.

Sampson, M. G., and Grassino, A. (1983). Neuromechanical properties in obese patients during carbon dioxide rebreathing. *Am. J. Med.* **75**: 81–90.

Santamaria, J., and Ruiz, C. (1988). Diaphragm elevation in stroke. *Eur. Neurol.* **28**:81–83.

Sawicka, E. H., and Branthwaite, M. A. (1987). Respiration during sleep in kyphoscoliosis. *Thorax* **42**:801–808.

Sawicka, E. H., Branthwaite, M. A., and Spencer, G. T. (1983). Respiratory failure after thoracoplasty: treatment by intermittent negative-pressure ventilation. *Thorax* **38**:433–435.

Scanlon, P. D., Loring, S. H., Pichurko, B. M., McCool, F. D., Slutsky, A. S., Sarkarati, M., and R. Brown. (1989). Respiratory mechanics in acute quadriplegia. *Am. Rev. Respir. Dis.* **139**:615–620.

Scharf, S. M., Feldman, N. T., Goldman, M. D., Hart, H. Z., Bruce, E., and Ingram, R. H., Jr. (1978). Vocal cord closure: a cause of upper airway obstruction during controlled ventilation. *Am. Rev. Respir. Dis.* **117**: 391–397.

Schiavi, E. A., Roncoroni, A. J., and Puy, R. J. M. (1984). Isolated bilateral diaphragmatic paralysis with interstitial lung disease. *Am. Rev. Respir. Dis.* **129**:337–339.

Schmidt-Nowara, W. W., and Altman, A. R. (1984). Atelectasis and neuromuscular respiratory failure. *Chest* **85**:792–795.

Schmidt-Nowara, W. W., Samet, J. M., and Rosario, P. A. (1983). Early and late pulmonary complications of botulism. *Arch. Intern. Med.* **143**: 451–456.

Senanayake, N., and Karalliedde, L. (1987). Meurotoxic effects of organophosphorus insecticides. *N. Engl. J. Med.* **316**:761–763.

Shackleford, S. R., Smith, D. E., Zarins, C. K., Rice, C. L., and Virgilio, R. W. (1976). The management of flail chest. A comparison of ventilatory and nonventilatory treatments. *Am. J. Surg.* **132**:759–762.

Shannon, D., Riseborough, E., and Kazemi, H. (1971). Ventilation perfusion relationships following correction of kyphoscoliosis. *JAMA* **217**:579–584.

Sharp, J., Henry, J., Sweany, S., Meadows, W., and Pietras, R., (1964). The total work of breathing in normal and obese men. *J. Clin. Invest.* **43**:728–739.

Sharp, J. T., Druz, W., and Kondragunta, V., (1986). Diaphragmatic responses to body position changes in obese patients with obstructive apnea. *Am. Rev. Respir. Dis.* **133**:32–37.

Shneerson, J. M. (1978). The cardiorespiratory response to exercise in thoracic scoliosis. *Thorax* **33**:457–463.

Shoemaker, R., Palmer, G., Brown, J. W., and King, H. (1981). Aggressive treatment of acquired phrenic nerve paralysis in infants and small children. *Ann. Thorac. Surg.* **32**:254–259.

Siebens, A. A., Kirby, N. A., and Poulos, D. A. (1964). Cough following transection of spinal cord at C-6. *Arch. Phys. Med. Rehab il.* **45**:1–8.

Silver, J. R. (1963). The oxygen cost of breathing in tetraplegic patients. *Paraplegia* **1**:204–214.

Silverstein, D., Michlin, B., Sobel, H. J., and Lavietes, M. H. (1983). Right ventricular failure in a patient with diabetic neuropathy (myopathy) and central alveolar hypoventilation. *Respiration* **44**:460–465.

Simonds, A. K., Parker, R. A., and Branthwaite, M. A. (1989). The effect of intermittent positive-pressure hyperinflation in restrictive chest wall disease. *Respiration* **55**:136–143.

Simonneau, E., Vivien, A., Sartene, R., Sartene, Kunstlinger, F., Samii, K., Noviant, Y., and Duroux, P. (1983). Diaphragm dysfunction induced by upper abdominal surgery. *Am. Rev. Respir. Dis.* **128**:899–903.

Sinha, R., and Bergofsky, E. H. (1972). Prolonged alteration of lung mechanics in kyphoscoliosis by positive pressure hyperinflation. *Am. Rev. Respir. Dis.* **106**:47–57.

Skatrud, J., Iber, C., McHugh, W., Rasmussen, H., and Nichols, D. (1980). Determinants of hypoventilation during wakefulness and sleep in diaphragmatic paralysis. *Am. Rev. Respir. Dis.* **121**:587–593.

Smith, P., Gold, A., Meyers, D., Haponik, E., and Bleecker, E. (1985). Weight loss in mildly to moderately obese patients with obstructive sleep apnea. *Ann. Intern. Med.* **103**:850–855.

Smith, P. E. M., Calverley, P. M. A., and Edwards, R. H. T. (1988a). Hypoxemia during sleep in Duchenne muscular dystrophy. *Am. Rev. Respir. Dis.* **137**:884–888.

Smith, P. E. M., Coakley, J. H.., and Edwards, R. H. T. (1988b). Respiratory muscle training in Duchenne muscular dystrophy. *Muscle Nerve* **11**:784.

Smith, P. E. M., Edwards, R. H. T., and Calverley, P. M. A. (1989). Ventilation and breathing pattern during sleep in Duchenne muscular dystrophy. *Chest* **96**:1346–1351.

Smyth, R. J., Chapman, K. R., Wright, T. A., Crawford, J. S., and Rebuck, A. S. (1984). Pulmonary function in adolescents with mild idiopathic scoliosis. *Thorax* **39**:901–904.

Solliday, N. H., Gaensler, E. A., Schwaber, J. R., and Parker, T. F. (1974). Impaired central chemoreceptor function and chronic hypoventilation many years following poliomyelitis. *Respiration* **31**:177–192.

Spiteri, M. A., Mier, A. K., Brophy, C. J., Pantin, C. F. A., and Green, M. (1985). Bilateral diaphragm weakness. *Thorax* **40**:631–632.

Steljes, D. G., Kryger, M. H., Kirk, B. W., and Millar, T. W. (1990). Sleep in postpolio syndrome. *Chest* **98**:133–140.

St. Louis, M. E., Peck, S. H. S., Bowering, D., Barry, G., Morgan, B. S. A., Blatherwick, J., Banerjee, S., Kettyls, G. D. M., Black, W. A., Milling, M. E., Hauschild, A. H. W., Tauxe, R. V., and Blake, P. A. (1988). Botulism from chopped garlic: delayed recognition of a major outbreak. *Ann. Intern. Med.* **108**:363–368.

Stokes, D. C., Pyeritz, R. E., Wise, R. A., Fairclough, D., and Murphy, E. A. (1988). Spirometry and chest wall dimensions in achondroplasia. *Chest* **93**:364–369.

Stokes, D. C., Wohl, M. E. B., Wise, R. A., Pyeritz, R. E., and Fairclough, D. L. (1990). The lungs and airways in achondroplasia. Do little people have little lungs? *Chest* **98**:145–152.

Stone, D. J., and Keltz, H. (1963). The effect of respiratory muscle dysfunction on pulmonary function. *Am. Rev. Respir. Dis.* **88**:621–629.

Streeten, E. A., de la Monte, S. M., and Kennedy, T. P. (1986). Amyloid infiltration of the diaphragm as a cause of respiratory failure. *Chest* **89**: 760–762.

Sugerman, H., Fairman., R., Baron, P., and Kwentus, J. (1986). Gastric surgery for respiratory insufficiency of obesity. *Chest* **90**:81–86.

Suratt, P., Wilhoit, S., Hsiao, H., Atkinson, R., and Rochester, D. (1984). Compliance of chest wall in obese subjects. *J. Appl. Physiol.* **57**:403–407.

Suratt, P., McTier, R., Findley, L., Pohl, S., and Wilhoit, S. (1987). Changes in breathing and the pharynx after weight loss in obstructive sleep apnea. *Chest* **92**:631–637.

Sutton, F., Zwillich, C., Creagh, E., Pierson, D., and Weil, J. (1975). Progesterone for outpatient treatment of pickwickian syndrome. *Ann. Intern. Med.* **83**:476–479.

Swank, S., Lonstein, J., Moe, J., Winter, R., and Bradford, D. (1981). Surgical treatment of adult scoliosis. *J. Bone Joint Surg.* **63**:268–287.

Szeinberg, A., Tabachnik, W., Rashed, N., McLaughlin, F. J., England, S., Bryan, C. A., and Levison, H. (1988). Cough capacity in patients with muscular dystrophy. *Chest* **94**:1232–1235.

Tassinari, C. A., Bernardina, B. D., Cirignotta, F., and Ambrosetto, G. (1972). Apnoeic periods and the respiratory related arousal patterns during sleep in the Pickwickian syndrome. A polygraphic study. *Bull. Physio-pathol. Resp.* **8**:1087–1102.

Thomas, A. N., Blaidsdell, F. W., Lewis, F. R., Jr., and Schlobohm, R. M. (1978). Operative stailization for flail chest after blunt trauma. *J. Thorac. Cardiovasc. Surg.* **75**:793:801.

Thomas, N. E., Passamonte, P. M., Sunderrajan, E. V., Andelin, J. B., and Ansbacher, L. E. (1984). Bilateral diaphragmatic paralysis as a possible paraneoplastic syndrome from renal cell carcinoma. *Am. Rev. Respir. Dis.* **129**:507–509.

Thomas, P., Cowen, E., Hulands, G., and Milledge, J. (1989). Respiratory function in the morbidly obese before and after weight loss. *Thorax* **44**:382–386.

Thompson, P. J., Dhillon, D. P., Ledingham, J., and Turner-Warwick, M. (1985). Shrinking lungs, diaphragmatic dysfunction, and systemic lupus erythematosus. *Am. Rev. Respir. Dis.* **132**:926–928.

Todd, T. R. J., and Shamji, F. (1985). Pathophysiology of chest wall trauma. In *The Thorax (Part B)*. Edited by C. Roussos and P. T. Macklem. Marcel Dekker, New York, Chapter 33, pp. 979–997.

Trinkle, J. K., Richardson, J. D., Franz, J. L., Grover, F. L., Arom, K. V., and Holmstrom, F. M. G. (1975). Management of flail chest without mechanical ventilation. *Ann. Thorac. Surg.* **19**:355–363.

Tsao, T. C-Y., Juang, Y-C., Chiang, Y-C., Tsai, Y-H., Lan, R-S., and Lee, C-H. (1991). Pneumonia preceding respiratory failure. A rare, easily misleading clinical manifestation in adult Arnold-Chiari malformation. *Chest* **99**:1294–1295.

Tzelepis, G. E., Ettensohn, D. B., Shapiro, B., and McCool, F. D. (1988). Unilateral absence of the diaphragm in an asymptomatic adult. *Chest* **94**:1301–1303.

Tzelepis, G. E., McCool, F. D., and Hoppin, F. G. Jr. (1989). Chest wall distortion in patients with flail chest. *Am. Rev. Respir. Dis.* **140**:31–37.

Urmey, W., Loring, S., Mead, J., Slutsky, A. S., Sarkarati, M., Rossier, A., and Brown, R. (1986). Upper and lower rib cage deformation during breathing in quadriplegia. *J. Appl. Physiol.* **60**:618–622.

Vanderlinden, R. G., Epstein, S. W., Hyland, R. L. H., Smythe, H. S., and Vanderlinden, L. D. (1988). Management of chronic ventilatory insufficiency with electrical diaphragm pacing. *Can. J.Neurol. Sci.* **15**:63–67.

Van Lunteren, E., Daniels, R., Deal, E. C., Jr., and Haxhiu, M. A. (1989). Role of costal and crural diaphragm and parasternal intercostals during coughing in cats. *J. Appl. Physiol.* **66**(1):135–141.

Vincken, W., Elleker, M. G., and Cosio, M. G. (1987). Determinants of respiratory muscle weakness in stable chronic neuromuscular disorders. *Am. J. Med.* **82**:53–58.

Weber, B., Smith, J. P., Briscoe, W. A., Friedman, S. A., and King, T. K. C. (1975). Pulmonary function in asymptomatic adolescents with idiopathic scoliosis. *Am. Rev. Respir. Dis.* **111**:389–397.

Weese-Mayer, D. E., Morrow, A. S., Brouillette, R. T., Ilbawi, M. N., and Hunt, C. E. (1989). Diaphragm pacing in infants and children. A life-table analysis of implanted components. *Am. Rev. Respir. Dis.* **139**:974–979.

Weinstein, S., Zavala, D., and Ponseti, I. (1981). Idiopathic scoliosis. *J. Bone Joint Surg.* **63**:702–712.

Weng, T. R., Schultz, G. E., Chang, C. H., and Nigro, M. A. (1985). Pulmonary function adn ventilatory response to chemical stimuli in familial myopathy. *Chest* **88**:488–495.

Wheeler, W. E., Rubis, L. J., Jones, C. W., and Harrah, J. D. (1985). Etiology and prevention of topical cardiac hypothermia-induced phrenic nerve injury and left lower lobe atelectasis during cardiac surgery. *Chest* **88**: 680–683.

Wicks, A. B., and Menter, R. R. (1986). Long-term outlook in quadriplegic patients with initial ventilator dependency. *Chest* **90**:406–410.

Wiers, P. W. J., LeCoultre, R., Dallinga, O. T., Van Dijl, W., Meinesz, A. F., and Sluiter, H. J. (1977). Cuirass respirator treatment of chronic respiratory failure in scoliotic patients. *Thorax* **32**:221–228.

Wilcox, P., Baile, E. M., Hards, J., et al. (1988a). Phrenic nerve function and its relationship to atelectasis after coronary artery bypass surgery. *Chest* **93**:693–698.

Wilcox, P. G., Morrison, N. J., Anzarut, A. R. A., and Pardy, R. L. (1988b). Lambert-Eaton myasthenic syndrome involving the diaphragm. *Chest* **93**:604–606.

Wilcox, P. G., Morrison, N. J., and Pardy, R. L. (1990a). Recovery of the ventilatory and upper airway muscles and exercise performance after type A botulism. *Chest* **98**:620–626.

Wilcox, P. G., Pare, P. D., and Pardy, R. L. (1990b). Recovery after unilateral phrenic injury associated with coronary artery revascularization. *Chest* **98**:661–666.

Wilson, D. O., Saunders, M. H., and Dauber, J. H. (1987). Abnormal ventilatory chemosensitivity and congenital myopathy. *Arch. Intern. Med.* **147**:1773–1777.

Witt, N. J., Zochodne, D. W., Bolton, C. F., Grand'Maison, F., Wells, G., Young, G. B., and Sibbald, W. J., (1991) Peripheral nerve function in sepsis and multiple organ failure. *Chest* **99**:176–184.

Woolf, C. R. (1990). Kyphoscoliosis and respiratory failure. A patient treated with assisted ventilation for 27 years. *Chest* **98**:1297–1298.

Wright, C. D., Williams, J. G., Ogilvie, A. M., and Donnelly, R. J. (1985). Results of diaphragmatic plication for unilateral diaphragmatic paralysis. *J. Thorac. Cardiovasc. Surg.* **90**:195–198.

Younger, D. S., Braun, N. M. T., Jaretzki, A., III, Penn, A. S., and Lovelace, R. E. (1984). Myasthenia gravis: determinants for independent ventilation after transsternal thymectomy. *Neurology* **34**:336–340.

Zochodne, D. D., Bolton, C. F., Wells, G. A., Gilbert, J. J., Hahn, A. F., Brown, J. D., and Sibbald, W. A. (1987). Critical illness polyneuropathy. A complication of sepsis and multiple organ failure. *Brain* **110**:819–842.

Zwillich, C., Sutton, F. D., Pierson, D. J., Creagh, E. M., and Weil, J. V. (1975). Decreased hypoxic ventilatory drive in the obesity-hypoventilation syndrome. *Am. J. Med.* **59**:343–348.

8

Rheumatological Diseases

UDAYA B. S. PRAKASH

Mayo Clinic, Mayo Medical Center, and Mayo Medical School
Rochester, Minnesota

I. Introduction

The terms "connective tissue diseases," "autoimmune diseases," "collagenoses," and "rheumatological diseases" are used interchangeably in clinical medicine. These diseases are a heterogeneous group of disorders frequently characterized by involvement of multiple organs by various degrees of inflammation. As a group, the collagenoses have no known etiological factors, although the inflammatory process in most of these entities is immunologically mediated, as shown by the presence of autoantibodies, rheumatoid factor, immune complexes, elevated erythrocyte sedimentation rate, and certain clinical characteristics. For the most part, the histological changes are nonspecific in all the rheumatological diseases. In diseases such as systemic lupus erythematosus (SLE), multiple criteria are used to arrive at the diagnosis (Davis et al., 1973; Tan et al., 1982; Trimble et al., 1974). Although vasculitis may be found in many of these disorders, they are not usually considered primary vasculitides. At times, however, it becomes difficult to separate the vasculitides from rheumatological diseases. The pulmonary manifestations of various vasculitides are covered in Chapter 9.

In each rheumatological disorder, it is common to see one major organ system affected to a greater extent than others. Moreover, it is not uncommon to see pulmonary manifestation as the presenting symptom or sign in many of these disorders, and in fact, in many of these diseases, pulmonary aspects assume a major role. This chapter will describe the pulmonary manifestations observed in rheumatoid arthritis (RA), SLE, scleroderma or progressive systemic sclerosis (PSS), polymyositis-dermatomyositis (PM-DM), mixed connective tissue disease (MCTD), and ankylosing spondylitis (AS). Because a recent issue in these series has covered in depth the research aspects and pathological changes of the lungs in rheumatological diseases (Cannon and Zimmerman, 1990), the major thrust of the discussion will be on the clinical aspects of these diseases with pertinent references to basic pathophysiology.

II. Rheumatoid Arthritis

RA is a chronic systemic inflammatory process characterized by nonsuppurative arthritis involving the diarthrodial joints with frequent involvement of tendons, ligaments, fascia, muscle, and bone. The American Rheumatism Association has established a set of criteria to diagnose RA. The prevalence of pleuropulmonary involvement in RA varies from 1.6% using chest roentgenogram alone to 47% utilizing DLCO (Hunninghake and Fauci, 1979). As a general rule, the pleuropulmonary involvement in RA is more common in those with active RA, although the pleuropulmonary findings may precede the onset of arthritic symptoms. Another peculiar feature of RA is the fact that middle-aged men are more likely than women to be affected by respiratory complications, where as the reverse is true of the arthritic manifestations.

A. Rheumatoid Pleurisy

Pleural involvement, the most common thoracic manifestation of RA, is found in nearly 50% of autopsy cases (Hunninghake and Fauci, 1979; Shiel and Prete, 1984). In clinical practice, however, it occurs in 8% of male patients and 16% of female patients (Hunninghake and Fauci, 1979). In a study of 309 patients with RA, chest roentgenographic evidence of pleural involvement was observed in 24% of men and 16% of women (Jurik et al., 1984). Nearly one-third of patients with rheumatoid pleurisy are asymptomatic, which contrasts to the painful pleurisy commonly observed in patients with SLE (Winslow et al., 1958). Pleurisy with effusion is more common in patients with active RA than in those with inactive disease (Fig. 1). Another clinically important feature is that pleural effusion may precede the onset of arthritic symptoms by months (Shiel and Prete, 1984). The pleural effusions are usually unilateral and small, but may be

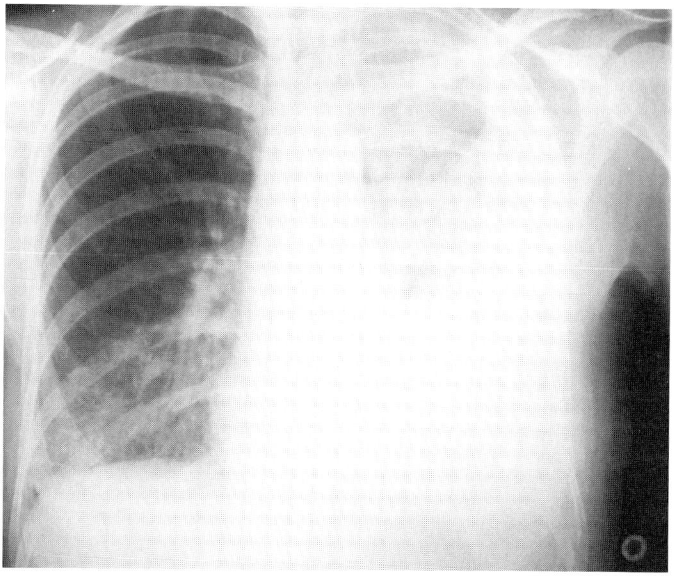

Figure 1 Chest roentgenograph demonstrating a large left pleural effusion in a woman with active rheumatoid arthritis. The pleural effusion became secondarily infected with *Pasteurella multocida* infection, requiring prolonged antibiotic therapy and pleural decortication.

persistent or recurrent. Chronic effusions persisting for months to years are not uncommon. One-third of rheumatoid pleural effusions are associated with other pulmonary processes (Hunninghake and Fauci, 1979).

Analysis of the pleural fluid reveals that it is typically an exudate, usually yellow and rarely bloody (Cervantes-Perez et al., 1980; Faurschou, 1984; Hunninghake and Fauci, 1979). Chronic effusions may appear opalescent green because of their high cholesterol content; this type of fluid has been described as "pseudochylothorax." The glucose content is very low (<30 mg/dl) in over 80% of patients (Hunninghake and Fauci, 1979; Shiel and Prete, 1984; Cervantes-Perez, et al., 1980). Pleural fluid hypoglycemia results both from selective blockage of glucose transport into the pleural space and from increased glucose use by the inflamed rheumatoid pleural mesothelial cells. The low glucose levels are nonspecific and also occur in pleural effusions secondary to malignant mesothelioma, tuberculosis, and empyema. The low pH of some rheumatoid pleural effusions is the result of localized acidosis resulting from blockage to the efflux of the end-products (lactate and CO_2) of glucose metabolism within the pleural space. Total complement levels in pleural fluid are low in 40% of patients (Hunder et al., 1972). High cholesterol levels are common in chronic pleural effusions associated with RA; some of the highest levels recorded have been in patients with RA (Staats et al., 1980). The presence of rheumatoid factor and the so-called RA cell (monocytes containing cytoplasmic inclusions representing phagocytized IgM in immune complex form) is nonspecific for the diagnosis of rheumatoid pleural effusion (Faurschou, 1984; Hunninghake and Fauci, 1979; Shiel and Prete, 1984).

B. Rheumatoid Lung

Rheumatoid lung denotes diffuse interstitial pneumonitis and fibrosis associated with RA. It is the most serious pleuropulmonary complication of RA (Hunninghake and Fauci, 1979). Chest roentgenograms show a compatible infiltrate in only 1.6–4.5% of patients (Hunninghake and Fauci, 1979; Jurik et al., 1984; Roschmann and Rothenberg, 1987), whereas the results of pulmonary function tests suggest restrictive lung disorder in more than one-third (Hunninghake and Fauci, 1979; Macfarlane et al., 1984; Roschmann and Rothenberg, 1987).

(A)

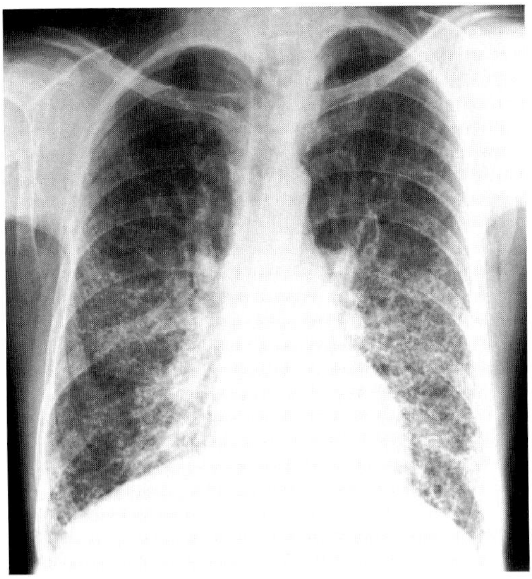

Figure 2 (A) Advanced case of rheumatoid lung seen on the chest roentgenograph of a middle-aged man with rheumatoid arthritis. The diffuse bilateral interstitial infiltrates with honeycombing, primarily affecting the lower two-thirds of the lung fields, are evident. (B) Localized view of the right lower lung region of the same patient 2 years earlier shows somewhat softer and feathery interstitial and alveolar infiltrates and no honeycombing.

Clinical, physiological, and histological features may mimic idiopathic pulmonary fibrosis (Keogh and Crystal, 1981). Cough and dyspnea are common symptoms, and clubbing has been described in up to 70% of patients (Roschmann and Rothenberg, 1987). Chest roentgenograms usually reveal a bibasilar interstitial process, micronodules, or honeycombing in late stages of the disease (Fig. 2). Up to 6% of patients with RA may develop a bilateral upper lobe process, reminiscent of the pulmonary abnormalities in ankylosing spondylitis (Macfarlane et al., 1984; McCann et al., 1983; and Roschmann and Rothenberg, 1987). Typically, the diffuse disease produces restrictive lung dysfunction, but the earliest physiological abnormality is diminished DLCO.

Lung biopsy in diffuse rheumatoid lung disease may show several abnormalities, depending on the stage of the disease. In one study of 40 patients with RA and an active pulmonary process, five histological patterns of pulmonary disease were identified: rheumatoid nodules, nonspecific interstitial pneumonitis, bronchiolitis obliterans with patchy organizing pneumonia, lymphoid hyperplasia, and cellular interstitial infiltrates (Yousem et al., 1985a). Nevertheless, each of these abnormalities by itself is nonspecific without clinical correlates. Bronchoalveolar lavage in patients with RA and established interstitial lung disease has shown abnormalities similar to those found in idiopathic pulmonary fibrosis (Garcia et al., 1986, 1987; Weiland et al., 1987; Gilligan et al., 1990). Some investigators have suggested that increased lymphocytosis of bronchoalveolar lavage fluid is associated with a good pulmonary prognosis

(B)

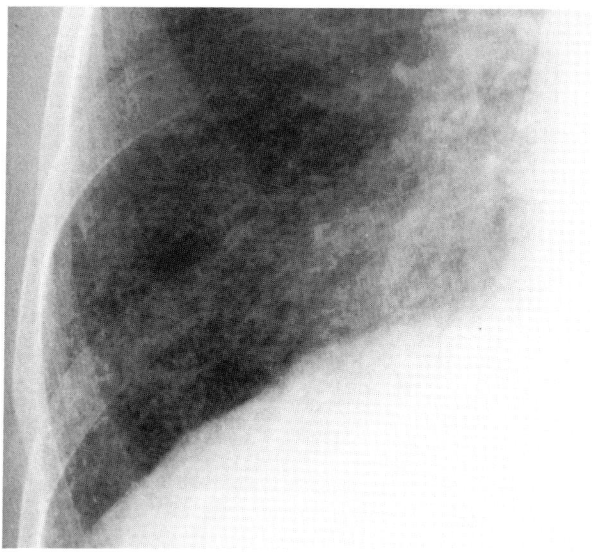

(Wallaert et al., 1990); this, however, has yet to be documented. Systemic corticosteroid therapy in its early stages may reverse the lung process.

C. Rheumatoid (Necrobiotic) Nodule

Rheumatoid nodules may occur within the lung parenchyma that are histologically identical to subcutaneous rheumatoid nodules (Shiel and Prete, 1984). These nodules are more likely to develop in men than women with seropositive RA, and they are known to precede the arthritic problems (Burke et al., 1977; Hunninghake and Fauci, 1979; Hull and Mathews, 1982; Nüsslein et al., 1987; Walters and Ojeda, 1986). The pulmonary nodules produce minimal symptoms and are often incidentally discovered (Fig. 3). The nodules may measure from a few millimeters to several centimeters and are usually bilateral, occur near pleuropulmonary surfaces, cavitate in two-thirds, and may rupture into pleural space to produce pneumothorax or empyema (Dumas et al., 1963; Macfarlane et al., 1984; Michalski et al., 1986; Portner and Gracie, 1966; Yates, 1963). Aspergillomas may develop in cavitary nodules (McConnochie et al., 1989). The necrobiotic nodules usually wax and wane with activity of the RA (Hunninghake

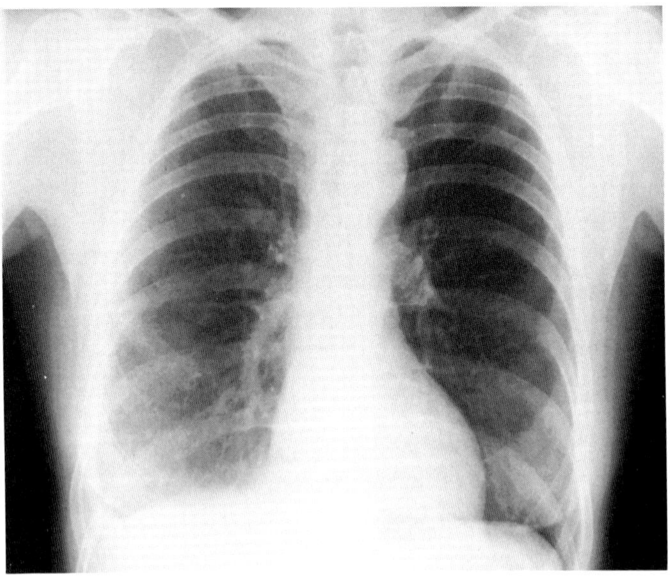

Figure 3 Rheumatoid nodules incidentally discovered in a woman with active rheumatoid arthritis. Well-defined round nodules measuring 1.5 cm can be seen in right suprahilar area and left lower lobe next to left cardiac border.

and Fauci, 1979), although they may resolve spontaneously despite continously active RA. The most common differential diagnosis of rheumatoid nodule is primary or metastatic lung cancer.

D. Rheumatoid Pneumoconiosis (Caplan's Syndrome)

Pneumoconiosis associated with rheumatoid nodules is called Caplan's syndrome. Originally described in coalworkers with rheumatoid arthritis, Caplan's syndrome is also found in persons with such conditions as silicosis, asbestosis, and aluminosis (Anttila et al., 1984; Caplan, 1953; Greaves, 1979). Caplan's syndrome is uncommon in the United States and most case reports have been from Europe (Wiedemann and Matthay, 1989). Caplan's syndrome is characterized by pulmonary nodules that measure 1–5 cm in diameter, evolve rapidly, and may undergo cavitation. These nodules may appear in crops and are frequently associated with other lung lesions (Fig. 4). Histological analysis will show features identical to those of rheumatoid nodules in addition to the presence of

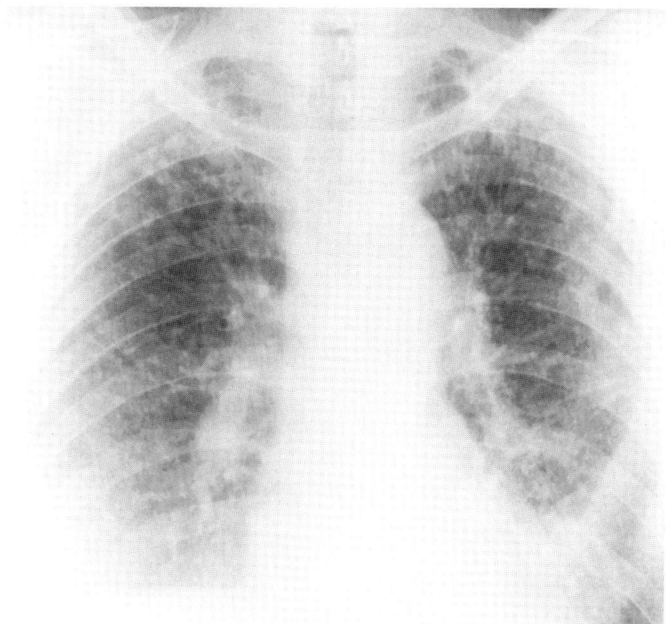

Figure 4 Caplan's syndrome in a patient exposed to silica demonstrating multiple nodules measuring 4–8 mm, predominantly located in the upper two-thirds of both lungs. Interstitial infiltrates are also noted in lower lung zones.

pneumoconiotic material in the center (Shiel and Prete, 1984). Occasionally, the nodules remain quiescent and heal by fibrosis.

E. Obstructive Airways Disease

Obstructive lung disease in RA is now a well-recognized phenomenon. Several prospective studies have demonstrated the presence of obstructive lung dysfunction in nearly one-third of patients with RA (Corrin et al., 1978; Geddes et al., 1977a, 1979; Herzog et al., 1981; Hills et al., 1979; Mountz et al., 1984; Passero and Myers, 1980; Sassoon et al., 1984). In one study of patients with active rheumatoid lung disease, 23% were found to have airflow obstruction by pulmonary function tests, and subsequent autopsy examination revealed the presence of severe bronchiolitis in these patients (Yousem et al., 1985b). Other pathological findings demonstrated follicular bronchiolitis/bronchitis in RA (Yousem et al., 1985b). Diminished mucociliary clearance has been demonstrated in patients with RA (Sutton et al., 1982). However, the combination of RA and smoking is associated with a much higher prevalence of obstructive lung disease than is either of these factors alone, and genetic predisposition to obstructive lung disease has been postulated as a contributing factor. The results of several studies have demonstrated that patients with RA and pulmonary involvement have a 50% incidence of non-MM (that is, MZ and MS) phenotypes of alpha-1-antitrypsin (Geddes et al., 1977b; Michalski et al., 1986; Roschmann and Rothenberg, 1987). Penicillamine and gold salts are used to treat RA, and because both these drugs are a known cause of bronchiolitis obliterans, this possibility should be considered in patients with RA who present with symptoms of airways obstruction.

F. Other Complications

Laryngeal rheumatoid nodules may occur in RA, but are rare. However, cricoarytenoid arthritis is recognized clinically in 25–35% of cases (Lawry et al., 1984) and is present in the majority of autopsies performed on patients with RA (Bienenstock et al., 1963; Lofgren and Montgomery, 1962). Chronic persistent sore throat and hoarseness are the main symptoms. Fixed obstruction at the laryngeal level may result in both inspiratory and expiratory difficulties. Laryngoscopy has demonstrated edema and erythema of the vocal apparatus, abnormal motion of vocal cords, and dysfunction of the arytenoids.

Pulmonary hypertension is uncommon, although several anecdotal cases have been described in the literature (Kay and Banik, 1977; Sharma et al., 1990). Alveolar hemorrhage is even more uncommon in RA, but the association has been described in six patients (Leatherman et al., 1982; Naschitz et al., 1989; Ognibene and Dito, 1965; Scott et al., 1981; Smith, 1966). Goodpasture's syndrome has also been reported in association with RA (Naschitz et al., 1989).

Pulmonary vasculitis is relatively uncommon in RA, although several cases have been reported and the presence of vasculitic lesions within the pulmonary capillaries may explain the alveolar hemorrhage (Scott et al., 1981; Leatherman et al., 1982).

G. Treatment and Prognosis

In the early stages of the evolving interstitial process, an initial response may be expected with corticosteroid therapy. The prognosis is poor, however, when the interstitial process is advanced. In one large series, such patients had a median survival of 3.5 years and a 5-year survival rate of 39% (Hakala, 1988). Rheumatoid bronchiolitis carries a poor prognosis. Corticosteroid and cytotoxic agents have been tried, but the response in chronic cases is poor. A point of clinical importance is that the cytotoxic agents such as gold, methotrexate, and cyclophosphamide can themselves produce pulmonary toxicity.

III. Systemic Lupus Erythematosus

SLE is a disease of unknown etiology characterized by immunologicaly mediated inflammation that affects multiple organs, including the skin, musculoskeletal, renal, and central nervous systems, and by the presence of multiple autoantibodies in the serum. Pleuropulmonary complications occur in 50–60% of patients with SLE, a higher percentage than in any other rheumatological disease (Hunninghake and Fauci, 1979; Turner-Stokes and Turner-Warwick, 1982). Intrathoracic manifestations of SLE include pleurisy with or without pleural effusion, lupus pneumonitis, atelectasizing pneumonitis, interstitial pneumonitis and fibrosis, pulmonary hemorrhage, diaphragmatic dysfunction, infections, pulmonary edema, obstructive lung disease, and pulmonary vasculitis. Histopathological abnormalities in pleuropulmonary tissues are nonspecific (Haupt et al., 1981).

A. Pleurisy

Pleural involvement is the most common and often the presenting manifestation of SLE, and has been found in 50–83% of patients at necropsy (Gross et al., 1972; Fayemi, 1975). Pathological changes in the pleura include infiltration by lymphocytes, mononuclear cells, and plasma cells, along with small-vessel vasculitis and various degrees of fibrosis (Bell and Lawrence, 1979; Purnell et al., 1955; Turner-Stokes and Turner-Warwick, 1982; Turner-Warwick, 1974). Painful pleurisy occurs in 50% of patients, and indeed pleuritic pain may be the initial symptom in many patients (Winslow et al., 1958). In fact, all young women who present with new-onset pleurisy or pleural effusion should be evaluated for SLE (Fig. 5). Another important differential diagnosis in such patients is the possibility of pulmonary embolism, because patients with SLE are at higher risk of thromboembolic phenomena owing to the presence of a circulating anticoagulant. Pleural effusions are usually small to moderate, bilateral in nearly 50% of patients, occasionally associated with small pericardial effusion, and frequently accompanied by dyspnea, cough, and fever (Good et al., 1983). Massive pleural effusions are rare in SLE (Good et al., 1983; Harvey et al., 1954; Winslow et al., 1958).

The pleural fluid is clear or serosanguineous (Good et al., 1983; Winslow et al., 1958); grossly bloody effusions are uncommon (Mulkey and Hudson, 1974; Passero and Myers, 1980). The fluid is almost always an exudate with varying numbers of leukocytes. The differential leukocyte count in SLE-associated pleural effusion is nonspecific and clinically unhelpful (Carr et al., 1970; Good et al., 1983). In contrast to the low pleural fluid glucose level in rheumatoid arthritis, the glucose level in patients with SLE is normal or high (Carr et al., 1970; Good et al., 1983; Hunder et al., 1972). Decreased and occasionally undetectable levels of total hemolytic complement as well as of C3

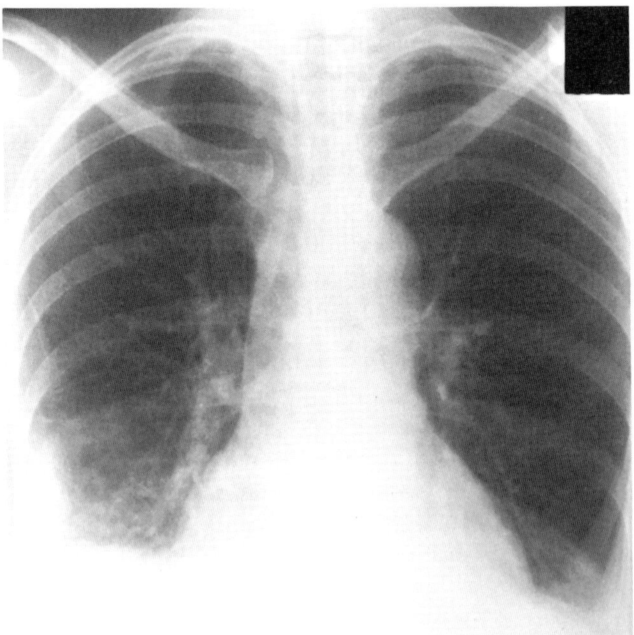

Figure 5 Chest roentgenograph of a young woman with systemic lupus erythematosus, initially manifested by bilateral pleural effusions and pericardial effusion.

and C4 components and increased immune complexes in the pleural fluid have been used as diagnostic tests of SLE-related pleurisy. Although these tests may corroborate the diagnosis of lupus pleuritis in nearly 80% of patients with pleural effusion, they are not diagnostic because similar findings have been described in rheumatoid pleural effusion and other disorders (Berendes and Miehkle, 1982; Good et al., 1983; Halla et al., 1980; Hunder et al., 1972, 1977). The presence of antinuclear antibody in the pleural fluid has also been reported to be helpful in the diagnosis of lupus pleuritis (Good et al., 1983). Lupus erythematosus cells have been found in from zero to more than 85% of lupus effusions (Berendes and Miehkle, 1973; Carr et al., 1970: Good et al., 1983); however, when present, these cells are highly specific for lupus pleuritis (Carr et al., 1970; Garnet et al., 1977; Good et al., 1983; Pandya et al., 1976). Pleural effusions are also common in drug-induced SLE (Hunder et al., 1972).

B. Pulmonary Hemorrhage

A study by Purnell et al. (1955) from the Mayo Clinic reported a high incidence of pulmonary hemorrhage discovered during autopsy examinations of patients with SLE. However, the clinical significance of this complication has only been recognized during the past decade (Churg et al., 1980; Eagen et al., 1978; Gould and Soriano, 1975; Marino and Pertschuk, 1981; Millman et al., 1981; Mintz et al., 1978). Now it has become increasingly clear that acute pulmonary alveolar hemorrhage is a common cause of mortality in these patients (Eagen et al., 1978; Matthay et al., 1975). Pulmonary hemorrhage is believed to be mediated by leukocytes, which are attracted by immune-complex deposits in the lungs, which cause leukocyte-mediated disruption of alveolar and capillary basement membrane integrity (Brentjens et al., 1977). Renal involvement by SLE may increase the risk of pulmonary hemorrhage. Pathological analysis of the lungs in cases of hemorrhage has shown abnormalities similar to those in lupus pneumonitis (Eagen et al., 1978), as well as a distinctive vasculitis of small vessels (Myers and Katzenstein, 1986).

Pulmonary hemorrhage may vary from subclinical to massive; significant hemoptysis is noted in 8–15% of patients (Eagen et al., 1978; Purnell et al., 1955; Mintz et al., 1978). Chronic subclinical pulmonary alveolar hemorrhage may lead to a clinical and pathological picture of pulmonary hemosiderosis (Abud-Mendoza et al., 1985 Byrd and Trunk, 1973; Kuhn, 1972). The onset of hemoptysis and progressive respiratory distress can be abrupt and the clinical presentation frequently resembles that of acute lupus pneumonitis (Churg et al., 1980; Eagen et al., 1978; Gould and Soriano, 1975; Marino and Pertschuk, 1981; Matthay et al., 1975; Miller et al., 1986; Millman et al., 1981; Mintz et al., 1978; Someren et al., 1983). Chest roentgenograms usually reveal bibasal, patchy, alveolar infiltrates (Fig. 6). The mortality from lupus-induced

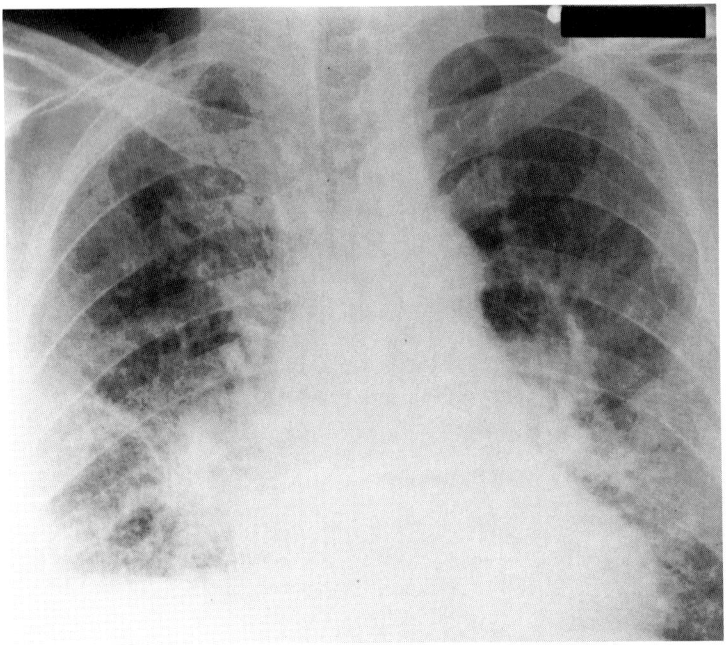

Figure 6 Diffuse alveolar hemorrhage manifesting as patchy bilateral alveolar infiltrates in a patient with systemic lupus erythematosus. The patient developed significant hemoptysis and renal dysfunction as a result of systemic lupus erythematosus.

pulmonary alveolar hemorrhage is in excess of 50%, and many of these patients die within several days of the onset of hemoptysis (Marino and Pertschuk, 1981; Mintz et al. 1978).

C. Interstitial Pneumonitis

Extensive interstitial fibrosis, as observed in patients with rheumatoid arthritis and scleroderma, is seldom seen in SLE. Patchy and irregular areas of interstitial pneumonitis and fibrosis develop in 15–45% of patients with SLE (Gross et al., 1972; Haupt et al., 1981; Bulgrin et al., 1960; Eisenberg et al., 1973; Holgate et al., 1976; Huang et al., 1965). Plate-like or discoid atelectatic areas are more common and usually occur in the lower two-thirds of the lung fields (Fig. 7) (Eisenberg et al., 1973). Infectious processes, particularly in patients who are on immunosuppressive therapy for SLE, are the most common cause of pulmonary parenchymal infiltrates (Haupt et al., 1981). However, sepsis and renal disease are more frequent causes of mortality in these patients than are pulmonary complications.

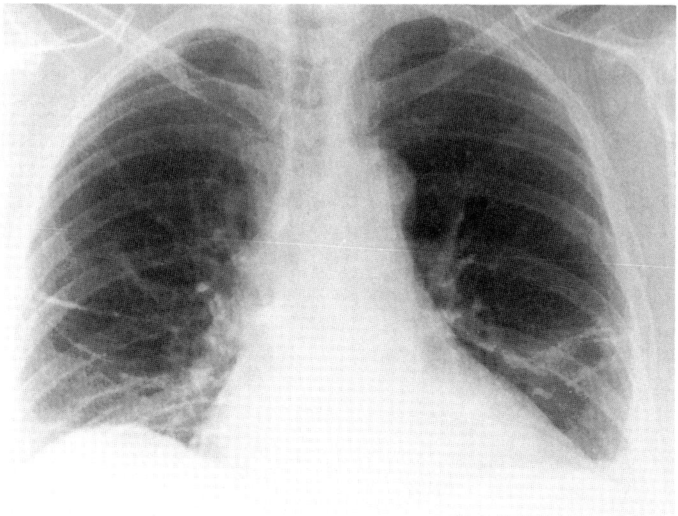

Figure 7 Chronic atelectasizing pneumonitis in a patient with chronic systemic lupus erythematosus. The chest roentgenograph demonstrates multiple platelike or discoid atelectatic areas in both lower lungs.

D. Pulmonary Thromboembolism

The SLE anticoagulant syndrome is characterized by a prolonged activated partial thromboplastin time, in association with otherwise normal clotting and platelet counts, and by the presence of anticardiolipin antibody and a false positive VDRL test (Espinoza and Hartmann, 1986). Recurrent thromboembolism and pulmonary emboli, which may be complicated by pulmonary hypertension, have been described in these patients (Asherson et al., 1983; Boey et al., 1983). Increasing experience with this condition suggests that long-term anticoagulant therapy is required to prevent venous thromboembolic phenomena (Asherson et al., 1985). Clinically significant pulmonary hypertension is relatively rare in SLE (Mahowald et al., 1985; Marchesoni et al., 1983; Perez and Kramer, 1981), but potential mechanisms that have caused it include progressive hypoxemia from interstitial fibrosis, chronic alveolar hemorrhage syndrome, vasculitis of small vessels, and recurrent pulmonary embolism.

E. Lupus Pneumonitis

Although the clinical syndrome of acute lupus pneumonitis has been described in several publications, it remains an uncommon feature of SLE (Cannon and Zimmerman, 1990; Matthay et al., 1975; Perez and Kramer, 1981; Pertschuk et al., 1977; Schwartzberg et al., 1984). The immediate postpartum period is considered to be a time of increased risk for acute lupus pneumonitis (Wiedemann and Matthay, 1989) because exacerbations of SLE during pregnancy and the postpartum period have been reported (Ainslie et al., 1979; Leikin et al., 1986; Myers et al., 1980). The acute lupus pneumonitis syndrome is characterized by the acute onset of dyspnea, high fever, and cough with occasional hemoptysis. Physical findings are minimal unless hypoxia is severe enough to cause cyanosis. Leukocytosis, elevated erythrocyte sedimentation rate, and significant hypoxemia may be apparent. Chest roentgenograms may reveal unilateral or bilateral diffuse or patchy lung infiltrates, predominantly in the lower lung zones with small pleural effusions (Fig. 8). Histologically, lupus pneumonitis reveals nonspecific changes that may include interstitial pneumonia, edema, and arteriolar thrombi. Vasculitis of major vessels is uncommon (Haupt et al., 1981; Hunninghake and Fauci, 1979; Matthay et al., 1975; Schleissner et al., 1976; Turner-Stokes and Turner-Warwick, 1982). Culture of lung specimens for pathogenic organisms is negative; however, because infections and other nonspecific pulmonary parenchymal abnormalities are more common in these patients, the diagnosis of lupus pneumonitis is one of exclusion (Hunter et al., 1980; Matthay et al., 1975; Pertschuk et al., 1977; Purnell et al., 1955).

F. Diaphragmatic Dysfunction

Diminished diaphragmatic function has been described in some patients with SLE (Gibson et al., 1977; Hoffbrand and Beck, 1965; Martens et al., 1983;

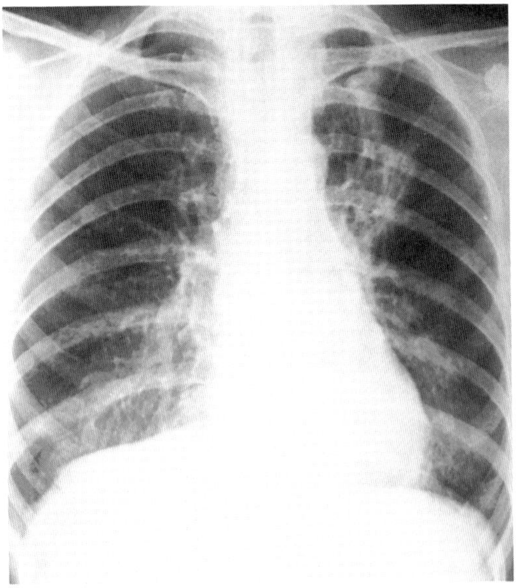

Figure 8 Chest roentgenograph of a patient with acute systemic lupus erythematosus and "lupus pneumonitis." An open lung biopsy revealed nonspecific pneumonitis; all cultures were negative.

Worth et al., 1988). The clinical significance of this finding is unclear, although this phenomenon may be responsible for the "unexplained dyspnea" in some patients with SLE (Fayemi, 1976). Many physicians have observed diaphragmatic elevation in patients with SLE, although the mechanisms responsible for the weakness are unknown; various possibilities include recurrent episodes of diaphragmatic pleurisy, basal atelectasis, and steroid myopathy. Some have described this phenomenon as the "shrinking lungs" syndrome (Fayemi, 1976). Most patients with lung involvement from SLE will demonstrate a restrictive type of pulmonary function abnormality, to which diaphragm dysfunction would contribute. This disorder does not appear to respond to corticosteroid therapy (Wiedemann and Matthay, 1989).

G. Other Complications

Although lung biopsies from patients with SLE may demonstrate areas of vasculitis, this abnormality is not characteristic of all lupus-induced pleuropulmonary processes. Because vasculitic lesions of large vessels and capillaries of the lung have been observed in less than half the patients (Fayemi, 1976; Gross et. al., 1972; Haupt et al., 1981; Purnell et al., 1955), it is clear that not all pleuropulmonary lesions in SLE are caused by vasculitis (Wiedemann and Matthay, 1989).

Obstruction to airflow is rare in SLE, although several anecdotal cases have been reported (Gold and Jennings, 1966; Huang and Lyons, 1966; Kallenbach et al., 1978). Bronchiolitis, noted in some patients, may be responsible for at least part of the airflow obstruction (Matthay et al., 1975; Pertschuk et al., 1977). Several cases of upper airway involvement from laryngeal inflammation have been reviewed (Wiedemann and Matthay, 1989).

Pulmonary function testing in patients with SLE usually reveals a restrictive type of dysfunction. The DLCO is characteristically reduced and the test is a reliable method to monitor patients with pulmonary parenchymal disease. Unless the diaphragmatic weakness is significant, maximal inspiratory and expiratory pressures are unlikely to exhibit severe abnormalities.

Drug-induced SLE is a clinically important syndrome, and the number of drugs known to cause SLE continues to increase (Cush and Goldings, 1985; Harmon and Portanova, 1982). Pleural and pulmonary involvement is common in drug-induced lupus, and pleural disease is especially common with certain drugs such as procainamide and hydralazine. The pleural fluid in this group of patients shows biochemical characteristics similar to the classic form of lupus. Withdrawal of the offending chemical usually results in resolution of symptoms and signs within days or weeks (Wiedemann and Matthay, 1989).

H. Treatment and Prognosis

Pleural effusion responds favorably to systemic corticosteroid therapy, with an occasional large effusion being refractory (Bell and Lawrence, 1979; Kaine,

1985). Lupus pneumonitis and the alveolar hemorrhage syndrome may respond to high-dose corticosteroid therapy. Cytotoxic agents have been used in patients refractory to corticosteroid therapy, but there is little evidence that they are more effective than cortisone alone (Eagen et al., 1978; Matthay et al., 1973, 1975). Sepsis and progressive renal dysfunction are the most frequent causes of mortality in patients with SLE, but acute pulmonary alveolar hemorrhage is also important. In patients with lupus pneumonitis, dramatic response can be expected following systemic corticosteroid therapy, although a review of 12 cases of lupus pneumonitis noted a mortality of about 50% (Wiedemann and Matthay, 1989).

IV. Scleroderma

Progressive systemic sclerosis (PSS), or scleroderma, is a systemic connective tissue disease characterized by a vascular disorder and excessive deposition of collagen and other matrix proteins in the skin and internal organs (LeRoy, 1981). The major pathological features of PSS that have been emphasized include vascular changes, immune dysfunction, and increased collagen synthesis (Claman, 1989). Pulmonary involvement from one or more of these alterations is common in patients with PSS (Steen et al., 1985a; Owens and Follansbee, 1987). Up to 80% have abnormal lungs at necropsy even though the patients were minimally symptomatic during life (D'Angelo et al., 1969; Weaver et al., 1968). Respiratory involvement may include pulmonary fibrosis, pulmonary hypertension with or without cor pulmonale, diffuse pulmonary calcification, aspiration pneumonia as a result of impaired swallowing from esophageal involvement, chest wall restriction from skin involvement, and scar cancer related to long-term fibrosis.

A. Pulmonary Fibrosis

Chronic progressive pulmonary fibrosis, the most common respiratory complication of PSS, occurs in up to two-thirds of patients. The histological appearances are identical to those of idiopathic pulmonary fibrosis (Harrison et al., 1990). In the early stages, alveolar edema with lymphocytic and monocytic infiltrates is seen. Later, severe fibrosis with honeycombing, cyst formation, and increased incidence of pneumothorax occur (Fig. 9). Although only one-third of patients with PSS have abnormal chest roentgenographic findings, more than 50% have exertional dyspnea and diminished DLCO. Asymptomatic patients with PSS demonstrate evidence of subclinical alveolitis as judged by the findings from bronchoalveolar lavage (Harrison et al., 1989; Wallaert et al., 1990). Additional studies have shown that increased pulmonary vascular leakage and neutrophilic alveolitis may be important early features of interstitial lung disease in PSS, and that these abnormalities are frequently associated with evidence of enhanced lung type II collagen synthesis (Harrison et al., 1990). Pulmonary

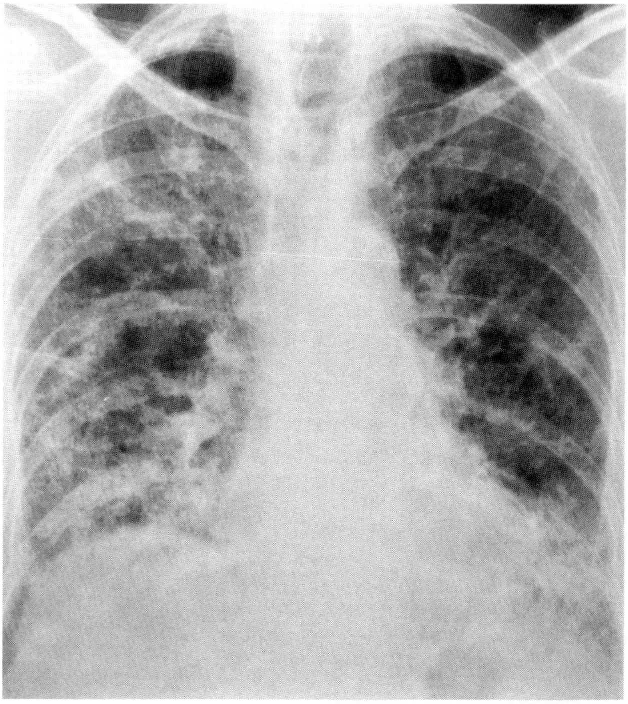

Figure 9 Chest roentgenograph of a patient with chronic scleroderma demonstrating extensive bilateral interstitial infiltrates. The patchy, asymmetrical distribution is noteworthy.

involvement tends to be particularly severe in patients with the CREST (calcinosis, Raynaud's phenomenon, esophageal involvement, sclerodactyly, and telangiectasia) variant of PSS.

Among groups of patients with various rheumatological diseases, those with PSS have undergone the most extensive pulmonary function testing. The most common abnormality is a slow, but relentlessly progressive restrictive dysfunction with diminished DLCO. The earliest abnormality is the diminished DLCO, and this test is also an important predictor of mortality (Bagg and Hughes, 1979; Owens et al., 1983). Several studies have shown that the presence of Raynaud's phenomenon is associated with lower DLCO (Ploysongsang and Foad, 1984; Ungerer et al., 1983).

B. Pulmonary Hypertension

Pulmonary hypertension occurs frequently in patients with PSS and is a major cause of mortality and morbidity (LeRoy, 1981). Pulmonary hypertension may develop as a result of chronic hypoxemia or from PSS-induced medial hypertrophy of the pulmonary arteries. The latter mechanism is independent of the arterial changes caused by chronic hypoxemia and is responsible for pulmonary hypertension in 35–60% of patients with PSS (Salerni et al., 1977; Stupi et al., 1986; Young and Mark, 1978). The incidence of pulmonary hypertension is particularly high in patients with the CREST variant of the disease (Stupi et al., 1986; Ungerer et al., 1983; Weaver et al., 1968; Young and Mark, 1978). Although there are a few case reports describing the responses to vasodilators, the overall results of treatment have been disappointing (Fudman and Kelling, 1985; Glikson et al., 1990; Niarchos et al., 1982; O'Brien et al., 1985). The incidence of renovascular pathology is high among patients with pulmonary vascular involvement.

C. Aspiration Pneumonia

Esophageal involvement, which is extremely common in patients with PSS, leads to esophageal dysfunction and acid reflux (Figs. 10 and 11). Aspiration of gastric contents secondary to esophageal reflux is believed to be one of the etiological factors in pulmonary fibrosis (Johnson et al., 1989).

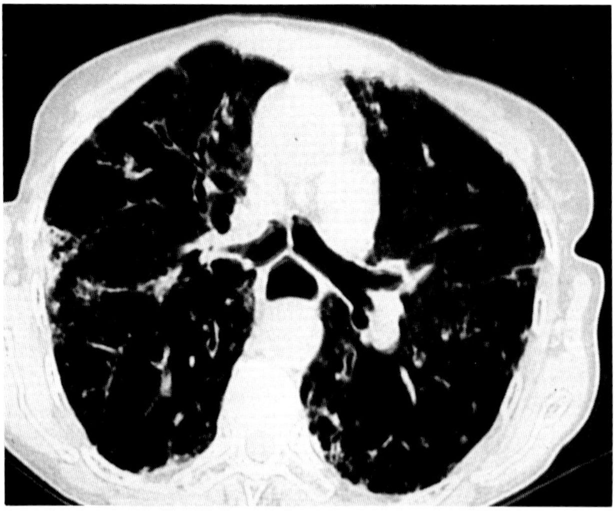

Figure 10 Computed tomography of the chest in a patient with scleroderma. Dilated esophagus, peripheral patchy pulmonary infiltrates, and traction bronchiectasis of right upper lobe bronchi are demonstrated.

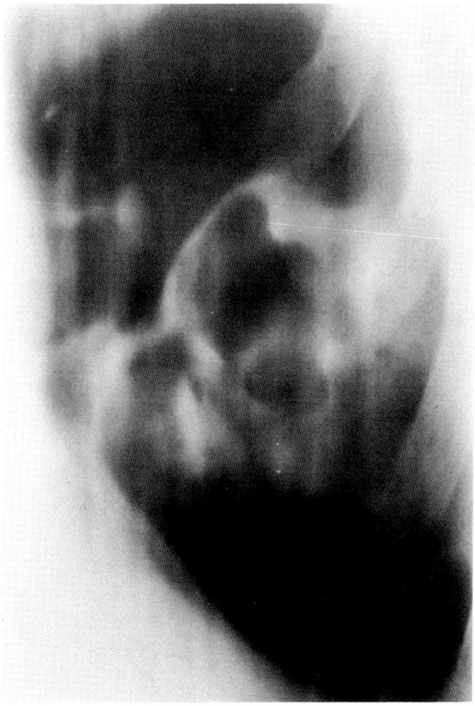

Figure 11 Localized view of the left lower lobe demonstrating a lung abcess in a patient with scleroderma. The lung abcess was a complication of aspiration pneumonia.

D. Other Complications

Other respiratory manifestations of PSS include diffuse pulmonary calcification in some patients with the CREST syndrome, resorption of ribs in chronic cases, and rare instances of pleural thickening. Although diffuse alveolar hemorrhage is now well known in patients with SLE and several vasculitides, it has seldom been described in PSS, with only two case reports in the literature (Griffin et al., 1990; Kallenbach et al., 1977).

Chronic PSS is reported to be associated with an increased risk of lung cancer (Peters-Golden et al., 1985; Rossi et al., 1985; Talbott and Barrocas, 1979, 1980). Although some have reported that the risk for developing bronchoalveolar carcinoma is increased (Tesluk, 1984), other histological types, including small-cell cancer, have been described in patients with chronic PSS (Sarma and Weilbaecher, 1985; Steen et al., 1985b; Winkelmann et al., 1988). It is not clear whether these cancers represent the so-called ''scar cancers'' or just incidental findings (Medsger, 1985).

Some of the uncommon thoracic manifestations of PSS reported in the literature include diaphargmatic dysfunction (Chausow et al., 1984; de Clerck et al., 1987), hemoptysis due to telangiectasia of the airways (Kim et al., 1988), and a syndrome resembling pulmonary hemosiderosis.

E. Treatment and Prognosis

Earlier reports showed that systemic corticosteroid therapy had no effect on the prognosis in patients with PSS. More recently, D-penicillamine has been used to prevent progression of the pulmonary complications (de Clerck et al., 1987; Medsger, 1987; Steen et al., 1985a), but the results of long-term, properly controlled trials are not available. When patients with PSS develop hypoxemia, supplemental oxygen therapy is the only treatment that provides relief of the dyspnea.

V. Polymyositis-Dermatomyositis

Polymyositis-dermatomyositis (PM-DM) is characterized by inflammation of skeletal muscles with resultant weakness of proximal muscles and a characteristic skin rash (heliotrope hue). The paraneoplastic variant of PM-DM should be differentiated from the idiopathic or autoimmune type (Plotz et al., 1989). The former may occur in up to 5–10% of patients with bronchogenic and other carcinomas (Callen 1982; Lakhanpal et al., 1986; Manchul et al., 1985). When elderly patients present with PM-DM, an underlying malignancy must be excluded before the diagnosis of autoimmune PM-DM is considered (Plotz et al., 1989). The discussion here pertains to the idiopathic or autoimmune variety of PM-DM. The idiopathic inflammatory myopathies are very uncommon, with no more than 5–10 cases per million persons per year in the United States (Plotz et al., 1989). The diagnosis is based on clinical features, elevation of creatine phosphokinase, electromyographic studies, and muscle biopsy. Pleuropulmonary involvement has been observed in up to 5% of patients with PM-DM (Bohan and Peter, 1975; Frazier and Miller, 1974; Hunninghake and Fauci, 1979) and precedes by 1–24 months the musculocutaneous signs and symptoms in approximately one-third of those who become involved (Bohan and Peter 1975). Of note is the observation that there is a lack of relationship between the severity and progression of the myositis and the severity of respiratory disease (Wiedemann and Matthay, 1989).

A. Interstitial Pneumonitis and Fibrosis

The most common pulmonary disorder is interstitial pneumonitis and fibrosis in the basal areas of the lungs, which occurs in 5–10% of patients (Plotz et al., 1989; Salmeron et al., 1981). It may present as acute pneumonitis with alveolar or mixed alveolar-interstitial infiltrates (Fig. 12). Even though not all patients

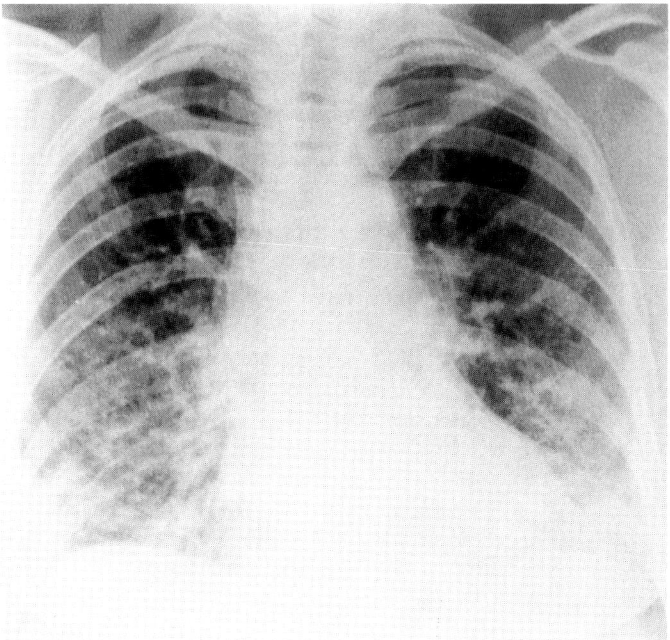

Figure 12 Chest roentgenograph of a patient with polymyositis-dermamyositis showing diffuse bilteral alveolar and interstitial infiltrates, with relative sparing of upper lung zones.

with PM-DM will demonstrate the anti-Jo-1 antibody in their serum, over 50% of patients with this antibody exhibit interstitial pulmonary disease (Arnett et al., 1981; Bernstein et al., 1984; Hochberg et al., 1984; Plotz et al., 1989; Wasicek et al., 1984). Bronchoalveolar lavage studies in affected patients have not identified a characteristic cellular pattern (Greene et al., 1987; Plotz et al., 1989). Respiratory disease presents as dyspnea, cough, and hypoxemia; symptoms related to gastroesophageal reflux may be the initial manifestation in some patients. The pathogenesis of the interstitial pneumonitis and fibrosis in PM-DM is unknown, but hypersensitivity mechanisms may play a role. Pathological analysis may reveal nonspecific fibrosis in addition to arteriolitis and desquamation of alveolar lining cells. A restrictive type of lung dysfunction is present in nearly 50% of patients.

B. Hypoventilation

With the involvement of proximal musculature, particularly the upper limb girdle, weakness of the respiratory muscles may ensue and result in progressive hypoventilation and respiratory failure. Muscle weakness may severely compromise the respiratory bellows mechanism, thereby producing restrictive disease and basal atelectasis. An ineffective cough increases the risk of bacterial pneumonia. Increasing hypercarbia is a poor prognostic sign in these patients.

C. Aspiration Pneumonitis

Esophageal involvement is common in patients with PM-DM. The clinical manifestations include uncoordinated peristalsis, esophageal reflux, odynophagia, and delayed gastric emptying (Horowitz et al., 1986). Bulbar involvement and dysfunction of the muscles of deglutition often lead to recurrent aspiration problems. Poor cough strength as a result of respiratory muscle weakness contributes to the development and progression of aspiration pneumonia. Clinical experience has shown that aspiration pneumonia is often the cause of death in these patients (Blumbergs et al., 1984; Medsger et al., 1971; Salmeron et al., 1982).

D. Treatment and Prognosis

Pulmonary involvement in PM-DM is usually progressive, and long-term response to corticosteroid therapy is poor even though the initial response may have been good (Henriksson and Sandstedt, 1982). However, patients who received high-dose therapy (prednisolone, 1–2 mg/kg/day) have shown improved morbidity (Bohan and Peter, 1975; Carpenter et al., 1977; Frazier and Miller, 1974; Winkelmann et al., 1968). Patients with acute onset of symptoms and pulmonary infiltrates appear to respond the best (Frazier and Miller, 1974). Many treatment programs, consisting of corticosteroid, azathioprine, methotrexate, total-body irradiation, and thymectomy, have been tried with varying rates of success (Plotz et al., 1989).

VI. Mixed Connective Tissue Disease

Clinicians had observed for many years that some patients exhibited features of more than one rheumatological disease and thus did not fit into the traditional classification. The laboratory tests to diagnose the well-established rheumatological entities in some of these patients were helpful, but not pathognomonic. Thus, when confronted with a patient who had clinical features of more than one of the rheumatological diseases, physicians often used the terms "overlap syndrome," "undifferentiated connective tissue disease," "sclerodermatomyositis," "RUPUS" (RA and SLE), or "lupoderma" (SLE and PSS) (Bennett, 1985; Ginsburg et al., 1983). The term "mixed connective tissue disease" (MCTD) was coined in 1972, based on the recognition that many patients with clinical features of SLE, PSS, and PM-DM had unusually high titers of a specific circulating antibody to an extractable nuclear ribonucleoprotein antigen (ENA) (Maddison et al., 1978; Sharp et al., 1972). The presence of high titers of antibody to ENA and the absence of antibodies to Sm antigen are thought to be specific for MCTD, although this has been questioned (Alarcón-Segovia and Palacios, 1981). Studies using T-lymphocyte characteristics have led to the belief that MCTD may be a distinct entity, but whether it is or not, the literature reveals many new publications on this topic and that more and more clinicians are accepting the diagnosis of MCTD (Reichlin, 1976; Sharp, 1982; LeRoy et al., 1980; Lemmer et al., 1982; Sharp and Anderson, 1980; Alarcón-Segovia, 1981). It appears that MCTD (also known as "Sharp's syndrome") will remain a disease entity in clinical practice for the foreseeable future. The etiology and prevalence of MCTD are unknown, but it is believed to be more common than PM-DM but less common than SLE. The majority of patients are women, and the average age at time of diagnosis is 37 years; no unusual ethnic or racial preponderance has been noted (Sharp and Singsen, 1985). Renal disease occurs in 10–20%, and some patients may require aggressive or prolonged pharmacological therapy (Grant et al., 1981; Nimelstein et al., 1980; Prakash et al., 1985; Sullivan et al., 1984; Wiener-Kronish et al., 1981).

Overall, pulmonary involvement has been described in 20–80% of patients with MCTD by two groups of investigators (Harmon et al., 1976; Vitali et al., 1985). A third, detailed prospective study of 34 patients with MCTD demonstrated pulmonary disease in 85% (Sullivan et al., 1984). In contrast, a retrospective analysis of 81 patients revealed pleuropulmonary manifestations in only 25% (Prakash et al., 1985). Many of the pleuropulmonary manifestations, both clinical and pathophysiological, are similar to those observed in SLE, PSS, and PM-DM (Prakash et al., 1985; Vitali et al., 1985).

A. Interstitial Fibrosis

Pathological features akin to idiopathic pulmonary fibrosis and characterized by alveolar septal infiltration by lymphocytes, plasma cells, and type III collagen have been demonstrated in patients with MCTD (Hurst et al., 1980; Sharp and Singsen, 1985; Wiener-Kronish et al., 1981). In one report on five patients, interstitial fibrosis with honeycomb formation and infiltration of alveolar septum by plasma cells and lymphocytes were the predominatnt pathological findings. Immunofluorescent stains for IgG, IgM, and IgA were negative. Mild, nonspecific interstitial fibrosis was observed in the prospective study already cited (Sullivan et al., 1984). Generally, the degree of fibrosis tends to be severe if the predominant clinical feature is PSS (Prakash, 1988). Abnormal pulmonary function tests and chest roentgenograms have been noted in 69% of patients without respiratory symptoms (Harmon et al., 1976). In a multicenter study of 100 patients with MCTD, impaired DLCO was noted in 67%, and restrictive lung volumes were observed in 50% (Sharp and Singsen, 1985). Chest roentgenographic changes similar to those in idiopathic pulmonary fibrosis have been described (Harmon et al., 1976; Silver et al., 1976).

A prospective evaluation of 34 patients with MCTD has shown decreased TLC in 41%, VC in 34%, and DLCO in 72% of the patients. Hypoxemia (Pao_2 lower than 10 mmHg of the predicted value) was observed in 21% of the patients. Of the four patients who died, three had a marked drop in DLCO over time. Chest roentgenographic abnormalities were present in 85% and consisted of small, irregular opacities in the lower and midlung fields (Sullivan et al., 1984). In a retrospective study of 81 patients, respiratory symptoms included dyspnea (16%), chest pain and tightness (7%), and cough (5%). Chest roentgenographs revealed abnormalities in 21%, the most common being an interstitial process in both lower lung fields (Fig. 13). Pulmonary function testing demonstrated a restrictive type of defect in 69% (Prakash et al., 1985). DLCO is the most sensitive single parameter in evaluating pulmonary dysfunction in MCTD (Derderian et al., 1985).

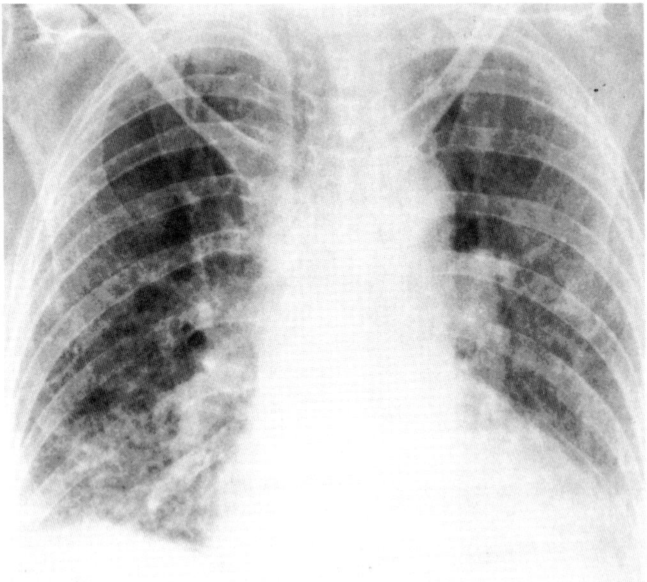

Figure 13 Chest roentgenograph of a patient with mixed connective tissue disease demonstrating bilateral interstitial infiltrates and blunting of left costophrenic angle due to small pleural effusion.

B. Pleural Effusion

Pleurisy is a common manifestation of MCTD. Although only 6% of patients in a retrospective study of 81 patients had pleural effusion (Prakash et al., 1985), 40% of patients in the prospective study were noted to have pleuritic pain (Sullivan et al., 1984). Pleural fluid shows the same characteristics as that in SLE. The effusions are usually small and resolve spontaneously (Hoogsteden et al., 1985).

C. Pulmonary Hypertension

The most serious complication of MCTD, progressive pulmonary hypertension, may be accompanied by severe vasculitic lesions (Alpert et al., 1983; Harmon et al., 1976; Jones et al., 1978; Wiener-Kronish et al., 1981). In the prospective evaluation of 34 patients, significant pulmonary hypertension was noted in 67% of the 15 patients studied (Sullivan et al., 1984). Moreover, the elevated pulmonary vascular resistance was associated with reduced DLCO in 9 of 10 patients. Analysis of lung biopsy specimens of one patient revealed muscular hypertrophy of small pulmonary arteries, and necropsy examination in three patients revealed right ventricular hypertrophy. Plexogenic angiopathy and chronic intimal thickening of medium-sized pulmonary arteries have been observed in patients with MCTD (Kobayashi et al., 1982; Wiener-Kronish et al., 1981). Fatal pulmonary hypertension has been reported in a number of patients (Graziano et al., 1983; Ueda et al., 1984).

In one report on five patients with MCTD, pulmonary vascular involvement was responsible for deaths in four. One patient had intimal thickening, focal fibrinoid necrosis, and positive immunofluorescent stains for IgG, C3, and C1q in medium-sized pulmonary arteries; three patients had disabling pulmonary hypertension (Wiener-Kronish et al., 1981). It is difficult to assess the role of vasculitic process in the origin of pulmonary hypertension in this group of patients.

D. Pulmonary Thromboembolism

The incidence of thromboembolic disease is high in SLE spite the presence of a circulating anticoagulant. Several similar cases of MCTD with circulating lupus anticoagulant and recurrent thromboemboli complicated by pulmonary embolism and pulmonary hypertension have been described (Alpert et al., 1983; Hainaut et al., 1986; Jones et al., 1978).

E. Aspiration Pneumonitis

Esophageal dysmotility is extremely common in both PSS and PM-DM. In patients with MCTD, barium esophagrams and esophageal manometry have been noted to be abnormal in 53% and 69% of patients, respectively (Prakash et al., 1985). Hypotonicity and dilatation of the esophagus are similar to those in PSS. These changes are responsible for the reflux and aspiration pneumonia. Although this aspect of MCTD has not received much attention, clinicians should be aware of this potentially lethal complication of MCTD (Fig. 14).

F. Other Complications

Pulmonary hemorrhage is a recognized complication of SLE, and the risk of hemorrhage increases with renal involvement. Similar abnormalities were reported in a 37-year-old woman with long-standing MCTD, who developed hemoptysis, bilateral pulmonary infiltrates, dyspnea, anemia, and acute renal failure secondary to immunologically mediated tubulointerstitial disease (Germain and Davidman., 1984). Although localized lesions are uncommon in MCTD, cavitary pulmonary nodules have been noted in five patients (Webb and Gamsu, 1981). Necropsy, bronchial brushing, or lung aspiration in three cases proved the nodules to be abscesses caused by bacteria in two and *Aspergillus* in one. One patient had pulmonary embolism and a necrotic pulmonary infarct. Generalized lymphadenopathy has been observed in 50% of patients with MCTD (Sullivan et al., 1984), and mediastinal lymphadenopathy has been described in two patients (Guit et al., 1985; Webb and Gamsu, 1981). Patients

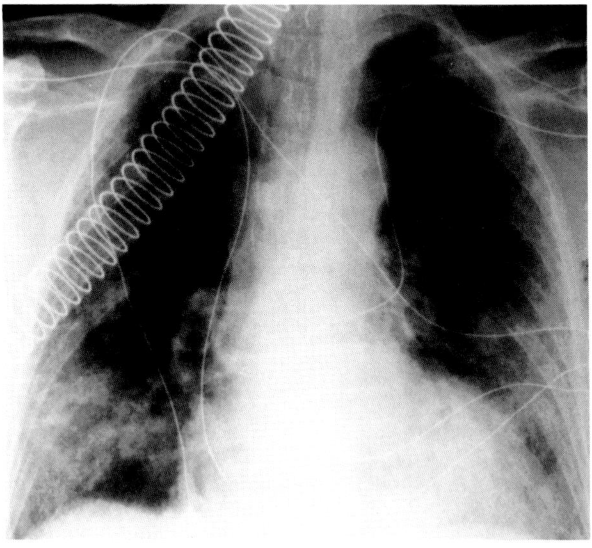

Figure 14 Bilateral aspiration pneumonia complicated by acute respiratory distress syndrome in a patient with mixed connective tissue disease.

receiving systemic corticosteroid and immunosuppressive therapy for MCTD are at risk to develop opportunistic infections (Bennett, 1980; Bennett and O'Connell, 1980).

Proximal myopathy with resultant weakness of respiratory muscles is another complication of PM-DM. If the features of PM-DM are prominent in MCTD, significant proximal muscle weakness may cause hypoventilatory respiratory failure. Diaphragmatic weakness has been described in a patient with MCTD (Martens and Demedts, 1982).

G. Treatment and Prognosis

Authors of early reports on MCTD suggested that corticosteroids were effective in reversing the pathological process (Bennett, 1985; Sharp et al., 1972). Subsequent experience, however, has shown that some patients do not respond to either corticosteroids or immunosuppressive agents, or both. Pleurisy usually responds well to corticosteroid therapy whereas pulmonary hypertension does not. Chlorambucil and cyclophosphamide have been tried with varying success (Sullivan et al., 1984; Wiener-Kronish et al., 1981). In the prospective study of 34 patients with MCTD, favorable responses were noted in two-thirds of the patients (Sullivan et al., 1984). Patients with predominantly PSS-like disease have demonstrated poor response (Prakash et al., 1985). Others have noted rapid deterioration and death despite corticosteroid and cytotoxic chemotherapy. In a retrospective study of 81 patients, six died during a 5-year follow-up period, two of whom had received corticosteroid. The causes of death included carcinoma of esophagus, aspiration pneumonia, pulmonary hypertension, cardiorespiratory arrest, and myocardial infarction.

VII. Ankylosing Spondylitis

Ankylosing spondylitis (AS), also known as rheumatoid spondylitis and Marie-Strümpell disease, is a chronic disorder of unknown etiology characterized by progressive inflammatory disease involving the axial spine and the adjacent soft tissues. The sacroiliac, hip, and shoulder are the most commonly affected joints. Males with AS predominate over females. The symptoms in most patients begin between the ages of 16 and 40 years. The disease may be inherited by a single autosomal dominant factor, with a 70% penetrance in males and a 10% in females. A high association exists between ankylosing spondylitis and the histocompatibility antigen HLA-B27. Extraskeletal manifestations affect many organs, and the abnormalities may include aortic valve incompetence, varying degrees of heart block, acute anterior uveitis, fever, anemia, fatigue, and weight loss. Pulmonary involvement has been reported in 2–70% of patients with AS (Rosenow et al., 1977). Respiratory problems include chest wall restriction due to ankylosis of costovertebral joints, fibrosis of the lung apices, and rare cases of apical cavitations.

A. Apical Fibrosis

Pulmonary complications are reported in 2–70% of patients with AS. In clinical practice, however, less than 5% exhibit respiratory problems (Bergofsky, 1979; Davies, 1972; Gacad and Hamosh, 1973; Rosenow et al., 1977; Scobie, 1971; Vale et al., 1974). In one large review of over 2000 patients with AS, pleuropulmonary manifestations were noted in only 1.3%, or 28 patients (Rosenow et al., 1977). The most common abnormality was fibrobullous apical lesions in 26 patients, followed by aspergilloma in five and pleural effusion with nonspecific pleuritis in three. An upper-lobe fibrotic process, nodular and linear lesions in the upper lobes, has been described in 14–30% (Chakera et al., 1975; Cruickshank, 1960). The process begins as linear infiltrates in the upper lung regions medially and then radiates laterally. The ''bamboo spine'' appearance of the spinal column and the linear fibrotic strands produce the ''telephone pole'' appearance on the chest roentgenograph. In chronic cases, the linear infiltrates are replaced by irregular nodular changes, which undergo cystic or cavitary changes (Fig. 15). Computed tomography has shown pleural thickening, bullous

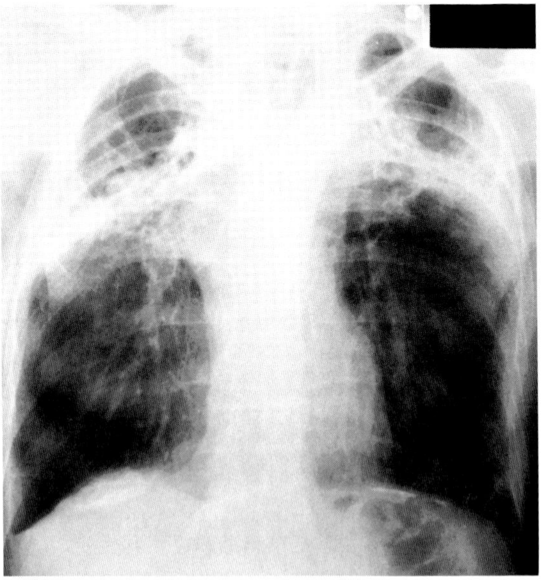

Figure 15 Advanced pulmonary abnormalities in a patient with chronic ankylosing spondylitis. Bilateral upper lung fibrosis, upward retraction of hila, cystic changes within the fibrotic areas, and bilateral diaphragmatic calcification demonstrated.

changes, mycetomas, parenchymal fibrosis, and bronchiectasis (Rumancik et al., 1984). Pulmonary histopathology has shown nonspecific fibrosis with lymphocytic infiltrates, dilated bronchi, and thin-walled bullae and cavities. The cavitary lesions may occasionally become infected by Aspergillus. *M. avium*-complex, or *M. kansasii* (Rosenow et al., 1977, Stiksa et al., 1976). Isolated cases of bilateral pleural effusion and interstitial pneumonitis are reported in the literature (Cohen et al., 1971; Kinnear and Shneerson, 1985).

B. Upper Airway Involvement

Fixation of cricoarytenoid apparatus with respiratory distress that necessitated tracheostomy has been described in four patients (Buszek et al., 1983). Some patients may develop calcification and ossification of cartilaginous structures in the upper airways. Removal of ossified arytenoid cartilage has been described in symptomatic patients (Libby et al., 1981). In all reported cases, laryngeal symptoms were present for several years before cricoarytenoid arthritis caused airway compromise (Bienenstock and Lanyi, 1977; Libby et al., 1981; Wojtulewski et al., 1973); accordingly, follow-up of these patients with periodic flow-volume curves is suggested.

C. Ankylosis of Thoracic Cage

The ankylosis of the costovertebral joints seldom produces pulmonary symptoms even though the pulmonary function tests are abnormal. Abnormalities noted include diminished TLC, VC, and DLCO. Increased RV and FRC are common findings, although in some studies FRC has been found to be decreased (Cruickshank, 1960; Feltelius et al., 1986; Stewart et al., 1976). Xenon-133 ventilation studies have shown diminished ventilation and volumes in the upper lobes (Stewart et al., 1976). The results of one study have implied that patients do not underventilate the upper regions of the lungs except in the presence of roentgenographically visible fibrosis (Parkin et al., 1982).

D. Other Complications

Ankylosing hyperostosis of cervical spines is known to cause dysphagia, foreign-body sensation, and aspiration. Bilateral vocal cord paralysis with airways obstruction has been described in some patients. The pathogenesis of these abnormalities is an infection of an ulcerated cricoid that, in turn, is produced by movement of the larynx over a large, sharp osteophyte (Hassard, 1984).

Cervical spondylosis can be associated with pressure symptoms in the neck. Dyspnea and paretic left hemidiaphragm relieved by laminectomy have been described in one patient (Buszek et al., 1983). Carcinoma of the lung has been observed in the upper lobes of patients with ankylosing spondylitis–associated lung disease (Ahern et al., 1982; Shankar, 1982). A small number of patients with AS develop diaphragmatic calcification (Figure 15). The mechanism of this little-known complication is obscure.

E. Treatment and Prognosis

Because most patients with AS are asymptomatic, aggressive therapy with corticosteroids is not indicated (Franssen et al., 1986). Skeletal symptoms usually respond to nonsteroidal anti-inflammatory agents. Depending on the symptoms, however, secondary problems such as aspergilloma and infected apical cysts may require appropriate treatment.

VIII. Summary

Respiratory involvement is common in rheumatological diseases. In many of the entities discussed above, pulmonary manifestations may preced the rheumatological signs and symptoms. Often the respiratory symptoms may be the presenting and most dramatic features of the disease. As a rule, pathological analyses of the lungs in the rheumatological disorders discussed above reveal nonspecific abnormalities, and as a result, lung biopsies are rarely indicated in patients with rheumatological diseases. Pulmonary function tests are helpful in assessing the degree of impairment and in follow-up of the pulmonary process. Corticosteroids are the mainstay of treatment in the majority of the rheumatological diseases, but the response of the pulmonary disease may vary depending on the acuteness of the pathological process.

References

Abud-Mendoza, C., Diaz-Jouanen, E., and Alarcón-Segovia, D. (1985). Fatal pulmonary hemorrhage in systemic lupus erythematosus. Occurrence without hemoptysis. *J. Rheumatol.* **12**:558–561.

Ahern, M. J., Maddison, P., Mann, S., and Scott, C. A. (1982). Ankylosing spondylitis and adenocarcinoma of the lung. *Ann. Rheum. Dis.* **41**: 292–294.

Ainslie, W. H., Jr., Britt, K., and Moshipur, J. A. (1979). Maternal death due to lupus pneumonitis in pregnancy. *Mt. Sinai J. Med.* **46**:494–499.

Alarcón-Segovia, D. (1981). Mixed conective tissue disease—a decade of growing pains. *J. Rheumatol.* **8**:535–540.

Alarcón-Segovia, D., and Palacios, R. (1981). Human postthymic precursor cells in health and disease. IV. Abnormalities in immunoregulatory T cell circuits in mixed connective tissue disease. *Arthritis Rheum.* **24**: 1486–1494.

Alpert, M. A., Goldberg, S. H., Singsen, B. H., Durham, J. B., Sharp, G. C., Ahmad, M., Madigan, N. P., Hurst, D. P., and Sullivan, W. D. (1983). Cardiovascular manifestations of mixed connective tissue disease in adults. *Circulation* **68**:1182–1193.

Anttila, S., Sutinen, S., Pääkkö, P., and Finell, B. (1984). Rheumatoid pneumoconiosis in a dolomite worker: a light and electron microscopic and x-ray microanalytical study. *Br. J. Dis. Chest* **78**:195–200.

Arnett, F. C., Hirsch, T. J., Bias, W. B., Nishikai, M., and Reichlin, M. (1981). The Jo-1 antibody system in myositis: relationships to clinical features and HLA. *J. Rheumatol.* **8**:925–930.

Asherson, R. A., Mackworth-Young, C. G., Body, M. L., Hull, R. G., Saunders, A., Gharavi, A. E., and Hughes, G. R. V. (1983). Pulmonary hypertension in systemic lupus erythematosus. *Br. Med. J.* **287**:1024–1025.

Asherson, R. A., Chan, J. K. H., Harris, E. N., Gharavi, A. E., and Hughes, G. R. V. (1985). Anticardiolipin antibody, recurrent thrombosis, and warfarin withdrawal. *Ann. Rheum. Dis.* **44**:823–825.

Bagg, L. R., and Hughes, T. D. (1979). Serial pulmonary function tests in progressive systemic sclerosis. *Thorax* **34**:224–228.

Bell, R., and Lawrence D. S. (1979). Chronic pleurisy in systemic lupus erythematosus treated with pleurectomy. *Br. J. Dis. Chest* **73**:314–316.

Bennett, R. M. (1985). Mixed connective tissue disease and other overlap syndromes. In *Textbook of Rheumatology*, 2nd ed., Vol. 1. Edited by W. N. Kelley, E. D. Harris, Jr., S. Ruddy, and C. B. Sledge. Saunders, Philadelphia, pp. 1115–1136.

Bennett, R. M., and O'Connell, D. J. (1980). Mixed connective tissue disease: a clinicopathologic study of 20 cases. *Semin. Arthritis Rheum.* **10**:25–51.

Berendes, J., and Miehlke, A. (1973). A rare ankylosis of the cricoarytenoid joints. *Arch. Otolaryngol.* **98**:63–65.

Bergofsky, E. H. (1979). Respiratory failure in disorders of the thoracic cage. *Am. Rev. Respir. Dis.* **119**:643–669.

Bernstein, R. M., Morgan, S. H., Chapman, J., Bunn, C. C., Mathews, M. B., Turner-Warwick, M., and Hughes, G. R. V. (1984). Anti-Jo-1 antibody: a marker for myositis with interstitial lung disease. *Br. Med. J.* **289**:151–152.

Bienenstock, H., and Lanyi, V. F. (1977). Cricoarytenoid arthritis in a patient with ankylosing spondylitis. *Arch. Otolaryngol.* **103**:738–739.

Bienenstock, H., Ehrich, G. E., and Freyberg, R. H. (1963). Rheumatoid arthritis of the cricoarytenoid joint: a clinicopathologic study. *Arthritis Rheum.* **6**:48–63.

Blumbergs, P. C. , Byrne, E., and Kakulas, B. A. (1984). Polymyositis presenting with respiratory failure. *J. Neurol. Sci.* **65**:221–229.

Boey, M. L., Colaco, C. B., Gharavi, A. E., Elkon, K. B., Loizou, S., and Hughes, G. R. V. (1983). Thrombosis in systemic lupus erythematosus:

striking association with the presence of circulating lupus anticoagulant. *Br. Med. J.* **287**:1021–1023.

Bohan, A., and Peter, J. B. (1975). Polymyositis and dermatomyositis. *N. Engl. J. Med.* **292**:344–347.

Brentjens, J., Ossi, E., Albini, B., Sepulveda, M., Kano, K., Sheffer, J., Vasilon, P., Marine, E., Baliah, T., Jockin, H., and Andres, G. (1977). Disseminated immune deposits in lupus erythematosus. *Arthritis Rheum.* **20**:962–968.

Bulgrin, J. G., Dubois, E. L., and Jacobson, G. (1960). Chest roentgenographic changes in systemic lupus erythematosus. *Radiology* **74**:42–49.

Burke, G. W., Carrington, C. B., and Grinnan, R. (1977). Pulmonary nodules and rheumatoid factor in the absence of arthritis. *Chest* **72**:538–540.

Buszek, M. C., Szymke, T. E., Honet, J. C., Raikes, J. A., Gass, H. H., Leuchter, W., and Bendix, S. A. (1983). Hemidiaphragmatic paralysis: an unusual complication of cervical spondylosis. *Arch. Phys. Med. Rehabil.* **64**:601–603.

Byrd, R. B., and Trunk, G. (1973). Systemic lupus erythematosus presenting as pulmonary hemosiderosis. *Chest* **64**:128–129.

Callen, J. P. (1982). Dermatomyositis and malignancy. *Clin. Rheum. Dis.* **8**:369–381.

Cannon, G. W., and Zimmerman, G. A. (1990). The Rheumatic patient with Lung Disease. Marcel Dekker, New York.

Caplan, A. (1953). Certain unusual radiological appearances in the chest of coal-miners suffering from rheumatoid arthritis. *Thorax* **8**:29–37.

Carpenter, J. R., Bunch, T. W., Engel, A. G., and O'Brien, P. C. (1977). Survival in polymyositis: corticosteroids and risk factors. *J. Rheumatol* **4**: 207–214.

Carr, D. T., Lillington, G. A., and Mayne, J. G. (1970). Pleural-filled glucose in systemic lupus erythematosus. *Mayo Clin. Proc.* **45**:409–412.

Cervantes-Perez, P., Toro-Perez, A. H., and Rodriguez-Jurado, P. (1980). Pulmonary involvement in rheumatoid arthritis. *JAMA* **243**:1715–1719.

Chakera, T. M. H., Howarth, F. H., Kendall, M. J., Lawrence, D. S., and Whitfield, A. G. W. (1975). The chest radiograph in ankylosing spondylitis. *Clin. Radiol.* **26**:455–459.

Chausow, A. M., Kane, T., Levinson, D., and Szidon, J. P. (1984). Reversible hypercapnic respiratory insufficiency in scleroderma caused by respiratory muscle weakness. *Am. Rev. Respir. Dis.* **130**:142:144.

Churg, A., Franklin, W., Chan, K. L., Kopp, E., and Carrington, C. B. (1980). Pulmonary hemorrhage and immune-complex deposition in the lung: complications in a patient with systemic lupus erythematosus. *Arch. Pathol. Lab. Med.* **104**:388–391.

Claman, H. N. (1989). On scleroderma: mast cells, endothelial cells, and fibroblasts. *JAMA* **262**:1206–1209.

Cohen, A. A., Natelson, E. A., and Fechner, R. E. (1971). Fibrosing interstitial pneumonitis in ankylosing spondylitis. *Chest* **59**:369–371.

Corrin, B., Turner-Warwick, M., Geddes, D. M., and Brewerton, D. A. (1978). Bronchiolitis obliterans: a new form of rheumatoid lung? (letter to the editor). *Chest* **73**:244.

Cruickshank, B. (1960). Pathology of ankylosing spondylitis. *Bull. Rheum. Dis.* **10**:211–214.

Cush, J. J., and Goldings, E. A. (1985). Southwestern Internal Medicine Conference: Drug-induced lupus: clinical spectrum and pathogenesis. *Am. J. Med. Sci.* **290**:36–45.

D'Angelo, W. A., Fries, J. F., Masi, A. T., and Schulman, L. E. (1969). Pathologic obervations in systemic sclerosis (scleroderma): a study of fifty-eight autopsy cases and fifty-eight matched controls. *Am. J. Med.* **46**:428–440.

Davies, D. (1972). Ankylosing spondylitis and lung fibrosis. *Q. J. Med.* **41**:395–417.

Davis, P., Atkins, B., Josse, R. G., and Hughes, G. R. V. (1973). Criteria for classification of SLE. *Br. Med. J.* **3**:88–89.

de Clerck, L. S., Dequeker, J., Francx, L., and Demedts, M. (1987). D-Penicillamine therapy and interstitial lung disease in scleroderma: a long-term followup study. *Arthritis Rheum.* **30**:643–650.

Derderian, S. S., Tellis, C. J., Abbrecht, P. H., Welton, R. C., and Rajagopal, K. R. (1985). Pulmonary involvement in mixed connective tissue disease. *Chest* **88**:45–48.

Dumas, L. W., Gregory, R. L., and Ozer, R. L. (1963). Case of rheumatoid lung with cavity formation. *Br. Med. J.* **1**:383–384.

Eagen, J. W., Memoli, V. A., Roberts, J. L., Matthew, G. R., Schwartz, M. M., and Lewis, E. J. (1978). Pulmonary hemorrhage in systemic lupus erythematosus. *Medicine* **57**:545–560.

Eisenberg, H., Dubois, E. L., Sherwin, R. P., and Balchum, O. J. (1973). Diffuse interstitial lung disease in systemic lupus erythematosus. *Ann. Intern. Med.* **79**:37–45.

Espinoza, L. R. and Hartmann, R. C. (1986). Significance of the lupus anticoagulant. *Am. J. Hematol.* **22**:331–337.

Faurschou, P. (1984). Decreased glucose in RA-cell-positive pleural effusion: correlation of pleural glucose, lactic dehydrogenase and protein concentration to the presence of RA-cells. *Eur. J. Respir. Dis.* **65**:272–277.

Fayemi, A. O. (1975). The lung in systemic lupus erythematosus: a clinicopathologic study of 20 cases. *Mt. Sinai J. Med.* **42**:110–118.

Fayemi, A. O. (1976). Pulmonary vascular disease in systemic lupus erythematosus. *Am. J. Clin. Pathol.* **65**:284–290.

Feltelius, N., Hedenström, H., Hillerdal, G., and Hällgren, R. (1986). Pulmonary involvement in ankylosing spondylitis. *Ann. Rheum. Dis.* **45**: 736–740.

Franssen, M. J. A. M., van Herwaarden, C. L. A., van de Putte, L. B. A., and Gribnau, F. W. J. (1986). Lung function in patients with ankylosing spondilitis: a study of the influence of disease activity and treatment with nonsteroidal antiinflammatory drugs. *J. Rheumatol.* **13**:936–940.

Frazier, A. R., and Miller, R. D. (1974). Interstitial pneumonitis in association with polymyositis and dermatomyositis. *Chest* **65**:403–407.

Fudman, E. J., and Kelling, D. G., Jr. (1985). Transient effect of nifedipine on pulmonary hypertension of systemic sclerosis. *J. Rheumatol.* **12**: 1191–1192.

Gacad, G., and Hamosh, P. (1973). The lung in ankylosing spondylitis. *Am. Rev. Respir. Dis.* **107**:286–289.

Garcia, J. G. N., Parhami, N., Killam, D., Garcia, P. L., and Keogh, B. A. (1986). Bronchoalveolar lavage fluid evaluation in rheumatoid arthritis. *Am. Rev. Respir. Dis.* **133**:450–454.

Garcia, J. G. N., James, H. L., Zinkgraf, S., Perlman, M. B., and Keogh, B. A. (1987). Lower respiratory tract abnormalities in rheumatoid interstitial lung disease: potential role of neutrophils in lung injury. *Am. Rev. Respir. Dis.* **136**:811–817.

Garnet, R. F., Jr., Atkinson, B. F., Bonner, H., and Wurzel, H. A. (1977). Rapid screening for lupus erythematosus cells using cytocentrifuge-prepared buffy coat monolayers. *Am. J. Clin. Pathol.* **67**:537–539.

Geddes, D. M., Corrin, B., Brewerton, D. A., Davies, R. J., and Turner-Warwick, M. (1977a). Progressive airway obliteration in adults and its association with rheumatoid disease. *Q. J. Med.* **46**:427–444.

Geddes, D. M., Webley, M., Brewerton, D. A., Turton, C. W., Turner-Warwick, M., Murphy, A. H., and Ward, A. M. (1977b). α_1-Antitrypsin phenotypes in fibrosing alveolitis and rheumatoid arthritis. *Lancet* **2**:1049–1051.

Geddes, D. M., Webley, M., and Emerson, P. A. (1979). Airways obstruction in rheumatoid arthritis. *Ann. Rheum. Dis.* **38**:222–225.

Germain, M. J., and Davidman, M. (1984). Pulmonary hemorrhage and acute renal failure in a patient with mixed connective tissue disease. *Am. J. Kidney Dis.* **3**:420–424.

Gibson, G. J., Edmonds, J. P., and Hughes, G. R. V. (1977). Diaphragm function and lung involvement in systemic lupus erythematosus. *Am. J. Med.* **63**:926–932.

Gilligan, D. M., O'Connor, C. M., Ward, K., Moloney, D., Bresnihan, B., and Fitzgerald, M. X. (1990). Bronchoalveolar lavage in patients with mild and severe rheumatoid lung disease. *Thorax* **45**:591–596.

Ginsburg, W. W., Conn, D. L., Bunch, T. W., and McDuffie, F. C. (1983). Comparison of clinical and serologic markers in systemic lupus erythematosus and overlap syndrome: a review of 247 patients. *J. Rheumatol.* **10**:235–241.

Glikson, M., Pollack, A., Dresner-Feigin R., Galun, E., and Rubinow, A. (1990). Nifedipine and prazosin in the management of pulmonary hypertension in CREST syndrome. *Chest* **98**:759–761.

Gold, W. M., and Jennings, D. B. (1966). Pulmonary function in patients with systemic lupus erythematosus. *Am. Rev. Respir. Dis.* **93**:556–567.

Good, J. T., Jr., King, T. E., Antony, V. B., and Sahn, S. A. (1983). Lupus pleuritis: clinical factors and pleural fluid characteristics with special reference to pleural fluid antinuclear antibodies. *Chest* **84**:714–718.

Gould, D. B., and Soriano, R. Z. (1975). Acute alveolar hemorrhage in lupus erythematosus. *Ann. Intern. Med.* **83**:836–837.

Grant, K. D., Adams, L. E., and Hess, E. V. (1981). Mixed connective tissue disease—a subset with sequential clinical and laboratory features. *J. Rheumatol.* **8**:587–598.

Graziano, F. M., Friedman, L. C., and Grossman, J. (1983). Pulmonary hypertension in a patient with mixed connective tissue disease: clinical and pathologic findings, and review of literature. *Clin. Exp. Rheumatol.* **1**:251–255.

Greaves, I. A. (1979). Rheumatoid ''pneumoconiosis'' (Caplan's syndrome) in an asbestos worker: a 17 years' follow-up. *Thorax* **34**:404–405.

Greene, N. B., Solinger, A. M., and Baughman, R. P. (1987). Patients with collagen vascular disease and dyspnea: the value of gallium scanning and bronchoalveolar lavage in predicting responce to steroid therapy and clinical outcome. *Chest* **91**:698–703.

Griffin, M. T., Robb, J. D., and Martin, J. R. (1990). Diffuse alveolar haemorrhage associated with progressive systemic sclerosis. *Thorax* **45**:903–904.

Gross, M., Esterly, J. R., and Earle, R. H. (1972). Pulmonary alterations in systemic lupus erythematosus. *Am. Rev. Respir. Dis.* **105**:572–577.

Guit, G. L., Shaw, P. C., Ehrlich, J., Kroon, H. M., and Oudkerk, M. (1985). Mediastinal lymphadenopathy and pulmonary arterial hypertension in mixed connective tissue disease. *Radiology* **154**:305–306.

Hainaut, P., Lavenne, E., Magy, J. M., and Lebacq, E. G. (1986). Circulating lupus type anticoagulant and pulmonary hypertension associated with mixed connective tissue disease. *Clin. Rheumatol.* **5**:96–101.

Hakala, M. (1988). Poor prognosis in patients with rheumatoid arthritis hospitalized for interstitial lung fibrosis. *Chest* **93**:748–752.

Halla, J. T., Schrohenloher, R. E., and Volanakis, J. E. (1980). Immune complexes and other laboratory features of pleural effusions: a comparison of rheumatoid arthritis, systemic lupus erythematosus, and other diseases. *Ann. Intern. Med.* **92**:748–752.

Harmon, C., Wolfe, F., Lillard, S., Held, C., Cordon, R., and Sharp, G. C. (1976). Pulmonary involvement in mixed connective tissue disease (MCTD) (abstract). *Arthritis Rheum.* **19**:801.

Harmon, C. E., and Portanova, J. P. (1982). Drug-induced lupus: clinical and serological studies. *Clin. Rheum. Dis.* **8**:121–135.

Harrison, N. K., Glanville, A. R., Strickland, B., Haslam, P. L., Corrin, B., Addis, B. J., Lawrence, R., Millar, A. B., Black, C. M., and Laurent, G. J. (1989). Pulmonary involvement in systemic sclerosis: the detection of early changes by thin section CT scan, bronchoalveolar lavage and ^{99m}Tc-DTPA clearance. *Respir. Med.* **83**:403–414.

Harrison, N. K., McAnulty, R. J., Haslam, P. L., Black, C. M., and Laurent, G. J. (1990). Evidence for protein oedema, neutrophil influx, and enhanced collagen production in lungs of patients with systemic sclerosis. *Thorax* **45**:606–610.

Harvey, A. M., Shulman, L. E., Tumulty, P. A., Conley C. L., and Schoenrich, E. H. (1954). Systemic lupus erythematosus: review of the literature and clinical analysis of 138 cases. *Medicine* **33**:291–437.

Hassard, A. D. (1984). Cervical ankylosing hyperostosis and airway obstruction. *Laryngoscope* **94**:966–968.

Haupt, H. M., Moore, G. W., and Hutchins, G. M. (1981). The lung in systemic lupus erythematosus: analysis of the pathologic changes in 120 patients. *Am. J. Med.* **71**:791–798.

Henriksson, K. G., and Sandstedt, P. (1982). Polymyositis—treatment and prognosis: a study of 107 patients. *Acta Neurol. Scand.* **65**:280–300.

Herzog, C. A., Miller, R. R., and Hoidal, J. R. (1981). Bronchiolitis and rheumatoid arthritis. *Am. Rev. Respir. Dis.* **124**:636–639.

Hills, E. A., Davies, S., and Geary, M. (1979). Frequency dependence of dynamic compliance in patients with rheumatoid arthritis. *Thorax* **34**:755–761.

Hochberg, M. C., Feldman, D., Stevens, M. B., Arnett, F. C., and Reichlin, M. (1984). Antibody to Jo-1 in polymyositis dermatomyositis: association with interstitial pulmonary disease. *J. Rheumatol.* **11**:663–665.

Hoffbrand, B. I., and Beck, E. R. (1965). "Unexplained" dyspnoea and shrinking lungs in systemic lupus erythematosus. *Br. Med. J.* **1**: 1273–1277.

Holgate, S. T., Glass, D. N., Haslam, P., Maini, R. N., and Turner-Warwick, M. (1976). Respiratory involvement in systemic lupus erythematosus: a clinical and immunological study. *Clin. Exp. Immunol.* **24**:385–395.

Hoogsteden, H. C., van Dongen, J. J. M., van der Kwast, T. H., Hooijkaas, H., and Hilvering, C. (1985). Bilateral exudative pleuritis, an unusual pulmonary onset of mixed connective tissue disease. *Respiration* **48**: 164–167.

Horowitz, M, McNeil, J. D., Maddern, G. J., Collins, P. J., and Shearman,, D. J. C. (1986). Abnormalities of gastric and esophageal emptying in polymyositis and dermatomyositis. *Gastroenterology* **90**:434–439.

Huang, C-T., and Lyons, H. A. (1966). Comparison of pulmonary func tion in patients with systemic lupus erythematosus, scleroderma, and rheumatoid arthritis. *Am. Rev. Respir. Dis.* **98**:865–875.

Huang, C-T., Hennigar, G. R., and Lyons, H. A. (1965). Pulmonary dysfunction in systemic lupus erythematosus. *N. Engl. J. Med.* **272**:288–293.

Hull, S., and Mathews, J. A. (1982). Pulmonary necrobiotic nodules as a presenting feature of rheumatoid arthritis. *Ann. Rheum. Dis.* **41**:21–24.

Hunder, G. G., McDuffie, F. C., and Hepper, N. G. G. (1972). Pleural fluid complement in systemic lupus erythematosus and rheumatoid arthritis. *Ann. Intern. Med.* **76**:357–363.

Hunder, G. G., McDuffie, F. C., Huston, K. A., Elveback, L. R., and Hepper, N. G. (1977). Pleural fluid complement, complement conversion, and immune complexes in immunologic and nonimmunologic diseases. *J. Lab. Clin. Med.* **90**:971–980.

Hunninghake, G. W., and Fauci, A. S. (1979). Pulmonary involvement in the collagen vascular diseases. *Am. Rev. Respir. Dis.* **119**:471–503.

Hunter, T., Arnott, J. E., and McCarthy, D. S. (1980). Features of systemic lupus erythematosus and sarcoidosis occurring together. *Arthritis Rheum.* **23**:364–366.

Hurst, D. J., Baker, W. M., and Gilbert, G. (1980). Lung collagen synthesis and type analysis in patients with mixed connective tissue disease (abstract). *Clin. Res.* **28**:744A.

Johnson, D. A., Drane, W. E., Curran, J., Cattau, E. L., Jr., Ciarleglio, C., Khan, A., Cotelingam, J., and Benjamin, S. B. (1989). Pulmonary disease in progressive systemic sclerosis: a complication of gastroesophageal reflux and occult aspiration? *Arch. Intern. Med.* **149**:589–593.

Jones, M. B., Osterholm, R. K., Wilson, R. B., Martin, F. H., Commers, J. R., and Bachmayer, J. D. (1978). Fatal pulmonary hypertension and resolving immune-complex glomerulonephritis in mixed connective tissue disease: a case report and review of the literature. *Am. J. Med.* **65**: 855–863.

Jurik, A. G., Davidsen, D., and Graudal, H. (1984). Prevalence of cardiac and aortic enlargement in rheumatoid arthritis and its relationship to some characteristics of the patients: a radiological and clinical study. *Rheumatol. Int.* **5**:15–19.

Kaine, J. L. (1985). Refractory massive pleural effusion in systemic lupus erythematosus treated with talc poudrage. *Ann. Rheum. Dis.* **44**:61–64.

Kallenbach, J., Prinsloo, I., and Zwi, S. (1977). Progressive systemic sclerosis complicated by diffuse pulmonary haemorrhage. *Thorax* **32**:767–770.

Kallenbach, J., Zwi, S., and Goldman, H. I. (1978). Airways obstruction in a case of disseminated lupus erythematosus. *Thorax* **33**:814–815.

Kay, J. M., and Banik, S. (1977). Unexplained pulmonary hypertension with pulmonary arteritis in rheumatoid disease. *Br. J. Dis. Chest* **71**:53–59.

Keogh, B. A., and Crystal, R. G. (1981). Chronic interstitial lung disease. In *Current Pulmonaology*. Edited by D. H. Simmons. Wiley, Chichester, pp. 237–240.

Kim, J. H., Follet, J. V., Rice, J. R., and Hampson, N. B. (1988). Endobronchial telangiectasias and hemoptysis in scleroderma. *Am. J. Med.* **84**:173–174.

Kinnear, W. J. M., and Shneerson, J. M. (1985). Acute pleural effusions in inactive ankylosing spondylitis. *Thorax* **40**:150–151.

Kobayashi, H., Sano, T., Ii, K., Hizawa, K., Yamanhoi, A., and Otsuka, T. (1982). Mixed connective tissue disease with fatal pulmonary hypertension. *Acta Pathol. Jpn.* **32**:1121–1129.

Kuhn, C. (1972). Systemic lupus erythematosus in a patient with ultrastructural lesions of the pulmonary capillaries previously reported in the *review* as due to idiopathic pulmonary hemosiderosis. *Am. Rev. Respir. Dis.* **106**: 931–932.

Lakhanpal, S., Bunch, T. W., Ilstrup, D. M., and Melton, L. J., III. (1986). Polymyositis-dermatomyositis and malignant lesions: does an association exist? *Mayo Clin. Proc.* **61**:645–653.

Lawry, G. V., Finerman, M. L., Hanafee, W. N., Mancuso, A. A., Fan, P. T., and Bluestone, R. (1984). Laryngeal involvement in rheumatoid arthritis: a clinical, laryngoscopic, and computerized tomographic study. *Arthritis Rheum.* **27**:873–882.

Leatherman, J. W., Sibley, R. K., and Davies, S. F. (1982). Diffuse intrapulmonary hemorrhage and glomerulonephritis unrelated to anti-glomerular basement membrane antibody. *Am. J. Med.* **72**:401–410.

Leikin, J. B., Arof, H. M., and Pearlman, L. M. (1986). Acute lupus pneumonitis in the postpartum period: a case history and review of the literature. *Obstet. Gynecol* **68**:29S–31S.

Lemmer, J. P., Curry, N. H., Mallory, J. H., and Waller, M. V. (1982). Clinical characteristics and course in patients with high titer anti-RNP antibodies. *J. Rheumatol.* **9**:536–542.

LeRoy, E. C. (1981). Scleroderma (systemic sclerosis). In *Textbook of Rheumatology*, Vol. II. Edited by W. N. Kelley, E. D. Harris, Jr., S. Ruddy, and C. B. Sledge. Saunders, Philadelphia, pp. 1211–1230.

LeRoy, E. C., Maricq, H. R., and Kahaleh, M. B. (1980). Undifferentiated connective tissue syndromes. *Arthritis Rheum.* **23**:341–343.

Libby, D. M., Schley, W. S., and Smith, J. P. (1981). Cricoarytenoid arthritis in ankylosing spondylitis: a cause of acute respiratory failure and cor pulmonale. *Chest* **80**:641–643.

Lofgren, R. H., and Montgomery, W. W. (1962). Incidence of laryngeal involvement in rheumatoid arthritis. *N. Engl. J. Med.* **267**:193–195.

Macfarlane, J. D., Franken, C. K., and van-Leeuwen, A. W. F. M. (1984). Progressive cavitating pulmonary changes in rheumatoid arthritis: a case report. *Ann. Rheum. Dis.* **43**:98–101.

Maddison, P. J., Mogavero, H., and Reichlin, M. (1978). Patterns of clinical disease associated with antibodies to nuclear ribonucleoprotein. *J. Rheumatol.* **5**:407–411.

Mahowald, M. L., Weir, E. K., Ridley, D. J., and Messner, R. P. (1985). Pulmonary hypertension in systemic lupus erythematosus: effect of vasodilators on pulmonary hemodynamics. *J. Rheumatol.* **12**:773–777.

Manchul, L. A., Jin, A., Pritchard, K. I., Tenenbaum, J., Boyd, N. F., Lee, P., Germanson, T., and Gordon, D. A. (1985). The frequency of malignant neoplasms in patients with polymyositis-dermatomyositis: a controlled study. *Arch. Intern. Med.* **145**:1835–1839.

Marchesoni, A., Messina, K., Carrieri, P., Sinigaglia, L., and Tosi, S. (1983). Pulmonary hypertension and systemic lupus erythematosus. *Clin. Exp. Rheumatol.* **1**:247–250.

Marino, C. T., and Pertschuk, L. P. (1981). Pulmonary hemorrhage in systemic lupus erythematosus. *Arch. Intern. Med.* **141**:201–203.

Martens, J., and Demedts, M. (1982). Diaphragm dysfunction in mixed connective tissue disease: a case report. *Scand. J. Rheumatol.* **11**:165–167.

Martens, J., Demedts, M., Vanmeenen, M. T., and Dequeker, J. (1983). Respiratory muscle dysfunction in systemic lupus erythematosus. *Chest* **84**:170–175.

Matthay, R. A., Hudson, L. D., and Petty, T. L. (1973). Acute lupus pneumonitis: response to azathioprine therapy. *Chest* **63**:117–120.

Matthay, R. A., Schwartz, M. I., Petty, T. L., Stanford, R. E., Gupta, R. C., Sahn, S. A., and Steigerwald, J. C. (1975). Pulmonary manifestations of systemic lupus erythematosus: review of twelve cases of acute lupus pneumonitis. *Medicine* **54**:397–409.

McCann, B. G., Hart, G. J., Stokes, T. C., and Harrison, B. D. W. (1983). Obliterative bronchiolitis and upper-zone pulmonary consolidation in rheumatoid arthritis. *Thorax* **38**:73–74.

McConnochie, K., O'Sullivan, M., Khalil, J. F., Pritchard, M. H., and Gibbs, A. R. (1989). Aspergillus colonization of pulmonary rheumatoid nodule. *Respir. Med.* **83**:157–160.

Medsger, T. A., Jr. (1985). Systemic sclerosis and malignancy—are they related? *J. Rheumatol.* **12**:1041–1043.

Medsger, T. A., Jr. (1987). D-Penicillamine treatment of lung involvement in patients with systemic sclerosis (scleroderma). *Arthritis Rheum.* **30**: 832–834.

Medsger, T. A., Jr., Robinson, H., and Masi, A. T. (1971). Factors affecting survivorship in polymyositis: a life-table study of 124 patients. *Arthritis Rheum.* **14**:249–258.

Michalski, J. P., McCombs, C. C., Scopelitis, E., Biundo, J. J., Jr., and Medsger, T. A., Jr. (1986). Alpha$_1$-antitrypsin phenotypes, including M subtypes, in pulmonary disease associated with rheumatoid arthritis and systemic sclerosis. *Arthritis Rheum.* **29**:586–591.

Miller, R. W., Salcedo, J. R., Fink, R. J., Murphy, T. M., and Magilavy, D. B. (1986). Pulmonary hemorrhage in pediatric patients with systemic lupus erythematosus. *J.* Pediatr. **108**:576–579.

Millman, R. P., Cohen, T. B., Levinson, A. I., Kelley, M. A., and Sachs, M. L. (1981). Systemic lupus erythematosus complicated by acute pulmonary hemorrhage: recovery following plasmapheresis and cytotoxic therapy (letter to the editor). *J. Rheumatol.* **8**:1021–1023.

Mintz, G., Galindo, L. F., Fernandez-Diez, J., Jimenez, F. J., Robles-Saavedra, E., and Enriquez-Casillas, R. D. (1978). Acute massive pulmonary hemorrhage in systemic lupus erythematosus. *J. Rheumatol.* **5**:39–50.

Mountz, J. D., Turner, R. A., Collins R. L., Gallup, K. R., Jr., and Semble, E. L. (1984). Rheumatoid arthritis and small airways function: effects of disease activity, smoking, and α_1-antitrypsin deficiency. *Arthritis Rheum.* **27**:728–736.

Mulkey, D., and Hudson, L. (1974). Massive spontaneous unilateral hemothorax in systemic lupus erythematosus. *Am. J. Med.* **56**:570–574.

Myers, J. L., and Katzenstein, A-L. A. (1986). Microangiitis in lupus-induced pulmonary hemorrhage. *Am. J. Clin. Pathol.* **85**:552–556.

Myers, S. A., Podczaski, E., and Freese, U. (1980). Acute lupus pneumonitis in the puerperium: a case report and literature review. *J. Reprod. Med.* **25**:285–289.

Naschitz, J. E., Yeshurun, D., Scharf, Y., Sajrawi, I., Lazarov, N. B., and Boss, J. H. (1989). Recurrent massive alveolar hemorrhage, crescentic glomerulonephritis, and necrotizing vasculitis in a patient with rheumatoid arthritis. *Arch. Intern. Med.* **149**:406–408.

Niarchos, A. P., Whitman, H. H., Goldstein, J. E., and Laragh, J. H. (1982). Hemodynamic effects of captopril in pulmonary hypertension of collagen vascular disease. *Am. Heart J.* **104**:834–838.

Nimelstein, S. H., Brody, S., McShane, D., and Holman, H. R. (1980). Mixed connective tissue disease: a subsequent evaluation of the original 25 patients. *Medicine* **59**:239–248.

Nüsslein, H. G., Rödl, W., Giedel, J., Missmahl, M., and Kalden, J. R. (1987). Multiple peripheral pulmonary nodules preceding rheumatoid arthritis. *Rheumatol. Int.* **7**:89–91.

O'Brien, J. T., Hill, J. A., and Pepine, C. J. (1985). Sustained benefit of verapamil in pulmonary hypertension with progressive systemic sclerosis. *Am. Heart J.* **109**:380–382.

Ognibene, A. J., and Dito, W. R. (1965). Rheumatoid disease with unusual pulmonary manifestations: pulmonary hemosiderosis, fibrosis, and concretions. *Arch. Intern. Med.* **116**:567–570.

Owens, G. R., and Follansbee, W. P. (1987). Cardiopulmonary manifestations of systemic sclerosis. *Chest* **91**:118–127.

Ownes, G. R., Fino, G. J., Herbert, D. L., Steen, V. D., Medsger, T. A., Pennock, B. E., Cottrell, J. J., Rodnan, G. P., and Rogers, R. M. (1983). Pulmonary function in progressive systemic sclerosis: comparison of CREST syndrome variant with diffuse scleroderma. *Chest* **84**:546–550.

Pandya, M. R., Agus, B., and Grady, R. F. (1976). In vivo LE phenomenon in pleural fluid (letter to the editor). *Arthritis Rheum.* **19**:962–963.

Parkin, A., Robinson, P. J., and Hickling, P. (1982). Regional lung ventilation in ankylosing spondylitis. *Br. J. Radiol.* **55**:833–836.

Passero, F. C., and Myers, A. R. (1980). Hemopneumothorax in systemic lupus erythematosus. *J. Rheumatol.* **7**:183–186.

Perez, H. D., and Kramer, N. (1981). Pulmonary hypertension in systemic lupus erythematosus: report of four cases and review of the literature. *Semin. Arthritis Rheum.* **11**:177–181.

Pertschuk, L. P., Moccia, L. F., Rosen, Y., Lyons, H., Marino, C. M., Rashford, A. A., and Wollschlager, C. M. (1977). Acute pulmonary complications in systemic lupus erythematosus: immunofluorescence and light microscopic study. *Am. J. Clin. Pathol.* **68**:553–557.

Peters-Golden, M., Wise, R. A., Hochberg, M., Stevens, M. B., and Wigley, F. M. (1985). Incidence of lung cancer in systemic sclerosis. *J. Rheumatol.* **12**:1136–1139.

Plotz, P. H., Dalakas, M., Leff, R. L., Love, L. A., Miller, F. W., and Cronin, M. E. (989). Current concepts in the idiopathic inflammatory myopathies: polymyositis, dermatomyositis, and related disorders. *Ann. Intern. Med.* **111**:143–157.

Ploysongsang, Y., and Foad, B. S. I. (1984). Lung function tests in connective tissue diseases associated with Raynaud's phenomenon. *Respiration* **46**: 222—230.

Portner, M. M., and Gracie, W. A., Jr. (1966). Rheumatoid lung disease with cavitary nodules, pneumothorax and eosinophilia. *N. Engl. J. Med.* **275**:697–700.

Prakash, U. B. S.(1988). Pulmonary manifestations in mixed connective tissue disease. *Semin. Respir. Med.* **9**:318–324.

Prakash, U. B. S., Luthra, H. S., and Divertie, M. B. (1985). Intrathoracic manifestations in mixed connective tissue disease. *Mayo Clin. Proc.* **60**:813–821.

Purnell, D. C., Baggenstoss, A. H., and Olsen, A. M. (1955). Pulmonary lesions in disseminated lupus erythematosus. *Ann. Intern. Med.* **42**: 619–628.

Reichlin, M. (1976). Problems in differentiating SLE and mixed connective-tissue disease (editorial). *N. Engl. J. Med.* **295**:1194–1195.

Roschmann, R. A., and Rothenberg, R. J. (1987). Pulmonary fibrosis in rheumatoid arthritis: a review of clinical features and therapy. *Semin. Arthritis Rheum.* **16**:174–185.

Rosenow, E. C., III, Strimlan, C. V., Muhm, J. R., and Ferguson, R. H. (1977). Pleuropulmonary manifestations of ankylosing spondylitis. *Mayo Clin. Proc.* **52**:641–649.

Rossi, G. A., Bitterman, P. B., Rennard, S. I., Ferrans, V. J., and Crystal, R. G. (1985) Evidence for chronic inflammation as a component of the interstitial lung disease associated with progressive systemic sclerosis. *Am. Rev. Respir. Dis.* **131**:612–617.

Rumancik, W. M., Firooznia, H., Davis, M. S., Jr., Leitman, B. S., Golimbu, C., Rafii, M., and McCauley, D. I. (1984). Fibrobullous disease of the upper lobes: an extraskeletal manifestation of ankylosing spondylitis. *J. Comput. Tomogr.* **8**:225–229.

Salerni, R., Rodnan, G. P., Leon, D. F., and Shaver, J. A. (1977). Pulmonary hypertension in the CREST syndrome variant of progressive systemic sclerosis (scleroderma). *Ann. Intern. Med.* **86**:394–399.

Salmeron, G., Greenberg, S. D., and Lidsky, M. D. (1981). Polymyositis and diffuse interstitial lung disease: a review of the pulmonary histopathologic findings. *Arch. Intern. Med.* **141**:1005–1010.

Sarma, D. P., and Weilbaecher, T. G. (1985). Systemic scleroderma and small cell carcinoma of the lung. *J. Surg. Oncol.* **29**:28–30.

Sassoon, C. S., McAlpine, S. W., Tashkin, D. P., Baydur, A., Quismorio, F. P., and Mongan, E. S. (1984). Small airways function in nonsmokers with rheumatoid arthritis. *Arthritis Rheum.* **27**:1218–1226.

Schleissner, L. A., Sheehan, W. W., and Orselli, R. C. (1976). Lupus erythematosus in a patient with amyloidosis, adrenal insufficiency, and subsequent immunoblastic sarcoma: demonstration of the LE phenomenon in the lung. *Arthritis Rheum.* **19**:249–254.

Schwartzberg, M., Lieberman, D. H., Getzoff, B., and Ehrlich, G. E. (1984). Systemic lupus erythematosus and pulmonary vascular hypertension. *Arch. Intern. Med.* **144**:605–607.

Scobie, B. A. (1971). The lungs in ankylosing spondylitis. *Br. Med. J.* **4**:560.

Scott, D. G. I., Bacon, P. A., and Tribe, C. R. (1981). Systemic rheumatoid vasculitis: a clinical and laboratory study of 50 cases. *Medicine* **60**: 288–297.

Shankar, P. S. (1982). Ankylosing spondylitis with fibrosis and carcinoma of the lung. *CA* **32**:177–179.

Sharma, S., Vaccharajani, A., and Mandke, J. (1990). Severe pulmonary hypertension in rheumatoid arthritis. *Int. J. Cardiol.* **26**:220–222.

Sharp, G. C. (1982). Anti-nRNP and anti-Sm antibodies. *Arthritis Rheum.* **25**:757–760.

Sharp, G. C., and Anderson, P. C. (1980). Current concepts in the classification of connective tissue diseases: overlap syndromes and mixed connective tissue disease (MCTD). *J. Am. Acad. Dermatol.* **2**:269–279.

Sharp, G. C., and Singsen, B. H. (1985). Mixed connective tissue disease. In *Arthritis and Allied conditions: A Textbook of Rheumatology*, 10th ed. Edited by D. J. McCarty. Lea & Febiger, Philadelphia, pp. 962–970.

Sharp, G. C., Irvin, W. S., Tan, E. M., Gould, R. G., and Holman, H. R. (1972). Mixed connective tissue disease—an apparently distinct rheumatic disease syndrome associated with a specific antibody to an extractable nuclear antigen (ENA). *Am. J. Med.* **52**:148–159.

Shiel, W. C., Jr., and Prete, P. E. (1984). Pleuropulmonary manifestations of rheumatoid arthritis. *Semin. Arthritis Rheum.* **13**:235–243.

Silver, T. M., Farber, S. J., Bole, G. G., and Martel, W. (1976). Radiological features of mixed connective tissue disease and scleroderma-systemic lupus erythematosus overlap. *Radiology* **120**:269–275.

Smith, B. S. (1966). Idiopathic pulmonary haemosiderosis and rheumatoid arthritis. *Br. Med. J.* **1**:1403–1404.

Someren, A. O., Honig, E., Gaffney, E., and Hewan-Lowe, K. (1983). Massive asphyxiating pulmonary hemorrhage and glomerulonephritis in a 41-year-old woman. *South. Med. J.* **76**:775–781.

Staats, B. A., Ellefson, R. D., Budahn, L. L., Dines, D. E., Prakash, U. B. S., and Offord, K. (1980). The lipoprotein profile of chylous and nonchylous pleural effusions. *Mayo. Clin. Proc.* **55**:700–704.

Steen, V. D., Owens, G. R., Fino, G. J., Rodnan, G. P., and Medsger, T. A., Jr. (1985a). Pulmonary involvement in systemic sclerosis (scleroderma). *Arthritis Rheum.* **28**:759–767.

Steen, V. D., Owens, G. R., Redmond, C., Rodnan, G. P., and Medsger, T. A., Jr. (1985b). The effect of D-penicillamine on pulmonary findings in systemic sclerosis. *Arthritis Rheum.* **28**:882–888.

Stewart, R. M., Ridyard, J. B., and Pearson, J. D. (1976). Regional lung function in ankylosing spondylitis. *Thorax* **31**:433–437.

Stiksa, G., Eklundh, G., Riebe, I., and Simonsson, B. G. (1976). Bilateral pulmonary aspergilloma in anklosing spondylitis treated with transthoracic intracavitary instillations of antifungal agents. *Scand. J. Respir. Dis.* **57**:163–170.

Stupi, A. M., Steen, V. D., Owens, G. R., Barnes, E. L., Rodnan, G. P., and Medsger, T. A. (1986). Pulmonary hypertension in the CREST syndrome variant of systemic sclerosis. *Arthritis Rheum.* **29**:515–523.

Sullivan, W. D., Hurst, D. J., Harmon, C. E., Esther, J. H., Agia, G. A., Maltby, J. D., Lillard, S. B., Held, C. N., Wolfe, J. F., Sunderrajan, E. V., Maricq, H. R., and Sharp, G. C. (1984). A prospective evaluation emphasizing pulmonary involvement in patients with mixed connective tissue disease. *Medicine* **63**:92–107.

Sutton, P. P., Kadir, N., Pavia, D., Sheahan, N. F., and Clarke, S. W. (1982). Lung mucociliary clearance in rheumatoid disease. *Ann. Rheum. Dis.* **41**:47–51.

Talbott, J. H., and Barrocas, M. (1979). Progressive systemic sclerosis (PSS) and malignancy, pulmonary and non-pulmonary. *Medicine* **58**:182–207.

Talbott, J. H., and Barrocas, M. (1980). Carcinoma of the lung in progressive systemic sclerosis: a tabular review of the literature and a detailed report of the roentgenographic changes in two cases. *Semin. Arthritis Rheum.* **9**:191–217.

Tan, E. M., Cohen, A. S., Fries, J. F., Masi, A. T., McShane, D. J., Rothfield, N. F., Schaller, J. G., Talal, N., and Winchester, R. J. (1982). The 1982 revised criteria for the classification of systemic lupus erythematosus. *Arthritis Rheum.* **25**:1271–1277.

Tesluk, H. (1984). Progressive systemic sclerosis and pulmonary cancer (letter to the editor). *Arch. Pathol. Lab. Med.* **108**:7–8.

Trimble, R. B., Townes, A. S., Robinson, H., Kaplan, S. B., Chandler, R. W., Hanissian, A. S., and Masi, A. T. (1974). Preliminary criteria for the classification of systemic lupus erythematosus (SLE): evaluation in early diagnosed SLE and rheumatoid arthritis. *Arthritis Rheum.* **17**:184–188.

Turner-Stokes, L., and Turner-Warwick, M. (1982). Intrathoracic manifestations of SLE. *Clin. Rheum. Dis.* **8**:229–242.

Turner-Warwick, M. (1974). Immunological aspects of systemic diseases of the lungs. *Proc. R. Soc. Med.* **67**:541–547.

Ueda, N., Mimura, K., Maeda, H., Sugiyama, T., Kado, T., Kobayashi, K., and Fukuzaki, H. (1984). Mixed connective tissue disease with fatal pulmonary hypertension and a review of literature. *Virchows Arch. (A)* **404**:335–340.

Ungerer, R. G., Tashkin, D. P., Furst, D., Clements, P. J., Gong, H., Jr., Bein, M., Smith, J. W., Roberts, N., and Cabeen, W. (1983). Prevalence and clinical correlates of pulmonary arterial hypertension in progressive systemic sclerosis. *Am. J. Med.* **75**:65–74.

Vale, J. A., Pickering, J. G., and Scott, G. W. (1974). Ankylosing spondylitis and upper lobe fibrosis and cavitation. *Guys Hosp. Rep.* **123**:97–119.

Vitali, C., Tavoni, A., Viegi, G., Begliomini, E., Agnesi, A., and Bombardieri, S. (1985). Lung involvement in Sjögren's syndrome: a comparison between patients with primary and with secondary syndrome. *Ann. Rheum. Dis.* **44**:455–461.

Wallaert, B., Dugas, M., Dansin, E., Perez, T., Marquette, C. H., Ramon, P., Tonnel, A. B., and Voisin, C. (1990). Subclinical alveolitis in immunological systemic disorders. Transition between health and disease? *Eur. Respir. J.* **3**:1206–1216.

Walters, M. N-I, and Ojeda, V. J., (1986). Pleuropulmonary necrobiotic rheumatoid nodules: a review and clinicopathological study of six patients. *Med. J. Aust.* **144**:648–651.

Wasicek, C. A., Reichlin, M., Montes, M., and Raghu, G. (1984). Polymyositis and interstitial lung disease in a patient with anti-Jo-$_1$ prototype. *Am. J. Med.* **76**:538–544.

Weaver, A. L., Diverite, M. B., and Titus, J. L. (1968). Pulmonary scleroderma. *Dis. Chest* **54**:490–498.

Webb, W. R., and Gamsu, G. (1981). Cavitary pulmonary nodules with systemic lupus erythematosus: differential diagnosis. *AJR* **136**:27–31.

Weiland, J. E., Garcia, J. G., Davis, W. B., and Gadek, J. E. (1987). Neutrophil collagenase in rheumatoid interstitial lung disease. *J. Appl. Physiol.* **62**:628–633.

Wiedemann, H. P., and Matthay, R. A. (1989). Pulmonary manifestations of the collagen vascular diseases. *Clin. Chest Med.* **10**:677–722.

Wiener-Kronish, J. P., Solinger, A. M., Warnock, M. L., Churg, A., Ordonez, N., and Golden, J. A. (1981). Severe pulmonary involvement in mixed connective tissue disease. *Am. Rev. Respir. Dis.* **124**:499–503.

Winkelmann, R. K., Mulder, D. W., Lambert, E. H., Howard, F. M., Jr., and Diessner, G. R. (1968). Course of dermatomyositis polymyositis: comparison of untreated and cortisone-treated patients. *Mayo Clin. Proc.* **43**: 545–556.

Winkelmann, R. K., Flach, D. B., and Unni, K. K. (1988). Lung cancer and scleroderma. *Arch. Dermatol. Res.* **280**(suppl):S15–S18.

Winslow, W. A., Ploss, L.N., and Loitman, B. (1958). Pleuritis in systemic lupus erythematosus: its importance as an early manifestation in diagnosis. *Ann. Intern. Med.* **49**:70–88.

Wojtulewski, J. A., Sturrock, R. D., Branfoot, A. C., and Hart, F. D. (1973). Cricoarytenoid arthritis in ankylosing spondylitis. *Br. J. Med.* **3**:145–146.

Worth, H., Grahn, S., Lakomek, H. J., Bremer, G., and Goeckenjan, G. (1988). Lung function disturbances versus respiratory muscle fatigue in patients with systemic lupus erythematosus. *Respiration* **53**:81–90.

Yates, D. A. (1963). Cavitation of a rheumatoid lung nodule. *Ann. Phys. Med.* **7**:105–106.

Young, R. H., and Mark, G. J. (1978). Pulmonary vascular changes in scleroderma. *Am. J. Med.* **64**:998–1004.

Yousem, S. A., Colby, T. V., and Carrington, C. B. (1985a). Follicular bronchitis/bronchiolitis. *Hum. Pathol.* **16**:700–706.

Yousem, S. A., Colby, T. V., and Carrington, C. B. (1985b). Lung biopsy in rheumatoid arthritis. *Am. Rev. Respir. Dis.* **131**:770–777.

9

Vasculitides

UDAYA B. S. PRAKASH

Mayo Clinic, Mayo Medical Center, and Mayo Medical School
Rochester, Minnesota

I. Introduction

The vasculitides, collagen tissue diseases, and rheumatological diseases are frequently discussed together in clinical medicine. Although many of the rheumatological diseases or collagenoses show vasculitic changes in tissue specimens, they are not usually considered primary vasculitides. At times, however, it is difficult to separate the vasculitides from rheumatological diseases. This chapter is devoted to disorders generally considered primary vasculitic syndromes. The pulmonary manifestations of rheumatological diseases are discussed in Chapter 8.

The vasculitides are a heterogeneous group of disorders characterized by varying degrees of inflammation and necrosis of the arteries in particular and sometimes of other vessels. Arteries and veins of all sizes and capillaries in different locations throughout the body may become involved by the pathological process. Most of the vasculitides have no known etiological factors. Immunological mechanisms, absence or deficiency of certain chemical mediators in the body, and fungal infections, especially from *Aspergillus* and *Mucor* species, are known to be associated with vasculitides. The presence of rheumatoid factor, circulating immune complexes, and elevated erythrocyte sedimentation rate, the recent discovery of antineutrophil cytoplasmic antibodies, the presence of certain characteristic pathological changes, and the absence of serum complement components may help in establishing the diagnosis of many of these entities.

The many attempts at classification of the vasculitides have been frustrating, because no single classification has proved clinically useful. The diagnostic criteria for various vasculitides, published in 1990, by the American College of Rheumatology (ACR) should prove helpful to clinicians (Arend et al., 1990; Bloch et al., 1990; Calabrese et al., 1990; Fries et al., 1990; Hunder et al, 1990a, b; Leavitt et al., 1990; Lie et al., 1990; Lightfoot et al., 1990; Masi et al., 1990; Mills et al., 1990). This multicenter study gathered data on 1020 patients with various types of vasculitides from 48 centers in the United States and Canada over a 5-year period. Of these, 807 patients met the criteria established for the diagnosis of several types of vasculitis. Removed from the study were 213 patients of whom 141 had vasculitis secondary to underlying rheumatological diseases. The classification criteria based on these studies, which are described and referenced later, are available for the following diseases: Wegener's granulomatosis (WG), Churg-Strauss syndrome (CSS), hypersensitivity vasculitis (HSV), Henoch-Schönlein purpura (HSP), giant cell (temporal) arteritis (GCA), Takayasu arteritis (TA), and other vasculitides of unspecified type.

It is common to see multiple organ involvement in each of the vasculitides. As in many of the rheumatological diseases, one major organ system may be affected to a greater extent than others. Moreover, it is not uncommon for pulmonary manifestations to be the reason for presentation nor for the pulmonary aspects to assume a major role in many of these disorders. This chapter will describe the pulmonary features of the vasculitides noted above as well as of hypocomplementemic urticarial vasculitis (HUV), Behçet disease (BD), and other miscellaneous vasculitides. The discussion will emphasize the clinical aspects of these diseases with pertinent references to basic pathophysiology; the interested reader is referred to a recent issue of this Lung Biology series that covers in depth the research aspects and pathological findings in the rheumatological diseases (Cannon and Zimmerman, 1990).

II. Wegener's Granulomatosis

First described in 1936, Wegener's granulomatosis (WG) is a distinct type of systemic vasculitis characterized by a clinicopathological complex of necrotizing granulomatous vasculitis of the upper and lower respiratory tract, glomerulonephritis, and variable degrees of small-vessel vasculitis (Churg, 1983; Fauci and Wolff, 1973; Fauci et al., 1983; Leavit et al., 1990; Liebow, 1973; Wegener, 1936). The term "limited WG" was introduced by Carrington and Liebow (1966) to describe WG involving the respiratory system but without glomerulonephritis. Clinical experience has shown that many patients with limited WG do indeed develop renal involvement during the course of their disease and that if renal biopsies are obtained in these patients, most will show abnormalities. The original criteria (Wegener's triad) set down to make the diagnosis of WG included necrotizing granulomas of the upper or lower respiratory tract or both, generalized focal necrotizing vasculitis involving both arteries and veins in the lungs and other organs, and focal necrotizing glomerulitis (Godman and Churg, 1954). WG is considered to be a necrotizing granulomatous disorder rather than a true vasculitis (Lie et al., 1990). Pathological features may include granulomatosis and necrotizing granuloma combined with vasculitis. The granuloma may be discrete or confluent. Fibrinoid necrosis, microabscesses, focal vasculitis, thrombosis, and fibrous obliteration of the vascular lumen may be seen. Although eosinophilic infiltrates are seen in tissue samples, peripheral blood eosinophilia is not a feature of WG.

Abnormal laboratory tests in patients with WG include elevated erythrocyte sedimentation rate, normochromic normocytic anemia, thrombocytosis, positive rheumatoid factor, and elevation of immunoglobulins and circulating immune complexes. However, all these abnormalities are nonspecific and indicate only a systemic inflammatory disease (Fauci et al., 1983). During the past decade, the identification of antineutrophil cytoplasmic antibodies (cANCA or pANCA) in the majority of patients with WG has helped in establishing the diagnosis in atypical or unusual cases of systemic vasculitis (Specks et al., 1989; Cross and Lillington, 1989). Three main patterns of cytoplasmic fluorescence are recognized: granular with central accentuation, perinuclear, and homogeneous. The granular pattern (cANCA) is reported to be specific for WG, whereas the other patterns have been noted with other vasculitides and collagen diseases (Specks and DeRemee, 1990). The titers of cANCA correlate with activity of the disease. However, it must be stressed that sensitivity varies with disease activity, and the specificity of the test depends on the nature of the controls chosen for analysis (Leavitt et al., 1990). The ACR studies did not include these tests in the diagnostic classification of WG, but judging from the experience to date (Falk et al., 1990; Jennette and Falk, 1990), it is likely that these tests will become important diagnostic criteria.

In the ARC study, 10.5% of 807 patients with various vasculitides had WG. The mean age at onset of symptoms of WG was 45.2 years. Male-to-female ratio was 2:1 and 91% of patients were white (Leavitt et al., 1990). Initial symptoms are nonspecific and may include vague symptoms of systemic illness, such as fever, malaise, weight loss, arthralgias, and myalgias (Fauci et al., 1983). Renal involvement with focal segmental glomerulonephritis is a hallmark of WG. The other organs affected by WG and the incidence of their involvement are as follows: skin (40–50%), eyes (43%), arthralgias (58%) but frank arthritis (28%), and neurological involvement occurs in approximately 25% (Fauci and Wolff, 1973; Fauci et al., 1983; Haynes et al., 1977; Noritake et al., 1987; Reed et al., 1963; Wolff et al., 1974). The cardiovascular system may also be affected.

A. Upper Airway Disease

Head and neck symptoms are the initial complaints in 90% of patients. Sinus pain, rhinorrhea, purulent or bloody nasal discharge, nasal mucosal drying and crust formation, epistaxis, and otitis media are common. Paranasal sinus involvement is associated with deep facial pain. Nasal septal perforation and ulceration of the vomer are important signs of WG (McDonald et al., 1974). A superimposed bacterial infection, particularly from *Staphylococcus aureus*, may lead to purulent nasal discharge. The increased incidence of bacterial infection is secondary to a breakdown in the mucosal barrier and the failure to clear secretions. Aphthous lesions of the nasal and oral mucosa may be seen. Inflammation and destruction of the nasal cartilages may lead to a "saddle nose deformity." This is usually a subacute or more often a chronic complication; this type of abnormality can also be seen in relapsing polychondritis.

Ulcerating lesions of larynx and trachea may be present in 30% of untreated cases, and subglottic stenosis is seen in 5–8% of treated patients. Because symptoms tend to be insidious in onset and slowly progressive, inspiratory and expiratory flow volume loops may aid in assessing the impairment of the upper airway.

B. Pulmonary Involvement

The lower respiratory tract is affected in more than 60% of patients with WG. Involvement of the lower respiratory tract alone is classified as "limited WG" (Carrington and Liebow, 1966). Respiratory symptoms comprise mainly hemoptysis, dyspnea, and cough. The clinical presentation can vary from subacute to rapidly progressive respiratory failure. The majority of the patients present with pulmonary symptoms associated with nodular infiltrates on chest roentgenograph (Fauci et al., 1983; Leavitt and Fauci, 1986). The ACR study noted hemoptysis in 98% of patients and abnormal chest roentgenographs in 65% (Leavitt et al., 1990). This compares with the 71% incidence of pulmonary infiltrates noted among 85 patients studied at the National Institutes of Health (Fauci et al., 1983). A review of 80 patients reported from three separate studies showed the distribution of chest roentgenographic abnormalities as follows: unilateral (55%), bilateral (45%), infiltrates (63%), nodules (31%), infiltrates with cavitation (8%), and nodules with cavitation (10%) (Matthews and Cupps, 1990). Chest roentgenographs reveal rounded opacities ranging from a few millimeters to several centimeters. The nodules are commonly bilateral and one-third contain cavities, which are irregular in outline, thick-walled, and possess a shaggy inner lining (Fig. 1). Solitary nodules may occur in 30–40% of

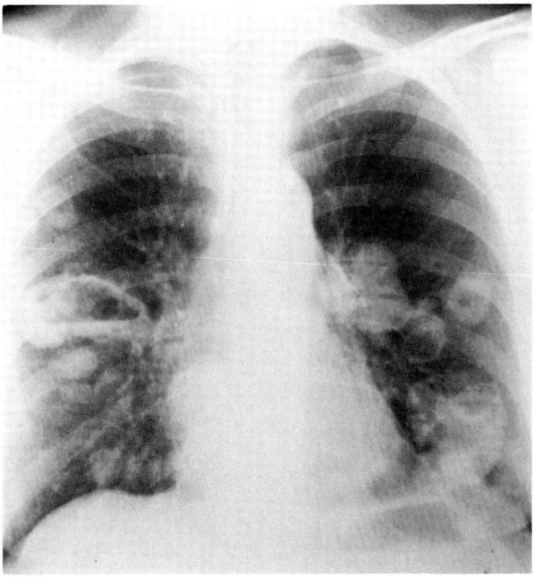

Figure 1 Chest roentgenograph of a patient with Wegener's granulomatosis demonstrating bilateral nodules of varying sizes; many are cavitated.

individuals with WG (Young, 1989). Pneumonic infiltrates, lobar consolidation, and pleural effusions can also be seen (Fig. 2). Diffuse alveolar infiltrates may indicate alveolar hemorrhage. Pure interstitial infiltrates are uncommon.

A recent study of the pulmonary pathological features in 87 open lung biopsies from 67 patients with WG reported the following observations: 72% had classical WG with renal involvement and 28% had limited WG without renal involvement. Pulmonary findings included interstitial fibrosis (26%), alveolar hemorrhage (49%), tissue eosinophils (100%), organizing intraluminal fibrosis (70%), endogenous lipoid pneumonia (59%), lymphoid aggregates (37%), and a variety of bronchial/bronchiolar lesions, including acute and chronic bronchiolitis (51% and 64%, respectively), follicular bronchiolitis (28%), and bronchiolitis obliterans (31%) (Travis et al., 1991).

The differential diagnosis in patients who present with clinical and pathological features suggestive of WG should include infectious diseases, especially mycobacteria, fungi, and helminths, which can cause systemic illness, pulmonary infiltrates, and histological evidence of granulomatous vasculitis that mimics WG (Fauci et al., 1983; Leavitt and Fauci, 1986). The ACR classification criteria included four features, namely, nasal inflammation, abnormal chest roentgenograph, abnormal urinary sediment, and granulomatous inflammation on biopsy; interestingly, in the absence of biopsy, hemoptysis was used as a "surrogate criterion," presumably because of the high incidence (98%) of hemoptysis (Leavitt et al., 1990). In contrast, the NIH study recorded hemoptysis

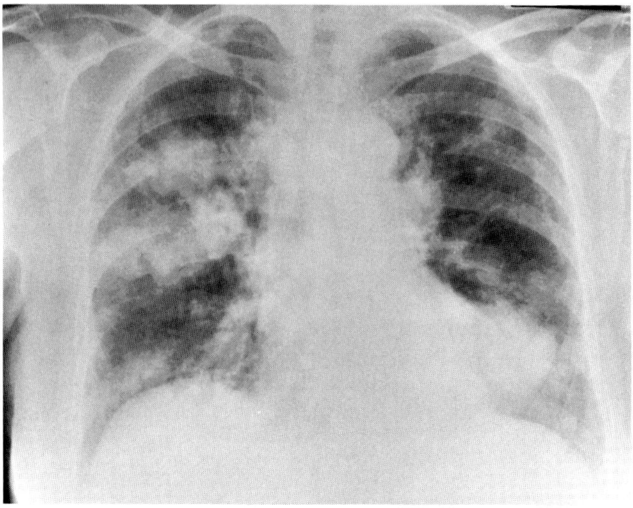

Figure 2 Bilateral soft mass-like lesions and patchy alveolar infiltrates in a patient with acute Wegener's granulomatosis.

in only 18% (Fauci et al., 1983). Overall, pulmonary involvement was seen in 94%, paranasal disease in 91%, and nasal and pharyngeal involvement in 64% (Leavitt et al., 1990). At present, it is unlikely that clinicians will commence high-dose corticosteroid therapy or cyclophosphamide without documentation of the diagnosis by a tissue biopsy.

As indicated, limited WG may not be a distinct entity because many patients with obvious respiratory involvement may also have clinically undetectable renal lesions. Without a renal biopsy, it is difficult to state emphatically that a patient with pulmonary manifestations has limited WG. Although the original description of limited WG reported that these patients have an excellent prognosis (Carrington and Liebow, 1966), it is important to treat them aggressively.

C. Alveolar Hemorrhage

Diffuse lung hemorrhage from necrotizing capillaritis is reported to occur in 5–45% of biopsy- or autopsy-documented cases (Colby, 1989; Leavitt et al., 1990; Travis et al., 1989). Massive pulmonary alveolar hemorrhage is occasionally seen in these patients and often presents as a life-threatening problem (Fig. 3) (Myers and Katzenstein, 1987; Travis et al., 1989, 1990a). When diffuse alveolar hemorrhage occurs, other causes of pulmonary alveolar hemorrhage syndrome should be considered in the differential diagnosis (Leatherman et al., 1984). In the presence of renal dysfunction and urinary sediment abnormalities,

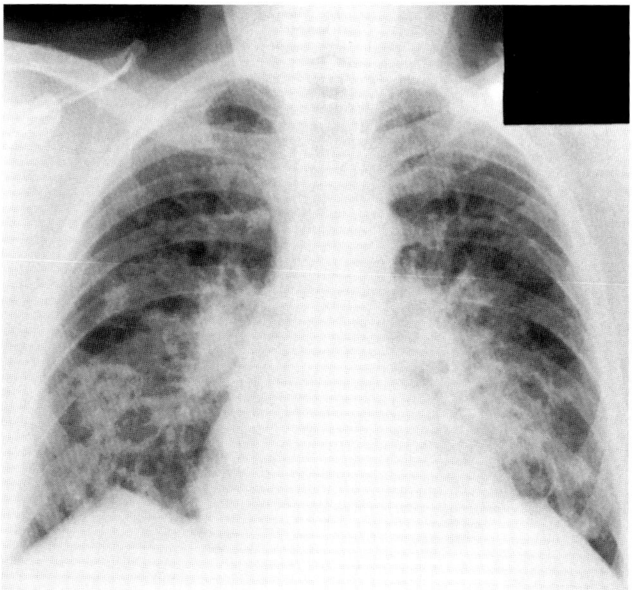

Figure 3 Wegener's granulomatosis with bilateral alveolar hemorrhage manifested roentgenologically by diffuse alveolar infiltrates and clinically by significant hemoptysis and renal failure.

the differentiation of WG from antiglomeruler antibody disease becomes difficult. Biopsy and special immunoflourescent studies may be necessary to establish the diagnosis.

D. Tracheobronchial Stenosis

Endotracheal or endobronchial involvement from WG occurs in a significant number of patients (Bohlman et al., 1984). Recently, I saw a middle-aged man who presented with a large, obstructing, neoplastic-like lesion in the trachea with no other involvement from WG. Nd:YAG laser therapy had to be used to provide relief of his dyspnea. All biopsies from the tracheal lesion were indicative of WG. His cANCA was strongly positive, indicating the active phase of disease. Hemoptysis in such cases may arise from mucosal ulcerations in the tracheobronchial tree, and bronchoscopic examination usually reveals extremely friable mucosa that bleeds profusely on instrumentation. In patients with subacute disease, these areas may undergo narrowing from concentric fibrosis.

Benign-appearing stenoses of the tracheobronchial tree are more likely in chronic cases and in patients whose disease is stable (Fig. 4). The NIH study

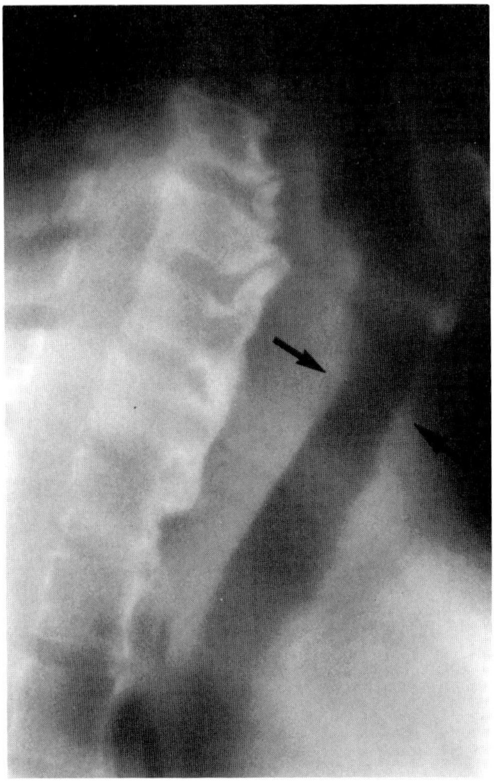

Figure 4 Lateral tomography of the trachea in a patient with chronic Wegener's granulomatosis showing mild subglottic tracheal stenosis (arrows).

reported that 14% of 85 patients had endobronchial disease at some point during their illness, and subglottic stenosis was present in 7% (Fauci et al., 1983). To assess the pulmonary dysfunction, pulmonary function tests have been used in follow-up of patients with WG (Rosenberg et al., 1980).

E. Treatment and Prognosis

Corticosteroids in combination with cyclophosphamide are effective in most patients with WG. The normal initial dosage of these two drugs is 1–2 mg/kg/day of each orally. Complete response can be expected in more than 90% of patients thus treated (Fig. 5) (Fauci et al., 1983). In milder cases, corticosteroids alone may produce remission. However, many patients will require prolonged treatment with smaller doses of corticosteroids and/or cyclophosphamide. Interestingly, some physicians have reported improvement of the disease following the use of an antimicrobial agent, trimethoprim-sulfamethoxazole (DeRemee et al., 1985). Subglottic stenosis may require surgical therapy (DeRemee, 1991). In some patients with chronic main bronchial stenoses, we have tried bronchoscopic dilation with excellent response. Others have used CO_2 laser to treat subglottic stenosis (Strange et al., 1990). Relapse of pulmonary WG is usually associated with viral or bacterial infections.

III. Churg-Strauss Syndrome

Also known as allergic granulomatosis and angiitis, Churg-Strauss syndrome (CSS) is distinct from hypersensitivity vasculitis (HSV) and polyarteritis nodosa (PAN). Churg and Strauss (1951) described 13 cases of severe asthma with a "strikingly uniform clinical picture including fever, hypereosinophilia, and vascular abnormality in various organ systems"; all but two patients died of the illness. The 11 fatal cases, which were located through autopsy files, had originally been categorized as PAN. In 1981, Churg and Strauss broadened the concept of CSS to include eosinophilic pneumonitis, eosinophilic nonnecrotizing angiitis, bronchocentric granulomatosis, allergic granuloma, and necrotizing angiitis. Subsequently, others portrayed CCS as an overlap syndrome that included hypereosinophilic disease (Löffler's syndrome), systemic vasculitides (PAN and HSV), and WG (Lanham et al., 1984). The understanding of the disease is further complicated by the observation that CSS has been described in association with such varied diseases as systemic lupus erythematosus, rheumatoid arthritis, lymphoma, leukemia, multiple myeloma, subacute bacterial endocarditis, chronic acute hepatitis, and chronic ulcerative colitis (Finan and Winkelmann, 1983), and in many patients, the clinical and pathological features overlap those of WG and PAN (Lie et al., 1990). Although many publications have appeared on this entity, CSS remains an uncommon disease. Over a period of 25 years (1950–1974), only 30 cases of CSS were identified at the Mayo Clinic (Chumbley et al., 1977). In the ACR study of 807 patients with various vasculitic syndromes, CSS constituted only 2.5% (Bloch et al., 1990).

CSS is characterized by pulmonary and systemic vasculitis, extravascular granulomas, and eosinophilia, which occur almost exclusively in patients with asthma or a history of allergy. It may occur in limited form in isolated organs or tissues and has been observed in some patients with connective tissue diseases or autoimmune disorders. The two diagnostically essential lesions of CSS are granulomatous or nongranulomatous angiitis and extravascular necrotizing granulomas, usually with eosinophilic infiltrates (Lie et al., 1990). The angiitis is disseminated and involves pulmonary and systemic arteries and veins. In contrast to WG, extrapulmonary lesions are found more commonly in the gastrointestinal tract, spleen, and heart than in the kidney (Lie et al., 1990). In the Mayo Clinic series of 30 cases, only one patient had renal failure (Chumbley et al., 1977). Hypereosinophilia and elevation of IgE are common (Churg, 1983;

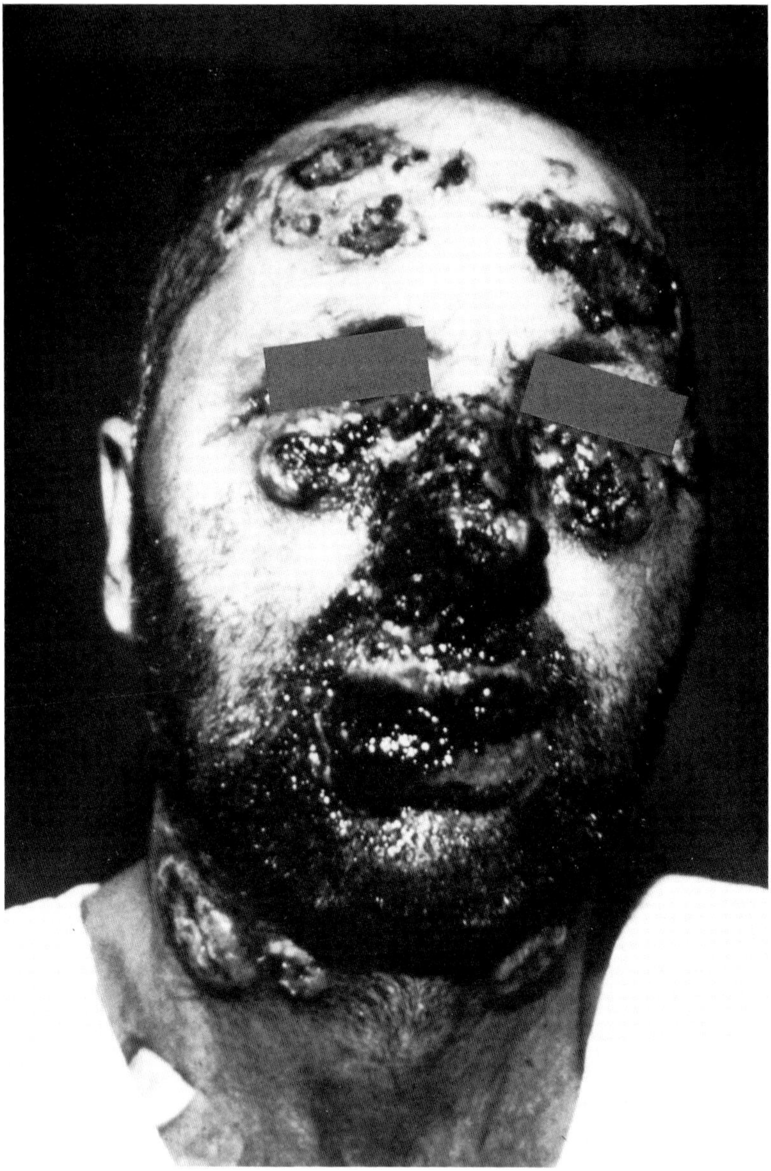

(A)

Figure 5 (A) Severe skin involvement in a patient with Wegener's granulomatosis. (B) Dramatic resolution of skin lesions several weeks after therapy. Scars can be seen in areas of previous lesions. (Photographs courtesy of Dr. Richard A. DeRemee.)

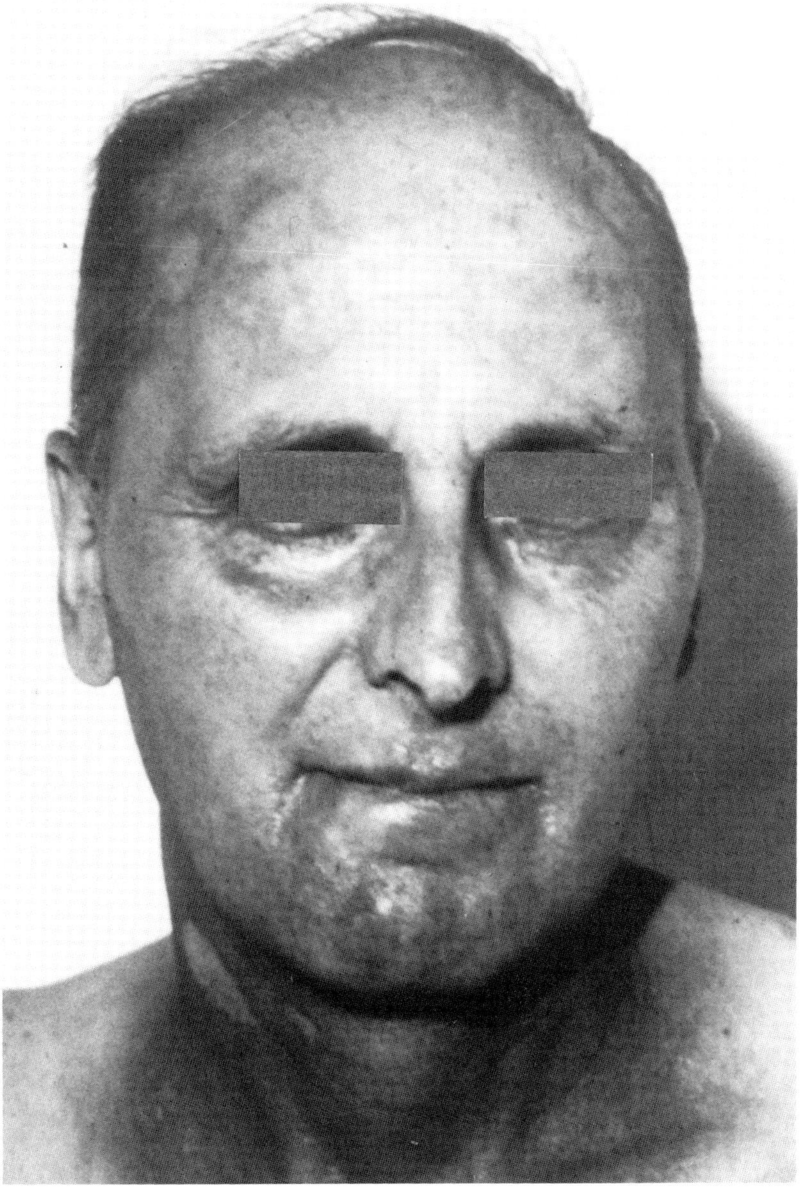

(B)

Churg and Strauss, 1951; Olsen et al., 1980; Varriale et al., 1964). The so-called "Churg-Strauss granulomas" of cutaneous and subcutaneous tissues lack diagnostic specificity (Fig. 6), because approximately 50% of these lesions occur in systemic diseases other than CSS (Lie, 1986).

A. Upper Airway Involvement

The patients described in the earlier reports were younger than the 20 patients studied by the ACR, who had a mean age of 50 years at the onset of CSS (Masi et al., 1990). Allergic rhinitis, nasal polyps, nasal mucosal crusting, and septal perforation are seen in over 70% of patients (Churg, 1983; Churg and Strauss, 1951; Olsen et al., 1980; Varriale et al., 1964). Nasal polyps in particular are the major clinical findings in the upper respiratory tract of patients with CSS. In the ACR report on 20 patients with CSS, all had chronic paranasal sinus pain or tenderness, 18 had seasonal allergy, and 14 had opacification of paranasal sinuses (Masi et al., 1990). Also in contrast to WG, disease of the trachea is seldom seen in CSS.

B. Pulmonary Involvement

The predominant pulmonary manifestation is asthma, which was described in all patients in three large series (Churg and Strauss, 1951; DeRemee, 1991; Lanham et al., 1984). As in the original description (Churg and Strauss, 1951), the 15 patients in the Mayo Clinic series who died had asthma for a mean interval of only 3 years prior to the onset of vasculitis; the mean duration of asthma among the remaining 15 survivors was 13 years (Chumbley et al., 1977). In 1984, a phasic pattern of CSS was described as initial allergic rhinitis, evolving into asthma, followed by peripheral blood eosinophilia, eosinophilic tissue infiltrates, and, ultimately, vasculitis (Lanham et al., 1984). In the ACR report on 20 patients with CSS, 19 had asthma, all had transitory pulmonary infiltrates on the chest roentgenogram, and peripheral blood eosinophilia and mono- or polyneuritis multiplex was noted in all (Masi et al., 1990).

One review of 138 patients from the literature, in addition to 16 patients of the authors, revealed the following: the mean age of the patients (84 males) was 28 years at the onset of allergic rhinitis, 35 years at the onset of asthma, and 38 years when vasculitis was diagnosed. The mean peak eosinophil count was 12.9×10^9/L ($1.5–29 \times 10^9$/L), anemia was present in 83%, granulomas in about 40%, tissue eosinophilia in approximately 50%, and vasculitis in more than 70%. The patients who died within a year of onset of vasculitis had a mean interval of 4.2 years between the onset of asthma and vasculitis, whereas those surviving longer than a year had a mean interval of 6.6 years. Respiratory failure was the cause of death in only 2%, although 8% died from status asthmaticus. The major causes of death were cardiac failure (48%), renal failure (18%),

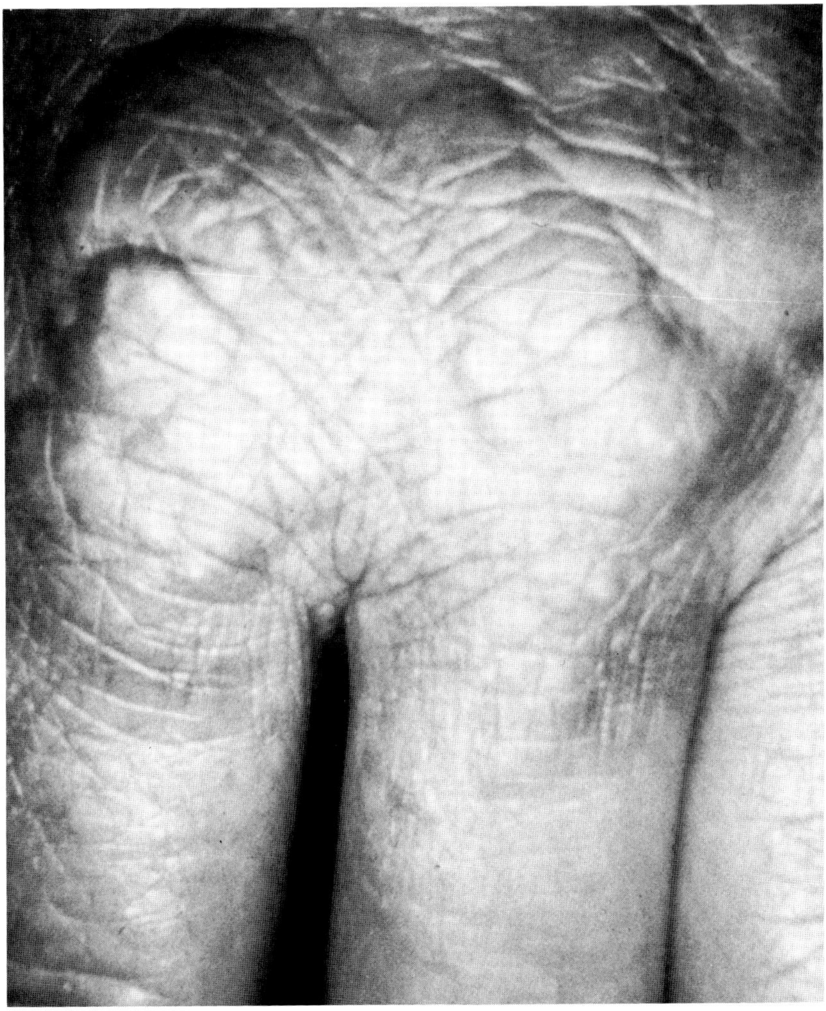

Figure 6 Photograph showing skin changes over the dorsal aspects of metacarpophalangeal joints in a patient with Churg-Strauss syndrome. The biopsy of these nodular lesions revealed "Churg-Strauss" granulomas with intense eosinophilic infiltrates.

cerebral hemorrhage (16%), and gastrointestinal hemorrhage in 8% (Lanham et al., 1984). Massive pulmonary hemorrhage is described in CSS, but the true incidence of this complication is unknown (Clutterbuck and Pusey, 1987).

Chest roentgenographic abnormalities are described in over 60% of patients with CSS (Fig. 7); the findings have included patchy and occasionally

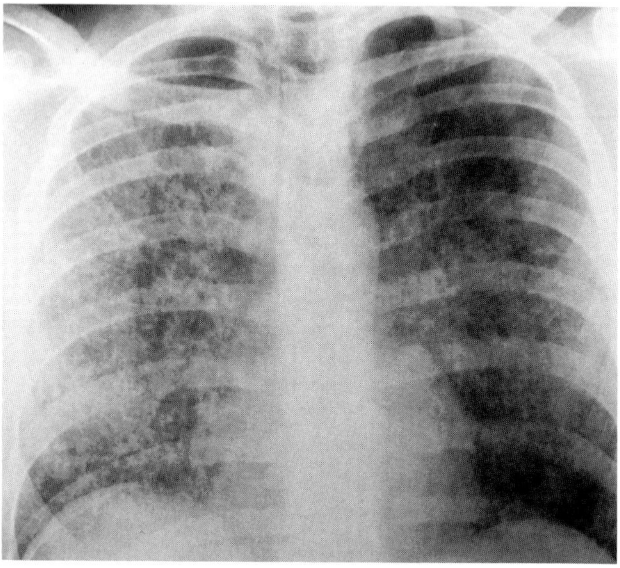

Figure 7 Chest roentgenograph in acute Churg-Strauss syndrome with bilateral diffuse soft ("feathery") alveolar infiltrates.

diffuse alveolar-interstitial infiltrates in the perihilar area with a predilection for the upper two-thirds of the lung fields (Chumbley et al., 1977). Small areas of cavitation occur rarely. Nodular changes seen in WG are uncommon in CSS but may be seen (Fig. 8). Pleural effusion has been noted (Erzurum et al., 1989).

The major differential diagnoses in asthmatic patients who become refractory to standard bronchodilator therapy should include CSS and, more likely, allergic bronchopulmonary aspergillosis.

C. Treatment and Prognosis

High mortality was commonly noted in the precorticosteroid era. None of the 20 patients studied in the ACR report died from CSS (Masi et al., 1990). Dramatic response can be expected from high-dose systemic corticosteroid therapy, which should be instituted as soon as the diagnosis of CSS is established.

IV. Henoch-Schönlein Purpura

Also referred to as anaphylactoid purpura, Henoch-Schönlein purpura (HSP) was first described by Schönlein (1837), who described the syndrome of acute purpura and arthritis in children, and then by Henoch (1874), who reported the

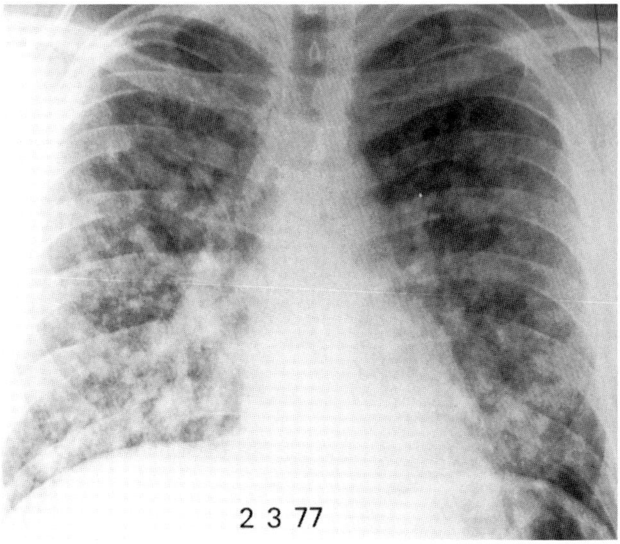

Figure 8 Dense bilateral nodular infiltrates in a patient with Churg-Strauss syndrome.

occurrence of colicky abdominal pain and nephritis. Although HSP occurs more commonly in children below the age of 10 years, an adult form of the disease is also well documented (Cream et al., 1970; Editorial, 1971). Among the 807 cases of vasculitis studied by the ARC, there were 85 (10.5%) cases of HSP (Bloch et al., 1990). The mean age of the patients was 17.4 years, nearly two-thirds were younger than 16 years, and 46 were males and 39 were females (Mills et al., 1990).

Histological examination shows acute vasculitis of arterioles and venules in the superficial dermis and the bowel. Proliferative and necrotizing glomerulonephritis is generally mild and self-limiting (Lie et al., 1990). Although immunofluorescence microscopy has shown IgA to be plentiful, and usually the only type of immunoglobulin in the skin and renal tissues, the suggestion that its presence be used as a specific diagnostic test has been refuted (Levinsky and Barratt, 1979; Lie, 1988b). Elevations in serum IgA- and IgG-containing complexes are present in adults. Necrotizing glomerulonephritis seen in HSP is also seen in patients with systemic lupus erythematosus, Goodpasture syndrome, WG, PAN, and infective endocarditis. At times it is extremely difficult to arrive at a precise diagnosis despite extensive investigations, including biopsies and even autopsy (Furlong et al., 1987; Goldstein et al., 1986; Parfrey et al., 1985).

The clinical triad of purpura, arthritis, and abdominal pain is seen in approximately 80% of patients with HSP. Palpable purpura, commonly distributed over the buttocks and lower extremities (Fig. 9), and fever are usually the first signs of HSP. Arthralgias and abdominal pain may precede, accompany, or follow the rash. Joint involvement is characteristically oligoarticular, transient, affects large joints, and with pain out of proportion to objective evidence of synovitis (Mills et al., 1990). Peritonitis and melena are common.

A. Pulmonary Involvement

Pulmonary alveolar hemorrhage, perihilar patchy opacities, and reticulonodular changes have been observed (Drogendijk and Schlesinger, 1961; Fiegler and Siemoneit, 1981; Jacome, 1967; Parfrey et al., 1985). A case of a young female presenting with pulmonary hemorrhage has been reported (Payton et al., 1987). However, among the 85 cases of HSP studied by the ARC, no pulmonary involvement was described (Mills et al., 1990). My review of English literature suggests that pulmonary involvement in HSP is distinctly rare.

B. Treatment and Prognosis

With high-dose corticosteroid therapy (0.5–1.0 mg/kg/day), a full recovery is the rule in HSP. Relapses of purpura, abdominal pain, and arthritis may be observed over 3–6 weeks before a complete resolution occurs (Mills et al., 1990).

V. Giant Cell (Temporal) Arteritis

A form of vasculitis of unknown etiology, giant-cell (temporal) arteritis (GCA), has also been described in association with polymyalgia rheumatica. However, the relationship between these two entities remains uncertain (Cohen and Ginsburg, 1990). The histological features of GCA are variable, but typical findings include lymphocytic infiltration with fragmentation of the internal elastic lamina, granulomatous inflammation, histiocytes, and multinucleated giant cells. GCA usually affects persons in middle age and older. There has been an increase in the annual incidence of GCA, with rates of 24.1 cases per 100,000 persons per year in the mid-1980s (Hunder, 1990). In the multicenter studies organized by the ACR, GCA was the most common form of vasculitis and was observed in 214 (26.5%) of 807 patients with various types of vasculitides (Bloch et al., 1990).

The onset of clinical illness is gradual, with the development of nonspecific constitutional symptoms such as low-grade fever, malaise, and weight loss followed by more specific symptoms such as jaw claudication and sudden loss of vision. Headache is the most common symptom in GCA. It is variable but often severe. Amaurosis fugax is observed in 20% and visual loss in 10% (Caselli et al., 1988). There are no specific laboratory tests available to diagnose GCA.

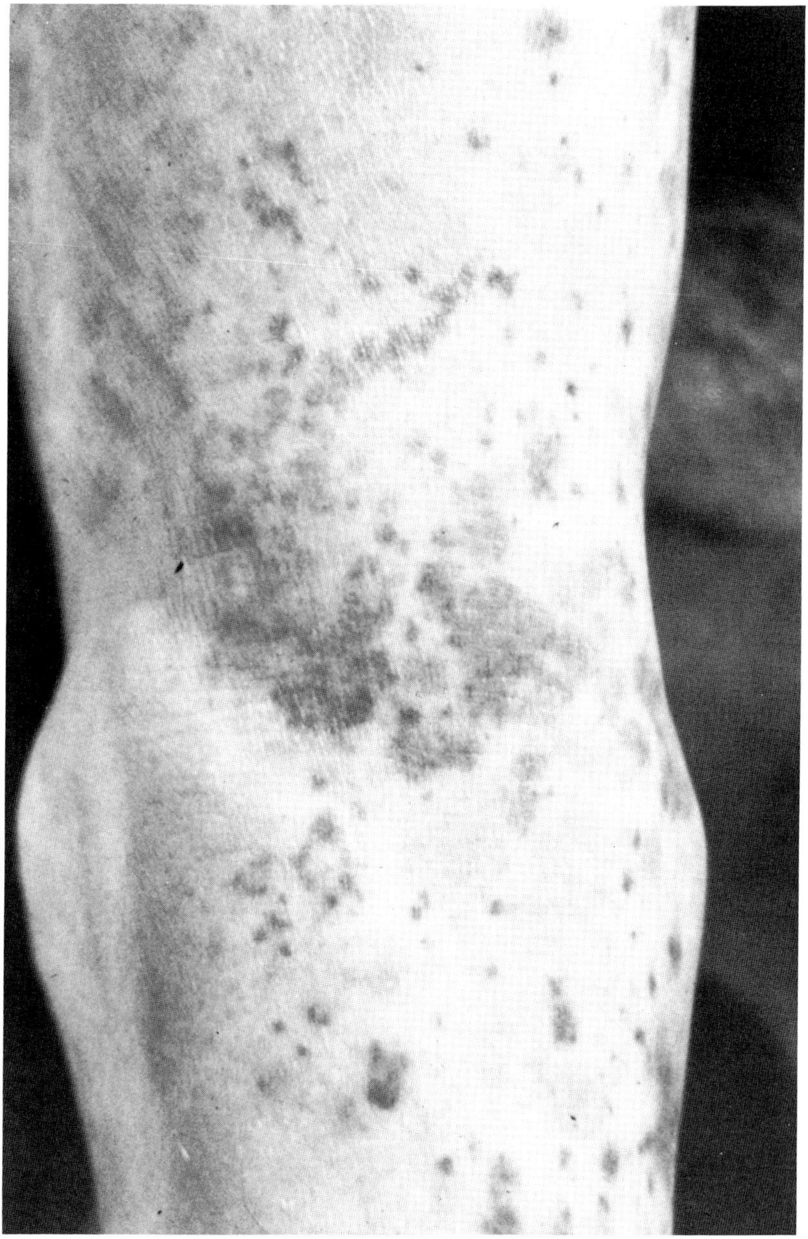

Figure 9 Photograph of the skin over the popliteal fossa of a patient with Henoch-Schönlein purpura shows palpable purpuric lesions.

The classic pathological features of GCA are seen in approximately 60% of temporal artery biopsies (Lie et al., 1990).

A. Pulmonary Involvement

Respiratory involvement in GCA was not recognized until 1984, when a report was published on 16 patients with GCA who had prominent symptoms related to the respiratory tract, including cough, sore throat, and hoarseness. These symptoms were the initial finding in 10 patients and obscured the diagnosis in some instances; the abnormalities resolved quickly when corticosteroids were given. The authors of this study estimated that 9% of patients with GCA have prominent respiratory tract symptoms, which are the initial manifestation in 4%, and suggested that GCA should be considered in any older patient with a new cough or throat pain without obvious cause (Larson et al., 1984). Further analysis in a population-based study of patients with GCA noted respiratory symptoms in up to 30% of 94 patients (Machado et al., 1988).

Acritidis et al. (1988) studied the pulmonary function of 26 nonsmoking patients with GCA and/or polymyalgia rheumatica and compared the findings with those of 28 age- and sex-matched nonsmoking control subjects; isolated small-airways disease was detected in 46.2% of patients, but the abnormalities were not significantly different from those of the controls. Obstructive, restrictive, and diffuse interstitial lung disease were seen in one, three, and two patients, respectively, but was absent in the control population. All the patients had normal chest roentgenographs (Acritidis et al., 1988).

Pulmonary nodules, interstitial infiltrations, pulmonary artery occlusion, and aneurysms have been described in patients with GCA (Bradley et al., 1984; Dennison et al., 1985; Glover et al., 1987; Kramer et al., 1987). In one report of two patients with biopsy-proven temporal arteritis, one patient presented with multinodular pulmonary lesions, whereas the second had a diffuse interstitial pattern. Both patients responded well to corticosteroid treatment (Kramer et al., 1987). One case has been reported of diffuse vasculitis in which pulmonary involvement with asthma, eosinophilic interstitial infiltrates, and small nodules were seen in association with jaw claudication, and GCA giant cells were found on biopsy (Amato et al., 1989). In addition, a patient with GCA preceded by pulmonary vascular disease has been reported (Doyle et al., 1988), and a patient with GCA with focal necrosis as well as granulomatous inflammation of large- and medium-sized pulmonary arteries at autopsy has also been reported (Ladanyi and Fraser, 1987). GCA limited to large pulmonary arteries has also been noted (Kramer et al., 1987).

B. Treatment and Prognosis

Almost all patients with GCA respond favorably to systemic corticosteroids therapy. Among the patients reported in the literature quoted above, uniform resolution of pulmonary complications was observed following corticosteroid therapy. There are reports of chronic or progressive pulmonary infiltrates in patients with GCA.

VI. Behçet's Disease

Behçet's disease (BD) is a chronic, relapsing, multisystemic, inflammatory disorder characterized by aphthous stomatitis along with two or more of the following: aphthous genital ulcerations, uveitis, cutaneous nodules or pustules (Fig. 10), synovitis, or meningoencephalitis (Behçet, 1937; Lakhanpal et al., 1985; O'Duffy, 1990). The prevalence rate in Japan (1:16,000 is roughly equivalent to the rate in the United States (1:20,000), although the disease runs a more severe course in the Japanese and in patients from the eastern Mediterranean area (O'Duffy, 1990). HLA-B5 and its subtype-B51 are 3–6 times more likely in patients with BD compared to controls, and the presence of B51 antigen may predict a severe course (O'Duffy, 1990). Histological examination of mucocutaneous lesions is not always convincing for vasculitis. When seen, the vasculitic lesions may demonstrate varying intensity with lymphocytic and plasma cell invasion and deposition of IgM and C_3 in the dermal vessels (O'Duffy, 1990). Vasculitis occurs in both arteries and veins.

Occlusion of major vessels and aneurysms has been described in 10–37% of patients with BD (Decroix, 1969; Lakhanpal et al., 1985; O'Duffy, 1990). Superficial and deep vein thromboses of upper and lower extremities and thrombosis of inferior and superior vena cava are detected in 7–37% of patients with BD, and these complications are more common than in patients with systemic lupus erythematosus (Chajek and Fainaru, 1975; Kansu et al., 1972; O'Duffy, 1990). In contrast, renal involvement in BD is rare.

A. Pulmonary Involvement

An earlier review of the literature disclosed pulmonary involvement in only 13 cases (Petty et al., 1977). Major hemoptysis due to pulmonary vasculitis was the most serious complication, and 4 of the 13 patients developed massive-

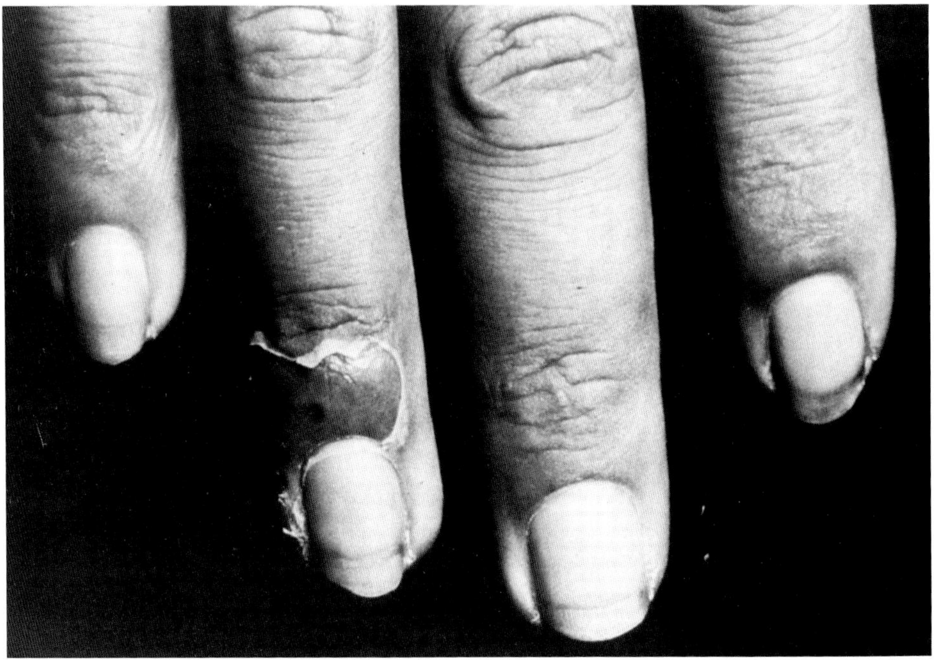

Figure 10 Typical skin lesion in a patient with Behçet's disease demonstrates periungual peeling of dermis associated with formation of pustule and ulceration; orogenital lesions were also present.

hemoptysis. In a later review of 28 patients with BD and pulmonary complications, a definite clinical pattern with hemoptysis, fever, chest pain, and dyspnea was noted in all (Efthimiou et al., 1986). Pulmonary disease was typically associated with active disease at other sites, and patients often complained of hemoptysis. Thrombophlebitis and hemoptysis seemed to be more common in men. Serious hemoptysis, although initially responsive to therapy with corticosteroids, tended to recur. Significant hemoptysis was common, and in 39%, death was caused by hemoptysis. All deaths due to hemoptysis occurred within 6 years of the onset of disease. Another analysis of 49 patients with pulmonary involvement from BD revealed that recurrent episodes of dyspnea, cough, chest pain ,and hemoptysis were the primary clinical signs, mainly in young men and that these features appeared 3.6 years after the first manifestation of BD. Fever, elevated erythrocyte sedimentation rate, and anemia were common, and chest roentgenographs demonstrated pulmonary infiltrates, pleural effusions, and prominent pulmonary arteries. Pulmonary artery aneurysms were seen in 7 of 13 patients in whom angiography was done (Raz et al., 1989).

Histopathological analysis in this study showed vasculitis of pulmonary vessels of various sizes, which was often associated with thrombosis, destruction of the elastic laminae, aneurysms, and arterial-bronchial fistula (Raz et al., 1989). In addition, pulmonary emboli and aphthous lesions of the tracheobronchial tree were noted. Recurrent pneumonia (Petty et al., 1977) and bronchial obstruction from mucosal involvement have been described (Gibson et al., 1982). Other studies have observed mucoid degeneration and intimal thickening of larger elastic pulmonary arteries, with medial hyperplasia, intimal fibroplasia, and angiomatoid lesions in muscular pulmonary arteries (Davies, 1973). Immunopathological studies suggest that the underlying pulmonary vasculitis is a result of circulating immune complexes (Gamble et al., 1979). This vasculitis is most likely responsible for the venous thromboses, pulmonary embolism and infarction, and pulmonary hemorrhage.

Multiple pulmonary artery aneurysms communicating with the bronchi should be suspected in any patient with BD having hemoptysis (Barberis et al., 1987; Hamza, 1987; Lie, 1988a; Raz et al., 1989; Shimizu et al., 1979). As a result of the very high incidence of thromboses of deep veins of the extremities and the venae cavae, the risk of developing pulmonary embolism is also high in patients with BD (Chajek and Fainaru, 1975; Kansu et al., 1972; Lakhanpal et al., 1985; O'Duffy, 1990). Nevertheless, it should be stressed that ventilation-perfusion scans are misleading in these patients and anticoagulant therapy for presumed pulmonary embolism may result in disastrous consequences (Gibson et al., 1982; O'Duffy, 1990). Pulmonary arteriography is diagnostic and should be considered in any patient with BD who presents with hemoptysis (Raz et al. 1989). Computed tomography has been suggested as a less invasive test to diagnose pulmonary artery aneurysms (Winer-Muram and Gavant, 1989).

Chest roentgenography in patients with BD may demonstrate patchy interstitial infiltrations, rounded opacities, and lobar consolidations (Fig. 11). Cavitation and pleural involvement are less common. Proximal perihilar opacities are due to the lobular or segmental pulmonary artery aneurysms (Grenier et al., 1981; Petty et al., 1977). Recently, tuberculosis has been reported in three patients with BD (Efthimiou et al., 1988).

B. Treatment and Prognosis

Although corticosteroids are palliative in all phases of BD, occurrence of sudden death in corticosteroid-treated patients has led some authorities to conclude that these drugs alone may be insufficient (O'Duffy, 1990). Other drugs, such as colchicine, chlorambucil, methotrexate, and azathioprine, may be needed for chronic treatment. It has been recommended that anticoagulant therapy be avoided in the presence of pulmonary arteritis (O'Duffy, 1990). Once diffuse pulmonary infiltration and massive hemoptysis occur, the prognosis is poor (Cadman et al., 1976). An analysis of 49 patients with pulmonary involvement from BD revealed 16 deaths, 15 from fatal pulmonary hemorrhage; 80% died within 2 years after the development of pulmonary disease (Raz et al., 1989).

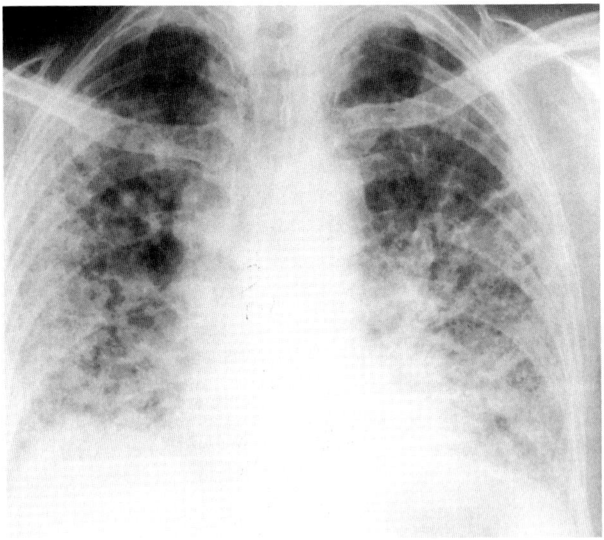

Figure 11 Pulmonary hemorrhage in a patient with Behçet's disease revealing extensive bilateral alveolar infiltrates; hemoptysis was the main sympton.

VII. Takayasu's Arteritis

Also described as "pulseless disease," Takayasu's arteritis (TA) is a chronic inflammatory disease of unknown etiology that primarily affects the aorta and its major branches (including the proximal coronary arteries and renal arteries) and the elastic pulmonary arteries (Fries et al., 1990; Hall and Buchbinder, 1990; Lie et al., 1990; Takayasu, 1908). The ACR study of 807 patients with various vasculitides revealed that 63 (7.8%) had TA (Bloch et al., 1990). Pulseless disease and aortic arch syndrome are classic manifestations, but claudication and renovascular hypertension may be the more disabling complications of the disease.

A. Pulmonary Involvement

Pulmonary artery involvement is common, having been observed in 50% of cases, with lesions generally localized to medium and large arteries (Lie et al., 1990; Lupi et al., 1975). One publication described three patients with classic TA, which affected the aorta and its major branches, all of whom were found to have a unique small pulmonary arteriopathy characterized by the deficiency of the outer media, with capillary ingrowth and thickened, fibrosed intima. Other distinct pathological features include granulomatous arteritis, transmural inflammation, patchy destruction of the medial musculoelastic lamellae, and lymphoplasmacytic infiltrates confined to the media with variable number of giant cells. Healing and healed arteritis will show progressive intimal and adventitious fibrosis and extensive scarring of the media (Lie et al., 1990). These abnormalities lead to pulmonary arterial occlusion and stenoses, which are found in the majority of cases.

The results of a retrospective study of 180 perfusion lung scans of 120 patients with TA revealed abnormalities in 76% of the patients. Early abnormalities occurred in the upper lobes, whereas the middle and lower lobes were involved at later stages of the disease. There was a weak correlation between scan abnormalities and spirometric and arterial blood gas findings (Umehara et al., 1991). Examination of the pulmonary arterial anatomy in 42 patients with TA, by intravenous digital subtraction angiography, has shown pulmonary arterial involvement in 14.3% of patients even though the pulmonary involvement was not suspected clinically in any patient, and the chest roentgenographs were abnormal in only two patients (Sharma et al., 1990). Pulmonary angiography in 59 patients has shown abnormalities in the form of arterial occlusions in 86%, whereas the chest roentgenographs were abnormal in 68% (Yamato et al., 1986).

Diffuse unilateral involvement of the right pulmonary artery associated with fistulas between the right coronary artery and the right pulmonary artery and between the right bronchial artery and the right pulmonary artery was reported in a woman with TA (Horimoto et al., 1991). Pulmonary-bronchial artery fistula has been described (Halon et al., 1987).

Pulmonary hypertension as the presenting manifestation of TA has been demonstrated in a small number of patients (Haas and Stiehm, 1986; Hayashi et al., 1986; Rose et al., 1984). A patient with Takayasu's arteritis was reported to have interstitial pulmonary fibrosis (Greene et al., 1986).

B. Treatment and Prognosis

Systemic corticosteroids therapy has resulted in symptomatic remission within days to weeks (Hall and Buchbinder, 1990). In patients with significant vascular disease, surgical correction may provide palliation (Chauvaud et al., 1987; Jakob et al., 1990). The cause of death in TA is usually vascular in origin, such as rupture of aneurysm, myocardial infarction, cardiac failure, or cerebrovascular accident (Hall and Buchbinder, 1990).

VIII. Other Vasculitic Syndromes

A. Urticarial Vasculitis

Urticarial vasculitis (UV) is characterized by urticarial lesions (Fig. 12), pruritus and arthralgias in 60%, arthritis in 28%, abdominal pain in 25%, and glomerulonephritis in 15%; the lesions begin as urticarial wheals and/or papules like the usual urticaria. Less common associations with UV include uveitis, episcleritis, fever, angioedema, and seizures (Gibson and Su, 1990). Elevated erythrocyte sedimentation rate is present in two-thirds and hypocomplementemia in 38% (Aboobaker and Greaves, 1986; Gibson and Su, 1990; Jones et al., 1983). Many of the pulmonary complications described have been in patients with the hypocomplementemic variety of UV.

Although there has been no documentation of vasculitis in the pulmonary vasculature in HV, many of these patients develop chronic obstructive pulmonary disease. In some studies, up to 62% of patients with hypocomplementemic UV developed chronic obstructive pulmonary disease (Sanchez et al., 1982; Schwartz et al., 1982). However, many of these patients have been smokers. One report on 16 patients with UV noted a significant degree of chronic obstructive pulmonary disease in 8 of 10 smokers studied, one of whom died of this complication. In three patients, severe chronic obstructive pulmonary disease developed at a young age after cigarette smoking for a relatively low number of pack-years. Lung disease probably results from the interaction of two major risk factors, namely, smoking and an immunologically mediated process that has not been identified (Baer et al., 1985; Schwartz et al., 1982).

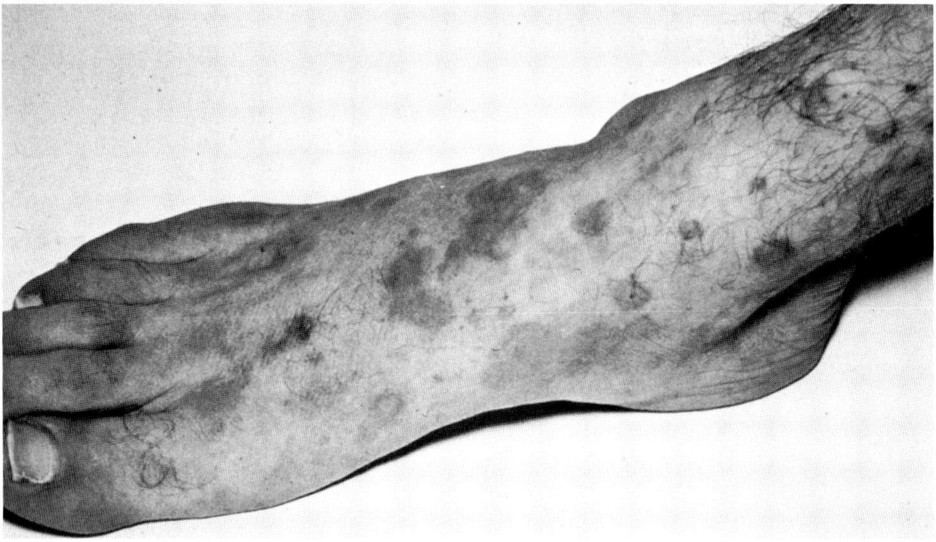

Figure 12 Hypocomplementemic urticarial vasculitis manifesting the urticarial lesions over the dorsum of the right foot in a patient who also demonstrated severe obstructive lung disease.

B. Leukocytoclastic Vasculitis

Leukocytoclastic vasculitis is synonymous with necrotizing vasculitis and is defined as fibrinoid necrosis of the vessel walls with leukocytoclasis of the inflammatory cells in the wall of the vessel (Gibson and Su, 1990). Leukocytoclastic vasculitis may be associated with a number of inflammatory, autoimmune, and malignant diseases. The most common presentation is in the form of palpable purpura.

The pulmonary complications that have been described include patchy pneumonitis due to vasculitis of the pulmonary venous system. A patient has been reported in whom hemoptysis and pleuritic chest pains were associated with clinical findings of leukocytoclastic vasculitis; an open lung biopsy revealed leukocytoclastic vasculitis of the pulmonary venules. Interestingly, this patient also had chronic obstructive pulmonary disease (Falk, 1984). Leukocytoclastic vasculitis and pneumonitis induced by metformin has been reported in one patient (Klapholz et al., 1986).

C. Eosinophilia Myalgia Syndrome

Dietary intake of L-tryptophan tablets was linked to an epidemic of eosinophilic myalgia syndrome (EMS) in New Mexico (CDC, 1989). As of April 1990, more than 1400 cases of EMS had been reported to the Centers for Disease Control (Catton et al., 1991). EMS may be a toxic reaction to contaminant(s) in this over-the-counter preparation used for various health reasons. Clinical manifestations of EMS include myalgias, fatigue, muscle weakness, arthralgias, edema of the extremities, skin rash, oral and vaginal ulcers, scleroderma-like changes, ascending neuropathy, and peripheral blood eosinophilia (Banner and Borochovitz, 1991; Catton et al., 1991; CDC, 1989; Clauw et al., 1990; Strumpf et al., 1991; Tazelaar et al., 1990; Travis et al., 1990b).

Pulmonary complaints were present in approximately 60% of patients with EMS (Catton et al., 1991). Pulmonary complications in EMS have consisted of pulmonary infiltrates associated with severe pulmonary distress and progressive hypoxemia, pleural effusion, diffuse bilateral reticulonodular infiltrates, and pulmonary hypertension (Banner and Borochovitz, 1991; Catton et al., 1991; Travis et al., 1990).

Analyses of lung biopsy specimens in patients with EMS have shown interstitial and perivascular infiltrates, fibrointimal hyperplasia of small vessels in the pulmonary vasculature, alveolar exudate made up of eosinophils and histiocytes, and changes characteristic of hypersensitivity pneumonitis (Banner and Borochovitz, 1991; Catton et al., 1991; Strumpf et al., 1991; Travis et al., 1990).

In one report of five histologically documented cases of EMS, all patients were women ranging in age from 34 to 65 years, and all presented with respiratory symptoms that began after 1–9 months of L-tryptophan therapy. Peripheral eosinophilia was present in four patients, as were bilateral interstitial infiltrates on chest roentgenography. One patient had a normal chest roentgenogram. Lung biopsies were done in all patients, and biopsy specimens showed a vasculitis and perivasculitis associated with a mild chronic interstitial pneumonitis and eosinophilia. Three patients had clinical and/or histological evidence of pulmonary hypertension, and one had a follicular bronchiolitis. Four patients recovered promptly with steroid therapy and discontinuation of L-tryptophan therapy, and one patient had minimal symptomatic improvement (Tazelaar et al., 1990).

D. Essential Mixed Cryoglobulinemia

Essential mixed cryoglobulinemia (EMC) is characterized by recurrent episodes of purpura, arthralgias, weakness, and multiorgan involvement. Pathological features are similar to those in leukocytoclastic vasculitis. Elevated rheumatoid factor and cryoglobulin are frequent findings. Pulmonary insufficiency, Sjögren's syndrome-like illness with lung involvement (Fig. 13), fibrosing alveolitis, and bronchiectasis have been described in isolated cases (Chejfec et al., 1981; Erhardt et al., 1979; Singer et al., 1986). Pulmonary function tests in 19 patients (17 women) with a mean age of 49.6 years) with EMC showed a decrease in DLCO and decrease in maximal expiratory flow at 50% of FVC, TLC, and FRC (Bombardieri et al., 1979; Viegi et al., 1989).

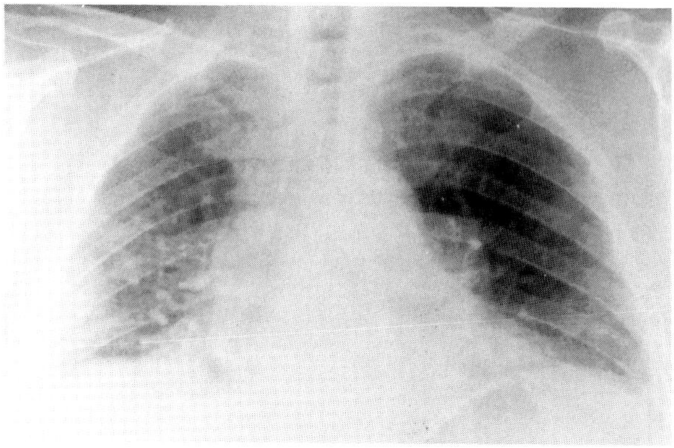

Figure 13 Chest roentgenograph of a patient with mixed cryoglobulinemia showing patchy pneumonitis in the right mid- and lower lung zones.

E. Polyarteritis Nodosa

Polyarteritis nodosa (PAN) is characterized by a necrotizing arteritis of small and medium-sized muscular arteries that affects multiple organ systems (Lightfoot et al., 1990). It is important to recognize that PAN seldom involves the lungs. The earlier literature described vasculitis in the bronchial and pulmonary vasculature, but many of the patients had granulomatous lesions with eosinophilic infiltrates (Rose and Spencer, 1957; Sweeney and Baggenstoss, 1949; Wilson and Alexander, 1945). In retrospect, it appears that the majority of the patients diagnosed as having pulmonary PAN indeed had CSS (Fig. 14). Nevertheless, the recent publications continue to describe patients with "pulmonary involvement in PAN" (Carratalá et al., 1989; Haworth et al., 1985; Komadina and Houk, 1989; Nguyen, 1991).

The ACR study on 807 patients with various vasculitides observed PAN in 118 (14.6%) patients, but no pulmonary complications were described in any of the patients (Bloch et al., 1990; Lightfoot et al., 1990). The difficulty of differentiating PAN from CSS has been pointed out by noting that several reports reiterate the serious risk of major pulmonary hemorrhage from microscopic polyarteritis of the lung, which probably represents a forme fruste of CSS (Lightfoot, 1991).

F. Secondary Vasculitis

Many of the rheumatological diseases demonstrated secondary vasculitic process in the tissues involved. Certain infectious processes, particularly mycoses, may cause secondary vasculitis. When confronted with vasculitic lesions, the

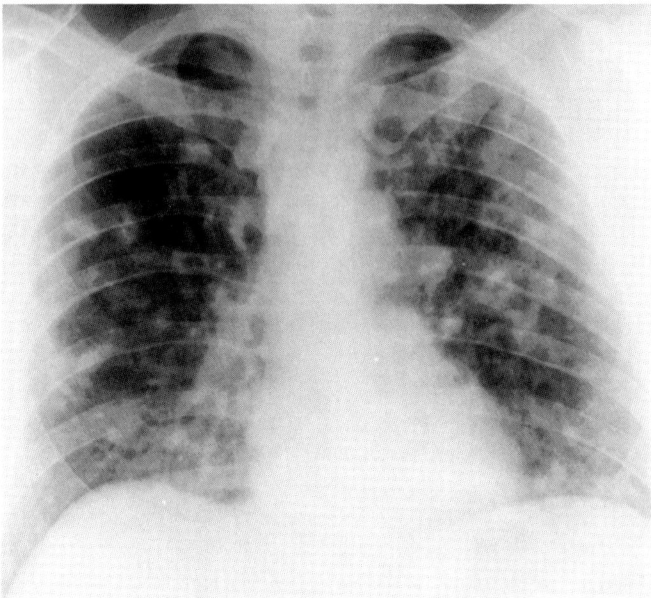

Figure 14 Chest roentgenograph (taken in 1960) of a patient with the diagnosis of polyarteritis nodosa. A recent review of clinical records in this patient suggested the diagnosis of Churg-Strauss syndrome.

well-known etiological agents such as drugs and chemicals should be considered (Seiden et al., 1990; Vaillant et al., 1990).

IX. Summary

Because of the rarity of vasculitides, physicians in clinical practice seldom consider vasculitides in the differential diagnosis of pulmonary problems. As in many of the rheumatological diseases, pulmonary signs and symptoms can be the presenting manifestations of a systemic vasculitis. The respiratory involvement may vary from mild to life-threatening respiratory distress. In contrast to the rheumatological diseases, lung biopsy in patients with pulmonary involvement from vasculitis is more likely to provide the diagnosis. Nevertheless, it is important to stress that there are many vasculitides that have nonspecific pathological features. In such cases, the clinical features and certain laboratory tests may aid in establishing the definitive diagnosis. Lymphomatoid granulomatosis is one of the entities that is sometimes classified as a vasculitis because of its clinical and morphological features. However, it should be classified as a lymphoproliferative disease and considered as such.

As discussed above, certain laboratory tests may point toward the diagnosis of vasculitis, but none of the tests, by itself, will establish the diagnosis. Chest roentgenographs also lack specific features, and clinical correlation is essential. The results of pulmonary function tests will vary depending on the extent of lung involvement. The majority of vasculitides respond favorably to high-dose corticosteroid therapy. Cytotoxic agents are important therapeutic adjuncts.

References

Aboobaker, J., and Greaves, M. W. (1986). Urticarial vasculitis. *Clin. Exp. Dermatol.* **11**:436–444.

Acritidis, N. C., Andonopoulos, A. P., Galanopoulou, V., Drosos, A. A., and Constantopoulos, S. H. (1988). Pulmonary function of nonsmoking patients with giant cell arteritis and/or polymyalgia rheumatica; a controlled study. *Clin. Rheumatol.* **7**:231–236.

Amato, M. B., Barbas, C. S. V., Delmonte, V. C., and Carvalho, C. R. R. (1989). Concurrent Churg-Strauss syndrome and temporal arteritis in a young patient with pulmonary nodules. *Am. Rev. Respir. Dis.* **139**: 1539–1542.

Arend, W. P., Michel, B. A., Bloch, D. A., Hunder, G. G., Calabrese, L. H., Edworthy, S. M., Fauci, A. S., Leavitt, R. Y., Lie, J. T., Lightfoot, R. W., Jr., Masi, A. T., McShane, D. J., Mills, J. A., Stevens, M. B., Wallace, S. L., and Zvaifler, N. J. (1990). The American College of Rheumatology 1990 criteria for the classification of Takayasu arteritis. *Arthritis Rheum.* **33**:1129–1134.

Baer, A. N., McCurley, T., Glick, A. D., and Sergent, J. S. (1985). Evidence for immunologically mediated pulmonary injury in the hypocomplementemic urticarial vasculitis syndrome (letter to the editor). *J. Am. Acad. Dermatol.* **13**:509–511.

Banner, A. S., and Borochovitz, D. (1991). Acute respiratory failure caused by pulmonary vasculitis after L-tryptophan ingestion. *Am. Rev. Respir. Dis.* **143**:661–664.

Barberis, M., Casadio, C., and Borghini, U. (1987). Massive haemoptysis in Behçet syndrome: case report. *Respiration* **52**:303–307.

Behçet, H. (1937). Über rezidivierende, aphthöse, durch ein Virus vesursachte Geschwüre am Mund, am Auge und an den Genitalien. *Dermatol. Wochenschr.* **105**:1152–1157.

Bloch, D. A., Michel, B. A., Hunder, G. G., McShane, D. J., Arend, W. P., Calabrese, L. H., Edworthy, S. M., Fauci, A. S., Fries, J. F., Leavitt, R. Y., Lie, J. T., Lightfoot, R. W., Jr., Masi, A. T., Mills, J. A., Stevens, M. B., Wallace, S. L., and Zvaifler, N. J. (1990). The American College of Rheumatology 1990 criteria for the classification of vasculitis: Patients and methods. *Arthritis Rheum.* **33**:1068–1073.

Bohlman, M. E., Ensor, R. E., and Goldman, S. M. (1984). Pulmonary Wegener's granulomatosis of the trachea: radiologic manifestations. *South. Med. J.* **77**:1318–1319.

Bombardieri, S., Paoletti, P., Ferris., C., Di Munno, O., Fornai, E., and Giuntini, C. (1979). Lung involvement in essential mixed cryoglobulinemia. *Am. J. Med.***66**:748–756.

Bradley, J. D., Pinals, R. S., Blumenfeld, H. B., and Poston, W. M. (1984). Giant cell arteritis with pulmonary nodules. *Am. J. Med.* **77**:135–140.

Cadman, E. C., Lundberg, W. B., and Mitchell, M. S. (1976). Pulmonary manifestations in Behçet syndrome: case report and review of the literature. *Arch. Intern. Med.* **136**:944–947.

Calabrese, L. H., Michel, B. A., Bloch, D. A., Arend, W. P., Edworthy, S. M., Fauci, A. S., Fries, J. F., Hunder, G. G., Leavitt, R. Y., Lie, J. T., Lightfoot, R. W., Jr., Masi, A. T., McShane, D. J., Mills, J. A., Stevens, M. B., Wallace, S. L., and Zvaifler, N. J. (1990). The American College of Rheumatology 1990 criteria for the classification of hypersensitivity vasculitis. *Arthritis Rheum.* **33**:1108–1113.

Cannon, G. W., and Zimmerman, G. A., eds. (1990). *The Rheumatic Patient with Lung Disease*. Lung Biology in Health and Disease, Vol. 45. Dekker, New York.

Carratalá, J., Vidaller, A., Maña, J., Manresa, F., and Fernández-Nogués, F. (1989). Polyarteritis nodosa associated with idiopathic pulmonary fibrosis: report of two cases (letter to the editor). *Ann. Rheum. Dis.* **48**: 876–877.

Carrington, C. B., and Liebow, A. A. (1966). Limited forms of angiitis and granulomatosis of Wegener's type. *Am. J. Med.* **41**:497–527.

Caselli, R. J., Hunder, G. G., and Whisnant, J. P. (1988). Neurologic disease in biopsy-proven giant cell (temporal) arteritis. *Neurology* **38**:352—359.

Catton, C. K., Elmer, J. C., Whitehouse, A. C., Clode, J. B., and Hustrulid, R. I. (1991). Pulmonary involvement in the eosinophilia-myalgia syndrome. *Chest* **99**:327–329.

Centers for Disease Control (1989). Eosinophilia-myalgia syndrome—New Mexico. *MMWR* **38** (45):765–767.

Chajek, T., and Fainaru, M. (1975). Behçet's disease. Report of 41 cases and review of the literature. *Medicine* (*Baltimore*) **54**:179–196.

Chauvaud, S., Mace, L., Brunewald, P., Tricot, J. L., Camilleri, J. P., and Carpentier, A. (1987). Takayasu's arteritis with bilateral pulmonary artery stenosis: successful surgical correction. *J. Thorac. Cardiovasc. Surg.* **94**:246–250.

Chejfec, G., Lichtenberg, L., Lertratanakul, Y., Lange, C., Baerwaldt, M., and Gould, V. E. (1981). Respiratory insufficiency in a patient with mixed cryoglobulinemia. *Ultrastruct. Pathol.* **2**:295–302.

Chumbley, L. C., Harrison, E. G., Jr., and DeRemee, R. A. (1977). Allergic granulomatosis and angiitis (Churg-Strauss syndrome): report and analysis of 30 cases. *Mayo Clin. Proc.* **52**:477–484.

Churg, A. (1983). Pulmonary angiitis and granulomatosis revisited. *Hum. Pathol.* **14**:868–883.

Churg, J., and Strauss, L. (1951). Allergic granulomatosis, allergic angiitis, and periarteritis nodosa. *Am. J. Pathol.* **27**:277–301.

Churg, J., and Strauss, L. (1981). Case 46-1980: interstitial eosinophilic pneumonitis, pleuritis, and angiitis (letter to the editor). *N. Engl. J. Med.* **304**:611.

Clauw, D. J., Nashel, D. J., Umhau, A., and Katz, P. (1990). Tryptophan-associated eosinophilic connective-tissue disease: a new clinical entity? *JAMA* **263**:1502–1506.

Clutterbuck, E. J., and Pusey, C. D. (1987). Severe alveolar haemorrhage in Churg-Strauss syndrome. *Eur. J. Respir. Dis.* **71**:158–163.

Cohen, M. D., and Ginsburg, W. W. (1990). Polymyalgia rheumatica. *Rheum. Dis. Clin. North Am.* **16**:325–339.

Colby, T. V. (1989). Diffuse pulmonary hemorrhage in Wegener's granulomatosis. *Semin. Respir. Med.* **10**:136–140.

Cream, J. J., Gumpel, J. M., and Peachy, R. D. G. (1970). Schönlein-Henoch purpura in the adult:a study of anaphylactoid or Schönlein-Henoch purpura. *Q. J. Med.* **39**:461–484.

Cross, C. E., and Lillington, G. A. (1989). Serodiagnosis of Wegener's granulomatosis: pathobiologic and clinical implications. *Mayo Clin. Proc.* **65**:119–122.

Davies, J. D. (1973). Behçet's syndrome with haemoptysis and pulmonary lesions. *J. Pathol.* **109**:351–356.

Decroix, A. G. (1969). Thoracic manifestations of Behçet's syndrome (abstract). *Thorax* **24**:380.

Dennison, A. R., Watkins, R. M., and Gunning, A. J. (1985). Simultaneous aortic and pulmonary artery aneurysms due to giant cell arteritis. *Thorax* **40**:156–157.

DeRemee, R. A. (1991). Wegener's granulomatosis. In *Immunologically Mediated Pulmonary Diseases*. Edited by J. P. Lynch, III and R. A. DeRemee. Lippincott, Philadelphia, pp. 250–273.

DeRemee, R. A., McDonald, T. J., and Weiland, L. H. (1985). Wegener's granulomatosis: observations on treatment with antimicrobial agents. *Mayo Clin. Proc.* **60**:27–32.

Doyle, L., McWilliam, L., and Hasleton, P. S. (1988). Giant cell arteritis with pulmonary involvement. *Br. J. Dis. Chest* **82**:88–92.

Drogendijk, A. C., and Schlesinger, F. G. (1961). Anatomical findings in a case of Schöenlein-Henoch syndrome. *Acta Med. Scand.* **169**:525–535.

Editorial (1971). Schönlein-Henoch purpura. *Br. Med. J.* **1**:416–417.

Efthimiou, J., Johnston, C., Spiro, S. G., and Turner-Warwick, M., (1986). Pulmonary disease in Behçet's snydrome. *Q. J.* Med. **58**:259–280.

Efthimiou, J., Hay, P. E., Spiro, S. G., and Lane, D. J. (1988). Pulmonary tuberculosis in Behçet's syndrome. *Br. J. Dis. Chest* **82**:300–304.

Erhardt, C. C., Mumford, P., and Maini, R. N. (1979). The association of cryoglobulinaemia with nodules, vasculitis and fibrosing alveolitis in rheumatoid arthritis and their relationship to serum C1q binding activity and rheumatoid factor. *Clin. Exp. Immunol.***38**:405–413.

Erzurum, S. C., Underwood, G. A., Hamilos, D. L., and Waldron, J. A. (1989). Pleural effusion in Churg-Strauss syndrome. *Chest* **95**:1357–1359.

Falk, D. K. (1984). Pulmonary disease in idiopathic urticarial vasculitis. *J. Am. Acad. Dermatol.* **11**:346–352.

Falk, R. J., Hogan, S., Carey, T. S., Jennette, J. C., and the Glomerular Disease Collaborative Network (1990). Clinical course of anti-neutrophil cytoplasmic autoantibody-associated glomerulonephritis and systemic vasculitis. *Ann. Intern. Med.* **113**:656–663.

Fauci, A. S., and Wolff, S. M. (1973). Wegener's granulomatosis: studies in eighteen patients and a review of the literature. *Medicine* (*Baltimore*) **52**:535–561.

Fauci, A. S., Haynes, B. F., Katz, P., and Wolff, S. M. (1983). Wegener's granulomatosis: prospective clinical and therapeutic experience with 85 patients for 21 years. *Ann. Intern. Med.* **98**:76–85.

Fiegler, V. W., and Siemoneit, K. D. (1981). Schöenlein-Henoch syndrome. *Fortschr. Geb. Roentgenstr. Nuklearmed.* **134**:269–272.

Finan, M. C., and Winkelmann, R. K. (1983). The cutaneous extravascular necrotizing granuloma (Churg-Strauss granuloma) and systemic disease: a review of 27 cases. *Medicine* (*Baltimore*) **62**:142–158.

Fries, J.F., Hunder, G.G., Bloch, D.A., Michel, B.A., Arend, W.P., Calabrese, L.H., Fauci, A.S., Leavitt, R.Y., Lie, J.T., Lightfoot, R.W., Jr., Masi, A.T., McShane, D. J., Mills, J. A., Stevens, M. B., Wallace, S. L., and Zvaifler, N. J. (1990). The American College of Rheumatology 1990 criteria for the classification of vasculitis: summary. *Arthritis Rheum.* **33**:1135–1136.

Furlong, T. J., Ibels, L. S., and Eckstein, R. P. (1987). The clinical spectrum of necrotizing glomerulonephritis. *Medicine* (*Baltimore*) **66**:192–201.

Gamble, C. N., Wiesner, K. B., Shapiro, R. F., and Boyer, W. J. (1979). The immune complex pathogenesis of glomerulonephritis and pulmonary vasculitis in Behçet's disease. *Am. J. Med.* **66**:1031–1039.

Gibson, J. M., O'Hara, M. D., Beare, J. M., and Stanford, C. F. (1982). Bronchial obstruction in a patient with Behçet's disease. *Eur. J. Respir. Dis.* **63**:356–360.

Gibson, L. E., and Su, W. P. D. (1990). Cutaneous vasculitis. *Rheum. Dis. Clin. North Am.* **16**:309–324.

Glover, M. U., Muñiz, J., Bessone, L., Carta, M., Casellas, J., and Maniscalco, B. S. (1987). Pulmonary artery obstruction due to giant cell arteritis. *Chest* **91**:924–925.

Godman, G. C., and Churg, J. (1954). Wegener's granulomatosis: pathology and review of the literature. *Arch. Pathol.* **58**:533–553.

Goldstein, J., Weil, J., and Liel, Y. (1986). Intrapulmonary hemorrhages and immune complex glomerulonephritis masquerading as Goodpasture's syndrome. *Hum. Pathol.* **17**:754–757.

Greene, N. G., Baughman, R. P., and Kim, C. K. (1986). Takayasu's arteritis associated with interstitial lung disease and glomerulonephritis. *Chest* **89**:605–606.

Grenier, P., Bletry, O., Cornud, F., Godeau, P., and Nahum, H. (1981). Pulmonary involvement in Behçet disease. *AJR* **137**:565–569.

Haas, A., and Stiehm, E. R. (1986). Takayasu's arteritis presenting as pulmonary hypertension. *Am. J. Dis. Child.* **140**:372–374.

Hall, S., and Buchbinder, R. (1990). Takayasu's arteritis. *Rheum. Dis. Clin. North Am.* **16**:411–422.

Halon, D. A., Turgeman, Y., Merdler, A., Hardoff, R., and Sharir, T. (1987). Coronary artery to bronchial artery anastomosis in Takayasu's arteritis. *Cardiology* **74**:387–391.

Hamza, M. (1987). Large artery involvement in Behçet's disease. *J. Rheumatol.* **14**:554–559.

Haworth, S. J., Savage, C. O., Carr, D., Hughes, J. M. B., and Rees, A. J. (1985). Pulmonary haemorrhage complicating Wegener's granulomatosis and microscopic polyarteritis. *Br. Med. J.* [*Clin. Res.*] **290**: 1775–1778.

Hayashi, K., Nagasaki, M., Matsunaga, N., Hombo, Z., and Imamura, T. (1986). Initial pulmonary artery involvement in Takayasu arteritis. *Radiology* **159**:401–403.

Haynes, B. F., Fishman, M. L., Fauci, A. S., and Wolff, S. M. (1977). The ocular manifestations of Wegener's granulomatosis: fifteen years experience and review of the literature. *Am. J. Med.* **63**:131–140.

Henoch, E. H. (1874). Uber ein eigenthumliche form von purpura. *Berl. Klin. Wochenschr.* **11**:641–643.

Horimoto, M., Igarashi, K., Aoi, K., Okamoto, K., and Takenaka, T. (1991). Unilateral diffuse pulmonary artery involvement in Takayasu's arteritis associated with coronary-pulmonary artery fistula and bronchial-pulmonary artery fistula: a case report. *Angiology* **42**:73–80.

Hunder, G. G. (1990). Giant cell (temporal) arteritis. *Rheum. Dis. Clin. North Am.* **16**:399–409.

Hunder, G. G., Arend, W. P., Bloch, D. A., Calabrese, L. H., Fauci, A. S., Fries, J. F., Leavitt, R. Y., Lie, J. T., Lightfoot, R. W., Jr., Masi, A. T., McShane, D. J., Michel, B. A., Mills, J. A., Stevens, M. B., Wallace, S. L., and Zvaifler, N. J. (1990a). The American College of Rheumatology 1990 criteria for the classification of vasculitis: introduction. *Arthritis Rheum.* **33**:1065–1067.

Hunder, G. G., Bloch, D. A., Michel, B. A., Stevens, M. B., Arend, W. P., Calabrese, L. H., Edworthy, S. M., Fauci, A. S., Leavitt, R. Y., Lie, J. T., Lightfoot, R. W., Jr., Masi, A. T., McShane, D. J., Mills, J. A., Wallace, S. L., and Zvaifler, N. J. (1990b). The American College of Rheumatology 1990 criteria for the classification of giant cell arteritis. *Arthritis Rheum.* **33**:1122:1128.

Jacome, A. F. (1967). Pulmonary hemorrhage and death complicating anaphylactoid purpura. *South. Med. J.* **60**:1003–1004.

Jakob, H., Volb, R., Stangl, G., Reifart, N., Rumpelt, H. J., and Oelert, H. (1990). Surgical correction of a severely obstructed pulmonary artery bifurcation in Takayasu's arteritis. *Eur. J. Cardiothorac. Surg.* **4**:456–458.

Jennette, J. C., and Falk, R. J., (1990). Antineutrophil cytoplasmic autoantibodies and associated diseases: a review. Am. *J. Kidney Dis.* **15**:517–529.

Jones, R. R., Bhogal, B., Dash, A., and Schifferli, J. (1983). Urticaria and vasculitis: a continuum of histological and immunopathological changes. *Br. J. Dermatol.* **108**:695–703.

Kansu, E., Özer, F. L., Akalin, E., Güler, Y., Zileli, T., Tanman, E., Kaplaman, E., and Müftüoğlu, E. (1972). Behçet's syndrome with obstruction of the venae cavae. *Q. J. Med.* **41**:151–168.

Klapholz, L., Leitersdorf, E., and Weinrauch, L. (1986). Leucocytoclastic vasculitis and pneumonitis induced by metformin. *Br. Med. J.* [*Clin. Res.*] **293**:483.

Komadina, K. H., and Houk, R. W. (1989). Polyarteritis nodosa presenting as recurrent pneumonia following splenectomy for hairy-cell leukemia. *Semin. Arthritis Rheum.* **18**:252–257.

Kramer, M. R., Melzer, E., Nesher, G., and Sonnenblick, M. (1987). Pulmonary manifestations of temporal arteritis. *Eur. J. Respir. Dis.* **71**: 430–433.

Ladanyi, M., and Fraser, R. S. (1987). Pulmonary involvement in giant cell arteritis. *Arch. Pathol. Lab. Med.* **111**:1178–1180.

Lakhanpal, S., Tani, K., Lie, J. T., Katoh, K., Ishigatsubo, Y., and Ohokubo, T. (1985). Pathologic features of Behçet's syndrome: a review of Japanese autopsy registry data. *Hum. Pathol.* **16**:790–795.

Lanham, J. G., Elkon, K. B., Pusey, C. D., and Hughes, G. R. (1984). Systemic vasculitis with asthma and eosinophilia: a clinical approach to the Churg-Strauss syndrome. *Medicine (Baltimore)* **63**:65–81.

Larson, T. S., Hall, S., Hepper, N. G. G., and Hunder, G. G. (1984). Respiratory tract symptoms as a clue to giant cell arteritis. *Ann. Intern. Med.* **101**:594–597.

Leatherman, J. W., Davies, S. F., and Hoidal, J. R. (1984). Alveolar hemorrhage, syndromes: diffuse microvascular lung hemorrhage in immune and idiopathic disorders. *Medicine (Baltimore)* **63**:343–361.

Leavitt, R. Y., and Fauci, A. S. (1986). Pulmonary vasculitis. *Am. Rev. Respir. Dis.* **134**:149–166.

Leavitt, R. Y., Fauci, A. S., Bloch, D. A., Michel, B. A., Hunder, G. G., Arend, W. P., Calabrese, L. H., Fries, J. F., Lie, J. T., Lightfoot, R. W., Jr., Masi, A. T., McShane, D. J., Mills, J. A., Stevens, M. B., Wallace, S. L., and Zvaifler, N. J. (1990). The American College of Rheumatology 1990 criteria for the classification of Wegener's granulomatosis. *Arthritis Rheum.* **33**:1101–1107.

Levinsky, R. J., and Barratt, T. M. (1979). IgA immune complexes in Henoch-Schönlein purpura. *Lancet* **2**:1100–1103.

Lie, J. T. (1986). The classification of vasculitis and a reappraisal of allergic granulomatosis and angiitis (Churg-Strauss syndrome). *Mt. Sinai J. Med.* **53**:429–439.

Lie, J. T. (1988a). Cardiac and pulmonary manifestations of Behçet syndrome. *Pathol. Res. Pract.* **183**:347–352.

Lie, J. T. (1988b). Systemic and isolated vasculitis: a rational approach to classification and pathologic diagnosis. *Pathol. Annu.* **24**:25–114.

Lie, J. T., and members and consultants of the American College of Rheumatology Subcommittee on Classification of Vasculitis (1990). Illustrated histopathologic classification criteria for selected vasculitis syndromes. *Arthritis Rheum.* **33**:1074–1087.

Liebow, A. A. (1973). Pulmonary angiitis and granulomatosis. *Am. Rev. Respir. Dis.* **108**:1–18.

Lightfoot, R. W., Jr. (1991). Churg-Strauss syndrome and polyarteritis nodosa. *Curr. Opin. Rheumatol.* **3**:3–7.

Lightfoot, R. W., Jr., Michel, B. A., Bloch, D. A., Hunder, G. G., Zvaifler, N. J., McShane, D. J., Arend, W. P., Calabrese, L. H., Leavitt, R. Y., Lie, J. T., Masi, A. T., Mills, J. A., Stevens, M. B., and Wallace, S. L. (1990). The American College of Rheumatology 1990 criteria for the classification of polyarteritis nodosa. *Arthritis Rheum.* **33**:1088–1093.

Lupi, E., Sánchez, G. T., Horwitz, S., and Gutierrez, F. (1975). Pulmonary artery involvement in Takayasu's arteritis. *Chest* **67**:69–74.

Machado, E. B. V., Michet, C. J., Ballard, D. J., Hunder, G. G., Beard, C. M., Chu, C-P., and O'Fallon, W. M. (1988). Trends in incidence and clinical presentation of temporal arteritis in Olmsted County, Minnesota, 1950–1985. *Arthritis Rheum.* **31**:745–749.

Masi, A. T., Hunder, G. G., Lie, J. T., Michel, B. A., Bloch, D. A., Arend, W. P., Calabrese, L. H., Edworthy, S. M., Fauci, A. S., Leavitt, R. Y., Lightfoot, R. W., Jr., McShane, D. J., Mills, J. A., Stevens, M. B., Wallace, S. L., and Zvaifler, N. J. (1990). The American College of Rheumatology 1990 criteria for the classification of Churg-Strauss syndrome (allergic granulomatosis and angiitis). *Arthritis Rheum.* **33**:1094–1100.

Matthews, S., and Cupps, T. R. (1990). Systemic vasculitis. *Lung Biol. Health Dis.* **45**:329:350.

McDonald, T. J., DeRemee, R. A., Kern, E. B., and Harrison, E. G., Jr. (1974). Nasal manifestations of Wegener's granulomatosis. *Laryngoscope* **84**:2101–2112.

Mills, J. A., Michel, B. A., Bloch, D. A., Calabrese, L. H., Hunder, G. G., Arend, W. P., Edworthy, S. M., Fauci, A. S., Leavitt, R. Y., Lie, J. T., Lightfoot, R. W., Jr., Masi, A. T., McShane, D. J., Stevens, M. B., Wallace, S. L., and Zvaifler, N. J. (1990). The American College of Rheumatology 1990 criteria for the classification of Henoch-Schönlein purpura. *Arthritis Rheum.* **33**:1114–1121.

Myers, J. L., and Katzenstein, A.-L. A. (1987). Wegener's granulomatosis presenting with massive pulmonary hemorrhage and capillaritis. *Am. J. Surg. Pathol.* **11**:895–898.

Nguyen, V. D. (1991). A rare cause of splenic infarct and fleeting pulmonary infiltrates: polyarteritis nodosa. *Comput. Med. Imaging Graph.* **15**:61–65.

Noritake, D. T., Weiner, S. R., Bassett, L. W., Paulus, H. E., and Weisbart, R. (1987). Rheumatic manifestations of Wegener's granulomatosis. *J. Rheumatol.* **14**:949–951.

O'Duffy, J. D. (1990). Vasculitis in Behçet's disease. *Rheum. Dis. Clin. North Am.* **16**:423–431.

Olsen, K. D., Neel, H. B., III, DeRemee, R. A., and Weiland, L. H. (1980). Nasal manifestations of allergic granulomatosis and angiitis (Churg-Strauss syndrome), *Otolaryngol. Head Neck Surg.* **88**:85–89.

Parfrey, P. S., Hutchinson, T. A., Jothy, S., Cramer, B. C., Martin, J., Hanley, J. A., and Seely, J. F. (1985). The spectrum of diseases associated with necrotizing glomerulonephritis and its prognosis. *Am. J. Kidney Dis.* **6**:387–396.

Payton, C. D., Allison, M. E. M., and Boulton-Jones, J. M. (1987). Henoch Schönlein purpura presenting with pulmonary haemorrhage. *Scott. Med. J.* **32**:26–27.

Petty, T. L., Scoggin, C. H., and Good, J. T. (1977). Recurrent pneumonia in Behçet's syndrome: roentgenographic documentation during 13 years. *JAMA* **238**:2529–2530.

Raz, I., Okon, E., and Chajek-Shaul, T. (1989). Pulmonary manifestations in Behçet's syndrome. *Chest* **95**:585–589.

Reed, W. B., Jensen, A. K., Konwaler, B. E., and Hunter, D. (1963). The cutaneous manifestations in Wegener's granulomatosis. *Acta Derm. Venereol. (Stockh.)* **43**:250–264.

Rose, A. G., Halper, J., and Factor, S. M. (1984). Primary arteriopathy in Takayasu's disease. *Arch. Pathol. Lab. Med.* **108**:644–648.

Rose, G. A., and Spencer, H. (1957). Polyarteritis nodosa. *Q. J. Med.* **26**: 43–81.

Rosenberg, D. M., Weinberger, S. E., Fulmer, J. D., Flye, M. W., Fauci, A. S., and Crystal, R. G. (1980). Functional correlates of lung involvement in Wegener's granulomatosis: use of pulmonary function tests in staging and follow-up. *Am. J. Med.* **69**:387–394.

Sanchez, N. P., Winkelmann, R. K., Schroeter, A. L., and Dicken, C. H. (1982). The clinical and histopathologic spectrums of urticarial vasculitis: study of forty cases. *J. Am. Acad. Dermatol.* **7**:599–605.

Schönlein, H. (1837). *Allgemeine und Specielle Pathologie und Therapie*, Vol. 2, 3rd ed. Herisau, Wurzburg.

Schwartz, H. R., McDuffie, F. C., Black, L. F., Schroeter, A. L., and Conn, D. L. (1982). Hypocomplemententemic urticarial vasculitis: association with chronic obstructive pulmonary disease. *Mayo Clin. Proc.* **57**:231–238.

Seiden, M. V., O'Donnell, W. J., Weinblatt, M., and Licht J. (1990). Vasculitis with recurrent pulmonary hemorrhage in a long-term survivor after autologous bone marrow transplantation. *Bone Marrow Transplant.* **6**: 345–347.

Sharma, S., Kamalakar, T., Rajani, M., Talwar, K. K., and Shrivastava, S. (1990). The incidence and patterns of pulmonary artery involvement in Takayasu's arteritis. *Clin. Radiol.* **42**:177–181.

Shimizu, T., Ehrlich, G. E., Inaba, G., and Hayashi, K. (1979). Behçet disease (Behçet syndrome). *Semin. Arthritis Rheum.* **8**:223–260.

Singer, D. R. J., Venning, M. C., Lockwood, C. M., and Pusey, C. D. (1986). Cryoglobulinaemia: clinical features and response to treatment. *Ann. Med. Intern. (Paris)* **127**:251–253.

Specks, U., and DeRemee, R. A. (1990). Granulomatous vasculitis: Wegener's granulomatosis and Churg-Strauss syndrome. *Rheum. Dis. Clin. North Am.* **16**:377–397.

Specks, U., Wheatley, C. L., McDonald, T. J., Rohrbach, M. S., and DeRemee, R. A. (1989). Anticytoplasmic autoantibodies in the diagnosis and follow-up of Wegener's granulomatosis. *Mayo Clin. Proc.* **64**: 28–36.

Strange, C., Halstead, L., Baumann, M., and Sahn, S. A. (1990). Subglottic stenosis in Wegener's granulomatosis: development during cyclophosphamide treatment with response to carbon dioxide laser therapy. *Thorax* **45**:300–301.

Strumpf, I. J., Drucker, R. D., Anders, K. H., Cohen, S., and Fajolu, O. (1991). Acute eosinophilic pulmonary disease associated with the ingestion of L-tryptophan-containing products. *Chest* **99**:8–13.

Sweeney, A. R., and Baggenstoss, A. H. (1949). Pulmonary lesions in periarteritis nodosa. *Proc. Staff Meet. Mayo Clin.* **24**:35–43.

Takayasu, M. (1908). Case with unusual changes of the central vessels in the retina. *Acta Soc. Ophthalmol.* **12**:554–557.

Tazelaar, H. D., Myers, J. L., Drage, C. W., King, T. E., Jr., Aguayo, S., and Colby, T. V. (1990). Pulmonary disease associated with L-tryptophan-induced eosinophilic myalgia syndrome: clinical and pathologic features. *Chest* **97**:1032–1036.

Travis, W. D., Carpenter, H. A., and Lie, J. T. (1989). Capillaritis and pulmonary hemorrhage in Wegener's granulomatosis (letter to the editor). *Am. J. Surg. Pathol.* **13**:78–79.

Travis, W. D., Colby, T. V., Lombard, C., and Carpenter, H. A. (1990a). A clinicopathologic study of 34 cases of diffuse pulmonary hemorrahge with lung biopsy confirmation. *Am. J. Surg. Pathol.* **14**:1112–1125.

Travis, W. D., Kalafer, M. E., Robin, H. S., and Luibel, F. J. (1990b). Hypersensitivity pneumonitis and pulmonary vasculitis with eosinophilia in a patient taking an L-tryptophan preparation. *Ann. Intern. Med.* **112**: 301–303.

Travis, W. D., Hoffman, G. S., Leavitt, R. Y., Pass, H. I., and Fauci, A. S. (1991). Surgical pathology of the lung in Wegener's granulomatosis: review of 87 open lung biopsies from 67 patients. *Am. J. Surg. Pathol.* **15**:315–333.

Umehara, I., Shibuya, H., Nakagawa, T., and Numano, F. (1991). Comprehensive analysis of perfusion scintigraphy in Takayasu's arteritis. *Clin. Nucl. Med.* **16**:352–357.

Vaillant, L., Pengloan, J., Blanchier, D., De Muret, A., and Lorette, G. (1990). Iododerma and acute respiratory distress with leucocytoclastic vasculitis following the intravenous injection of contrast medium. *Clin. Exp. Dermatol.* **15**:232–233.

Varriale, P., Minogue, W. F., and Alfenito, J. C. (1964). Allergic granulomatosis: case report and review of literature. *Arch. Intern. Med.* **113**: 235–240.

Viegi, G., Fornai, E., Ferri, C., Di Munno, O., Begliomini, E., Vitali, C., Melocchi, F., Bombardieri, S., and Paoletti, P. (1989). Lung function in essential mixed cryoglobulinemia: a short-term follow-up. *Clin. Rheumatol.* **8**:331–338.

Wegener, F. (1936). Über generalisierte, septische Gefäßerkrankungen. *Verh. Dtsch. Ges. Pathol.* **29**:202–210.

Wilson, K. S., and Alexander, H. L. (1945). The relationship of periarteritis nodosa to bronchial asthma and other forms of human hypersensitiveness. *J. Lab. Clin. Med.* **30**:195–203.

Winer-Muram, H. T., and Gavant, M. L. (1989). Pulmonary CT findings in Behçet disease. *J. Comput. Assist. Tomogr.* **13**:346–347.

Wolff, S. M., Fauci, A. S., Horn, R. G., and Dale, D. C. (1974). Wegener's granulomatosis. *Ann. Intern. Med.* **81**:513–525.

Yamato, M., Lecky, J. W., Hiramatsu, K., and Kohda, E. (1986). Takayasu arteritis: radiographic and angiographic findings in 59 patients. *Radiology* **161**:329–334.

Young, K. R., Jr. (1989). Pulmonary-renal syndromes. *Clin. Chest Med.* **10**:655–675.

10

Dermatological Diseases

UDAYA B. S. PRAKASH

Mayo Clinic, Mayo Medical Center, and Mayo Medical School
Rochester, Minnesota

I. Introduction

Dermatological manifestations of internal diseases are well known in clinical practice. Many of the benign internal diseases manifest themselves in the form of dermatological problems. Among the malignant diseases, pulmonary neoplasms are a well-known cause of cutaneous paraneoplastic syndromes, such as dermatomyositis, acanthosis nigricans, and bullous pemphigoid, which are often the first sign of the underlying malignancy. Several vasculitic syndromes and collagen diseases produce significant skin abnormalities; many of these are discussed in Chapters 8 and 9 on rheumatological diseases and vasculitides. This chapter will include discussions about the pulmonary manifestations of "primary" dermatological disorders, a term used to indicate that the disease under consideration presents with dermatological lesions. Some miscellaneous disease entities with skin manifestations are also considered.

II. Yellow Nail Syndrome

The term "yellow nail syndrome" (YNS) was first used in 1964 to describe the association of yellow discoloration of the fingernails and lymphedema in 13 patients (Samman and White, 1964). Affected nails were thickened, excessively curved along both axes, very slow growing, and of yellowish-gray hue; both the cuticle and lunula were usually absent and onychyolysis was frequently evident. Lower limb lymphangiography in most patients revealed hypoplasia or aplasia of the lymphatics, similar to that occurring in primary lymphedema (Müller et al., 1979; Samman and White, 1964). A review of the reported findings of 97 patients with YNS in 1986 indicated that most patients developed the disease in early middle age and that the male-to-female ratio was 1:1.6 (Nordkild et al., 1986); however, YNS has been described in an 8-year-old (Magid et al., 1987). Further experience with more than 150 patients described in the literature has shown the association of yellow nails with pleural effusion, bronchiectasis, and lymphedema of the breasts (Dilley et al., 1968; Hiller et al., 1972). The toenails as well as the fingernails can be discolored (Fig. 1, see Color Plate, facing p. 478). The etiology of this disorder is unknown, although a few cases seemed to follow episodes of pneumonia (Venencie and Dicken, 1984). The lymphedema is believed to be secondary to congenital atresia or hypoplasia of the lymphatics. Nail discoloration may precede or follow pleural effusion and lymphedema (Beer et al., 1978), but its mechanism is unknown. Most patients with YNS do not notice the nail discoloration, because its onset is subtle, and it is found only in slightly more than half the patients. Histopathological changes in the nail matrix and bed demonstrate dense fibrous tissue that replaces subungual stroma with numerous ectatic, endothelium-lined vessels that are similar the pleura abnormalities in YNS. Based on these findings, it is hypothesized that primary stromal sclerosis may lead to lymphatic obstruction (DeCoste et al., 1990).

The recurrent pleural effusions may also be secondary to lymphatic hypoplasia. To examine this possibility by looking at the pleural fluid kinetics, investigators measured the rate of pleural fluid turnover by using radioiodinated albumin to trace the efflux of fluid by lymphatics. The rate of pleural lymphatic flow in patients with YNS was low in comparison to previous estimates obtained by the same method in a variety of other conditions.The results were consistent with the postulate that accumulation of pleural fluid in YNS is due to defective lymphatic drainage rather than excess production (Runyon et al., 1979; Mambretti-Zumwalt et al., 1980). Histological analysis has shown the pleura to be thickened with fibrosis and chronic inflammatory infiltration, and dilatation of lymphatic capillaries in the visceral pleura. Electron microscopy confirmed the presence of ectatic lymphatic capillaries, thereby suggesting a downstream obstruction to the lymph drainage (Solal-Celigny et al., 1983). It has been suggested that the pathology is not confined to the lymphatic system, but also involves the blood vessels because the capillaries in the conjunctival and nail beds show decreased diameter (Ben-Yehuda et al., 1986).

Pleural effusion may precede the onset of nail changes by several years (Ryan et al., 1981). The respiratory symptoms are dependent on the size of the pleural effusion and the severity of bronchiectasis. Pleural effusions range from small, unilateral, and asymptomatic to large, bilateral (Fig. 2), recurrent, and debilitating (Beer et al.,1978); The fluid can be an exudate or a transudate. Pleural fluid glucose level may be reduced in some (Angelillo and O'Donohue, 1979). Empyema thoracis has been reported as a complication of YNS (Lodge et al., 1989)

The increased incidence of bronchiectasis and sinus infections in patients with YNS is well known (Hiller et al., 1972; Camilleri, 1990; Hassard et al., 1984; Moran and Larkworthy, 1976; Nakielna et al., 1976); at times, the bronchiectasis is limited to the upper lung zones (McNicholas et al., 1984). The mechanism that renders patients with this syndrome susceptible to respiratory infections is not known. Ciliary beat frequency measured in two patients was within normal limits (12 Hz) (Miro et al., 1990).

Other clinical manifestations reported in YNS include keratosis obturans involving the external ear and excess cerumen (Armitage et al., 1990; Moran and Larkworthy, 1976), chylous ascites (Tan, 1989; Duhra et al., 1985), hypoalbuminemia (Sahi and Bansal, 1988), chyluria (Toal et al., 1988), intestinal lymphangiectasia (Ocaña et al., 1988; Duhra et al., 1985), pericardial effusion (Wakasa et al., 1987), giant-cell interstitial infiltrates (Gupta et al., 1986),

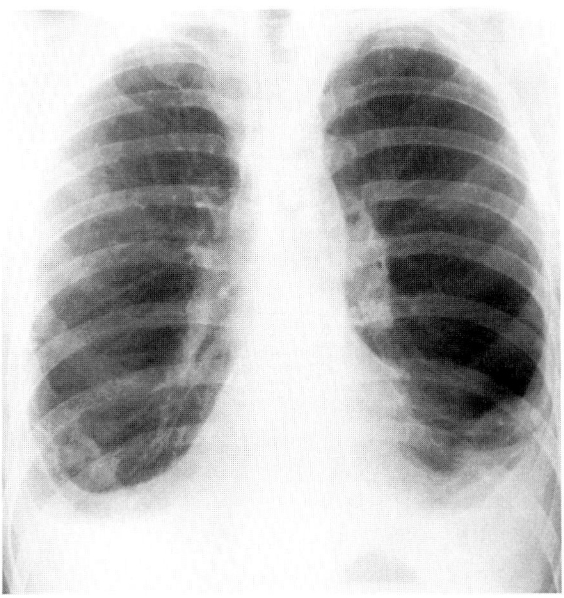

Figure 2 Chest roentgenograph of a patient with yellow nail syndrome shows bilateral pleural effusions.

lymphedema of the eyelids (Maisels and Korachi, 1985), nephrotic syndrome (Cockram and Richards, 1979), and Raynaud's phenomenon (Awerbuch, 1976).

Interestingly, one report of eight patients with proved diagnoses of acquired immunodeficiency syndrome (AIDS) and *Pneumocystis carinii* pneumonia mentioned yellow discoloration of the distal portions of the nails in four patients, with some showing ridging, loss or decrease in size of lunulae, and opaqueness (Chernosky and Finley, 1985). YNS is reported to have developed in three patients with rheumatoid arthritis (Mattingly and Bossingham, 1979), and has occurred in two siblings with mental retardation (Kamatani et al., 1978).

Although several cases of YNS in association with carcinomas of breast, lung, and larynx are described, it is not clear that YNS is a paraneoplastic syndrome (Guin and Ellman, 1979; Gupta et al., 1986; Mambretti-Zumwalt et al., 1980; Thomas and Sidhu, 1987); the nail changes are related to lymphatic obstruction that, in turn, is caused by the underlying malignancy. Nevertheless, it is of interest that the nail abnormalities resolved after treatment of the malignancy (Guin and Elleman, 1979; Gupta et al., 1986). One case of YNS following penicillamine therapy and resolution after the discontinuation of the drug is reported (Ilchyshyn and Vickers, 1983).

Large, recurrent, or debilitating pleural effusions may require repeated thoracentesis, pleuroperitoneal shunting, medical or surgical pleurodesis, or pleurectomy (Beer et al., 1978; Brofman et al., 1990; David et al., 1986). There are reports of successful treatment of the nail changes with topical vitamin E solution (Ayres and Mihan, 1973; Norton, 1985; Williams et al., 1991). Treatment of the pulmonary disease has resulted in normalization of the nails (Pavlidakey et al., 1984). In contrast, spontaneous resolution of the nail abnormalities without a change in respiratory status has also been noted (DeCoste et al., 1990). Chylous effusion are more difficult to treat. A case of chylous ascites in YNS is described that was treated successfully with dietary restriction of fat and supplements of medium-chain triglycerides (Tan, 1989).

III. Neurofibromatosis

Neurofibromatosis (von Recklinghausen's disease) (NF) is a relatively common disease of variably expressive autosomal dominant inheritance characterized by café-au-lait spots, freckling, and neurofibromas of skin and internal organs. Its incidence is 1 per 3000; about half the cases occur sporadically. Maldevelopment of neural crest cells is responsible for the skin lesions. The number of cutaneous neurofibromas varies greatly from one afflicted person to another and may be enormous (Fig. 3). Large plexiform neurofibromas may develop along peripheral nerves and involve deeper tissues. Extracutaneous (visceral) involvement may not be apparent during life unless it produces symptoms (Unger et al., 1984; Peterson and Ferguson, 1984).

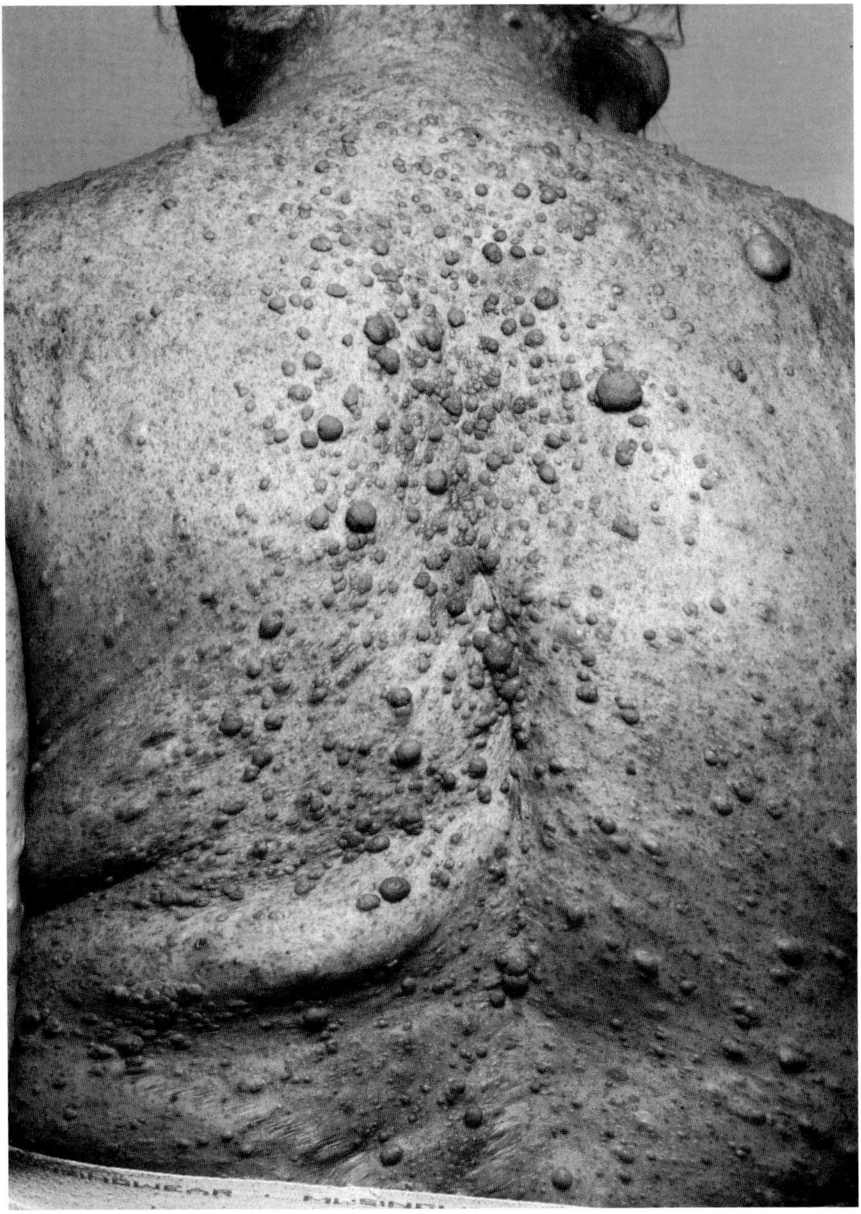

Figure 3 Skin over the back of a patient with neurofibromatosis reveals typical skin lesions; multiple neurofibromata of varying sizes can be seen.

Pulmonary disease is observed in nearly 10–15 percent of affected individuals (Massaro and Katz, 1966; Webb and Goodman, 1977; Riccardi, 1981; Davies, 1963). Although NF is a congenital disorder, the pulmonary manifestations become evident in adulthood. Diffuse interstitial fibrosis develops in approximately 20%of patients over the age of 35 years (Unger et al., 1984). The pulmonary parenchymal process has been attributed to a mesenchymal defect resulting in primary deposition of collagen (Aughenbaugh, 1984). The pathological features are similar to those in idiopathic pulmonary fibrosis (Massaro and Katz, 1966). Ultrastructural studies have shown fragmentation of collagen fibers in the lung (Patchefsky et al., 1973). Lung involvement in a patient with cutaneous neurofibromatosis who was evaluated by radionuclide scanning techniques has shown diminished perfusion and ventilation to apices of both lungs (Prediletto et al., 1987). Bullous lung disease may occur alone or in combination with diffuse pulmonary fibrosis (Hardcastle and Hendricks, 1984). Pulmonary fibrosis is usually seen in the basal areas of the lungs, whereas the bullous lesions occur predominantly in the apical areas (Fig. 4) (Klatte et al., 1976; Webb

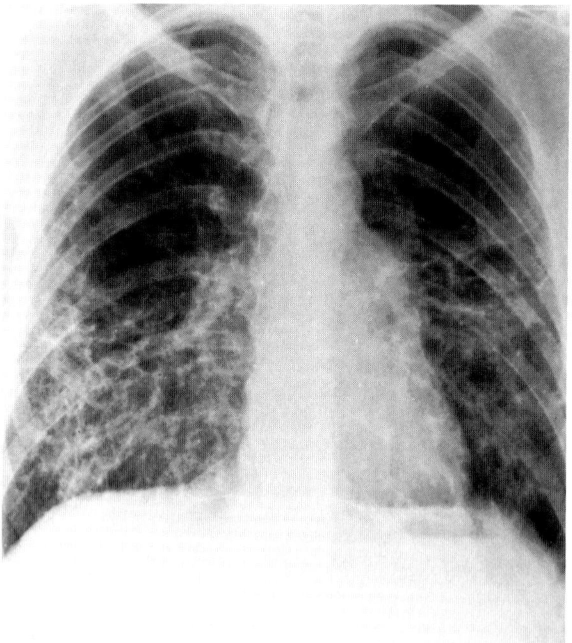

Figure 4 Chest roentgenograph of a patient with neurofibromatosis reveals bullous changes in both upper lung zones and interstitial process with honeycombing in both lower lung fields.

and Goodman, 1977). Cystic lung disease resembling honeycomb lung has also been described (Massaro et al., 1965). The clinical manifestations are usually mild and consist only of exertional dyspnea, but a restrictive pattern of pulmonary function and diminished diffusing capacity may be observed (Webb and Goodman, 1977).

Intrathoracic neurofibromas and meningoceles may be associated with the cutaneous form of NF, but these are usually undetected because they seldom produce symptoms (Unger et al., 1984). However, when these lesions are located in the posterior mediastinum (Fig. 5), as they commonly are, they may present as "dumbbell" tumors with intraspinal extension (Hardcastle and Hendricks, 1984). Computed tomography or magnetic resonance imaging of the involved spinal area is helpful in assessing the anatomical relationships of such tumors. Primary pulmonary parenchymal neurofibromas are rare (Unger et al., 1984; Petersen and Ferguson, 1984). Benign neurogenic tumors arising in the trachea are rare. One report described a patient with NF who presented with shortness of breath caused by endotracheal neurofibroma (Lossos et al., 1988). Hoarseness may result from recurrent laryngeal nerve involvement (Aughenbaugh, 1984).

A primary or secondary malignancy in the lung was overlooked in two patients with generalized NF due to roentgenographic confusion caused by

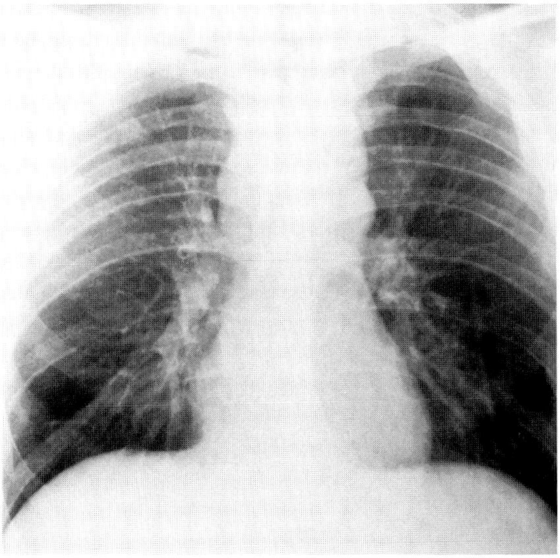

Figure 5 Chest roentgenograph of a patient with neurofibromatosis demonstrates mediastinal widening due to multiple neurogenic tumors in the posterior mediastinum.

overlying cutaneous lesions (Schabel et al., 1980). Increased incidence of malignancy, ranging from malignant tumors of the central nervous system to Wilms' tumor, rhabdomyosarcoma, leukemia, and pheochromocytoma, is well documented (Aughenbaugh, 1984). In 5% of patients with NF, the neurofibromas, regardless of their location, can undergo malignant degeneration and commonly metastasize to the lungs (Aughenbaugh, 1984). ''Scar'' cancer of the lung has also been reported as a complication of chronic pulmonary involvement in NF (De Scheerder et al., 1984).

IV. Tuberous Sclerosis

Also known as Bourneville's disease (Bourneville, 1880), tuberous sclerosis (TS) is an autosomal dominant disease of mesodermal development characterized clinically by epilepsy and mental retardation and pathologically by congenital tumors and malformations of the brain, skin, and viscera. The classic triad consists of adenoma sebaceum, mental retardation, and seizures. Cutaneous manifestations, in addition to adenoma sebaceum or dermal angiofibroma (Fig. 6), include ash leaf spots, shagreen patches, and periungual fibromas. Ash leaf spots, or hypopigmented macules, are the earliest dermatological manifestation of TS. Shagreen patches, seen in about half the patients with TS, are hamartomas of the connective tissue, are usually located over the lumbosacral area, and appear as rough, yellow leathery plaques. Periungual fibromas, seen in 15–20%, are benign, pink-colored fibrous neoplasms that develop adjacent to nails during adolescence. Poliosis, or hypopigmentation of the scalp hair or eyelashes, is also seen (Monaghan et al., 1981; Cassidy, 1984). Noncutaneous manifestations include either a seizure disorder or electroencephalographic abnormalities, or both, in 80–90% of patients, mental retardation of a wide range of severity, hamartomatous lesions of the central nervous system, retinal phakomas, angiomyolipomas of the kidney, renal and bone cysts,and cardiac rhabdomyomas (Cassidy, 1984; Gomez et al., 1982; Lie, 1991; Monaghan et al., 1981). Only 25% of affected children live beyond their twentieth year (Harris et al., 1969).

Pulmonary involvement is seen in less than 1% of patients. Most of the patients with pulmonary manifestations are women of childbearing age between the ages of 18 and 34 years (Dwyer et al., 1971; Lagos and Gomez, 1967; Lie, 1991). Pulmonary involvement has been described in a mother and daughter from a family with TS for four generations (Slingerland et al., 1989). Pulmonary involvement in males is very rare (Foresti et al., 1990). Dyspnea on exertion is the most common pulmonary symptom and may progress to the point of disability. Diffuse pulmonary interstitial fibrosis may progress to honeycombing and cyst formation (Fig. 7), spontaneous pneumothorax, and corpulmonale. A

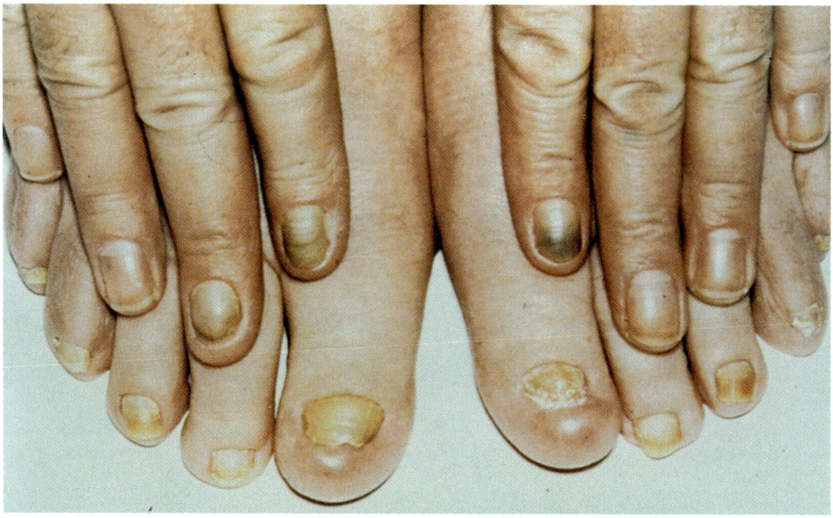

Figure 1 Nails of fingers and toes demonstrating the typical nail changes in yellow nail syndrome.

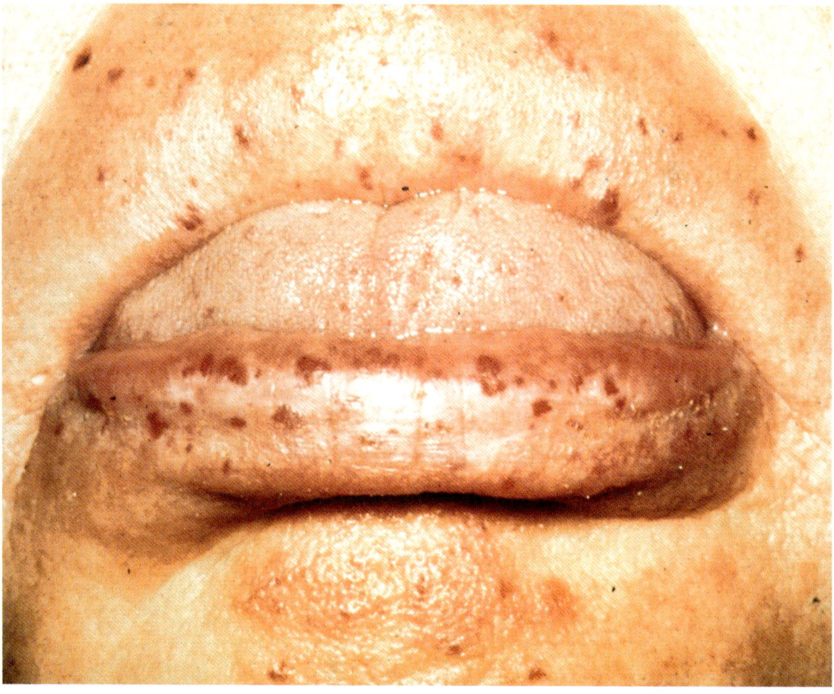

Figure 8 Lips and tongue of a patient with hereditary hemorrhagic telangiectasia show typical telangiectatic lesions over the skin and mucosa.

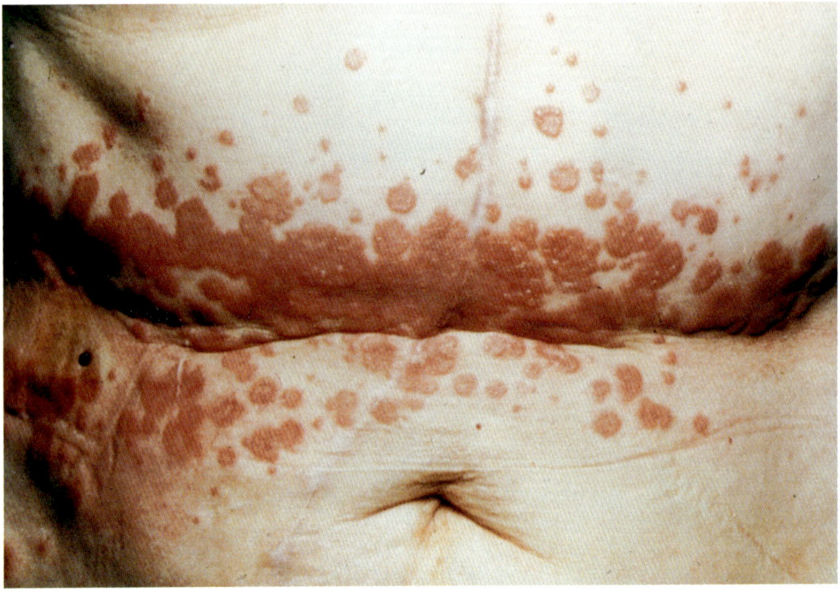

Figure 18 Abdomen of a patient with erythema multiforme shows the reddish macules, papules, and vesicles. The most characteristic skin lesion, known as a target or a bull's-eye lesion, can be seen in some of the individual lesions.

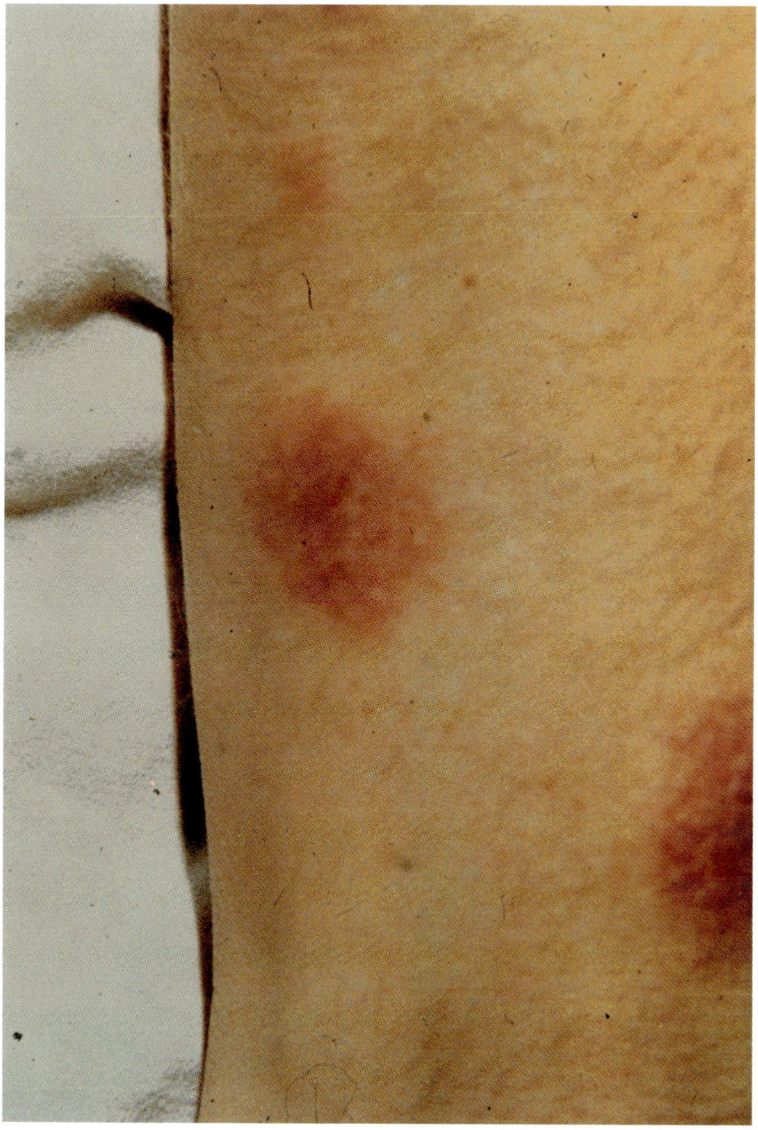

Figure 20 Lower leg of a patient with typical lesions of erythema nodosum.

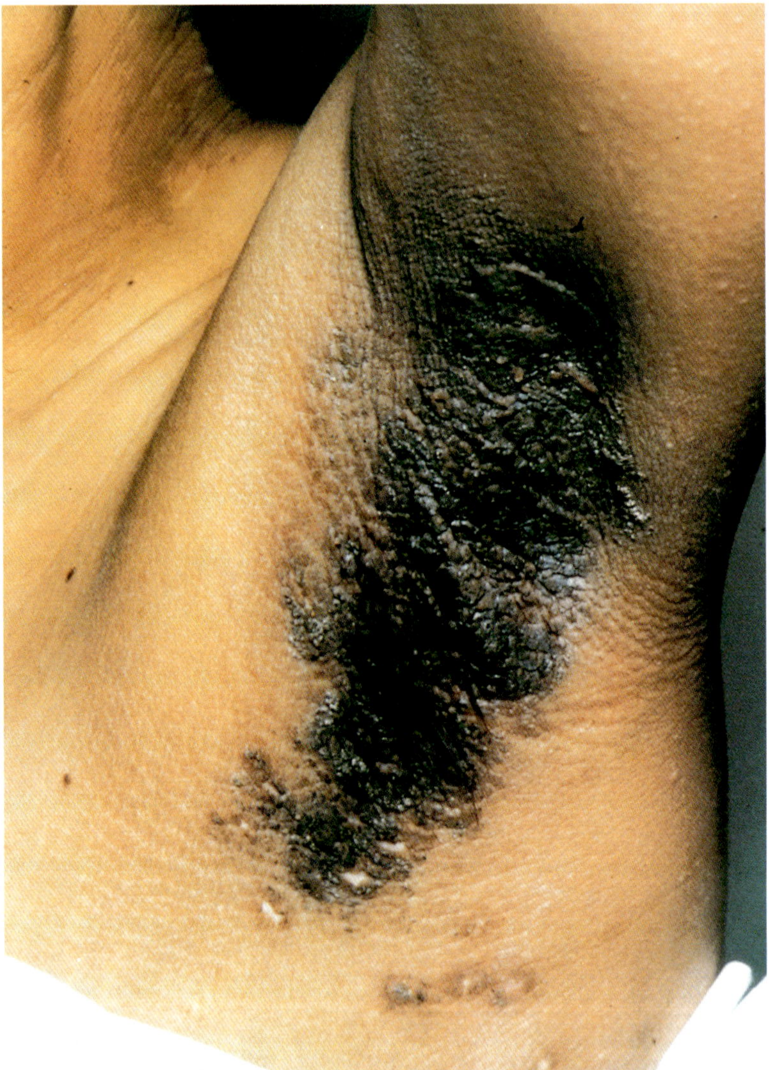

Figure 22 Left axilla of a patient with typical appearance of acanthosis nigricans.

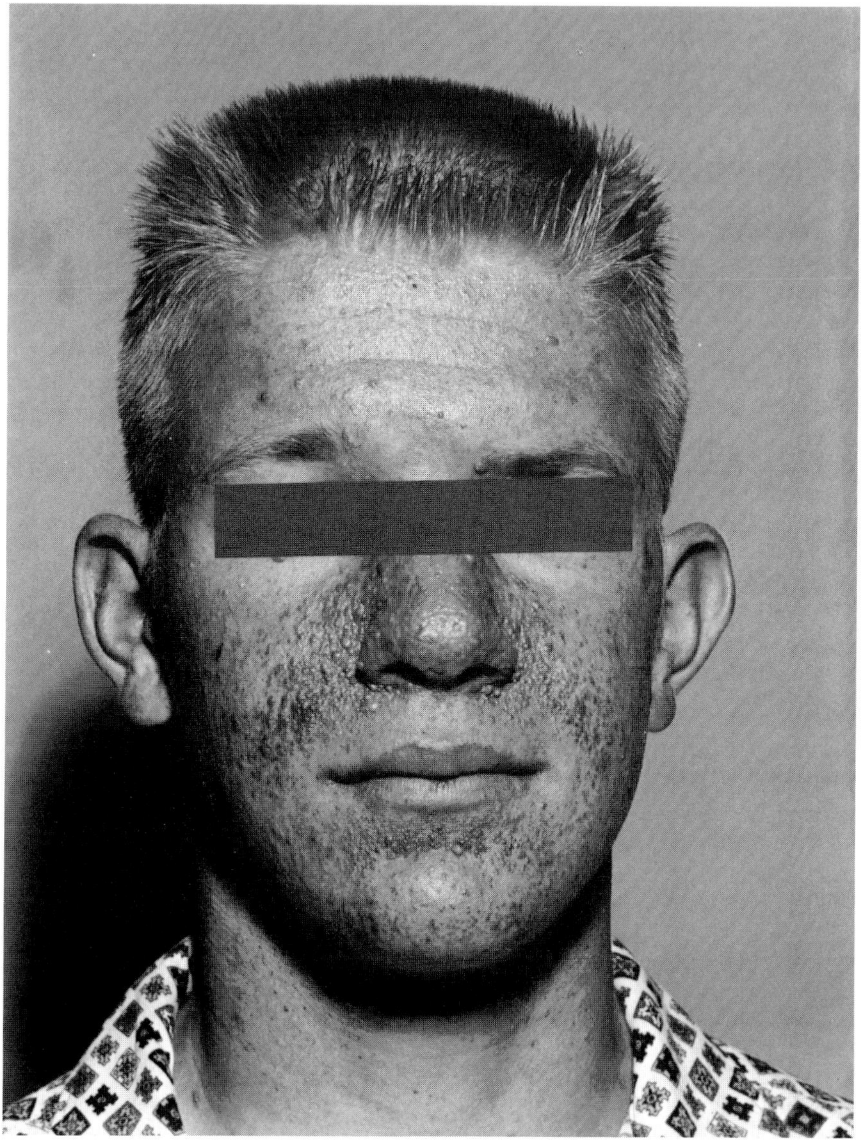

Figure 6 Patient with tuberous sclerosis with typical adenoma sebaceum involving bilateral nasolabial regions and the skin under the lower lip.

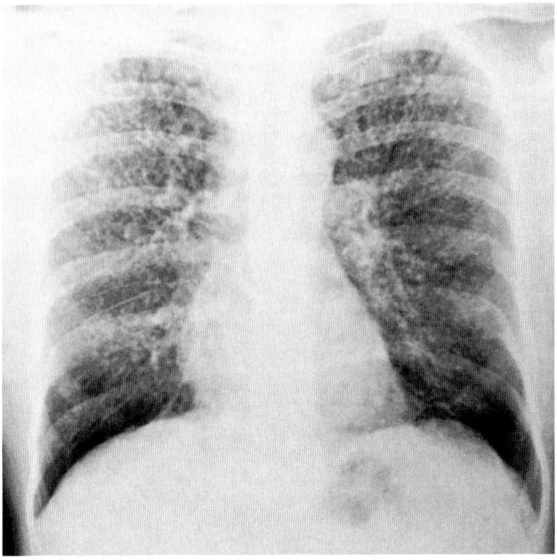

Figure 7 Chest roentgenograph of a patient with tuberous sclerosis shows extensive nodular infiltrates with areas of honeycombing. Although diffuse, the infiltrates are more pronounced in the upper three-fourths of lung fields.

review of the literature revealed 19 patients with tuberous sclerosis who also had spontaneous pneumothorax (Aughenbaugh, 1984; Babcock and Snyder, 1982; Liberman et al., 1984); eight died from the complication. Chylous pleural effusion has been noted in patients with TS, and may have been secondary to mediastinal lymphadenopathy, which was noted on computed tomography, and associated lymphatic obstruction (Foresti et al., 1990). Severe pulmonary hypertension has been observed in patients with TS (Józwiak, 1990b; Wagener et al., 1989). Nevertheless, pulmonary involvement, which is usually accompanied by involvement of other organs (Harris et al., 1969), has been reported to be associated with a more benign course, compared to TS without pulmonary manifestation (Hauck et al., 1990).

Chest roentgenograms in tuberous sclerosis reveal a pattern of diffuse interstitial infiltrates. Reticulonodular charges and pleural effusions are found in the early stages. Spontaneous pneumothorax is common. Thin-section computed tomographic scans of lungs in TS have shown thin-walled cysts less than 20 mm in diameter scattered at random in all parts of the lungs, with normal-appearing lung tissue between cysts. CT findings correlate better with DLCO than do chest roentgenographs (Lenoir et al., 1990).

Pulmonary function tests have shown that small airways are narrowed and collapsed because of the surrounding emphysema, and that the airspace lesions are more important than muscular proliferation in the walls of small airways in producing airflow limitation (Sobonya et al., 1985). Lung volume is increased (Corrin et al., 1975). Pathological examination of the lungs show multiple cysts measuring a few millimeters in diameter (Miledge et al., 1966); their walls are formed of smooth-muscle cells identical to pulmonary lymphangioleiomyomatosis. Cystic disease of the lungs with focal adenomatoid proliferation is among the least common pathological stigmata of tuberous sclerosis. It tends to develop in adult life, occurs more commonly among female patients who do not have mental retardation and epileptic seizures, and may be rapidly fatal after the onset of respiratory symptoms (Lie et al., 1980). Mesodermal tumors containing smooth muscle and other structures are seen more frequently (Harris et al., 1969; Stovin et al., 1975).

Lymphangioleiomyomatosis is considered by some to be a forme fruste of tuberous sclerosis (Capron et al., 1983; Józwiak, 1990a; Luna et al., 1985), although the presence of hormonal (estrogen, progesterone) receptors, which are found in many patients with pulmonary lymphangioleiomyomatosis, may differentiate it from TS. Ultrastructural morphology of the lung in tuberous sclerosis has shown that the findings are identical to those in lymphangioleiomyomatosis (Capron et al., 1983; Carrington et al., 1977). Because many patients with pulmonary lymphangioleiomyomatosis have responded to hormones, pulmonary tuberous sclerosis has been treated similarly (Westermann et al., 1986).

V. Hereditary Hemorrhagic Telangiectasia

Popularly known by its eponym, Osler-Weber-Rendu disease, hereditary hemorrhagic telangiectasia (HHT) is an autosomal dominantly inherited disorder characterized by telangiectasias of the skin and mucous membranes (Fig. 8, see Color Plate, facing p. 478) and intermittent bleeding from vascular abnormalities. The calculated period prevalence of simultaneous HHT and pulmonary arteriovenous fistula in the decade 1964–1974 in one Scandinavian county (429,207 inhabitants) was 2.6 per 100,000 (Vase et al., 1985). The male-to-female ratio is 1:2 (Sammons, 1959; Peery, 1987). Telangiectasias of the skin and oral, nasal, and conjunctival mucosa become evident in the second and third decades of life. They appear bright red, punctate, or linear, and blanch upon pressure. Gastrointestinal bleeding occurs in approximately 15% (Alper and Kegel, 1987).

HHT is the most common cause of pulmonary arteriovenous fistulas, which occur in approximately 20% of patients with the genetic defect (Revill and Matts, 1958). A study of 91 affected individuals belonging to different generations of a large family revealed that 15% had associated pulmonary arteriovenous fistulas (Hodgson et al., 1959). Roentgenograms have shown that the majority of these fistulas are located in the lower lobes and that they are multiple in a third of patients (Gomes and Bernatz, 1970; Sanders and Martt, 1962). Characteristically, they appear on plain roentgenograms as oval or round, homogeneous, nodular lesions from a few millimeters to several centimeters in diameter. These fistulas may continue to enlarge over long periods, sometimes as long as 24 years (Vase et al., 1985; Teragaki et al., 1988). Tomograms of the lesion usually disclose an artery entering the fistula and a vein leaving it (Fig. 9). Angiographic examination may be required and it confirms the diagnosis in virtually all cases (Fig. 10). One case of spontaneous pneumothorax

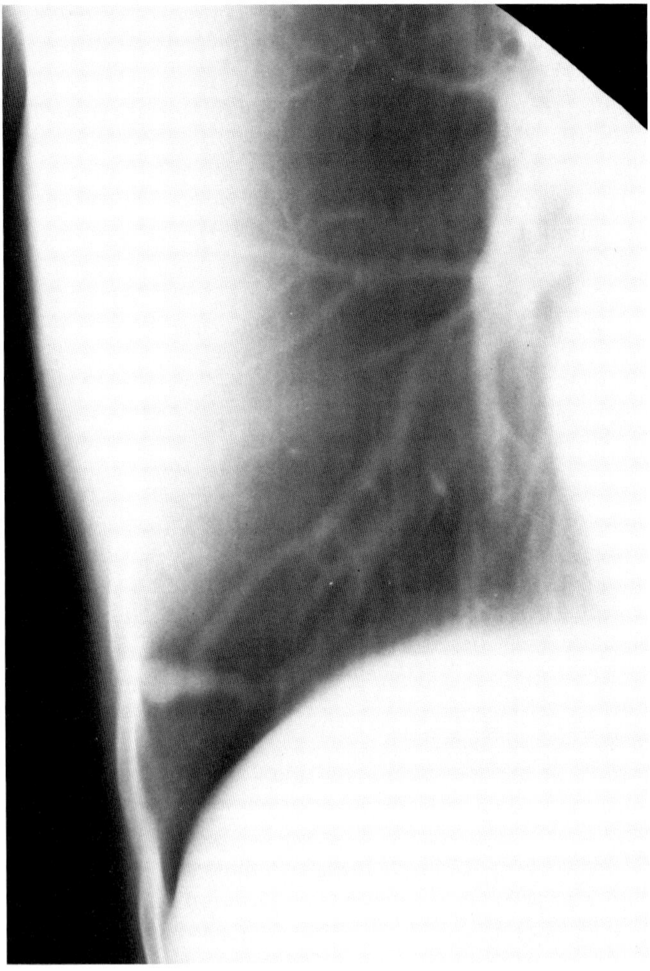

Figure 9 Localized tomography of a pulmonary arteriovenous malformation in a patient with hereditary hemorrhagic telangiectasia exhibits the arteriovenous malformation as well as the afferent and efferent blood vessels.

and another of hemothorax secondary to intrapleural rupture of an arteriovenous fistula have been reported (Kintzer et al., 1978; Shashy et al., 1985).

The severity of pulmonary symptoms, which often occur in the third and fourth decades of life, depends on the degree of right-to-left shunting of blood. Dyspnea is present in nearly 60% of patients, but hemoptysis is the most common presenting symptom (Gomes and Bernatz, 1970). Physical examination may reveal cyanosis, clubbing of the fingers, and a systolic or continuous bruit over the site of the fistula (Gomes and Bernatz, 1970). Endobronchial telangiectases, although described in the literature, are distinctly rare (Lincoln and Shigeoka, 1988). Catheterization studies show diminished arterial oxygen

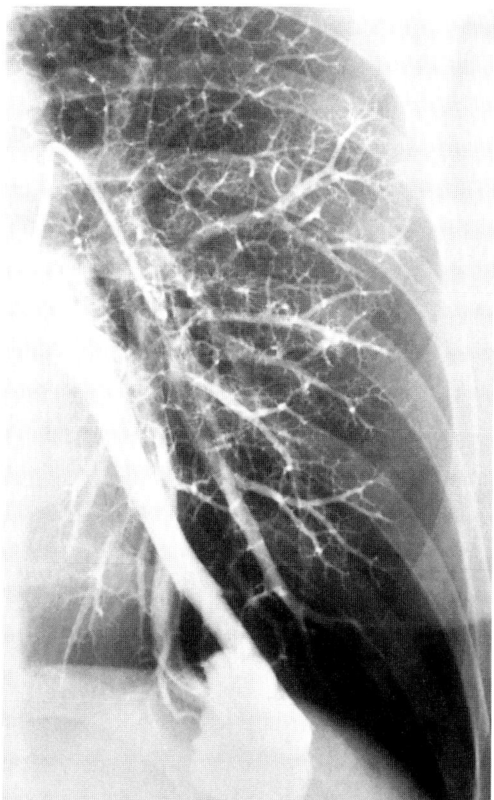

Figure 10 Localized view of the pulmonary arteriogram in a patient with hereditary hemorrhagic telangiectasia reveals a large solitary arteriovenous malformation in the left lower lobe, partially obscured by the left diaphragm.

tension and saturation but normal pulmonary arterial pressure (Sanders and Martt, 1962). Contrast echocardiography with indocyanine green dye may reveal a characteristic flow pattern (Shub et al., 1976), but this finding does not indicate either the number or location of the fistulas.

Brain and systemic abscesses are potentially serious complications in patients with HHT (Gelfand et al., 1988; Momma et al., 1990). Although neurological complications are seen in up to 30%, brain abscess is estimated to develop in approximately 1% of patients with HHT (Press and Ramsey, 1984; White et al., 1988). Brain abscess can be the initial clinical manifestation in previously asymptomatic pulmonary arteriovenous fistula. A review of the clinical courses of 31 episodes of brain abscess and one episode of meningitis in patients with HHT revealed that obtundation, headache, visual disturbances, hemiplegia, and seizures were the most common presenting features (Press and Ramsey, 1984). Leukocytosis and fever were present in a minority of cases and all blood cultures were sterile. Anaerobic and microaerophilic streptococci were the most common pathogens found in the brain abscesses. Thirteen patients died; those patients whose abscesses were not drained and those with delayed diagnosis had a higher mortality rate (Press and Ramsey, 1984). Hewes et al. (1985) reported that four of five patients with asymptomatic small or moderate-size pulmonary arteriovenous malformation presented with stroke secondary to paradoxical embolism. Another report on 67 patients with pulmonary arteriovenous malformations secondary to HHT recorded clinical histories of strokes and transient ischemic attack in 37% (White et al., 1988). A review of the literature in 1990 revealed 52 reported cases of these complications (Momma et al., 1990). Among the more than 200 reported patients with HHT and central nervous system involvement, 61% had complications secondary to a pulmonary arteriovenous fistula, whereas 36% of the patients had vascular malformations of the brain and spinal cord as the presumed cause (Román et al., 1978).

Other complications include high-output congestive heart failure and portosystemic encephalopathy from hepatic arteriovenous malformations. Disseminated intravascular coagulation was recorded in 51% of 47 patients with documented HHT (Bick, 1981).

The current treatment includes pulmonary artery embolization using coils and other intravascular devices (Hatfield and Fried, 1981). Multiple embolizations are necessary in many patients because new fistulas often appear after successful treatment of earlier ones (Fig. 11). In one report of a 10-year experience with embolization in 76 patients, 67 (88%) of whom had HHT, 276 pulmonary arteriovenous malformations were occluded by balloon embolotherapy. Improvements in physiological parameters remained stable for 5 years, complications were minimal, and no patient required surgery. Another study evaluated the effects of percutaneous transcatheter steel coil embolization on pulmonary function and exercise capacity in 11 patients with pulmonary arteriovenous malformations secondary to HHT. The physiological parameters were measured

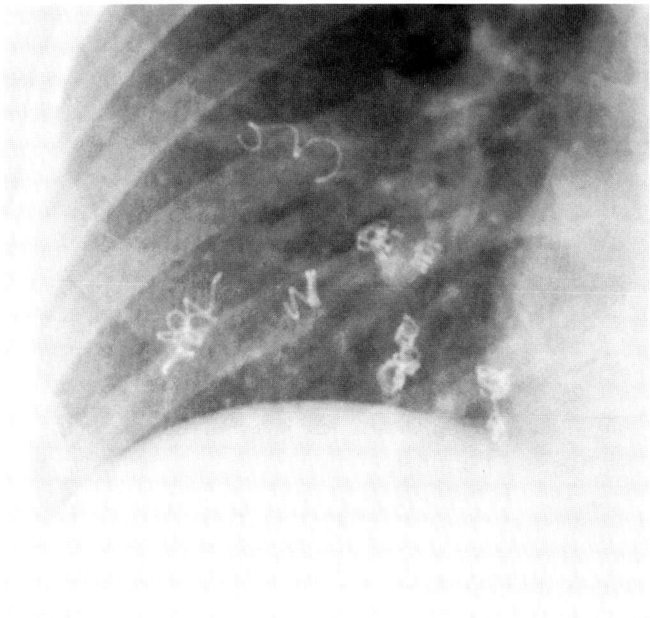

Figure 11 Localized roentgenographic view of right lower lobe in a patient with hereditary hemorrhagic telangiectasia. Multiple embolization coils used to treat recurrent pulmonary arteriovenous malformations are shown.

before and 2–6 months after treatment. Lung function tests before intervention showed normal VC and FEV_1/FVC ratios, reduced DLCO (mean 71% predicted, range 36–123%), a resting supine SaO_2 of 86% (range 67–95%) and mean shunt fraction of 33% (range 15–47%). Exercise capacity was well preserved. Following therapy, the mean shunt fraction decreased from 33 to 19% and resting SaO_2 improved from 86 to 92%. There was no change in VC, but a consistent improvement in DLCO was seen. There were no long-term complications following embolization (Chilvers et al., 1990). Although embolization is the initial treatment of choice, large arteriovenous fistulas may require surgical resection (Brown et al., 1982; Dines et al., 1983). The life expectancy of patients with HHT is not reduced provided treatable complications are promptly diagnosed and treated.

VI. Cutis Laxa (Generalized Elastolysis)

Cutis laxa (CL) is a rare and unique systemic disorder of connective tissue in which the elastic fibers suddenly become fragmented, disorganized, and fewer in number; this attrition results in such entities as cutis laxa, emphysema, aortic aneurysms, and bowel diverticula, depending on the organ system involved, i.e., skin, lung, vasculature, or gastrointestinal tract (Harris et al., 1978). CL is a distinct entity from Ehlers-Danlos syndrome, pseudoxanthoma elasticum, and Marfan's syndrome. Both congenital (X-linked recessive) and acquired varieties of this disorder have been described (Beighton, 1972; Byers et al., 1976; Hajjar and Joyner, 1968; Reed et al., 1971; Van Maldergem et al., 1988). The genetic origin in late cases (acquired) is uncertain. The congenital and acquired varieties are identical clinically, morphologically, and pathologically. Histological findings are characterized by the disappearance of elastic fibers of the skin. The cutaneous abnormalities in cutis laxa seem to result mainly from a developmental defect of the elastic network in the papillary dermis (Ledoux-Corbusier, 1983). The skin changes are associated with the appearance of early senility (Fig. 12) (Ferreira and Spina, 1973).

The lungs rank only second to the skin as the most commonly affected organ (Harris et al., 1978). The most common and serious pulmonary problem associated with cutis laxa is panlobular emphysema (Fig. 13) (Turner-Stokes

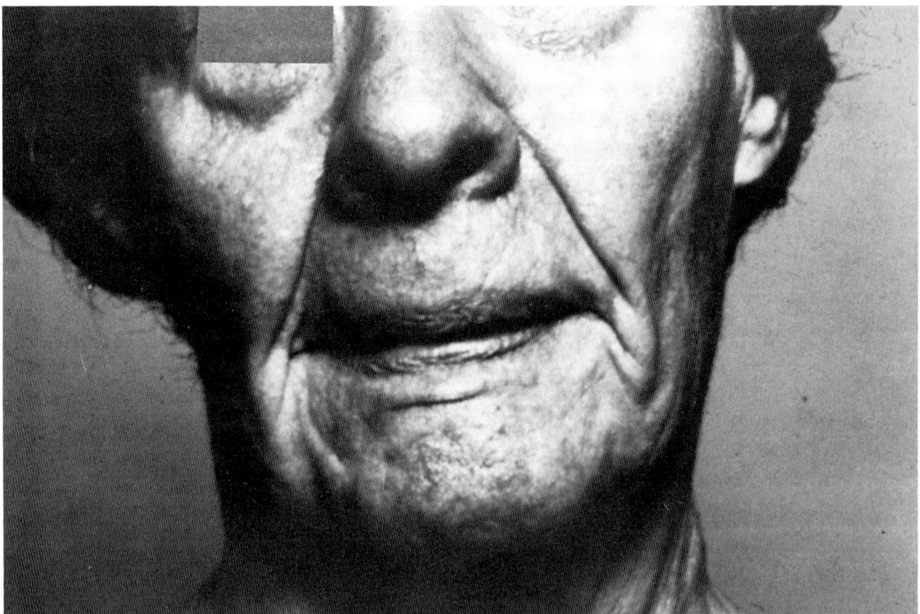

Figure 12 Lower part of the face of a patient with generalized elastolysis. The "aged" appearance of this 43-year-old woman is due to the loss of skin elasticity resulting in looseness of the skin and increasing skin folds giving raise to "lugubrious" skin.

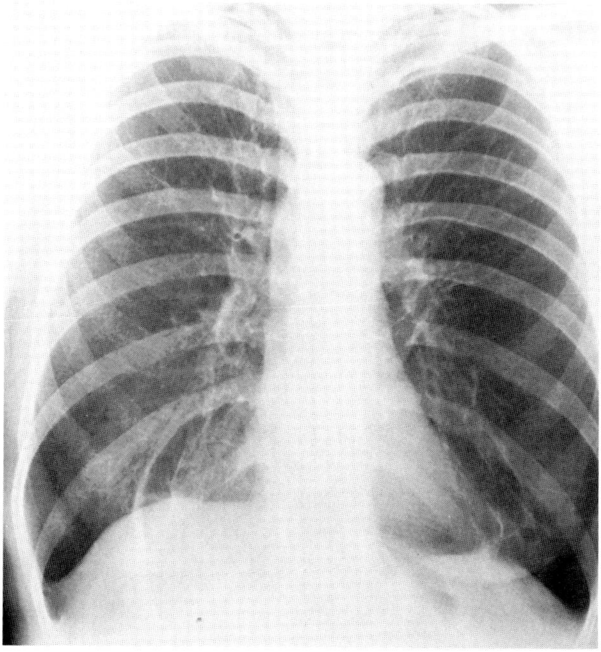

Figure 13 Chest roentgenograph of the patient in Figure 12. Hyperinflation and bullous changes of lower lobes are evident. Pulmonary function tests revealed severe obstructive pulmonary disease and examination of the serum showed normal level and phenotype of alpha$_1$-antitrypsin.

et al., 1983); in the congenital variety especially, emphysema with cor pulmonale is the most common cause of death, markedly elevated activity of an elastase-like serum enzyme has been observed in some patients with cutis laxa (Anderson et al. 1984). A review of the literature disclosed 31 cases of congenital and 17 cases of acquired cutis laxa (Prakash and Rosenow, 1989). In each variety, the incidence of emphysema was 50%. Other pulmonary complications reported are pneumothorax, pulmonary fibrosis, pulmonary artery stenosis, eventration of the diaphragm, recurrent pulmonary infections, bronchiectasis, tracheobronchomegaly, and thoracic-aortic aneurysms (Hayden et al., 1968; Prakash and Rosenow, 1989; Weir et al., 1977).

VII. Ehlers-Danlos Syndrome

Ehlers-Danlos syndrome (EDS) is a group of inherited disorders in which connective-tissue diseases result from disorganization of collagen fibers

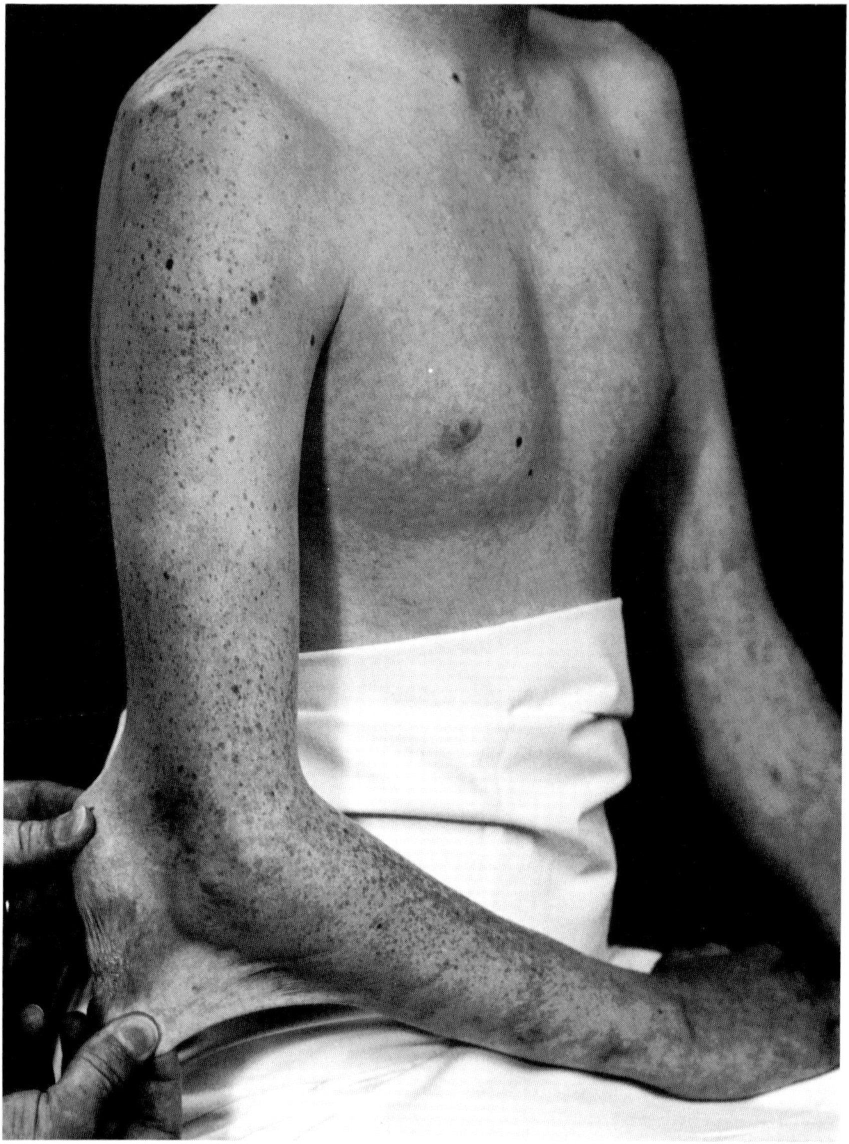

Figure 14 Loose skin in a patient with Ehler-Danlos syndrome. Hyperextensibility of the joints was also present.

(Barabas, 1967). EDS is clinically characterized by abnormal skin flaccidity (Fig. 14), hyperextensibility of the joints, bleeding tendencies, atrophic scars, easy skin bruising, and pseudotumors.

Pulmonary involvement in EDS results from weakness of collagen, particularly type III collagen, in the lungs. Ultrastructural and biochemical analysis of the lung tissue in EDS has revealed markedly decreased type III collagen; moreover, fibroblasts cultured from the abnormal lung produce less than normal type III procollagen relative to type I procollagen. Electron microscopic examination of lung specimens has shown dilated endoplasmic reticulum of the firbroblasts with normal collagen (Baumer and Hankey, 1980). Pulmonary complications described in patients with EDS include pneumothorax from bullous lung disease (Smit et al., 1978) and severe panacinar emphysema (Cavanaugh and Cooper, 1976; Cupo et al., 1981). Transient pulmonary cysts have been observed with Ehlers-Danlos syndrome (Buamer and Hankey, 1980). EDS-related weakness of the pulmonary arterial wall has resulted in rupture and hemoptysis (Ayers et al., 1981); however, of the six subtypes of EDS, which can usually be clinically differentiated, only types 1 and 4 are reported to be associated with a substantial risk of arterial rupture (Pearl and Spicer, 1981). Pulmonary artery regurgitation and pulmonary valvular stenosis are also described (Lees et al., 1969; Leier et al., 1980; Marquez et al., 1978), and spontaneous dissection of the aorta may occur (Beighton, 1968). Bronchiectasis resulting from weakened bronchial walls has been reported (Fraser and Paré, 1979). Tracheobronchomegaly (Fig. 15), similar to that in Mounier-Kuhn syndrome, has been noted in a patient with EDS (Cavanaugh and Cooper, 1976).

VIII. Pseudoxanthoma Elasticum

Pseudoxanthoma elasticum is a disorder characterized by fragmentation and calcification of elastic fibers in the skin, blood vessels, and retina (Altman et al., 1974). Both autosomal dominant and recessive forms have been described. The basic defect is unknown. One patient with pseudoxanthoma elasticum has been reported in whom a lung biopsy showed widespread deposition of calcium in the walls of some arteries, arterioles, and venules, with swollen, short, irregularly clumped elastic fibers and irregularity of the elastic laminae (Jackson and Loh, 1980).

IX. Oculocutaneous Albinism

Also known by the eponym Hermansky-Pudlak syndrome, oculocutaneous albinism (OCA) is an autosomal recessive disorder characterized by oculocutaneous tyrosinase-positive albinism, platelet pool disease with moderate bleeding

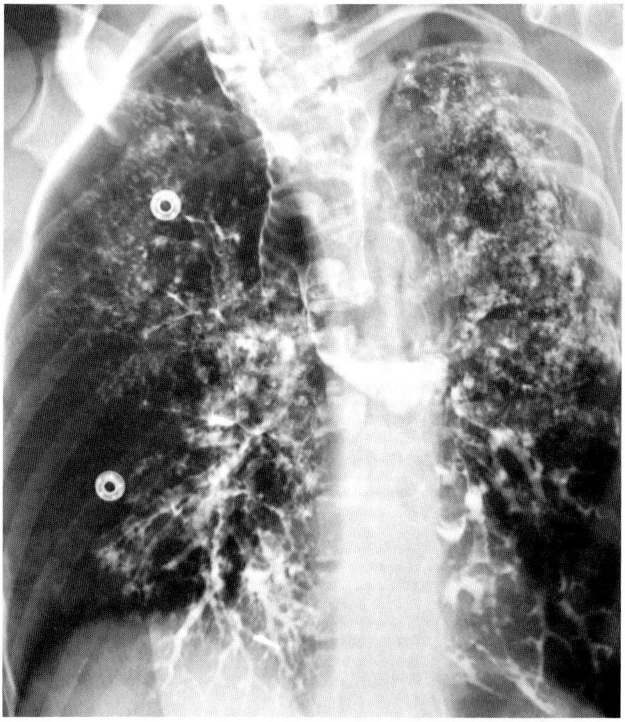

Figure 15 Bronchographic examination in a patient with severe tracheobronchomegaly (sometimes described as Mounier-Kuhn syndrome) and bronchiectasis and slight clinical suggestion of Ehler-Danlos syndrome.

tendency, and ceroid-like inclusions in the reticuloendothelial system (Davies and Tuddenham, 1976; Depinho and Kaplan, 1985; Garay et al., 1979). Ceroid is believed to be a product of oxidation and polymerization of unsaturated lipids. The number of reported and/or known cases of OCA has been estimated at 200 patients worldwide (DePinho and Kaplan, 1985). The most striking feature of OCA on physical examination is the oculocutaneous albinism. However, the most frequent clinical problem is bleeding, and epistaxis is the most common bleeding manifestation (Depinho and Kaplan, 1985).

Pulmonary involvement is fairly common in OCA. More than 20 patients with a process similar to idiopathic pulmonary fibrosis have been described (Garay et al., 1979). It usually begins in the third or fourth decade of life and presents with constant nonproductive cough and progressive dyspnea. Even though men and women are equally affected by OCA, the incidence of pulmonary disease is twice as high in women as in men. The age of onset of pulmonary fibrosis extends from 20 to 44 years. Dyspnea can develop abruptly over several weeks or gradually over years, and the disease can progress to end-stage fibrosis and death. The pulmonary pathology in OCA is consistent with oxidant damage, as it resembles the morphological abnormalities seen with pulmonary oxygen toxicity. Bronchoalveolar lavage studies have shown that pulmonary alveolar macrophages contain characteristic ceroid-like material (White et al., 1984). Elevated levels of immunoglobulins, numbers of IgG- and IgA-secreting cells, and normal percentages of helper and suppressor T cells have been noted in these patients. Brown-pigmented histiocytes have been demonstrated in the pulmonary alveolar spaces (Sastre et al., 1987). Since the pulmonary fibrosis in patients with OCA is an irreversible, progessive process, symptomatic treatment is the only option.

Pulmonary ceroidosis occurs in many of the approximately 30 disorders in which systemic or localized deposition of ceroid occurs (Sastre et al., 1987). Sea-blue histiocytosis syndrome is an example of ceroidosis, and lung involvement is present in 11% of patients (Tachibana et al., 1979). Deposition of ceroid-like pigment in the alveolar macrophages was noted in eight patients with gastric carcinoma (Maeda, 1967). Idiopathic pulmonary ceroidosis may represent pulmonary alveolar deposition of ceroid-like material in the absence of clinical or biochemical data characteristic of any specific ceroid storage disease (Takahashi et al., 1978; Sastre et al., 1987).

X. Nonsuppurative Panniculitis

Sometimes referred to as Weber-Christian disease, nonsuppurative panniculitis (NSP) is characterized by cutaneous nodular fat necrosis of the panniculus adiposum. NSP is clinically characterized by tender, erythematous subcutaneous nodules over the extremities and trunk (Fig. 16).

In a review by Federman et al. (1976) pulmonary involvement was reported in only five cases. Pulmonary manifestations include pulmonary fat emboli and infarcts, lipogranulomatous pneumonitis with nodules measuring 0.8–3 cm in diameter (Schoen et al., 1958), and fluffy roentgenographic densities bilaterally (Federman et al., 1976). Recurrent pneumonia and pleural effusion (Fig. 17) also occur (Sorenson et al., 1986). Interestingly, deficiency of alpha$_1$-antitrypsin has been found in some patients with acute panniculitis (Rubinstein et al., 1977). There is no report of emphysematous lung disease occurring as a result of this abnormality.

XI. Erythema Multiforme

Erythema multiforme (EM) is a systemic disease characterized by fever, generalized eruptions of red or violaceous macules similar to urticaria, papules, vesicles, or bullae, and involvement of various internal organs. The most

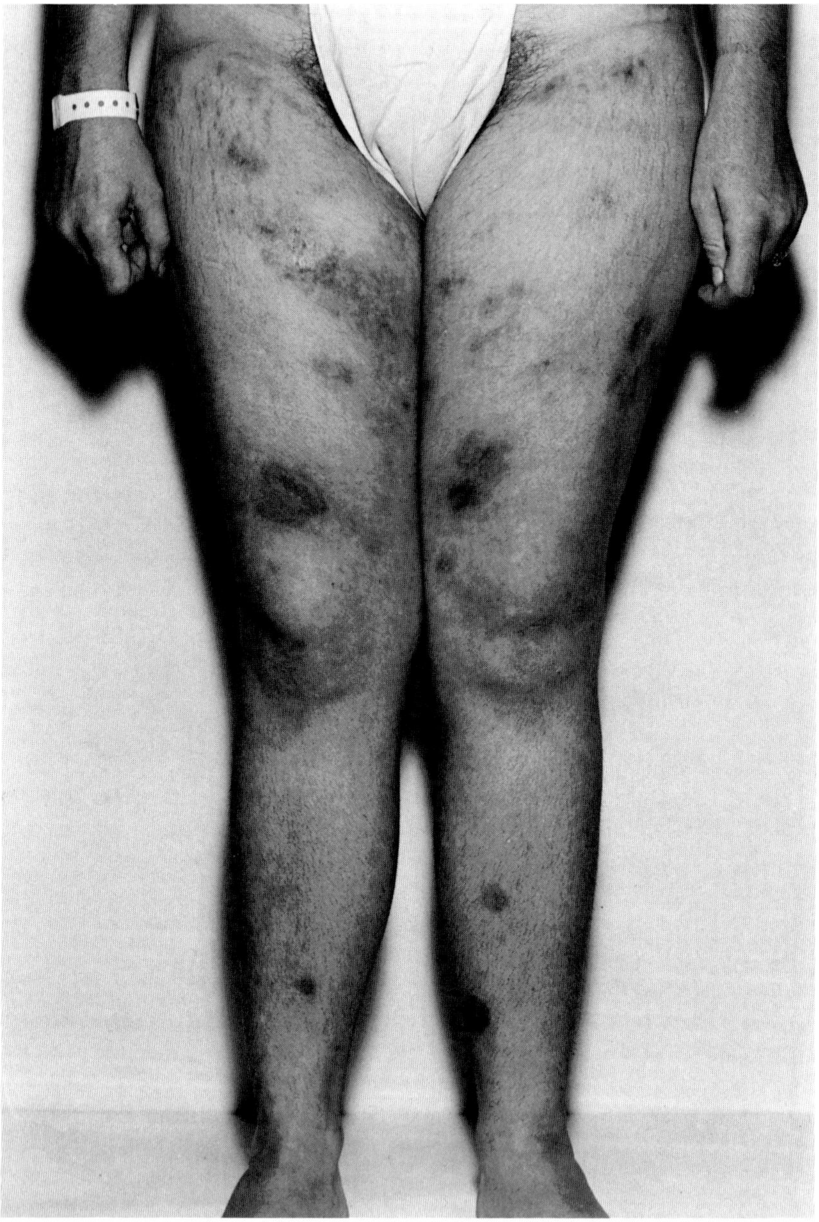

Figure 16 Female patient with nonsuppurative panniculitis (Weber-Christian disease) with cutaneous nodular fat necrosis of the panniculus adiposum; the syndrome is clinically characterized by tender, erythematous subcutaneous nodules over the extremities and trunk.

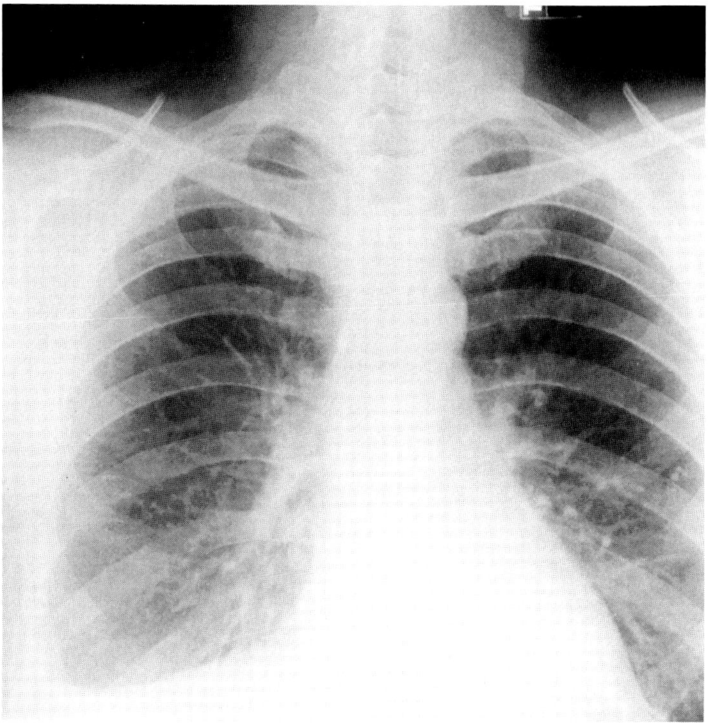

Figure 17 Chest roentgenograph in a patient with nonsuppurative panniculitis shows right-sided pleural effusion.

characteristic skin lesion is known as a target, or bull's-eye (Fig. 18, see Color Plate, facing p. 478). A more severe form of EM is referred to as the Stevens-Johnson syndrome, in which mucocutaneous ulcerations are seen (Stevens and Johnson, 1922).

An association of EM with pulmonary infection caused by *Mycoplasma pneumoniae* is well documented (Fleming et al., 1967); however, an even more common association is with bacterial pneumonias caused by streptococci, *pseudomonas*, the pneumococcus, *Legionella*, and *Hemophilus influenzae* (Fig. 19) (Schwartz and Clendenning, 1985). EM has also been described in patients with histoplasmosis and blastomycosis (Drake, 1985; Medeiros et al., 1966). Other etiologies of EM include penicillin, antipyretics, barbiturates, and sulfonamide. Several pulmonary manifestations have been described, including patchy bronchopneumonic infiltrates, miliary lesions, massive pneumonic consolidations, hilar lymphadenopathy, and, rarely, pleural effusions (Beerman and Kirshbaum, 1985). Clinical respiratory manifestations consist of

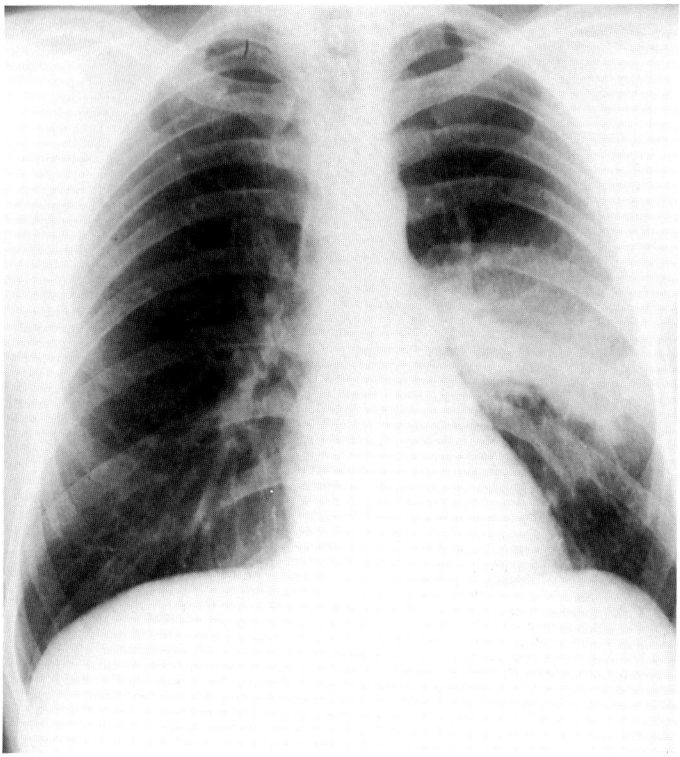

Figure 19 Chest roentgenograph demonstrating pneumonitis of left midlung field in a patient with erythema multiforme. *Hemophilus influenzae* was isolated from the sputum, and the pulmonary and skin lesions resolved after appropriate treatment.

laryngotracheobronchitis, cough, hemoptysis, dyspnea, and cyanosis. Savill et al. (1988) published a report of a 46-year-old white woman with active systemic lupus erythematosus who developed a skin rash 8 hr after intravenous urography with the nonionic contrast medium iopamidol; severe Stevens-Johnson syndrome with erythema multiforme, intrahepatic cholestasis, pulmonary infiltrates, and acute renal failure ensued, which led to her death.

XII. Erythema Nodosum

Erythema nodosum (EN) is a self-limited disease characterized by inflammatory nodules in the dermis and subcutaneous tissues, usually on the extensor aspects of the legs (Fig. 20, see Color Plate, facing p. 478). It is a type of panniculitis clinically manifested by pain in the anterior tibial area followed by development of tender pink nodules on the shins. The lesions resolve over a period of several weeks. The clinical appearance is so characteristic that biopsy is rarely required. Presumably, EN is a hypersensitivity reaction to a wide variety of underlying systemic disorders, especially drug reactions and viral, bacterial, and fungal infections. The etiology is unknown in approximately half the patients (Bullock, 1986).

In the United States, mycoses, particularly histoplasmosis and coccidioidomycosis (Fig. 21), are common causes of EN (Joffe, 1960; Savill et al., 1988). Pulmonary blastomycosis associated with EN has been described (Miller et al., 1982). EN was observed in 12% of 305 children with postprimary tuberculosis (Derham, 1956), but is rare today. The presence of EN in all these infections denotes a good prognosis, because the presence of EN signifies development of hypersensitivity. In a study of 88 cases of tularemia in northern Finland (Syrjälä et al., 1984), pulmonary involvement was noted in 27% of the patients. EN, either alone or in combination with some other skin eruption, was

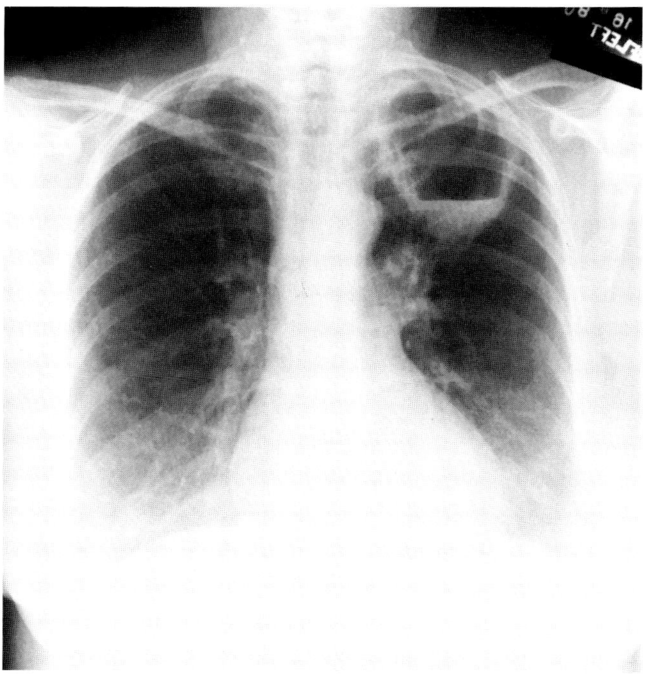

Figure 21 Chest roentgenograph exhibits a cavitated lesion in the left upper lobe of a patient with erythema nodosum; cultures from the lung lesion grew *Coccidioides immitis*.

encountered in 28% of all the patients, but EN was seen more often in patients with pulmonary tularemia than in other types of the disease.

Sarcoidosis is one of the common diseases not infrequently associated with EN. In a large series of patients with sarcoidosis, 13% had EN (Winterbauer et al., 1973), which in the early stages can be a presenting manifestation (Crawley, 1950). In one study of 188 patients with dermal sarcoidosis, 13% were found to have EN (Veien et al., 1987). As in mycotic infections and tuberculosis, the presence of EN sarcoidosis has been shown to be associated with good prognosis (Milman and Selroos, 1990). An acute onset of sarcoidosis with erythema nodosum also indicateds a good prognosis and a high likelihood of spontaneous resolution (Sharma, 1990). The generally good prognosis of erythema nodosum, acute arthritis, and bilateral hilar lymphadenopathy was confirmed in a computerized, retrospective study of 818 patients with sarcoidosis (Neville et al., 1983), although 16% of the patients who presented with these manifestations pursued a chronic course. Bronchoalveolar lavage in patients who had an acute inflammatory onset of sarcoidosis with EN has demonstrated both a high proportion of T lymphocytes and a high lymphocyte helper: suppressor (CD4:CD8) ratio that decrease after resolution of erythema nodosum (Ward et al., 1989). EN and non-Hodgkin's lymphoma, the latter presenting as a solitary pulmonary nodule, have been reported (Reverter et al., 1987).

XIII. Acanthosis Nigricans

Acanthosis nigricans (AC) is an uncommon dermopathy characterized by hyperpigmentation and epidermal hypertrophy (Fig. 22, see Color Plate, facing p. 478). (Brown and Winkelmann, 1968). The malignant type of acanthosis nigricans is associated, in 90% of cases, with either adenocarcinoma of the stomach or some other intra-abdominal malignancy (Curth et al., 1962). Dermal changes appear before clinical evidence of the carcinoma in 20% of patients, and the two appear together in approximately 60%. Acanthosis nigricans may be the initial manifestation of bronchogenic carcinoma (Knowles and Smith, 1960). Adenocarcinoma (Fig. 23) is the most likely lung cancer to be associated with acanthosis nigricans, but alveolar cell carcinoma has also been noted (Menzies et al., 1988). The prognosis associated with malignancy and acanthosis nigricans is poor, and progressive skin changes are said to be associated with a higher mortality.

Although acanthosis nigricans is the most well-recognized dermatological manifestation of visceral malignancy, several other less well-known disorders are also associated with cancer. Bowen's disease is a chronic dermatosis characterized by the development of in situ epidermoid carcinoma of the skin

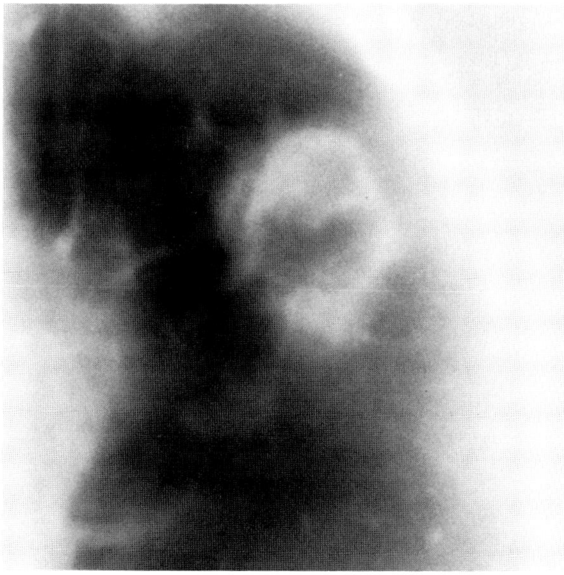

Figure 23 Tomographic view of left upper lobe of the patient shown in Figure 22 reveals a cavitated mass; biopsy showed primary adenocarcinoma of the lung.

(Bowen, 1912). In some cases, Bowen's disease is related to arsenic exposure and has been complicated by carcinoma of the lung (Goldman, 1973). Porphyria cutanea tarda (Nyman, 1972), tylosis or hyperkeratosis palmaris et plantaris (Powell and Mackey, 1981; Schwindt et al., 1970), acquired hypertrichosis lanuginosa (Shee and Graham, 1981), pemphigoid (Abadir, 1967), tripe palms (Cohen et al., 1989), and epidermolysis bullosa (Almeyda, 1972) are additional dermatoses that have been associated with bronchogenic carcinoma and that occasionally precede the onset of the malignancy. In a case-control study of 66 lung cancer patients, 71% exhibited palmar keratoses, in contrast to only 36% of control subjects (Cuzick et al., 1984). The prevalence of keratoses increased with age and was higher in men than women. There were no distinguishing features in the keratoses found in patients from those in controls. The association of intrathoracic malignancy with sympathetic neurological complications, particularly Horner's syndrome, is well recognized as a paraneoplastic syndrome. Another manifestation, unilateral hyperhidrosis of the thoracic cage, has been described in several patients (Lindsay et al., 1986), and, in most cases, has been localized to the same side as the tumor. It has been postulated that direct irritation of nerves may excite the autonomic efferent fibers. In some, excision of a cervical rib has abolished the hyperhidrosis. The presence of this symptom carries a poor prognosis.

XIV. Mastocytosis

Systemic mastocytosis, or mast cell disease, is an uncommon disorder characterized by urticaria pigmentosa, hepatosplenomegaly, osteosclerotic bone lesions, and diarrhea, nausea, vomiting, and flushing. Pulmonary manifestations include interstitial pulmonary disease (Roberts et al., 1968) and extensive peribronchial and alveolar infiltration with mast cells (Mutter et al., 1963).

XV. Malignant Atrophic Papulosis

Malignant atrophic papulosis (Degos' disease) is a rare, multisystemic disease with characteristic cutaneous lesions and gastrointestinal symptoms. The disease has been rapidly fatal in many cases. The initial manifestation is the appearance of crops of asymptomatic oval cutaneous lesions, ranging from 2 mm to 8 mm in diameter. A review (Pierce and Smith, 1978) of 60 reported cases of Degos' disease found that 17 included intrathoracic lesions, most of which were found incidentally at autopsy. The most common intrathoracic findings were pleuritis and pericarditis. Bilateral hemorrhagic pleural effusions, pleural plaques, pulmonary infarcts, and pulmonary abscess were also noted in these patients.

XVI. Miscellaneous Dermatoses

A. Epidermolysis Bullosa Dystrophica

This condition is a rare inherited skin disorder that generally presents in newborns. It is characterized by noninflammatory bullous lesions that can sometimes involve the respiratory mucosa and cause respiratory distress (Thompson et al., 1980). A patient with epidermolysis bullosa dystrophica was reported to have chronic stridor due to localized subglottic edema and inflammatory membrane formation in the trachea (Shackelford et al., 1982). Postmortem studies in a 29-month-old boy who died from laryngeal obstruction secondary to epidermolysis bullosa letalis revealed marked mucosal inflammation and swelling of the seromucinous glands in the supraglottic airway (Glossop et al., 1984). The laryngeal cysts were different in nature from the cutaneous bullae. Bullous pemphigoid (Fig. 24) may be associated with bronchogenic carcinoma.

B. Blue Rubber Nevus Syndrome (Bean's Syndrome)

This rare disorder consists of rubbery blue hemangiomas of the skin and gastrointestinal tract associated with bleeding (Bean, 1958). Subsequent authors have

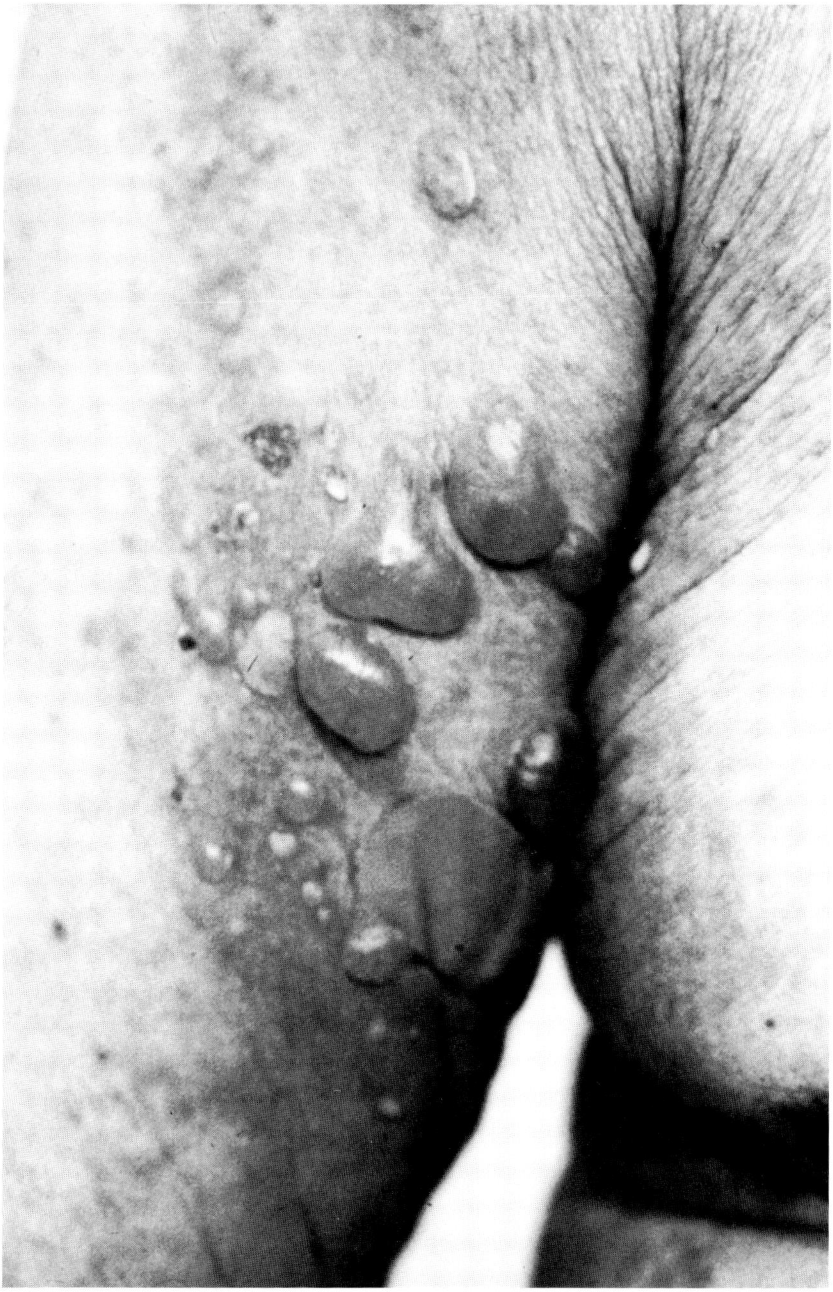

Figure 24 Right upper medial arm of a patient with typical changes of bullous pemphigoid.

described hemangiomas of other organs. Patients with pleural hemangiomas complicated by hemothorax have been described (Langleben et al., 1989). Pleural angiomas detected by histological studies have shown typical skin findings.

C. Anhidrotic Ectodermal Dysplasia

A hereditary, usually X-linked disorder characterized by deficient sweating, sparse hair, and deficient teeth, anhidrotic ectoderman dysplasia, is reported to predispose to severe bronchitis (Beahrs et al., 1971). The frequent upper respiratory infections in these patients have been attributed to scanty mucus and deficient cilia. Total absence of mucous glands in the tracheobronchial tree has been noted in children with this disorder (De Jager, 1965; Capitano et al., 1968). An increased prevalence of asthma has also been reported (Reed et al., 1970).

D. Acute Febrile Neutrophilic Dermatosis (Sweet's Syndrome)

Sweet's syndrome is an uncommon, recurrent, often dramatic skin disorder characterized by painful, plaque-forming inflammatory papules. These are usually associated with fever, arthralgia, and peripheral leukocytosis. Nearly one-fifth of the patients with Sweet's syndrome have associated malignancies, especially hematological disorders (Takimoto et al., 1991). Patchy pulmonary parenchymal infiltrates have been observed on chest roentgenograms. An open lung biopsy in one patient revealed chronic interstitial pneumonitis, minimal fibrosis, and a marked intra-alveolar neutrophilic infiltrate, which was similar to the findings of skin biopsy. Pulmonary infiltrates resolved with corticosteroid therapy (Lazarus et al., 1986). In other cases (Gibson et al., 1985; Takimoto et al., 1991), open lung biopsy revealed generalized interstitial edema, neutrophilic interstitial and alveolar exudates, recent hemorrhages, and hyperplasia of type I and II cells.

E. Pyoderma Gangrenosum

Pyoderma gangrenosum is a painful, chronic, destructive, and ulcerating skin disease of unknown etiology. The occurrence of this disorder in intestinal diseases is well known. In a report on 86 patients with this disease, inflammatory bowel disease was present in 36% (Powell et al., 1985). Asthma or chronic obstructive pulmonary disease was noted in 5%. Pulmonary abscess has been described in a patient with pyoderma gangrenosum (Vignon-Pennamen et al., 1989). The relationship between pyoderma gangrenosum and pulmonary disease is unclear.

F. Chronic Mucocutaneous Candidiasis

This rare disorder can be complicated by laryngeal, bronchial, and esophageal candidiasis. Symptoms include hoarseness, hemoptysis, and dysphagia

(Kobayashi et al., 1980). Severe bronchiectases following recurrent bronchpneumonia has been described in a patient with this disorder (Brägger et al., 1989). Immunological investigations revealed IgG2/IgG4 subclass deficiency and absence of antibodies against pneumococcal and *Hemophilus* polysaccharide. Extensive studies of a pediatric patient with mucocutaneous candidiasis and recurrent pulmonary infections disclosed a severe defect in cell-mediated immunity but normal humoral immune responses (Kirkpatrick et al., 1976).

G. Cogan's Syndrome

Cogan's syndrome is a disorder of undetermined etiology characterized by nonsyphilitic interstitial keratitis, audiovestibular symptoms, and systemic manifestations such as an elevated sedimentation rate, fever, anemia, leukocytosis, and thrombocytosis. Serious outcomes include deafness, vasculitis, aortic insufficiency, blindness, and death. In about 40% of patients, an upper respiratory tract infection precedes the onset of the syndrome. Among the 78 patients reported in the literature (Vollertson et al., 1986), transient pulmonary infiltrates

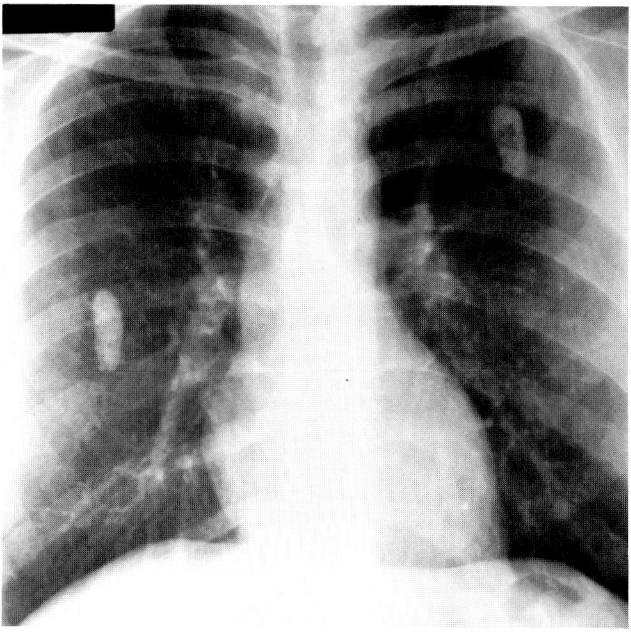

Figure 25 Chest roentgenograph of a patient with bilateral calcified lesions. Both lesions were located in the skin and were thought to be secondary to previous skin infection from dracunculosis.

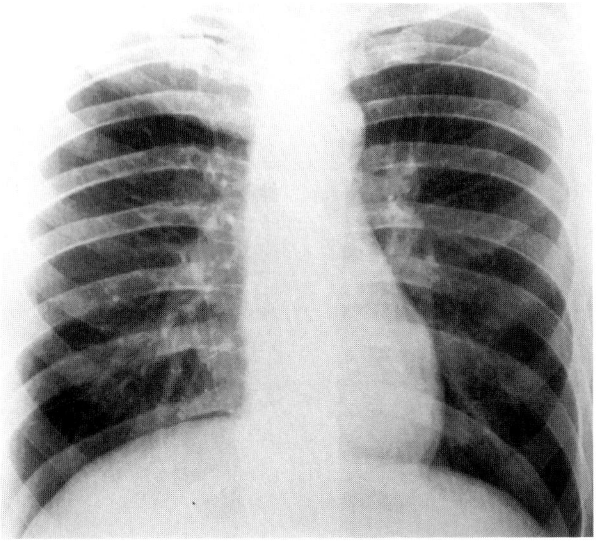

Figure 26 Chest roentgenograph displays an apparent density in the right apical region. This abnormality was in fact due to a skin graft over the chest wall.

and pleuritis were noted in 9 and 5%, respectively. Recurrent pulmonary infiltrations were observed that have not previously been described in connection with this syndrome.

H. Chest Wall Lesions

Dermatological lesions situated in the chest wall may appear as densities in the chest roentgenogram (Figs. 25–27) and cause diagnostic concerns. Many of these cutaneous lesions are erroneously diagnosed as intrapulmonary lesions, and needlessly extensive and expensive investigations, including computed tomography, have been performed to evaluate them. Good physical examination with posteroanterior stereo and lateral chest roentgenograms should aid in excluding an intrathoracic location for these lesions.

XVII. Summary

This chapter has described some of the common dermatological disorders in which pulmonary signs and symptoms are present. The diseases of the skin discussed are of varied etiology and pathogenesis, and many of the dermatological findings represent cutaneous manifestations of pulmonary disorders. However, it

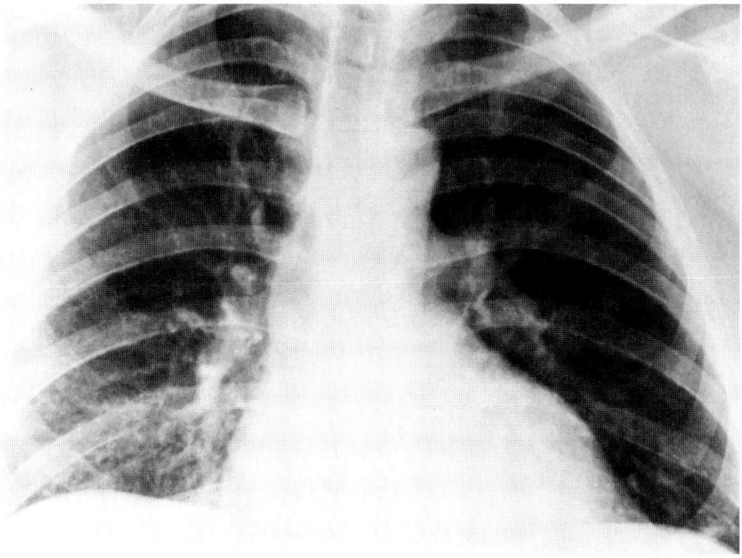

Figure 27 This chest roentgenograph suggests unilateral hyperlucency of left lung. This apparent abnormality was caused by the absence of left pectoral muscle.

is difficult to categorize each disease as belonging to either the respiratory or dermatological system. In fact, many of the dermatological and pulmonary manifestations discussed above are the complications of a primary disease that originates in an entirely different organ system and that may manifest itself in the skin or lungs simultaneously or at different time intervals.

References

Abadir, R. (1967). Pemphigoid, bronchial neoplasm and radiotherapy. *Proc. R. Soc. Med.* **60**:1271–1272.

Almeyda, J. (1972). Epidermolysis bullosa associated with neoplasm of the bronchus. *Br. J. Dermatol.* **87**:70–71.

Alper, J., and Kegel, M. (1987). Skin signs in pulmonary disease. *Clin. Chest Med.* **8**:299–311.

Altman, L. K., Fialkow, P. J., Parker, F., and Sagebiel, R. W. (1974). Pseudoxanthoma elasticum: an undiagnosed genetically heterogeneous disorder with protean manifestations. *Arch. Intern. Med.* **134**:1048–1054.

Anderson, C. E., Finklestein, J. Z., Nussbaum, E., Larson, E. J., Halpern, R., Uitto, J., and Tanaka, K. R. (1984). Association of hemolytic anemia and early-onset pulmonary emphysema in three siblings. *J. Pediatr.* **105**:247–251.

Angelillo, V. A., and O'Donohue, W. J., Jr. (1979). Yellow nail syndrome with reduced glucose level in pleural fluid. *Chest* **75**:83–85.

Armitage, J. M., Lane, D. J., Stradling, J. R., and Burton, M. (1990). Ear involvement in the yellow nail syndrome. *Chest* **98**:1534–1535.

Aughenbaugh, G. L. (1984). Thoracic manifestations of neurocutaneous disease. *Radiol. Clin. North Am.* **22**:741–756.

Awerbuch, M. S. (1976). The yellow nail syndrome, bronchiectasis and Raynaud's disease—a relationship. *Med. J. Aust.* **2**:829–830.

Ayers, J., Rees, J., and Cochrane, G. M. (1981). Haemoptysis and non-organic upper airways obstruction in a patient with previously undiagnosed Ehlers-Danlos syndrome. *Br. J. Dis. Chest* **75**:309–310.

Ayres, S., Jr., and Mihan, R. (1973). Yellow nail syndrome: response to vitamin E. *Arch. Dermatol.* **108**:267–268.

Babcock, T. L., and Synder, B. A. (1982). Spontaneous pneumothorax associated with tuberous sclerosis. *J. Thoracic Cardiovasc. Surg.* **83**:100–104.

Barabas, A. P. (1967). Heterogeneity of the Ehlers-Danlos syndrome: description of three clinical types and a hypothesis to explain the basic defect(s). *Br. Med. J.* **2**:612–613.

Baumer, J. H., and Hankey, S. (1980). Transient pulmonary cysts in an infant with the Ehlers-Danlos syndrome. *Br. J. Radiol.* **53**:598–599.

Beahrs, J. O., Lillington, G. A., Rosan, R. C., Russin, L., Lindgren, J. A., and Rowley, P. T (1971). Anhidrotic ectodermal dysplasia: predisposition to bronchial disease. *Ann. Intern. Med.* **74**:92–96.

Bean, W. B. (1958). *Vascular Spiders and Related Lesions of the Skin.* Charles C. Thomas, Springfield, IL, pp. 178–185.

Beer D. J., Pereira, W., Jr., and Snider, G. L. (1978). Pleural effusion associated with primary lymphedema: a perspective on the yellow nail syndrome. *Am. Rev. Respir. Dis.* **117**:595–599.

Beerman, H., and Kirshbaum, B. A. (1961). Some associated pulmonary and cutaneous diseases: a review of recent literature. *Am. J. Med. Sci.* **242**:494–517.

Beighton, P. (1968). Lethal complications of the Ehlers-Danlos syndrome. *Br. Med. J.* **3**:656–659.

Beighton, P. (1972). The dominant and recessive forms of cutis laxa. *J. Med. Genet.* **9**:216–221.

Ben-Yehuda, A., Ben-Chetrit, E., and Eliakim, M. (1986). Yellow nail syndrome: case report and review of the literature. *Isr. J. Med. Sci.* **22**:117–119.

Bick, R. L. (1981). Hereditary hemorrhagic telangiectasia and disseminated intravascular coagulation: a new clinical syndrome. *Ann. NY Acad. Sci.* **370**:851–854.

Bourneville, D. M. (1880). Sclerose tuereuse des circonvolutions cerebrales: idiotie et epilepsie hemiplegique. *Arch. Neurol.* (*Paris*) **1**:81–91.

Bowen, J. T. (1912). Precancerous dermatoses: a study of two cases of chronic atypical epithelial proliferation. *J. Cutan. Dis.* **30**:241–255.

Brägger, C., Seger, R. A., Aeppli, R., Hallè, F., and Hitzig, W. H. (1989). IgG_2/IgG_4 subclass deficiency in a patient with chronic mucocutaneous candidiasis and bronchiectases. *Eur. J. Pediatr.* **149**:168–169.

Brofman, J. D., Hall, J. B., Scott, W., and Little, A. G. (1990). Yellow nails, lymphedema and pleural effusion: treatment of chronic pleural effusion with pleuroperitoneal shunting. *Chest* **97**:743–745.

Brown, J., and Winkelmann, R. K. (1968). Acanthosis nigricans: a study of 90 cases. *Medicine* **47**:33–51.

Brown, S. E., Wright, P. W., Renner, J. W., and Riker, J. B. (1982). Staged bilateral thoracotomies for multiple pulmonary arteriovenous malformations complicating hereditary hemorrhagic telangiectasia. *J. Thorac. Cardiovasc. Surg.* **83**:285–289.

Bullock, W. E. (1986). The clinical significance of erythema nodosum. *Hosp. Pract.* [*Off.*] **15**(21):102E–102H, 102K–102L, 102Q–102R.

Byers, P. H., Narayanan, A. S., Bornstein, P., and Hall, J. G. (1976). An X-linked form of cutis laxa due to deficiency of lysyl oxidase. *Birth Defects* **12**(5):293–298.

Camilleri, A. E. (1990). Chronic sinusitis and the yellow nail syndrome. *J. Laryngol. Otol.* **104**:811–813.

Capitano, M. A., Chen, J. T. T., Arey, J. B., and Kirkpatrick, J. A. (1968). Congenital anhidrotic ectodermal dysplasia. *Am. J. Roentgenol.* **103**: 168–172.

Capron, F. Ameille, J., Leclerc, P., Mornet, P., Barbagellata, M., Reynes, M., and Rochemaure, J. (1983). Pulmonary lymphangioleiomyomatosis and Bourneville's tuberous sclerosis with pulmonary involvement: the same disease? *Cancer* **52**:851–855.

Carrington, C. B., Cugell, D. W., Gaensler, E. A., Marks, A., Redding, R. A., Schaaf, J. T., and Tomasian, A. (1977). Lymphangioleiomyomatosis: physiologic-pathologic-radiologic correlations. *Am. Rev. Respir. Dis.* **116**:977–995.

Cassidy, S. B. (1984). Tuberous sclerosis in children: diagnosis and course. *Compr. Ther.* **10**(11):43–48.

Cavanaugh, M. J., and Cooper, D. M. (1976). Chronic pulmonary disease in a child with the Ehlers-Danlos syndrome. *Acta. Paediatr. Scand.* **65**:679–684.

Chernosky, M. E., and Finley, V. K. (1985). Yellow nail syndrome in patients with acquired immunodeficiency disease. *J. Am. Acad. Dermatol.* **13**: 731–736.

Chilvers, E. R., Whyte, M. K. B., Jackson, J. E., Allison, D. J., and Hughes, J. M. B. (1990). Effect of percutaneous transcatheter embolization on pulmonary function, right-to-left shunt, and arterial oxygenation in patients with pulmonary arteriovenous malformations. *Am. Rev. Respir. Dis.* **142**:420–425.

Cockram, C. S., and Richards, P. (1979). Yellow nails and nephrotic syndrome. *Br. J. Dermatol.* **101**:707–709.

Cohen, P. R., Grossman, M. E., Almeida, L., and Kurzrock, R. (1989). Tripe palms and malignancy. *J. Clin. Oncol.* **7**:669–678.

Corrin, B., Liebow, A. A., and Friedman, P. J. (1975). Pulmonary lymphangiomyomatosis. *Am. J. Pathol.* **79**:348–382.

Crawley, F. E. (1950). Erythema nodosum as initial manifestation of Boeck's sarcoidosis. *Br. Med. J.* **2**:1362–1364.

Cupo, L. N., Pyeritz, R. E., Olson, J. L., McPhee, S. J., Hutchins, G. M., and McKusick, V. A. (1981). Ehlers-Danlos syndrome with abnormal collagen fibrils, sinus of Valsalva aneurysms, myocardial infarction, panacinar emphysema and cerebral heterotopias. *Am. J. Med.* **71**:1051–1058.

Curth, H. O., Hilberg, A. W., and Machacek, G. F. (1962). The site and histology of the cancer associated with malignant acanthosis nigricans. *Cancer* **15**:364–382.

Cuzick, J., Harris, R., and Mortimer, P. S. (1984). Palmar keratoses and cancers of the bladder and lung. *Lancet* **1**:530–533.

David, I., Crawford, F. A., Jr., Hendrix, G. H., Harley, R. A., and Tucker, T. (1986). Thoracic surgical implications of the yellow nail syndrome. *J. Thorac. Cardiovasc. Surg.* **91**:788–793.

Davies, B. H., and Tuddenham, E. G. D. (1976). Familial pulmonary fibrosis associated with oculocutaneous albinism and platelet function defect: a new syndrome. *Q. J. Med.* **45**:219–232.

Davies, P. D. B. (1963). Diffuse pulmonary involvement in von Recklinghausen's disease: a new syndrome. *Thorax* **18**:198.

DeCoste, S. D., Imber, M. J., and Baden, H. P. (1990). Yellow nail syndrome. *J. Am. Acad. Dermatol.* **22**:608–611.

De Jager, H. (1965). Congenital anhidrotic ectodermal dysplasia: case report. *J. Pathol. Bacteriol.* **90**:321–322.

Depinho, R. A., and Kaplan, K. L. (1985). The Hermansky-Pudlak syndrome: report of three cases and review of pathophysiology and management considerations. *Medicine* **64**:192–202.

Derham, R. J. (1956). Postprimary intrathoracic tuberculosis in childhood: with special reference to its sequelae. *Tex. State J. Med.* **52**:583.

De Scheerder, I., Elinck, W., Van Renterghem, D., Cuvelier, C., Tasson, J., and Van Der Straeten, M. (1984). Desquamative interstitial pneumonia and scar cancer of the lung complicating generalised neurofibromatosis. *Eur. J. Respir. Dis.* **65**:623–626.

Dilley, J. J., Kierland, R. R., Randall, R. V., and Shick, R. M. (1968). Primary lymphedema associated with yellow nails and pleural effusions. *JAMA* **204**:670–673.

Dines, D. E., Seward, J. B., and Bernatz, P. E. (1983). Pulmonary arteriovenous fistulas. *Mayo Clin. Proc.* **58**:176–181.

Drake, R. G., Jr. (1985). North American blastomycosis: a review. *J. Ky. Med. Assoc.* **83**:77–82.

Duhra, P. M., Quigley, E. M. M., and Marsh, M. N. (1985). Chylous ascites, intestinal lymphangiectasia and the "yellow-nail" syndrome. *Gut* **26**:1266–1269.

Dwyer, J. M., Hickie, J. B., and Garvan, J. (1971). Pulmonary tuberous sclerosis: report of three patients and a review of the literature. *Q. J. Med.* **40**:115–125.

Federman, Q., Abrams, R. M., and Lee, T. (1976). Pulmonary radiographic findings in a case of febrile, relapsing, nonsuppurative panniculitis (Weber-Christian disease). *Mt. Sinai J. Med.* **43**:174–179.

Ferreira, M. C., and Spina, V. (1973). A case of cutis laxa with abnormal copper metabolism. *Br. J. Plast. Surg.* **26**:283–286.

Fleming, P. C., Krieger, E., Turner, J. A. P., Watty, E. I., Quinn, P. A., and Bannatyne, R. M. (1967). Febrile mucocutaneous syndrome with respiratory involvement, associated with isolation of *Mycoplasma pneumoniae*. *Can. Med. Assoc. J.* **97**:1458–1459.

Foresti, V., Casati, O., Zubani, R., and Villa, A. (1990). Chylous pleural effusion in tuberous sclerosis. *Respiration* **57**:398–401.

Fraser, R. G., and Paré, J. A. P. (1979). *Diagnosis of Diseases of the Chest*, Vol. 3, 2nd ed. Saunders, Philadelphia, p. 1745.

Garay, S. M., Gardella, J. E., Fazzini, E. P., and Goldring, R. M. (1979). Hermansky-Pudlak syndrome: pulmonary manifestations of a ceroid storage disorder. *Am. J. Med.* **66**:737–747.

Gelfand, M. S., Stephens, D. S., Howell, E. I., Alford, R. H., and Kaiser, A. B. (1988). Brain abscess: association with pulmonary arteriovenous fistula and hereditary hemorrhagic telangiectasia: report of three cases. *Am. J. Med.* **85**:718–720.

Gibson, L. E., Dicken, C. H., and Flach, D. B. (1985). Neutrophilic dermatoses and myeloproliferative disease: report of two cases. *Mayo Clin. Proc.* **60**:735–740.

Glossop, L. P., Michaels, L., and Bailey, C. M. (1984). Epidermolysis bullosa letalis in the larynx causing acute respiratory failure: a case presentation and review of the literature. *Int. J. Pediatr. Otorhinolarygol.* **7:281–288.**

Goldman, A. L. (1973). Lung cancer in Bowen's disease. *Am. Rev. Respir. Dis.* **108**:1205–1207.

Gomes, M. M. R., and Bernatz, P. e. (1970). Arteriovenous fistulas: a review and ten-year experience at the Mayo Clinic. *Mayo Clin. Proc.* **45**:81–102.

Gomez, M. R., Kuntz, N. L., and Westmoreland, B. F. (1982). Tuberous sclerosis, early onset of seizures, and mental subnormality; a study of discordant homozygous twins. *Neurology* **32**:604–611.

Guin, J. D., and Elleman, J. H. (1979). Yellow nail syndrome: possible association with malignancy. *Arch. Dermatol.* **115**:734–735.

Gupta, A. K., Davies, G. M., and Haberman, H. F. (1986). Yellow nail syndrome. *Cutis* **37**:371–374.

Hajjar, B. A., and Joyner, E. N., III. (1968). Congenital cutis laxa with advanced cardiopulmonary disease. *J. Pediatr.* **73**:116–119.

Hardcastle, S. W., and Hendricks, M. L. (1984). Neurofibromatosis (von Recklinghausen's disease)—an unusual cause of parenchymal lung disease. *S. Afr. Med. J.* **66**:959–960.

Harris, J. O., Waltuck, B. L., and Swenson, E. W. (1969). The pathophysiology of the lungs in tuberous sclerosis: a case report and literature review. *Am. Rev. Respir. Dis.* **100**:379–387.

Harris, R. B., Heaphy, M. R., and Perry, H. O. (1978). Generalized elastolysis (cutis laxa). *Am. J. Med.* **65**:815–822.

Hassard, A. D., Martin, J., and Ross, J. B. (1984). Yellow nail syndrome and chronic sinusitis. *J. Otolaryngol.* **13**:318–320.

Hatfield, D. R., and Fried, A. M. (1981). Therapeutic embolization of diffuse pulmonary arteriovenous malformations. *AJR* **137**:861–863.

Hauck, R. W., König, G., Permanetter, W., Weiss, M., Wöckel, W., and Fruhmann, G. (1990). Tuberous sclerosis with pulmonary involvement. *Respiration* **57**:289–292.

Hayden, J. G., Talner, N. S., and Klaus, S. N. (1968). Cutis laxa associated with pulmonary artery stenosis. *J. Pediatr.* **72**:506–509.

Hewes, R. C., Auster, M., and White, R. I., Jr. (1985). Cerebral embolism—first manifestation of pulmonary arteriovenous malformation in patients with hereditary hemorrhagic telangiectasia. *Cardiovasc. Intervent. Radiol.* **8**:151–155.

Hiller, E., Rosenow, E. C., III, and Olsen, A. M. (1972). Pulmonary manifestations of the yellow nail syndrome. *Chest* **61**:452–458.

Hodgson, C. H., Burchell, H. B., Good, C. A., and Clagett, O. T. (1959). Hereditary hemorrhagic telangiectasia and pulmonary arteriovenous fistula: survey of a large family. *N. Engl. J. Med.* **261**:625–636.

Ilchyshyn, A., and Vickers, C. F. H. (1983). Yellow nail syndrome associated with penicillamine therapy. *Acta Derm. Venereol.* (*Stockh.*) **63**: 554–555.

Jackson, A., and Loh, C-L. (1980). Pulmonary calcification and elastic tissue damage in pseudoxanthoma elasticum. *Histopathology* **4**:607–611.

Joffe, B. (1960). An epidemic of coccidioidomycosis probably related to soil. *N. Engl. J. Med.* **262**:720–722.

Jóźwiak, S. (1990a). Pulmonary lymphangioleiomymatosis: a "forme fruste" of tuberous sclerosis? letter to the editor. *AJR* **155**:419.

Jóźwiak, S. (1990b). Severe pulmonary hypertension with diffuse smooth muscle proliferation of the lungs (letter to the editor). *Chest* **98**:250.

Kamatani, M., Rai, A., Hen, H., Hayashi, K., Aoki, T., Umeyama, K., and Takebayashi, J. (1978). Yellow nail syndrome associated with mental retardation in two siblings. *Br. J. Dermatol.* **99**:329–333.

Kintzer, J. S., Jones, F. L., and Pharr, W. F. (1978). Intrapleural haemorrhage complicating pulmonary arteriovenous fistula. *Br. J. Dis. Chest* **72**: 155–157.

Kirkpatrick, C. H., Ottenson, E. A., Smith, T. K., Wells, S. A., and Burdick, J. F. (1976). Reconstitution of defective cellular immunity with foetal thymus and dialysable transfer factor: long-term studies in a patient with chronic mucocutaneous candidiasis. *Clin. Exp. Immunol.* **23**:414–428.

Klatte, E. C., Franken, E. A., and Smith, J. A. (1976). The radiographic spectrum in neurofibromatosis. *Semin. Roentgenol.* **11**:17–33.

Knowles, J. H., and Smith, L. H., Jr. (1960). Extrapulmonary manifestations of bronchogenic carcinoma. *N. Engl. J. Med.* **262**:505–510.

Kobayashi, R. H., Rosenblatt, H. M., Carney, J. M., Byrne, W. J., Ament, M. E., Mendoza, G. R., Dudley, J. P., and Stiehm, E. R. (1980). *Candida* esophagitis and laryngitis in chronic mucocutaneous candidiasis. *Pediatrics* **66**:380–384.

Lagos, J. C., and Gomez, M. R. (1967). Tuberous sclerosis: reappraisal of a clinical entity. *Mayo Clin. Proc.* **42**:20–49.

Langleben, D., Wolkove, N., Srolovitz, H., Billick, R. C., and Sheiner, N. M. (1989). Hemothorax and hemopericardium in a patient with Bean's blue rubber bleb nevus syndrome. *Chest* **95**:1352–1353.

Lazarus, A. A., McMillan, M., and Miramadi, A. (1986). Pulmonary involvement in Sweet's syndrome (acute febrile neutrophilic dermatosis): preleukemic and leukemic phases of acute myelogenous leukemia. *Chest* **90**:922–924.

Ledoux-Corbusier, M. (1983). *Cutis laxa*, congenital form with pulmonary emphysema: an ultrastructural study. *J. Cutan. Pathol.* **10**:340–349.

Lees, M. H., Menashe, V. D., Sunderland, C. O., Morgan, C. L., and Dawson, P. J. (1969). Ehlers-Danlos syndrome associated with multiple pulmonary artery stenoses and tortuous systemic arteries. *J. Pediatr.* **75**:1031–1036.

Leier, C. V., Call, T. D., Fulkerson, P. K., and Wooley, C. F. (1980). The spectrum of cardiac defects in the Ehlers-Danlos syndrome, types I and III. *Ann. Intern. Med.* **92**:171–178.

Lenoir, S., Grenier, P., Brauner, M. W., Frija, J., Remy-Jardin, M., Revel, D., and Cordier, J. F. (1990). Pulmonary lymphangiomyomatosis and tuberous sclerosis: camparison of radiographic and thin-section CT findings. *Radiology* **175**:329–334.

Liberman, B. A., Chamberlain, D. W., and Goldstein, R. S. (1984). Tuberous sclerosis with pulmonary involvement. *Can. Med. Assoc. J.* **130**:287–289.

Lie, J. T. (1991). Cardiac, pulmonary, and vascular involvements in tuberous sclerosis. *Ann. NY Acad. Sci.* **615**:58–70.

Lie, J. T., Miller, R. D., and Williams, D. E. (1980). Cystic disease of the lungs in tuberous sclerosis: clinicopathologic correlation, including body plethysmographic lung function tests. *Mayo Clin. Proc.* **55**:547–553.

Lincoln, M. J., and Shigeoka, J. W. (1988). Pulmonary telangiectasia without hypoxemia. *Chest* **93**:1097–1098.

Lindsay, D. C., Freeman, J. G., and Record, C. O. (1986). Unilateral hyperhidrosis associated with underlying intrathoracic neoplasia. *Thorax* **41**:814–815.

Lodge, J. P. A., Hunter, A. M., and Saunders, N. R. (1989). Yellow nail syndrome associated with empyema. *Clin. Exp. Dermatol.* **14**:328–329.

Lossos, I. S., Breuer, R., and Lafair, J. S. (1988). Endotracheal neurofibroma in a patient with von Recklinghausen's disease. *Eur. Respir. J.* **1**:464–465.

Luna, C. M., Gené, R., Jolly, E. C., Nahmod, N., Defranchi, H. A., Patiño, G., and Elsner, B. (1985). Pulmonary lymphangiomyomatosis associated with tuberous sclerosis: treatment with tamoxifen and tetracycline-pleurodesis. *Chest* **88**:473–475.

Maeda, R. (1967). The origin and characteristics of ceroid. *Acta Pathol. Jpn.* **17**:439–456.

Magid, M., Esterly, N. B., Prendiville, J., and Fujisaki, C. (1987). The yellow nail syndrome in an 8-year-old girl. *Pediatr. Dermatol.* **4**:90–93.

Maisels, D. O., and Korachi, A. O. (1985). Lymphoedema of the eyelids in the yellow nail syndrome. *Br. J. Plast. Surg.* **38**:93–96.

Mambretti-Zumwalt, J., Seidman, J. M., and Higano, N. (1980). Yellow nail syndromw: complete triad with pleural protein turnover studies. *South. Med. J.* **73**:995–997.

Marquez, J., Juffé, A., Rufilanchas, J. J., Maitre, M., and Artaza, M. (1978). Successful correction of valvular and fibromuscular subpulmonary ring stenosis in a patient with Ehlers-Danlos syndrome. *J. Cardiovasc. Surg. (Torino)* **19**:271–276.

Massaro, D., and Katz, S. (1966). Fibrosing alveolitis: its occurrence, roentgenographic, and pathologic features in von Recklinghausen's neurofibromatosis. *Am. Rev. Respir. Dis.* **93**:934–942.

Massaro, D., Katz, S., Matthew, M. J., and Higgins, G. (1965). Von Recklinghausens's neurofibromatosis associated with cystic lung disease. *Am. J. Med.* **38**:233–240.

Mattingly, P. C., and Bossingham, D. H. (1979). Yellow nail syndrome in rheumatoid arthritis: report of three cases. *Ann. Rheum. Dis.* **38**:475–478.

McNicholas, W. T., Quigley, C., and FitzGerald, M. X. (1984). Upper lobe bronchiectasis in the yellow nail syndromwe report of a case. *Ir. J. Med. Sci.* **153**:394–395.

Medeiros, A. A., Marty, S. D., Tosh, F. E., and Chin, T. D. Y. (1966). Erythema nodosum and erythema multiforme as clinical manifestations of histoplasmosis in a community outbreak. *N. Engl. J. Med.* **274**:415–420.

Menzies, D. G., Choo-Kang, J., Buxton, P. K., and Campbell, I. W. (1988). Acanthosis nigricans associated with alveolar cell carcinoma. *Thorax* **43**:414–415.

Milledge, R. D., Gerald, B. E., and Carter, W. J. (1966). Pulmonary manifestations of tuberous sclerosis. *Am. J. Roentgenol.* **98**:734–738.

Miller, D. D., Davies, S. F., and Sarosi, G. A. (1982). Erythema nodosum and blastomycosis. *Arch. Intern. Med.* **142**:1839.

Milman, N., and Selroos, O. (1990). Pulmonary sarcoidosis in the Nordic countries 1950–1982. Epidemiology and clinical picture. *Sarcoidosis* **7**:50–57.

Miro, A. M., Vasudevan, V., and Shah, H. (1990). Ciliary motility in two patients with yellow nail syndrome and recurrent sinopulmonary infections. *Am. Rev. Respir. Dis.* **142**:890–891.

Momma, F., Ohara, S., Ohyama, T., Moto, A., Okada, H., and Harada, H. (1990). Brain abscess associated with congenital pulmonary arteriovenous fistula. *Surg. Neurol.* **34**:439–441.

Monaghan, H. P., Krafchik, B. R., MacGregor, D. L., and Fitz, C. R. (1981). Tuberous sclerosis complex in children. *Am. J. Dis. Child* **135**:912–917.

Moran, M. F., and Larkworthy, W. (1976). Upper respiratory problems in the yellow nail syndrome. *Clin. Otolaryngol.* **1**:333–336.

Müller, R.-P., Peters, P. E., Echternacht-Happle, K., and Happle, R. (1979). Roentgenographic and clinical signs in yellow nail syndrome. *Lymphology* **12**:257–261.

Mutter, R. D., Tannenbaum, M., and Ultmann, J. E. (1963). Systemic mast cell disease. *Ann. Intern. Med.* **59**:887–906.

Nakielna, E. M., Wilson, J., and Ballon, H. S. (1976). Yellow-nail syndrome: report of three cases. *Can. Med. Assoc. J.* **115**:46–48.

Neville, E., Walker, A. N., and James, D. G. (1983). Prognostic factors predicting the outcome of sarcoidosis: an analysis of 818 patients. *Q. J. Med.* **52**:525–533.

Nordkild, P., Kromann-Andersen, H., and Struve-Christensen, E. (1986). Yellow nail syndrome—the triad of yellow nails, lymphedema and pleural effusions: a review of the literature and a case report. *Acta Med. Scand.* **219**: 221–227.

Norton, L. (1985). Further observations on the yellow nail syndrome with therapeutic effects of oral alpha-tocopherol. *Cutis* **36**:457–462.
Nyman, C. R. (1972). Porphyria cutanea tarda, carcinoma of bronchus, rheumatoid arthritis, right hydronephrosis. *Proc. R. Soc. Med.* **65**:688–690.
Ocaña, I., Bejarano, E., Ruiz, I., Ribera, E., Pigrau, C., and Martinez-Vázquez, J. M. (1988). Intestinal lymphangiectasia and the yellow nail syndrome (letter to the editor). *Gastroenterology* **94**:858.
Patchefsky, A. S., Atkinson, W. G., Hoch, W. S., Gordon, G., and Lipshitz, H.I. (1973). Interstitial pulmonary fibrosis and von Recklinghausen's disease. An ultrastructural and immunofluorescent study. *Chest* **64**:459–464.
Pavlidakey, G. P., Hasimoto, K., and Blum, D. (1984). Yellow nail syndrome. *J. Am. Acad. Dermatol.* **11**:509–512.
Pearl, W., and Spicer, M. (1981). Ehlers-Danlos syndrome. *South. Med. J.* **74**:80–82.
Peery, W. H. (1987). Clinical spectrum of hereditary hemorrhagic telangiectasia (Osler-Weber-Rendu disease). *Am. J. Med.* **82**:989–997.
Petersen, J. M., and Ferguson, D. R. (1984). Gastrointestinal neurofibromatosis. *J. Clin. Gastroenterol.* **6**:529–534.
Pierce, R. N., and Smith, G. J. W. (1978). Intrathoracic manifestations of Degos' disease (malignant atrophic papulosis). *Chest* **73**:79–84.
Powell, F., and Mackey, J. P. (1981). Bronchial carcinoma and hyperkeratosis palmaris et plantaris. *Postgrad. Med. J.* **57**:57–59.
Powell, F. C., Schroeter, A. L., Su, W. P. D., and Perry, H. O. (1985). Pyoderma gangrenosum: a review of 86 patients. *Q. J. Med.* **55**:173–186.
Prakash, U. B. S., and Rosenow, E. C., III (1989). Unpublished data.
Prediletto, R., Viegi, G., and Bernard, P. (1987). Lung involvement in a patient with cutaneous neurofibromatosis evaluated by radioisotope techniques. *J. Nucl. Med. Allied Sci.* **31**:249–253.
Press, O. W., and Ramsey, P. G. (1984). Central nervous system infections associated with hereditary hemorrhagic telangiectasia. *Am. J. Med.* **77**:86–92.
Reed, W. B., Lopez, D. A., and Landing, B. (1970). Clinical spectrum of anhidrotic ectodermal dysplasia. *Arch. Dermatol.* **102**:134–143.
Reed, W. B., Horowitz, R. E., and Beighton, P. (1971). Acquired cutis laxa: primary generalized elastolysis. *Arch. Dermatol.* **103**:661–669.
Reverter, J. C., Coca, A., Font, J., and Ingelmo, M. (1987). Erythema nodosum and pulmonary solitary nodule as the first manifestations of a non-Hodgkin's lymphoma. *Br. J. Dis. Chest* **81**:397–399.
Revill, D., and Matts, S. G. F. (1958). Pulmonary arteriovenous aneurysm in hereditary telangiectasia. *Br. J. Tubercl.* **52**:222–224.
Riccardi, V. M. (1981). Von Recklinghausen neurofibromatosis. *N. Engl. J. Med.* **305**:1617–1627.

Roberts, P. L., McDonald, H. B., and Wells, R. F. (1968). Systemic mast cell disease in a patient with unusual gastrointestinal and pulmonary abnormalities. *Am. J. Med.* **45**:638–642.

Román, G., Fisher, M., Perl, D. P., and Poser, C. M. (1978). Neurological manifestations of hereditary hemorrhagic telangiectasia (Rendu-Osler-Weber disease): report of 2 cases and review of the literature. *Ann. Neurol.* **4**:130–144.

Rubinstein, H. M., Jaffer, A. M., Kudrna, J. C., Lertratanakul, Y., Chadrasekhar, A. J., Slater, D., and Schmid, F. R. (1977). Alpha$_1$-antitrypsin deficiency with severe panniculitis: report of two cases. *Ann. Intern. Med.* **86**:742–744.

Runyon, B. A., Forker, E. L., and Sopko, J. A. (1979). Pleural-fluid kinetics in a patient with primary lymphedema, pleural effusions, and yellow nails. *Am. Rev. Respir. Dis.* **119**:821–825.

Ryan, C. J., Rodgers, R. F., Unni, K. K., and Hepper, N. G. (1981). The outcome of patients with pleural effusion of indeterminate cause at thoracotomy. *Mayo Clin. Proc.* **56**:145–149.

Sahi, S. P., and Bansal, S. K. (1988). Yellow nail syndrome with persistent hypoalbuminaemia. *Br. J. Clin. Pract.* **42**:36–37.

Samman, P. D., and White, W. F. (1964). The "yellow nail" syndrome. *Br. J.* Dermatol. **76**:153–157.

Sammons, B. P. (1959). Arteriovenous fistula of the lung *Radiology* **72**: 710–715.

Sanders, J. S., and Martt, J. M. (1962). Mutiple small pulmonary arteriovenous fistulas: diagnosis by cardiac catheterization. *Circulation* **25**:383–389.

Sastre, J., Renedo, G., Mangado, N. G., Cabrera, P., and Lahoz, F. (1987). Pulmonary ceroidosis. *Chest* **91**:281–283.

Savill, J. S., Barrie, R., Ghosh, S., Muhlemann, M., Dawson, P., and Pusey, C. D. (1988). Fatal Stevens-Johnson syndrome following urography with iopamidol in systemic lupus erythematosus. *Postgrad. Med. J.* **64**:392–394.

Schabel, S. I., Schmidt, G. E., and Vujic, I. (1980). Overlooked pulmonary malignancy in neurofibromatosis. *J. Can. Assoc. Radio.* **31**:135–136.

Schoen, I., Reingold, I. M., and Meister, L. (1958). Relapsing nodular nonsuppurative panniculitis with lung involvment: clinical and autopsy findings, with notes on pathogenesis. *Ann. Intern. Med.* **49**:687–698.

Schwartz, B. K., and Clendenning, W. E. (1985). Bullous erythema multiforme associated with *Hemophilus influenzae pneumonia. Cutis* **36**:255–256.

Schwindt, W. D., Bernhardt, L. C., and Johnson, S. A. M. (1970). Tylosis and intrathoracic neoplasms. *Chest* **57**:590–591.

Shackelford, G. D., Bauer, E. A., Graviss, E. R., and McAlister, W. H. (1982). Upper airway and external genital involvement in epidermolysis bullosa dystrophica. *Radioloby* **143**:429–432.

Sharma, O. P. (1990). Sarcoidosis. *Dis. Mon.* **36**(9):469–535.

Shashy, S. S., Jones, B. C., and Kitchens, C. S. (1985). Spontaneous hemothorax in a patient with Osler-Weber-Rendu disease. *South. Med. J.* **78**:1393–1394.

Shee, C. D., and Graham, V. A. L. (1981). Acquired hypertrichosis lanuginosa and carcinoma of the bronchus. *Thorax* **36**:153–154.

Shub, C., Tajik, A. J., Seward, J. B., and Dines, D. E. (1976). Detecting intrapulmonary right-to-left shunt with contrast echocardiography: observations in a patient with diffuse pulmonary arteriovenous fistulas. *Mayo Clin. proc.* **51**:81–84.

Slingerland, J. M., Grossman, R. F., Chamberlain, D., and Tremblay, C. E. (1989). Pulmonary manifestations of tuberous sclerosis in first degree relatives. *Thorax* **44**:212–214.

Smit, J., Alberts, C., and Balk, A. G. (1978). Pneumothorax in the Ehlers-Danlos syndrome: consequence or coincidence. *Scand. J. Respir. Dis.* **59**:239–242.

Sobonya, R. E., Quan, S. F., and Fleishman, J. S. (1985). Pulmonary lymphangioleiomyomatosis: quantitative analysis of lesions producing airflow limitation. *Hum. Pathol.* **16**:1122–1128.

Solal-Celigny, P., Cormier Y., and Fournier M. (1983). The yellow nail syndrome: light and electron microscopic aspects of the pleura. *Arch. Pathol. Lab. Med.* **107**:183–185.

Sorensen, R. U., Abramowsky, C. R., and Stern, R. C. (1986). Ten-year course of early-onset Weber-Christian syndrome with recurrent pneumonia: a suggestion for pathogenesis. *Pediatrics* **78**:115–120.

Stevens, A. M., and Johnson, F. C. (1922). A new eruptive fever asociated with stomatitis and ophthalmia: Report of two cases in children. *Am. J. Dis. Child* **24**:526–533.

Stovin, P. G. I., Lum, L. C., Flower, C. D. R., Drake, C. S., and Beeley, M. (1975). The lungs in lymphangiomyomatosis and in tuberous sclerosis. *Thorax* **30**:497–509.

Syrjälä, H., Karvonen, J., and Salminen, A. (1984). Skin manifestations of tularemia: a study of 88 cases in northern Finland during 16 years (1967–1983). *Acta. Dermat. Venereol.* (*Stockh.*) **64**:513–516.

Tachibana, F., Hakozaki, H., Takahashi, K., Kojima, M., Enomoto, S., and Wada, J. (1979). Syndrome of the sea-blue histiocyte: the first cas report in Japan and review of the literature. *Acta Pathol. Jpn.* **29**:73–97.

Takahashi, K., Hakozaki, H., and Kojima, M. (1978). Idiopathic pulmonary ceroidosis. *Acta Pathol. Jpn.* **28**:301–311.

Takimoto, C. H., Warnock, M., and Golden, J. A. (1991). Sweet's syndrome with lung involvement. *Am. Rev. Respir. Dis.* **143**:177–179.

Tan, W. C. (1989). Dietary treatment of chylous ascites in yellow nail syndrome. *Gut* **30**:1622–1623.

Teragaki, M., Akioka, K., Yasuda, M., Ikuno, Y., Oku, H., Takeuchi, K., and Takeda, T. (1988). Hereditary hemorrhagic telangiectasia with growing pulmonary atreriovenous fistulas followed for 24 years. *Am. J. Med. Sci.* **295**:545–547.

Thomas, P. S., and Sidhu, B. (1987). Yellow nail syndrome and bronchial carcinoma (letter to the editor). *Chest* **92**:191.

Thompson, J. W., Ahmed, A. R., and Dudley, J. P. (1980). Epidermolysis bullosa dystrophica of the larynx and trachea: acute airway obstruction. *Ann. Otol. Rhinol. Laryngol.* **89**:428–429.

Toal, B. J., Doherty, C. C., and Johnston, S. R. (1988). Chyluria and the yellow nail syndrome. *Br. J. Urol.* **61**:360–361.

Turner-Stokes, L., Turton, C., Pope, F. M., and Green, M. (1983). Emphysema and cutis laxa. *Thorax* **38**:790–792.

Unger, P. D., Geller, S. A., and Anderson, P. J. (1984). Pulmonary lesions in a patient with neurofibromatosis. *Arch. Pathol. Lab. Med.* **108**:654–657.

Van Maldergem, L., Vamos, E., Liebaers, I., Petit, P., Vandevelde, G., Simonis-Blumenfrucht, A., Bouffioux, R., Kulakowski, S., Hanquinet, S., Van Durme, P., Laporte M., and Ledoux-Corbusier, M. (1988). Severe congenital cutis laxa with pulmonary emphysema: a family with three affected sibs. *Am. J. Med. Genet.* **31**:455–464.

Vase, P., Holm, M., and Arendrup, H. (1985). Pulmonary arteriovenous fistulas in hereditary hemorrhagic telangiectasia. *Acta Med. Scand.* **218**:105–109.

Veien, N. K., Stahl, D., and Brodthagen, H. (1987). Cutaneous sarcoidosis in Caucasians. *J. Am. Acad. Dermatol.* **16**:534–540.

Venencie, P-Y., and Dicken, C-H. (1984). Yellow nail syndrome: report of five cases. *J. Am. Acad. Dermatol.* **10**(2 Pt 1):187–192.

Vignon-Pennamen, M. D., Zelinsky-Gurung, A., Janssen, F., Frija, J., and Wallach, D. (1989). Pyoderma gangrenosum with pulmonary involvement. *Arch. Dermatol.* **125**:1239–1242.

Vollertson, R. S., McDonald, T. J., Younge, B. R., Banks, P. M., Stanson, A. W., and Ilstrup, D. M. (1986). Cogan's syndrome: 18 cases and a review of the literature. *Mayo Clin. Proc.* **61**:344–361.

Wagener, O. E., Roncoroni, A. J., and Barcat, J. A. (1989). Severe pulmonary hypertension with diffuse smooth muscle proliferation of the lungs: pulmonary tuberous sclerosis? *Chest* **95**:234–237.

Wakasa, M., Imaizumi, T., Suyama, A., Takeshita, A., and Nakamura, M. (1987). Yellow nail syndrome associated with chronic pericardial effusion. *Chest* **92**:366–367.

Ward, K., O'Connor, C., Odlum, C., and Fitzgerald, M. X. (1989). Prognostic value of bronchoalveolar lavage in sarcoidosis: the critical influence of disease presentation. *Thorax* **44**:6–12.

Webb, W. R., and Goodman, P. C. (1977). Fibrosing alveolitis in patients with neurofibromatosis. *Radiology* **122**:289–293.

Weir, E. K., Joffe, H. S., Blaufuss, A. H., and Beighton, P. (1977). Cardiovascular abnormalities in cutis laxa. *Eur. J. Cardiol.* **5**:255–261.

Westermann, C. J. J., Oostveen, A. C. M., Wagenaar, S. S., Hilvering, C., Overbeek, S. E., and Verheijen-Breemhaar, D. (1986). Pulmonary tuberous sclerosis treated with tamoxifen and progesterone. *Thorax* **41**:892–893.

White, D. A., Smith, G. J. W., Cooper, J. A. D., Jr., Glickstein, M., and Rankin, J. A. (1984). Hermansky-Pudlak syndrome and interstitial lung disease: report of a case with lavage findings. *Am. Rev. Respir. Dis.* **130**:138–141.

White, R. I., Jr., Lynch-Nyhan, A., Terry, P., Buescher, P. C., Farmlett, E. J., Charnas, L., Shuman, K., Kim, W., Kinnison, M., and Mitchell, S. E. (1988). Pulmonary arteriovenous malformations: techniques and long-term outcome of embolotherapy. *Radiology* **169**:663–669.

Williams, H. C., Buffham, R., and du-Vivier, A. (1991). Successful use of topical vitamin E solution in the treatment of nail changes in yellow nail syndrome. *Arch. Dermatol.* **127**:1023–1028.

Winterbauer, R. H., Belic, N., and Moores, K. D. (1973). A clinical interpretation of bilateral hilar adenopathy. *Ann. Intern. Med.* **78**:65.

11

Pulmonary Manifestations of Obstetric and Reproductive Tract Conditions

MICHAEL R. FLICK

School of Medicine, University of California, San Francisco,
and San Francisco General Hospital
San Francisco, California

I. Introduction

When the pulmonary manifestations of extrapulmonary conditions are tallied, the reproductive organs usually are not given much consideration. There is no general review of the pulmonary manifestations of obstetric and reproductive tract "diseases." This chapter aims to do just that. Pregnancy, of course, is not a disease at all, but rather a normal condition to which the lungs readily adapt. Because at some time in their lives half of all people may be pregnant, the pulmonary status in normal pregnancy is considered first. Following this, obstetric and reproductive tract manifestations in the pulmonary vascular bed, airways, lung parenchyma, and pleural space are discussed, in turn. Finally, various benign and malignant growths in the lungs that originate in the reproductive tract are reviewed. Rather than providing an exhaustive list of references, citations have been limited almost exclusively to reasonably accessible writings of the last decade. The reproductive system affects the lungs in interesting and important ways and therefore deserves consideration by anyone involved in the diagnosis and treatment of pulmonary diseases. What follows is a starting place for study.

II. Pulmonary Status in Normal Pregnancy

There was a comprehensive and still current review of pregnancy and the lung a decade ago (Weinberger et al., 1980), and more recent reviews have focused on pregnant women with respiratory problems (Noble et al., 1988) and on acute respiratory failure in pregnancy (Hollingsworth et al., 1989). Generally, most lung volumes are unaffected by pregnancy, except for functional residual capacity (FRC), which is decreased because both expiratory reserve (ERV) and residual (RV) volumes are smaller than in nonpregnant women. Airway resistance is decreased, and its reciprocal, airway conductance, is increased. Tidal volume is usually increased, which leads to hyperventilation and respiratory alkalosis (the pH is normal by renal compensation). Oxygen consumption ($\dot{V}O_2$) is also increased, as are both intravascular volume and cardiac output. Intravascular pressures in the pulmonary vascular bed are usually normal, but vascular reactivity is decreased. The quantity of interstitial water in the lungs may be increased, and there are often small postpartum pleural effusions. There are also, of course, metabolic, hormonal, and immunological changes affecting the lungs' working environment. These include: high levels of circulating estrogen and progesterone; increased plasma cortisol, human chorionic gonadotropin, and thyroid hormone; increased production of prostaglandins and cyclic nucleotides; and a decrease in cellular immunity.

Most pregnant women are young, healthy, and unaware of the pulmonary manifestations of their pregnancies other than common complaints of dyspnea (probably related to hyperventilation). When cardiopulmonary function is already compromised by preexisting disease, the natural course of pulmonary diseases may be altered and the mother-to-be at increased risk for complications of her pregnancy.

A. Gas Exchange

The most obvious manifestation of pregnancy is the enlarging uterus, which leads to increases in both the level of the diaphragm and the transverse diameter of the chest. Function of the diaphragm and chest wall musculature is unimpaired, and because tidal breathing is large, their excursions are increased (Gilroy et al., 1988; Weinberger et al., 1980). However, end-expiratory lung volume (FRC) is smaller and intrathoracic pressure less negative than when the woman is not pregnant. On physical examination, diaphragmatic elevation may be mistaken for lobar consolidation, and rales may be heard at the lung bases if atelectasis is present. Pregnancy is not analogous to morbid obesity, in which abdominal pressure is increased and inspiratory muscle motion is decreased.

The consequences of these mechanical changes are reflected in the results of various pulmonary function studies (Berry et al., 1989; Hollingworth et al.,

1989; Liberatore et al., 1984; Weinberger et al., 1980). The primary effects are on resting lung volumes. Beginning at about the fifth month of pregnancy and progressing to delivery, the end-expiratory volume of the lungs decreases. By term, FRC is reduced about 10–20%, owing to decreases in both ERV and RV. Because the strength of the diaphragm and thoracic musculature is unimpaired, vital capacity (VC) is usually unchanged. Total lung capacity, as the sum of RV and VC, is therefore decreased slightly owing to the reduction in residual volume of the lungs.

Large-airway function is not usually impaired by pregnancy, and forced expiratory volumes and their ratios are normal. Total pulmonary resistance may be decreased late in pregnancy, perhaps owing to relaxation of the smooth muscle in the tracheobronchial tree under hormonal influence. Lung compliance is probably unchanged.

Small-airway function is either normal or mildly impaired, depending on how it is tested. Measurements of closing volume or closing capacity in the last month of pregnancy have suggested airway closure either above or close to FRC during tidal breathing, an effect attributed primarily to the decrease in FRC. Additional evidence for such closure is an increase (about 5 mmHg) in the alveolar-arterial oxygen difference [(A-a)P_{O_2}] near term, which could be due to perfusion of areas of lung that are poorly ventilated because of small-airways closure during tidal breathing. However, small-airway dysfunction was not suggested in other studies of maximal expiratory flow-volume curves. In any case, the effect on Pa_{O_2} is quite modest (decreased $<5\%$ from peak values early in pregnancy, but still detectable when compared to Pa_{O_2} values in the nonpregnant state).

Diffusing capacity of the lungs for CO (DL_{CO}) may be unchanged or increased early, but is generally normal or slightly decreased during the second half of pregnancy. The relative contributions of the membrane and pulmonary capillary blood volume components to these changes in overall DL_{CO} are not well worked out. Changes have not correlated with pulmonary blood or alveolar volumes, or with hemoglobin or 17-β-estradiol concentrations.

Ventilation is generally increased in pregnancy, beginning before the uterus enlarges to any significant degree. Tidal volume increases, but respiratory rate is usually constant through pregnancy; consequently, expired volume ($\dot{V}_E$) is increased by as much as 50% when compared to the nonpregnant state. $\dot{V}O_2$ and metabolic rate are increased during pregnancy (about 20% and 15%, respectively), but not to the same extent as $\dot{V}_E$. The change in ventilation is believed to be an effect primarily of the sixfold increase in circulating progesterone during the course of pregnancy. Progesterone increases ventilation by increasing respiratory center sensitivity to CO_2. Increased circulating estrogen may add to this respiratory center stimulation by increasing the number of progesterone receptors (Brodeur et al., 1986; Pickett et al., 1989).

Hyperventilation results in decreased $P_{A_{CO_2}}$ and Pa_{CO_2}, with the Pa_{CO_2} reaching a plateau of 25–32 mmHg during pregnancy. This respiratory alkalosis is fully compensated by increased renal bicarbonate excretion, and therefore, blood pH is generally unaffected by pregnancy. As predicted from the alveolar air equation, hyperventilation causes $P_{A_{O_2}}$ to increase to over 100 mmHg, and this, in turn, raises Pa_{O_2}. A slight drop in Pa_{O_2} usually occurs near term, perhaps, as discussed, attributable to airway closure, but Pa_{O_2} generally remains in excess of nonpregnant values. Postural effects have been reported, with Pa_{O_2} lower in the supine than in the seated position in pregnancy. These effects are believed to be related to pressure on the diaphragm by the uterus while supine, which contributes to airway closure, inferior vena caval compression, and hemodynamic changes. During labor, there can be dramatic swings in Pa_{O_2} during vigorous expulsive Valsalva maneuvers, and during uterine contractions $\dot{V}O_2$ can triple and Pa_{CO_2} decrease still further.

The bottom line of these changes in ventilation is threefold: first, the lung is normally prepared to meet the challenges of pregnancy; second, a consequence of the reduced FRC is that the oxygen reserve within the lung is diminished (Byrne et al., 1987), and pregnant women can tolerate only very short periods of apnea (for example, when inducing anesthesia or intubating); and third, most women (60–70%) complain of dyspnea during their pregnancies. Because it is usually noted early and often improves as pregnancy progresses, mechanical factors associated with the enlarging uterus do not appear to play a role in the etiology of this sensation of breathlessness. Proposed mechanisms include awareness of hyperventilation, the decreased Pa_{CO_2}, or a ventilatory response that is inappropriate for the demand. The obvious problem can be that of ruling out more ominous, nonphysiological causes of dyspnea, such as infection, pulmonary edema or embolism, bronchospasm, barotrauma, or hypoxemia.

B. Vascular Bed

The lungs are passive participants in the major cardiovascular changes that accompany pregnancy (Cole and Sutton, 1989). Plasma volume increases 50–100% over nonpregnant values, and red cell volume increases 20–40% progressively throughout gestation. Increased total body water and exchangeable sodium occur in response to elevated renin and aldosterone levels, and other factors contributing to expanded volume include progesterone-induced relaxation of venous smooth muscle, the placenta acting as an arteriovenous fistula, and increased levels of prostaglandins, atrial natriuretic factor, erythropoietin, and prolactin. The "physiological anemia of pregnancy" results from the greater increase in plasma than in red cell volume.

Cardiac stroke volume and heart rate begin to increase early in pregnancy and cause resting cardiac output to increase to levels 30–50% above the nonpregnant state. There can be profound positional effects on the circulation, with lower cardiac output in the supine position when the gravid uterus compresses the inferior vena cava. The generally expanded and hyperkinetic circulation can produce a variety of physical findings in pregnancy, including, commonly, a third heart sound and, more variably, systolic murmurs due to tricuspid regurgitation and to increased blood flow in the breasts and mammary arteries, and supraclavicular murmurs can sometimes be heard over the brachiocephalic arteries. Data conflict with regard to small changes in systemic blood pressure during pregnancy, but systemic vascular resistance is generally decreased owing to the increased cardiac output. During labor and delivery, there are further increases in cardiac output with contractions, and there can be profound swings in systemic blood pressure and heart rate.

Because of the invasive nature of right heart catheterization, pulmonary vascular pressures have not been measured in many normal pregnant women. When they have been measured, the pressures have been normal (Barron, 1984; Cole and Sutton, 1989; Noble et al., 1988; Wasserstrum and Cotton, 1986). Pulmonary vascular resistance, the pressure difference across the pulmonary vascular bed divided by cardiac output, is therefore decreased, because the intravascular pressures are normal while cardiac output is increased.

Pulmonary vascular reactivity has been found to be decreased in most pregnant experimental animals (Cutaia et al., 1987; Fuchs et al., 1982; Moore and Reeves, 1980). The blunting of hypoxic vasoconstriction in the lungs may be a factor in the usual decline in Pa_{O_2} late in pregnancy (discussed above). The reason for this depressed reactivity of the pulmonary vascular bed has been suspected to be a combination of direct estrogen effects and enhanced release of vasodilator prostaglandins (Sylvester et al., 1985).

C. Interstitium

The only information about changes in lung water during pregnancy comes from a study of chest radiographs of 20 pregnant women, 35% of whom were said to have had radiological evidence of interstitial pulmonary edema during the early puerperium (MacLennan et al., 1987). However, the technique of scoring chest radiographs is not a very sensitive method of detecting increases in extravascular lung water (requiring an increase of 30–80% before radiographs become "abnormal"), and the scoring system might have been confounded by the increased intrathoracic blood volume, extra fat and water content of overlying subcutaneous tissues, and small lung volumes in normal pregnancy.

Nevertheless, there are reasons to suspect that the lungs might tend to be "wetter" in pregnancy. First, there is a general increase in connective-tissue water during pregnancy (MacLennan et al., 1987; Rutherford and Hands, 1989). Clinical peripheral edema is found in about 80% of healthy pregnant women, and there is no reason to suspect the lungs would be spared from the general increase in body water content. Second, plasma oncotic pressure may fall during pregnancy (Hollingsworth et al., 1989; Hughson et al.,1982; MacLennan et al., 1987), which would favor an increase in filtration in the lungs. Third, overall fluid filtration in the lungs is likely to be increased because the surface area for filtration is expanded by the increased blood volume and cardiac output. Fourth, the lung lymphatics, which are important for the removal of interstitial liquid and protein, may be affected by the general smooth-muscle relaxation in pregnancy. Finally, even if lung water volume were normal in pregnancy, it would be contained in a smaller than usual interstitial space because the lungs are at a smaller volume (and intrathoracic pressure is less negative). The forces favoring a "wetter" lung may be augmented at the time of delivery, when high intrathoracic pressures caused by Valsalva maneuvers during contractions could impede lymphatic function and raise the backpressure against which fluid is drained. Postpartum shifts in fluid volume might also contribute to formation of puerperal interstitial pulmonary edema. At delivery, blood volume remains expanded, but vena caval obstruction is released and vascular capacitance is suddenly decreased by the loss of the placenta and uterine contraction.

Knowing whether lung water actually is increased during pregnancy awaits development of a safe, accurate, sensitive method for measuring lung water. Until better information is available, it seems reasonable to suspect that the normal "safety factors" protecting the lungs against alveolar edema accumulation (Flick, 1988) are reduced in pregnancy and the early postpartum period.

D. Pleural Space

In one study, small pleural effusions were a common finding in the first 24 hrs after normal vaginal delivery (Hughson et al., 1982). Three-fourths of the effusions were bilateral, the rest unilateral with right- and left-sided effusions occurring with equal frequency. The protein composition of these effusions was not investigated, but they resolved uneventfully and were probably transudates. In another study, small pleural effusions were detected in 97% of women after vaginal delivery or cesarean section (Stark and Pollack, 1986). In addition to the reasons discussed above as to why fluid flow across the lungs might be increased during pregnancy and the puerperium, pleural pressure would be more negative when the distortions of the rib cage and diaphragm are released at delivery, thus tending to suck fluid into the pleural space.

III. Vascular Bed

Although pulmonary vascular manifestations of obstetric and reproductive tract conditions are rare, they account for a disproportionate share of maternal deaths (Hollingsworth et al., 1989; Weinberger et al., 1980). Pulmonary edema, pulmonary embolism, and pulmonary hypertension are the major complications.

Each can occur in both the pregnant and nonpregnant states. A current review focused on acute respiratory failure in pregnancy (Hollingsworth et al., 1989). A comprehensive review of cardiopulmonary pathophysiology is, of course, beyond the scope of this chapter. Four previous volumes in the Lung Biology in Health and Disease series have considered disorders of the pulmonary vascular bed in detail (Staub, 1978; Moser, 1979; Weir and Reeves, 1989; Scharf and Cassidy, 1989).

A. Pulmonary Edema

The pathophysiology of pulmonary edema and acute lung injury is discussed elsewhere in detail (Flick, 1988; Staub, 1978). Fluid flow out of the vascular space into the lungs is determined by the product of the hydrostatic and osmotic driving pressures in the microcirculation and the barrier permeability in those vessels. Thus, there are two distinct types of pulmonary edema: that due to alterations in the balance of pressures (increased pressure pulmonary edema) and that due to alterations in microvascular permeability (increased permeability pulmonary edema). These types are distinguishable by the protein concentration of the edema fluid flooding the lungs. When barrier permeability is normal, water passes into the lungs much more readily than proteins, and therefore the edema fluid in increased pressure pulmonary edema has a low protein concentration relative to that in plasma (generally <60%). In contrast, when the lungs are injured and barrier permeability is compromised, proteins leak easily into the extravascular space, and therefore increased permeability pulmonary edema fluid has almost the same protein concentration as plasma (generally >70%). Determination of the relative concentration of proteins in edema fluid (usually suctioned through an endotracheal tube) and plasma is the single most useful test for identifying the type of pulmonary edema (Flick, 1988). Because therapy differs between types, such information can be clinically relevant. Unfortunately, these measurements have not been reported very often, even though they can be made at the bedside with a hand-held refractometer. Measurements are most helpful early in the course of pulmonary edema, because fluid is cleared from the lungs more rapidly than proteins as edema resolves, which leads to an increase in the edema fluid protein concentration (Matthay and Wiener-Kronish, 1988).

Pressure-Driven Edema

There are four pressures driving fluid filtration in the lungs. Intravascular hydrostatic and interstitial osmotic pressure act to move fluid into the interstitium. These are opposed by interstitial hydrostatic and intravascular osmotic pressures, which act to move fluid into the vascular space. The most important of these pressures is the intravascular hydrostatic pressure, but the low intravascular osmotic pressure in pregnancy (Hollingsworth et al., 1989; Hughson et al., 1982; MacLennan et al., 1987) accentuates its effects.

Volume Overload

Overdistention of the pulmonary vascular bed causes a rise in vascular pressure and consequently can lead to pulmonary edema. Pregnant women may be especially vulnerable to volume overload because their vascular "tank" is already full (discussed above). Sodium and water retention can be augmented at the time of delivery by oxytocin and by volume and capacitance shifts (also discussed above). Iatrogenic volume overload is probably the most common cause of pulmonary edema near term and has been a serious complication of therapies to postpone delivery (discussed in more detail below). The diagnosis is often obvious from the clinical situation and must be suspected whenever intravenous fluids have been administered during pregnancy or delivery. Another possible iatrogenic source of volume overload can be escape into the maternal circulation of hypertonic saline used to induce abortion.

A rare cause of increased pressure pulmonary edema is peripartum cardiomyopathy (James and Healy, 1989; Rutherford and Hands, 1989; Veille, 1984), an idiopathic dilated cardiomyopathy associated with pregnancy. The disorder is more common in underdeveloped areas, such as Africa (where it may complicate up to 10% of pregnancies), than in the United States (where it complicates less than 1:1300–4000 deliveries). Peripartum cardiomyopathy is a diagnosis of exclusion, and unrecognized underlying cardiovascular disease can often be discovered by an assiduous search (Cunningham et al., 1986). Because of misdiagnosis, the true U.S. incidence may be closer to 1:15,000 deliveries than to the figures cited above. Patients typically present during the last trimester or in the early months after delivery with symptoms of biventricular congestive heart failure and embolic phenomena are common. Initial mortality can be high (25–50%), and the condition tends to recur with subsequent pregnancies, even if there was interim recovery.

Tocolytic Therapy

Pulmonary edema associated with the use of beta-adrenergic agents to inhibit labor (tocolytic therapy) was the subject of a recent review (Pisani and Rosenow, 1989). Less than 5% of pregnant women who receive tocolytic agents develop pulmonary edema, which becomes increasingly likely as therapy is prolonged and usually resolves rapidly when these agents are withdrawn and diuretics and oxygen are administered. Terbutaline, isoxsuprine, ritodrine, and salbutamol are most commonly used. They are believed to inhibit labor by increasing intracellular cyclic adenosine monophosphate, which in turn decreases the activity of myosin light-chain kinase, the rate-limiting enzyme leading to uterine contraction. Other effects of beta-receptor stimulation include tachycardia, vasodilation, hyperglycemia, hypokalemia, antidiuresis, and, of course, bronchodilation (Benedetti, 1986).

Pulmonary edema has not been a complication of asthma treatment with high doses of beta-sympathomimetic agents. Edema associated with these agents in pregnancy has occurred almost exclusively after tocolytic therapy has failed to arrest labor. The likely cause is congruence of factors promoting volume overload and resultant increased pressure pulmonary edema. As noted above, pregnant women are especially vulnerable because they are already on the edge of volume overload. Administration of tocolytic agents can push them over that edge in a variety of ways. First, beta-sympathomimetic agents cause vasodilation and tachycardia, which are treated with fluid loading, in addition to the obligatory volume load involved in administering tocolytic therapy. Second, beta-sympathomimetic agents promote volume overload by increasing sodium and water resorption under the influence of beta receptors in the proximal tubules, by increasing the secretion of antidiuretic hormone and plasma renin, and by decreasing renal blood flow and consequently glomerular filtration rate. Many of the afflicted women are also given steroids to accelerate fetal lung maturation in case labor cannot be halted, and mineralocorticoid activity adds to sodium and fluid retention. Third, hypotonic fluid overload and tocolytic therapy have been associated with a significant decrease in serum albumin concentration, which may lower the threshold for hydrostatic (increased pressure) pulmonary edema (mentioned above). Fourth, beta-sympathomimetic agents stimulate an already hyperkinetic circulation (discussed above) and may have direct cardiac effects, including increased myocardial stiffness; ischemia as a consequence of tachycardia and short, low-pressure diastole; and arrhythmias due to increased excitability of the heart and to accelerated conduction in the atrioventricular node. Although cardiac failure has not been shown to be the primary cause of pulmonary edema in tocolytic therapy (Benedetti, 1986; Wagner et al., 1981), subtle compromise of cardiac function might add to the precarious volume situation. Finally, infection may be the cause of the premature labor that is being treated, and the state of volume overload will be complicated by leaky capillaries (increased permeability pulmonary edema caused by infection is discussed in more detail below). Although pulmonary edema usually occurs during therapy, in some cases it may be delayed until after therapy has been stopped. A factor in these cases might be the increased venous tone expected when vasodilator beta-sympathomimetics are no longer being administered, resulting in volume shifts into the thorax, increased lung microvascular hydrostatic pressure, and therefore pulmonary edema.

There are two separate reports of high pulmonary edema fluid relative to plasma protein concentration in the setting of tocolytic therapy (Hawker, 1984; Russi et al., 1988). This, of course, would not be expected if the pulmonary edema associated with tocolytic therapy were purely of the increased pressure type, as discussed earlier in this chapter. These findings, however, might have been related to a delay in time at which the edema fluid was sampled or to underlying infection. Definitive characterization of the type of pulmonary edema associated with tocolytic therapy awaits more complete information about the protein concentration of pulmonary edema fluid from a broader sample of patients undergoing therapy for premature labor.

Eclampsia

In pregnancy complicated by preeclampsia or eclampsia, the basic problem is generalized arteriolar vasospasm, which does not, however, involve the pulmonary circulation. The result is peripheral edema, proteinuria, and hypertension (preeclampsia), and ultimately convulsions (eclampsia) (Sibai et al., 1987; Villar and Sibai, 1988; Wasserstrum and Cotton, 1986). The cause is unknown. The hypothesis of placental overproduction of vasoconstrictor metabolites of arachidonic acid does not appear credible without an explanation of why the pulmonary vascular bed is spared. Pulmonary edema is not frequent (about 2%) unless there is other, superimposed disease (risk rises to about 7%). A combination of causes can lead to pulmonary edema. First, there is the volume overload and low colloid osmotic pressure of pregnancy already discussed above. Although characteristic of preeclampsia-eclampsia is that intravascular volume is contracted relative to that in normal pregnancy, in the presence of contracted vasculature, fluid loading can rapidly result in pulmonary edema. Second, severe hypertension in these patients compromises cardiac function by increasing afterload, which may lead to increased pulmonary vascular pressures. Third, arteriolar vasospasm can result in oliguria, which compounds sodium and fluid retention. Finally, the usual therapy with magnesium sulfate to prevent convulsions has effects similar to those of beta-sympathomimetic therapy, such as hypotension and tachycardia, that require therapeutic volume expansion. Pulmonary edema is much more likely after than before delivery, perhaps as a result of the volume shifts that occur in the immediate postpartum period (discussed above).

The results of studies of 10 patients with severe preeclampsia complicated by pulmonary edema, who required invasive hemodynamic monitoring (Benedetti et al., 1985), showed that the administration of large volumes of fluid and consequent volume overload was the most common cause of pulmonary edema in this setting (accounting for pulmonary edema in half the patients). An increase in capillary permeability (30%), probably associated with sepsis, and cardiac failure (20%), probably a result of high systemic vascular resistance, also occurred. Pulmonary edema (4.5%) and pleural effusions (7%) have also been reported in a subset of severe preeclampsia described as the HELLP syndrome (named from the occurrence of *h*emolysis, *e*levated *l*iver enzymes, and *l*ow *p*latelet count) (Sibai et al., 1986). The major additional complication in these patients is frequent intravascular coagulopathy.

Permeability Edema

Acute lung injuries of diverse etiologies with resultant increased permeability pulmonary edema are often grouped under the rubric of the "adult respiratory distress syndrome" (ARDS). The general problem is discussed elsewhere in detail (Flick, 1988). Recent reports have collected cases of ARDS of various causes complicating pregnancy (Smith et al., 1990) and of pulmonary injury complicating antepartum pyelonephritis (Cunningham et al., 1987). Permeability edema is quite uncommon, occurring almost always in the last trimester, and from obstetric problems only in about 1:3900 pregnancies, and in 2% of pregnant women admitted to hospital for pyelonephritis (incidence about 1:5400 pregnancies). The mortality in the ARDS of diverse causes from various series, excluding patients who did not have obstetric causes, was 50%, but less than 7% of the women with pulmonary injury associated with pyelonephritis died.

Other than this excellent survival rate in the setting of pyelonephritis, which is probably due to the young age and good health of most pregnant women, there is nothing distinguishing increased permeability pulmonary edema resulting from obstetric and reproductive tract problems from that reported in general series. The underlying cause is usually infection. Obstetric foci have included chorioamnionitis, endometritis, and pelvic abscess. On a global scale, septic abortion is likely the most common cause, and endometritis is most common following operative delivery. Death can occur early, from fulminant shock, or late, from multiple organ system failure. In addition to obstetric infection, increased permeability pulmonary edema can be associated with tocolytic therapy (see above), eclampsia (see above), abruptio placentae, uterine hemorrhage or rupture, retained placenta, and trophoblastic disease (discussed below).

Lung injury and pulmonary edema from aspiration of gastric contents into the tracheobronchial tree was first described in women undergoing labor and delivery (so-called Mendelson's syndrome) (Mendelson, 1946), and it remains a significant cause of total maternal deaths (2%), accounting for 30–50% of maternal mortality associated with anesthesia (Hollingsworth et al., 1989; Noble et al., 1988). Factors contributing to an increased risk for aspiration of stomach contents in pregnancy include: increased intragastric pressure caused by compression by the gravid uterus; relaxation of the lower esophageal sphincter under the influence of progesterone; delayed gastric emptying during labor; and diminished laryngeal reflexes associated with analgesia. The greatest risk for aspiration during pregnancy—by far—is general anesthesia. It may not be possible to lower the incidence because anesthesia must often be induced for emergency cesarean section. It is prudent to assume that all pregnant women whose airways must be controlled will aspirate, and to use special care during induction, intubation, and extubation. While attention has been focused on the role of gastric acid in causing a chemical pneumonitis, aspiration of gastric contents with a high pH is not always benign. The lungs can be flooded by large volumes, which causes asphyxia rather than pneumonitis, or, alternatively, aspirated food particles can obstruct the airways or provoke an intense inflammatory responses.

Pulmonary emboli and infections (discussed in detail below) can also cause increased permeability pulmonary edema. An additional, but rare, cause has been direct toxicity or anaphylaxis associated with the use of 32% dextran 70 as the distending medium for hysteroscopy (Leake et al., 1987; Zbella et al., 1985).

Therapeutic Considerations

The therapy of pulmonary edemas has been discussed elsewhere in detail (Flick, 1988). Special therapeutic considerations in pregnancy arise from the presence of the dependent fetus, whose interests may not always be congruent with its mother's. Generally, therapy should be directed at the mother, because the fetus is most at risk from maternal decompensation. Attempted delivery of an unstable mother will often result in a distressed fetus and is usually best avoided unless the fetal compartment is a source of sepsis.

There are a few special considerations associated with intubation and mechanical ventilation in pregnancy (Hollingsworth et al., 1989). The indications are no different from those in nonpregnant patients. However, hyperemia associated with pregnancy can narrow the upper airway and increase the risk of trauma at intubation; for this reason, small endotracheal tubes are recommended and nasotracheal intubation should probably be avoided. As noted above, oxygen reserve may be limited by the decreased FRC, and apnea during intubation should be as brief as possible. Tidal volume can be selected using general guidelines based on lean body weight. Excessive ventilation should be avoided because alkalosis decreases uterine blood flow. In spontaneously breathing patients, intermittent mandatory ventilation (IMV) may produce less hyperventilation than assist modes, particularly during labor. Patients on IMV should also be able to assist with labor, allowing spontaneous vaginal delivery (Sosin et al., 1986). Morphine sulfate and pancuronium bromide can be used for sedation and paralysis without adverse fetal effects, except at delivery. Benzodiazepines are customarily avoided during the first trimester because of increased risk of congenital defects and should be avoided in hemodynamically unstable patients, regardless of whether they are pregnant or not, because these drugs can cause profound hypotension and their effects are, unlike morphine's, not readily reversible. There is no information about weaning pregnant patients from ventilators, but it may be best to position them in the left lateral decubitus position rather than in the usual seated position, to avoid venal caval compression.

The hemodynamic status in pregnancy complicated by severe pulmonary edema can be clinically uncertain, and in preeclampsia and eclampsia can be extremely variable. Therefore, invasive hemodynamic monitoring may be helpful in management (Clark and Cotton, 1988; Wasserstrum and Cotton, 1986). Fetal monitoring is also useful, especially when the mother is very ill and as the complexity of therapy must be increased. In situations where intravascular volume needs to be expanded, administration of packed red blood cells can be advantageous, both because erythrocytes tend to stay in the intravascular space and because oxygen-carrying capacity is thereby increased.

Special consideration should be given before administering vasoactive drugs. The placenta is not a protected vascular bed, and the uterine arterioles are very sensitive to exogenous vasopressors. Dopamine, dobutamine, and norepinephrine may cause decreased uterine blood flow. The first option to pursue when hypotension complicates pulmonary edema is to elevate the right hip so that the gravid uterus is moved away from the inferior vena cava. In pregnancy, the Trendelenburg position may actually decrease venous return because of vena cava compression. Hypotension unresponsive to reduction of uterine pressure on the inferior vena cava and fluid resuscitation (if appropriate) is best treated with beta-adrenergic agents, such as ephedrine or metaraminol, that tend to preserve uterine blood flow as well as increase maternal systemic pressure. Caution also must be used when administering vasodilators. Nitroprusside therapy may be complicated by fetal cyanide or thiocyanate toxicity, or by fetal bradycardia secondary to reduced maternal cardiac output unless maternal intravascular volume is first expanded.

The single most important therapeutic consideration in increased permeability pulmonary edema is to find and treat infection. In the presence of infection, it is unlikely that any therapy will be of much use unless the infection is identified and treated.

B. Pulmonary Embolism

The pathophysiology of pulmonary embolism is discussed elsewhere in detail (Moser, 1988). Obstruction of blood flow in the lungs results in an increase in alveolar dead space from regions of lung that remain ventilated but are not perfused. The reduction of vascular cross-sectional area in the lungs causes an increase in pulmonary vascular resistance and in the work the heart must do to move blood through the lungs. Pulmonary hypertension does not develop until 40–60% of the pulmonary vascular bed has been obstructed. The consequences of pulmonary vascular obstruction depend on how much the vascular cross-sectional area of the lungs is reduced. At one end of the spectrum, when the main pulmonary artery or large vessels are suddenly blocked, the primary effect is immediate failure of the right ventricle and possibly death. At the other end of the spectrum, when very small vessels are involved there may be no discernible effects. The respiratory response to vascular obstruction is usually tachypnea, and patients frequently complain of dyspnea. Hypoxemia develops due to some combination of ventilation-perfusion mismatching in those areas of the lungs where blood continues to flow, atelectasis, and heart failure.

Thromboembolism

The pulmonary manifestations of thromboembolism have been discussed in reviews of thromboembolic disease in pregnancy (Bolan, 1983; Rutherford and Phelan, 1986), and also in more general reviews of pregnancy and the lungs (Hollingsworth et al., 1989; Weinberger et al., 1980). Pulmonary thromboembolism can complicate not only pregnancy and the puerperium, but also surgery for cervical and uterine malignancy (Clarke-Pearson et al., 1983), oral contraceptive use (even if estrogen dose is low) (Helmrich et al., 1987), and abortion (Lawson et al., 1990).

Attention is usually focused on the hypercoagulable state in pregnancy and on the normal, low-grade, chronic, disseminated intravascular coagulation within the placental bed. However, the risk of thromboembolism is greatest in the postpartum rather than in the antepartum period. The risk is also increased by cesarean section (10-fold) and other surgical procedures during pregnancy and the early puerperium (including assisted delivery), by bed rest for complications of pregnancy, and by suppression of lactation with estrogens. Important risk factors appear to include venous stasis, injury to pelvic blood vessels, and increased production of fibrinogen, other clotting factors, and inhibitors of fibrinolysis as the body prepares for placental separation. Apart from these considerations during pregnancy and estrogen therapy, deep-vein thrombosis in apparently healthy patients can be a premonitory sign of occult reproductive tract cancers (Aderka et al., 1986).

Amniotic Fluid Embolism

Amniotic fluid embolism was the subject of two recent, comprehensive reviews (Clark, 1986b; Price et al., 1985) and has been discussed in general reviews of pregnancy and the lungs (Hollingsworth et al., 1989; Noble et al., 1988; Weinberger et al., 1980). It is not a common occurrence (about 1:40,000–60,000 deliveries), but with a mortality rate over 85%, it accounts for 10–15% of total maternal deaths. Although usually associated with delivery, it has been reported as early as 20 weeks' gestation and as late as 32 hr postpartum and has been associated with cesarean delivery, abortion (about 1:400,000), amniocentesis, and intrauterine pressure catheters.

Patients suddenly develop dyspnea, cyanosis, and profound hypotension. Those who survive the first hour (less than 75%) go on to develop pulmonary edema (up to 75%), hemorrhage (about 50%), and tonic-clonic seizures (10–20%). Hemodynamic measurements have shown left ventricular failure.

Laboratory studies often indicate disseminated intravascular coagulation. Clinically suspected amniotic fluid embolism is said to be confirmed at autopsy by finding mucin, fetal squamous cells, lanugo, vernix caseosa, or bile-containing meconium in the pulmonary vasculature. The diagnosis also has been made by finding debris of fetal origin in sputum or in blood aspirated from central venous or pulmonary arterial catheters. The presence of fetal debris in venous blood, however, is not pathognomonic, as it can be found in the pulmonary arterial blood of most pregnant women undergoing pulmonary artery catheterization for whatever reason (Clark, 1986b; Lee et al., 1986).

The pathogenesis and mechanism of amniotic fluid embolism are quite obscure. Entry of amniotic fluid into the maternal venous system involves its connection with the amniotic sac, which may occur when the uterus is instrumented or when the membranes rupture. Many cases involve placental abruption (up to 50%) or prior fetal death (40%), and in some cases the fetal head pushed against the cervix might act as a pump pushing amniotic fluid under high pressure into the lower uterus or cervix. How much fluid does or needs to enter the maternal circulation to initiate the clinical syndrome is unknown. Also unknown is how the syndrome is initiated. The results of studies in experimental animal models have been contradictory and confusing. In the only studies in primates, intravenous injections of amniotic fluid were entirely innocuous, and in other species, the amount of fluid that had to be injected to elicit responses was very large. No animal model has come close to replicating the human amniotic fluid embolism syndrome. Suggestions that humoral substances, such as leukotriene D_4 (Azegami and Mori, 1986) or complement (Hammerschmidt et al., 1984), contribute to the pathogenesis are not very convincing. The clinical syndrome is probably multifactorial, involving intravascular activation of the inflammatory response and coagulation cascade, humoral substances in amniotic fluid, vascular obstruction by debris, and perhaps direct toxic effects of amniotic fluid on the lungs and myocardium.

There are two reports in human amniotic fluid embolism of pulmonary edema fluid protein concentration relative to that in plasma. It is a split decision. In one case, the ratio was 55% (Girard et al., 1986), which indicates increased pressure pulmonary edema and which is consistent with the presence of acute left ventricular failure characteristic of the amniotic fluid embolism syndrome. But in the other case, the ratio was 96% (Masson et al., 1979), indicating increased permeability pulmonary edema. This edema fluid sample was collected early, and there was no evidence of infection.

A serious difficulty in understanding the amniotic fluid embolism syndrome, in addition to the lack of suitable animal models, is the tendency of the diagnosis to become a wastebasket for all cases of unexplained death in labor. Better information will be hard to come by owing to the syndrome's unpredictable, rapid, and catastrophic nature. It might be possible, however, to gain better understanding of at least the type of pulmonary edema involved if edema fluid were sampled early in more cases for measurement of protein concentration.

Air Embolism

Venous air embolism has been associated with normal labor, delivery of patients with placenta previa, criminal abortions using air, legal abortions by suction or dilation and evacuation, insufflation of the vagina during gynecological procedures, douching, and orogenital sex play (Hollingsworth et al., 1989; Kaufman et al., 1987; Lawson et al., 1990). The lungs can respond to air embolism in three ways. First, if large amounts of air collect in the right ventricle, its outflow tract can be obstructed and the patient may die quickly because no blood can flow into the lungs. Second, when air passes into the pulmonary circulation, the patient can suffer pulmonary hypertension and right heart failure if enough cross-sectional area is obstructed (as in thromboembolism, discussed above). Third, air in the pulmonary circulation (even in amounts not sufficient to cause hypertension) results in increased permeability pulmonary edema. Because air is resorbed from the vascular space into the alveoli, the problem tends to be short-lived. The mechanism of lung injury in air embolism is believed primarily to involve activation of inflammatory responses (Clark and Flick, 1984).

Diagnostic and Therapeutic Considerations

As in the case of pulmonary edema, special diagnostic and therapeutic considerations concerning thromboembolism in pregnancy arise from the presence of the fetus. Noninvasive diagnostic tests are preferred, but ^{125}I-labeled fibrinogen scanning is contraindicated because unbound ^{125}I crosses the placental barrier and collects in the fetal thyroid; ^{125}I has also been detected in breast milk. Adverse fetal effects have not been reported from ventilation (^{133}Xe) and perfusion (^{99m}Tc) lung scans.

Warfarin, with its small molecular weight, can cross the placenta and enter the fetal circulation. Its use in pregnancy is associated with a variety of congenital abnormalities, and there is a high risk of fetal hemorrhage in utero and with delivery. For these reasons, heparin is the anticoagulant of choice. Its high molecular weight prevents it from crossing the placenta, and it can be effectively self-administered over the long-term by subcutaneous injection. Thrombolytic therapy can also be used during pregnancy (streptokinase usually does not cross the placenta), but the danger of serious maternal bleeding is very high in the puerperium (due primarily to the raw surface area left behind when the placenta is extruded). If the lytic state must be rapidly reversed before delivery, aprotinin (Trasylol), which does not cross the placenta, is preferred over aminocaproic acid, which does.

There really are no therapeutic considerations for amniotic fluid embolism. The disorder is so swift and catastrophic, and knowledge so limited, that only heroic supportive measures can be advised. Heparin therapy in bleeding patients with disseminated intravascular coagulation is controversial and cannot be recommended. Air embolism is usually transient and self-limited unless the right ventricular outflow tract is obstructed, in which case the patient should be placed in the left lateral decubitus position to attempt to move air away from the outflow tract. Closed-chest cardiac massage may help move air into the lungs, and air might be aspirated with a pulmonary artery catheter. The difficulty, of course, is to think of the diagnosis in time to do anything about it.

C. Pulmonary Hypertension

Pulmonary hypertension, whatever the etiology, carries a grave prognosis during pregnancy (mortality about 50%) (Clark, 1986a; Dawkins et al., 1986; James and Healy, 1989; Weinberger et al., 1980). The increases in cardiac output and blood volume during pregnancy, labor, delivery, and the postpartum period are poorly tolerated in the presence of pulmonary hypertension and may precipitate acute right ventricular failure with severely decreased cardiac output and sudden death. Pregnancy is best avoided, and abortion is advised as the most appropriate management for women with pulmonary hypertension of any etiology, and even mild severity, who do get pregnant. If they choose to continue their pregnancies, bed rest, anticoagulation, and attendance by skilled obstetricians, cardiologists, and anesthesiologists are recommended, but may prove futile because of the dangers involved.

Primary (idiopathic) pulmonary hypertension is principally a disease of young women in their childbearing years. Whether and how this could be a pulmonary manifestation of pregnancy or of other conditions of the reproductive tract is unknown.

IV. Airways

The lungs respond to hormonal changes during the menstrual cycle in much the same way as in pregnancy, albeit to a lesser degree (Schoene et al., 1981; Takano, 1982; White et al., 1983). Thus, during the luteal phase, when progesterone concentration is high, hypoxic and hypercapneic ventilatory responses increase, whereas $P_{A_{CO_2}}$, Pa_{CO_2}, and maximal exercise O_2 consumption and CO_2 production decrease. Respiratory frequency is unchanged. The finding of increased resting mouth occlusion pressures, which are thought to be a reflection of the total neural output of the respiratory system, is consistent with the hypothesis that progesterone acts centrally to augment ventilation. Because $\dot{V}_E$ increases with no change in respiratory frequency, tidal volume must be increased.

Other changes noted in pregnancy may be overlooked in the menstrual cycle because they are quite modest or have not been systematically investigated.

A. Reactivity

Asthma

The effects of pregnancy on asthma and its management were the subject of two comprehensive reviews (Greenberger and Patterson, 1985; Turner et al., 1980) and have been discussed in general reviews of pregnancy and the lungs (Hollingsworth et al., 1989; Noble et al., 1988; Weinberger et al., 1980). Pregnancy makes asthma either better (30%), worse (20%), or has no effect (50%). Prediction of which will be the case is impossible, but patients with severe asthma antedating pregnancy often become worse, and whatever the effect in any given patient, it is likely to be repeated in her subsequent pregnancies. Because Pa_{CO_2} is normally lower in pregnancy, fatigue and imminent respiratory failure during acute attacks may be indicated by Pa_{CO_2} in the low to mid-30s (mmHg) (i.e., at lower Pa_{CO_2} than in the nonpregnant state).

The effect of the menstrual cycle on asthma has also been studied (Eliasson et al., 1986; Juniper et al., 1987; Weinmann et al., 1987). Most women report no change in their symptoms, although about a third complain of worsening in the premenstrual-menstrual period (often in conjunction with complaints of dysmenorrhea) (Eliasson et al., 1986). Airway responsiveness is unaffected by menses and oral contraceptives, and asthmatic symptoms are not related to progesterone or to airway responsiveness (Juniper et al., 1987).

Allergic Reactions

Human seminal plasma allergy has been reported as a cause of postcoital asthma (Blair and Parish, 1985; Shah et al., 1988). Desensitization was successful in one case (Blair and Parish, 1985).

B. Chronic Respiratory Diseases

Most pregnant women are young and in good health, but there are several recent reports of the effects of pregnancy in women with various chronic obstructive and restrictive lung diseases, including cystic fibrosis (Noble et al., 1988; Palmer et al., 1983), bronchiectasis (Thaler et al., 1986), and kyphoscoliosis and myasthenia gravis (Noble et al., 1988). Knowledge about pregnancy in women with borderline respiratory function and limited reserve is not very extensive (Weinberger et al., 1980), and how much function is needed to sustain a pregnancy in unknown. As could be expected, the most severely compromised patients fare worst. The largest experience is in cystic fibrosis (Palmer et al., 1983). Maternal and infant morbidity and mortality were high in women who were in poor condition or had severe disease, but other women's overall condition was little affected.

Patients with impaired respiratory systems may not be able to cope with the additional respiratory and cardiac demands of pregnancy, but there are no certain guidelines for advising such women. Those with baseline CO_2 retention or pulmonary hypertension (discussed above) probably face unacceptable risks.

C. Control of Breathing

Sex hormones affect the control of breathing. Compared to men, women have greater resting minute ventilation per millimeter of CO_2 produced and consequently lower PA_{CO_2}, lower tidal volume (even when corrected for body surface area), greater respiratory frequency, and lower hypoxic and hypercapneic ventilatory responses (White et al., 1983). Testosterone has been shown to increase $\dot{V}_{O_2}$, $\dot{V}_E$, and the hypoxic ventilatory response, but to have no effect on PA_{CO_2} or on the hypercapneic ventilatory response (White et al., 1985). How these effects might contribute to clinical observations that men and postmenopausal women suffer from sleep-disordered breathing much more frequently than do premenopausal women is not entirely clear. The hypoxic ventilatory responses of both men and women fall to their lowest levels during rapid-eye-movement sleep, but there is no difference between men and women in their ventilatory responses during sleep, owing to a steep fall in male ventilatory responsiveness but only a small fall in female ventilatory responsiveness (White et al., 1982).

D. Hemoptysis

Catamenial hemoptysis is recurrent hemoptysis associated with menstrual periods (Bateman and Morrison, 1990; Elliot et al., 1985; Grimm et al., 1988; Lawrence, 1988). Less than 20 cases have been reported. Endometrial tissue presumably arrives in the tracheobronchial tree by hematogenous dissemination and bleeds in response to hormonal stimulation. If the source of bleeding cannot be seen on routine chest roentgenograms, it may be possible to learn which side is involved by bronchoscopy at the time of bleeding and to locate the aberrant endometrium by thoracic computed tomography scanning. Therapeutic options include surgical resection or suppression of the endometrial tissue with progesterone or the antigonadotrophic agent danazol. The problem has also resolved following the menopause. Endometriosis is discussed further below (Section VI, "Pleural Space," and Section VII, "Growths"). Intermittent hemoptysis also occurs in lymphangiomyomatosis (Dishner et al., 1984; Taylor et al., 1990) (discussed below).

V. Lung Parenchyma

"Lung parenchyma" is used here in a very loose sense to refer to pulmonary manifestations of reproductive tract conditions that are generalized.

A. Infection

Pulmonary infections complicating pregnancy have been discussed in general reviews of pregnancy and the lungs (Hollingsworth et al., 1989; Noble et al., 1988; Weinberger et al., 1980). Tolerance of the fetal allograft may be mediated in part by suppression of the maternal immune response. There is evidence that maternal in vitro cell-mediated immune responses are diminished, particularly in the second and third trimesters (Lederman, 1984). Clinical immunosuppression is not profound. Pregnancy does not appear to increase the risk of acquiring viral infections, but there may be excess mortality during influenza pandemics. The mortality of pregnant women with varicella pneumonia has been reported to be more than double that of nonpregnant patients (45% versus 15–20%), and varicella-zoster infections appear to progress to pneumonia more frequently in women in their second and third trimesters than in in other women.

Effects of pregnancy are not limited to impairment of host immune factors. Increased 17-β-estradiol levels during pregnancy are a powerful growth stimulant to *Coccidioides immitis*. Both progesterone and testosterone also stimulate its growth (Catanzaro, 1984). The risk of dissemination of *C. immitis* primary lung infection (20% compared to 0.2% in nonpregnant patients) is highest during the third trimester of pregnancy and may be associated with a high mortality rate. Another effect of pregnancy unrelated to host immune responses is sequestration of malaria parasites in the placenta, which acts as a reservoir for their maturation. Resulting persistent parasitemia can lead to "malarial lung" (Petersen et al., 1988; Phillips, 1984; Warrell, 1987). This usually fatal condition is believed to be an increased permeability type of pulmonary edema.

The effect of pregnancy on tuberculosis has been the subject of controversy (Snider, 1984), but pregnancy does not appear to be a risk factor for tuberculosis. Tuberculin skin testing is probably valid throughout the course of pregnancy despite decreased in vitro lymphocyte reactivity to purified protein derivative (PPD). There is no solid evidence that pregnancy has an adverse effect on tuberculosis, and indications for chemotherapy and the basic principles of management in pregnant women are no different from those in nonpregnant patients.

B. Sarcoid

Two general reviews include discussions of sarcoidosis in pregnancy (Noble et al., 1988; Weinberger et al., 1980). The condition of most pregnant women with sarcoidosis remains unchanged or improves, but it can deteriorate (de Regt, 1987). The frequent ameliorating effect of pregnancy on sarcoidosis has been attributed to increased circulating corticosteroids and to suppressed immune responses. It is not possible to predict which patients will fare poorly, although it seems likely that women with the most severe cardiopulmonary compromise are at the highest risk.

C. Rare Diseases

There have been sporadic case reports of various rare pulmonary diseases complicated by pregnancy. Pregnancy had adverse effects on idiopathic pulmonary hemosiderosis (Michaeli et al., 1987) and on familial fibrosing alveolitis (Prichard and Musk, 1984). A patient with severe alveolar proteinosis suffered progressive clinical and respiratory deterioration during pregnancy, which was safely ameliorated with whole-lung bronchopulmonary lavage (Matuschak et al., 1984). The cardiopulmonary demands of pregnancy will probably be met with difficulty by any woman with antecedent severe underlying pulmonary disease of whatever etiology.

VI. Pleural Space

A. Pneumothorax/Pneumomediastinum

Catamenial pneumothoraces are recurrent pneumothoraces associated with menstrual periods. Less than 100 cases have been reported (Schoenfeld et al., 1986), and the syndrome accounted for less than 3% of the spontaneous pneumothoraces in an epidemiological study of Japanese women (Nakamura et al., 1986). The characteristic pattern is for a small, almost always right-sided (90%) pneumothorax to occur within 24–72 hr. of the onset of menstruation. However, a case has been reported in which pneumothoraces occurred at midcycle (Ghio and Crapo, 1988). Pneumothoraces have been prevented by suppressing ovulation, but a case was reported in which catamenial pneumothorax occurred both when the patient was taking contraceptives and when she was pregnant (Schoenfeld et al., 1986). Tubal ligation has cured some patients (Müller and Nelems, 1986). The pathogenesis of this syndrome is quite obscure, and there are numerous inventive, but unproven theories that attempt to explain how air finds its way into the pleural space coincident with the menses (Ghio and Crapo, 1988; Müller and Nelems, 1986; Schoenfeld et al., 1986). Some cases are associated with endometriosis (20–40%). Factors that could be involved include entry of air into the peritoneum from the fallopian tubes via the uterus when the cervix is open during menstruation, diaphragmatic lacunas and defects connecting the thoracic and peritoneal cavities, air trapping by tissue (endometrial and maybe even bronchial) swelling in response to humoral changes during the menstrual cycles, and local effects of cyclical bleeding, sloughing, and regeneration of ectopic endometrium. Therapeutic options included suppression of ovulation and pleural symphysis. Pneumothoraces can also be seen associated with lumphangiomyomatosis (Dishner et al., 1984; Taylor et al., 1990) (discussed below).

In addition to periodic pneumothoraces, catamenial pneumomediastinum without pneumothorax in association with endometriosis has been reported (Shahar and Angelillo, 1986). Spontaneous pneumomediastinum is also a rare complication of labor (Karson et al., 1984). The likely mechanism is either high pressure generated during Valsalva maneuvers causing alveoli to rupture or dissection from pneumoperitoneum generated when membranes are ruptured.

B. Effusions

Metastatic neoplasms originating from the breast (15–20%), the ovaries (10%), and, more uncommonly, the endometrium, cervix, or penis account for a significant proportion of malignant pleural effusions (Irani et al., 1987; Johnston, 1985). Patients with various ovarian neoplasms complicated by ascites can develop hydrothorax (Meigs-Salmon syndrome), as described by Matthay in Chapter 6, this volume. Transudates, often massive, are more frequent on the right side, but can be on the left or bilateral. Surgical removal of the pelvic tumor usually resolves the problem. Catamenial hemothorax (Hibbard et al., 1981) is a very rare cause of abnormal fluid collection in the pleural space. Chylous pleural effusions associated with lymphangiomyomatosis (discussed below) have also been reported (Dishner et al., 1984; Sheth et al., 1984; Taylor et al., 1990).

C. Pleuritic Pain

In addition to pleuritic chest pain associated with catamenial pneumothoraces (discussed above), recurrent pleuritic chest pain timed with menstruation can occur associated with thoracic endometriosis, even though no air enters the pleural space or mediastinum (Hibbard et al., 1981; Horsfield, 1989).

VII. Growths

A. Endometriosis

Pleural and parenchymal pulmonary endometriosis have been reviewed (Foster et al., 1981), and recent case reports of lung and chest cage endometriosis were collected in a general review of extrapelvic endometriosis (Markham et al., 1989). Pleural endometriosis is believed to be caused by spread of endometrial tissue from the pelvic cavity, probably following peritoneal fluid flow through diaphragmatic lacunas or rents. Disease is almost always on the right side. The major effects are catamenial pneumothorax, pain, and hemothorax (discussed above). Most patients have pelvic endometriosis. Pulmonary parenchymal endometriosis usually occurs in women without coexisting pelvic disease and is believed to arise from embolism of endometrial tissue. Most patients have previously been pregnant or have had pelvic surgical procedures. Disease is usually in the lower lobes. The major symptom is hemoptysis (discussed above). Treatment options are discussed elsewhere (Barbieri, 1988).

B. Lymphangiomyomatosis

Pulmonary lymphangiomyomatosis was the subject of recent reports (Dishner et al., 1984; Taylor et al., 1990). Known variously as lymphangiomyomatosis, lymphangioleiomyomatosis, or leiomyomatosis, this rare disease of unknown etiology occurs exclusively in women. Most are of reproductive age, and the disorder does not appear to develop in women while their estrogen levels are low. Hamartomatous, immature smooth muscle proliferates in the alveolar walls, bronchioles, venules, lymphatics, and hilar lymph nodes. The consequences are related to this overgrowth. Proliferation of airway and alveolar smooth muscle causes obstruction, air trapping, increased lung volumes, and reduced DL_{CO}. Pneumothorax is frequent, presumably on the basis of air trapping. Proliferation of smooth muscle in the walls of pulmonary veins causes obstruction, pulmonary hemorrhage, hemoptysis, and pulmonary hemosiderosis. Finally, proliferation of perilymphatic smooth muscle and infiltration of mediastinal lymph nodes causes lymphatic obstruction and chylothorax.

Interstitial infiltrates, lung cysts, bullae, and a honeycomb pattern have been described on chest roentgenograms. Computed tomography (CT) of the chest can be valuable in suggesting the diagnosis—numerous, thin-walled cysts (mostly <10 mm in diameter) are distributed throughout the lungs, and lymphangiomyomatosis can be distinguished from the cystic changes of either emphysema, which do not have well-formed walls, or pulmonary fibrosis, which are mainly peripheral in distribution (Taylor et al., 1990). Tissue diagnosis can be made from transbronchial lung biopsy; the pathologist should be alerted to the suspected diagnosis so that the characteristic changes will not be misinterpreted as generic fibrosis (Taylor et al., 1990).

The prognosis had been thought to be dismal, with most patients dying from progressive respiratory insufficiency within 10 years of onset of symptoms (Dishner et al., 1984). The latest report was more encouraging—almost 80% of a series of 38 patients were still living more than 8 years after the onset of disease (Taylor et al., 1990). Because lymphangiomyomatosis is rare, there are only anecdotal reports of success and failure of treatments. Some patients have responded to oophorectomy or hormonal manipulation with progesterone or estrogen. Exogenous estrogen, however, can also exacerbate the disease (Shen et al., 1987). Therapy with medroxyprogesterone acetate appears to be most promising, particularly in women with chylous effusions or chylous ascites (Taylor et al., 1990).

C. Trophoblastic Disease

Circulating trophoblasts are part of normal pregnancy (Clark, 1986b; Price et al., 1985). Trophoblastic emboli can result in acute pulmonary edema either before or after removal of benign hydatidiform mole (Huberman et al., 1982;

Orr et al., 1980). Chorionic neoplasms can originate in the placenta (gestational trophoblastic disease) or in the gonads of either sex (nongestational trophoblastic disease). Pulmonary metastases are very common (Kumar et al., 1988). They can disappear following removal of the primary tumor or in response to chemotherapy (Gordon et al., 1985). Delay in diagnosis is believed to account for a higher mortality rate associated with antecedent normal pregnancy.

D. Malignant Neoplasms

Various reproductive tract neoplasms can metastasize to the lungs. Breast in women and prostate in men are the most common, but the lungs can be invaded by malignant growths originating in any of the reproductive organs and in the germ cells. Special considerations in these tumors are the possibility that patients might respond to resection of pulmonary nodules (Fuller et al., 1985), gonadal ablation, or hormonal manipulations. A more detailed discussion is beyond the scope of this chapter.

VIII. Summary

This chapter in retrospect appears to have unconsciously adopted the conventional view that sees men as "normal" in both health and disease. Therefore, mostly women's health issues have been discussed. In the broad sense, all differences between men and women in the manifestations of pulmonary diseases could be attributed to obstetric and reproductive tract conditions. This is an important health issue for both men and women. Considerable information is available, but much more is needed about the pulmonary effects of the reproductive organs.

References

Aderka, D., Brown, A., Zelikovski, A., and Pinkhas, J. (1986). Idiopathic deep vein thrombosis in an apparently healthy patient as a premonitory sign of occult cancer. *Cancer* **57**:1846–1849.

Azegami, M. and Mori, N. (1986). Amniotic fluid embolism and leukotrienes. *Am. J. Obstet. Gynocol.* **155**:1119–1124.

Barberi, R. L. (1988). New therapy for endometriosis. *N. Engl. J. Med.* **318**:512–514.

Barron, W. M. (1984). The pregnant surgical patient: medical evaluation and management. *Ann. Intern. Med.* **101**:683–691.

Bateman, E. D., and Morrison, S. C. (1990). Catamenial haemoptysis from endobronchial endometriosis—a case report and review of previously reported cases. *Respir. Med.* **84**:157–161.

Benedetti, T. J. (1986). Life-threatening complications of betamimetic therapy for preterm labor inhibition. *Clin. Perinatol.* **13**:843–852.

Benedetti, T. J., Kates, R., and Williams, V. (1985). Hemodynamic observations in severe preeclampsia complicated by pulmonary edema. *Am. J. Obstet. Gynecol.* **152**:330–234.

Berry, M. J., McMurray, R. G., and Katz, V. L. (1989). Pulmonary and ventilatory responses to pregnancy, immersion, and exercise. *J. Appl. Physiol.* **66**:857–862.

Blair, H., and Parish, W. E. (1985). Asthma and urticaria induced by seminal plasma in a woman with IgE antibody and T-lymphocyte responsiveness to a seminal plasma antigen. *Clin. Allergy* **15**:117–130.

Bolan, J. C. (1983). Thromboembolic complications of pregnancy. *Clin. Obstet. Gynecol.* **26**:913–922.

Brodeur, P., Mockus, M., McCullough, R., and Moore, L. G. (1986). Progesterone receptors and ventilatory stimulation by progestin. *J. Appl. Physiol.* **60**:590–595.

Byrne, F., Oduro-Dominah, A., and Kipling, R. (1987). The effect of pregnancy on pulmonary nitrogen washout: a study of pre-oxygenation. *Anaesthesa* **42**:148–150.

Catanzaro, A. (1984). Pulmonary mycosis in pregnant women. *Chest* **86**: 14S–18S.

Clark, M., and Flick, M. R. (1984). Permeability pulmonary edema caused by venous air embolism. *Am. Rev. Respir. Dis.* **129**:633–635.

Clark, S. L. (1986a). Labor and delivery in the patient with structural cardiac disease. *Clin. Perinatol.* **13**:695–703.

Clark, S. L. (1986b). Amniotic fluid embolism. *Clin. Perinatol.* **13**:801–811.

Clark, S. L., and Cotton, D. B. (1988). Clinical indications for pulmonary artery catheterization in the patient with severe preeclampsia. *Am. J. Obstet. Gynecol.* **158**:453–458.

Clarke-Pearson, D. L., Jelovsek, F. R., and Creasman, W. T. (1983). Thromboembolism complicating surgery for cervical and uterine malignancy: incidence, risk factors, and prophylaxis. *Obstet. Gynecol.* **61**:87–94.

Cole, R. L., and Sutton, M. S. (1989). Normal cardiopulmonary adjustments to pregnancy: cardiovascular evaluation. *Cardiovasc. Clin.* **19**:37–56.

Cunningham, F. G., Pritchard, J. A., Hankins, G. D., Anderson, P. L., Lucas, M. J., and Armstrong, K. F. (1986). Peripartum heart failure: idiopathic cardiomyopathy or compounding cardiovascular events? *Obstet. Gynecol.* **67**:157–168.

Cunningham, F. G., Lucas, M. J., and Hankins, G. D. V. (1987). Pulmonary injury complicating antepartum pyelonephritis. *Am. J. Obstet. Gynecol.* **156**:797–807.

Cutaia, M., Friedrich, P., Grimson, R., and Porcelli, R. J. (1987). Pregnancy- and gender-related changes in pulmonary vascular reactivity. *Exp. Lung Res.* **13**:343–357.

Dawkins, K. D., Burke, C. M., Billingham, M. E., and Jamieson, S. W. (1986). Primary pulmonary hypertension and pregnancy. *Chest* **89**:383–388.

de Regt, R. H. (1987). Sarcoidosis and pregnancy. *Obstet. Gynecol.* **70**: 369–372.

Dishner, W., Cordasco, E. M., Blackburn, J., Demeter, S., Levin, H., and Carey, W. D. (1984). Pulmonary lymphangiomyomatosis. *Chest* **85**: 796–799.

Eliasson, O., Scherzer, H. H., and DeGraff, A. C. (1986). Morbidity in asthma in relation to the menstrual cycle. *J. Allergy Clin. Immunol.* **77**:87–94.

Elliot, D. L., Barker, A. F., and Dixon, L- M. (1985). Catamenial hemoptysis: new methods of diagnosis and therapy. *Chest* **87**:687–688.

Flick, M. R. (1988). Pulmonary edema and acute lung injury. In *Respiratory Medicine*. Edited by J. F. Murray and J. A. Nadel. Saunders, Philadelphia, pp. 1359–1409.

Foster, D. C., Stern, J. L., Buscema, J., Rock, J. A., and Woodruff, J. D. (1981). Pleural and parenchymal pulmonary endometriosis. *Obstet. Gynecol.* **58**:552–556.

Fuchs, K. I., Moore, L. G., and Rounds, S. (1982). Pulmonary vascular reactivity is blunted in pregnant rats. *J. Appl. Physiol.* **53**:703–707.

Fuller, A. F., Scannell, J. G., and Wilkens, E. W. (1985). Pulmonary resection for metastases from gynecologic cancers: Massachusetts General Hospital experience, 1943–1982. *Gynecol. Oncol.* **22**:174–180.

Ghio, A. J., and Crapo, R. O. (1988). Midcycle pneumothorax in a patient with catamenial pneumothoraces. *West. J. Med.* **149**:462–463.

Gilroy, R. J., Mangura, B. T., and Lavietes, M. H. (1988). Rib cage and abdominal volume displacements during breathing in pregnancy. *Am. Rev. Respir. Dis.* **137**:668–672.

Girard, P., Mal, H., Laine, J-F., Petitpretz, P., Rain, B., and Duroux, P. (1986). Left heart failure in amniotic fluid embolism. *Anesthesiology* **64**:262–265.

Gordon, A. N., Gershenson, D. M., Copeland, L. J., Saul, P. B., and Kavanagh, J. J. (1985). High-risk metastatic gestational trophoblastic disease. *Obstet. Gynecol.* **65**:550–556.

Greenberger, P. A., Patterson, R. (1985). Management of asthma during pregnancy. *N. Engl. J. Med.* **312**:897–902.

Grimm, M. H., Grady, K. J., and Golish, J. A. (1988). Bronchopulmonary endometriosis: a rare cause of hemoptysis. *South. Med. J.* **81**:1198–1199.

Hammerschmidt, D. E., Ogburn, P. L., and Williams, J. E. (1984). Amniotic fluid activates complement: a role in amniotic fluid embolism syndrome? *J. Lab. Clin. Med.* **104**:901–907.

Hawker, F. (1984). Five cases of pulmonary oedema associated with β_2-sympathomimetic treatment of premature labour. *Anaesth. Intens. Care* **12**:159–162.

Helmrich, S. P., Rosenberg, L., Kaufman, D. W., Strom, B., and Shapiro, S. (1987). Venous thromboembolism in relation to oral contraceptive use. *Obstet. Gynecol.* **69**:91–95.

Hibbard, L. T., Schumann, W. R., and Goldstein, G. E. (1981). Thoracic endometriosis: a review and report of two cases. *Am. J. Obstet. Gynecol.* **140**:227–232.

Hollingsworth, H. M., Pratter, M. R., and Irwin, R. S. (1989). Acute respiratory failure in pregnancy. *J. Intens. Care Med.* **4**:11–34.

Horsfield, K. (1989). Catamenial pleural pain. *Eur. Respir. J.* **2**:1013–1014.

Huberman, R. P., Fon, G. T., and Bein, M. E. (1982). Benign molar pregnancies: pulmonary complications. *AJR* **138**:71–74.

Hughson, W. G., Friedman, P. J., Feigin, D. S., Resnik, R., and Moser, K. W. (1982). Postpartum pleural effusion: a common radiologic finding. *Ann. Intern. Med.* **97**:856:858.

Irani, D. R., Underwood, R. D., Johnson, E. H., and Greenberg, S. D. (1987). Malignant pleural effusions: a clinical cytopathologic study. *Arch. Intern. Med.* **147**:1133–1136.

James, K. B., and Healy, B. P. (1989). Heart disease arising during or secondary to pregnancy. *Cardiovasc. Clin.* **19**:81–96.

Johnston, W. W. (1985). The malignant pleural effusion: a review of cytopathologic diagnoses of 584 specimens from 472 consecutive patients. *Cancer* **56**:905–909.

Juniper, E. F., Kline, P. A., Roberts, R. S., Hargreave, F. E., and Daniel, E. E. (1987). Airway responsiveness to methacholine during the natural menstrual cycle and the effect of oral contraceptives. *Am. Rev. Respir. Dis.* **135**:1039–1042.

Karson, E. M., Saltzman, D., and Davis, M. R. (1984). Pneumomediastinum in pregnancy: two case reports and a review of the literature, pathophysiology, and management. *Obstet. Gynecol.* **64**:39S–43S.

Kaufman, B. S., Kaminsky, S. J., Rackow, E. C., and Weil, M. H. (1987). Adult respiratory distress syndrome following orogenital sex during pregnancy. *Crit. Care Med.* **15**:703–704.

Kumar, J., Ilancheran, A., and Ratnam, S. S. (1988). Pulmonary metastases in gestational trophoblastic disease: a review of 97 cases. *Br. J. Obstet. Gynaecol.* **95**:70–74.

Lawrence, H. C. (1988). Pulmonary endometriosis in pregnancy. *Am. J. Obstet. Gynecol.* ***159***:733–734.

Lawson, H. W., Atrash, H. K., and Franks, A. L. (1990). Fatal pulmonary embolism during legal induced abortion in the United States from 1972 to 1985. *Am. J. Obstet. Gynecol.* **162**:986–990.

Leake, J. F., Murphy, A. A., and Zacur, H. A. (1987). Noncardiogenic pulmonary edema: a complication of operative hysteroscopy. *Fertil. Steril.* **48**:497–499.

Lederman, M. M. (1984). Cell-mediated immunity and pregnancy. *Chest* **86**:6S–9S.

Lee, W., Ginsburg, K. A., Cotton, D. B., and Kaufman, R. H. (1986). Squamous and trophoblastic cells in the maternal pulmonary circulation identified by invasive hemodynamic monitoring during the peripartum period. *Am. J. Obstet. Gynecol.* **155**:999–1001.

Liberatore, S. M., Pistelli, R., Patalano, F., Moneta, E., Incalzi, R. A., and Ciappi, G. (1984). Respiratory function during pregnancy. *Respiration* **46**:145–150.

MacLennan, F. M., MacDonald, A. F., and Campbell, D. M. (1987). Lung water during the puerperium. *Anaesthesia* **42**:141–147.

Markham, S. M., Carpenter, S. E., and Rock, J. A. (1989). Extrapelvic endometriosis. *Obstet. Gynecol. Clin. North Am.* **16**:193–219.

Masson, R. G., Ruggieri, J., and Siddiqui, M. M. (1979). Amniotic fluid embolism: definitive diagnosis in a survivor. *Am. Rev. Respir. Dis.* **120**:187–192.

Matthay, M. A., and Wiener-Kronish, J. P. (1988). Resolution of alveolar edema in man: is active transport an important mechanism? (abstract). *Am. Rev. Respir Dis.* **137** (suppl):228.

Matuschak, G. M., Owens, G. R., Rogers, R. M., and Tibbals, S. C. (1984). Progressive intrapartum respiratory insufficiency due to pulmonary alveolar proteinosis: amelioration by therapeutic whole-lung bronchopulmonary lavage. *Chest* **86**:496–499.

Mendelson, C. L. (1946). The aspiration of stomach contents into the lungs during obstetric anesthesia. *Am. J. Obstet. Gynecol.* **52**:191–205.

Michaeli, J., Kornberg, A., Menashe, M., Lugassy, G., and Mogle, P. (1987). Exacerbation of idiopathic pulmonary hemosiderosis in pregnancy. *Eur. J. Obstet. Gynecol. Reprod. Biol.* **25**:153–158.

Moore, L. G., and Reeves, J. T. (1980). Pregnancy blunts pulmonary vascular reactivity in dogs. *Am. J. Physiol.* **239**:H297–H301.

Moser, K., ed. (1979). *Pulmonary Vascular Diseases*. Lung Biology in Health and Disease, Vol. 14. Marcel Dekker, New York.

Moser, K. M. (1988). Pulmonary embolism. In *Respiratory Medicine*. Edited by J. F. Murray and J. A. Nadel. Saunders, Philadelphia, pp. 1299–1327.

Müller, N. L., and Nelems, B. (1986). Postcoital catamenial pneumothorax. Report of a case not associated with endometriosis and successfully treated with tubal ligation. *Am. Rev. Respir. Dis.* **134**:803–804.

Nakamura, H., Konishiike, J., Sugamura, A., and Takeno, Y. (1986). Epidemiology of spontaneous pneumothorax in women. *Chest* **89**:378–382.

Noble, P. W., Lavee, A. E., and Jacobs, M. M. (1988). Respiratory diseases in pregnancy. *Obstet. Gynecol. Clin. North Am.* **15**:391–428.

Orr, J. W., Austin, J. M., Hatch, K. D., Shingleton, H. M., Younger, J. B., and Boots, L. R. (1980). Acute pulmonary edema associated with molar pregnancies: a high-risk factor for development of persistent trophoblastic disease. *Am. J.* Obstet. *Gynecol.* **136**:412–415.

Palmer, J., Dillon-Baker, C., Tecklin, J. S., Wolfson, B., Rosenberg, B., Burroughs, B., Holsclaw, D. S., Scanlin, T. F. Huang, N. N., and Sewell, E. M. (1983). Pregnancy in patients with cystic fibrosis. *Ann. Intern. Med.* **99**:596–600.

Petersen, C., Slutkin, G., and Mills J. (1988). Parasitic infections. In *Respiratory Medicine*. Edited by J. F. Murray and J. A. Nadel. Saunders, Philadelphia, pp.950–985.

Phillips, R. E. (1984). Management of *Plasmodium falciparum* malaria. *Med. J. Aust.* **141**:511–517.

Pickett, C. K., Regensteiner, J. G., Woodard, W. D., and Hagerman, D. D. (1989). Progestin and estrogen reduce sleep-disordered breathing in postmenopausal women. *J. Appl. Physiol.* **66**:1656–1661.

Pisani, R. J., and Rosenow, E. C. (1989). Pulmonary edema associated with tocolytic therapy. *Ann. Intern. Med.* **110**:714–718.

Price, T. M., Baker, V. V., and Cefalo, R. C. (1985). Amniotic fluid embolism. Three case reports with a review of the literature. *Obstet. Gynecol. Surv.* **40**:462–475.

Prichard, M. G., and Musk, A. W. 91984). Adverse effect of pregnancy on familial fibrosing alveolitis. *Thorax* **39**:319–320.

Russi, E. W., Spaetling, L., Gmür, J., and Schneider, H. (1988). High permeability pulmonary edema (ARDS) during tocolytic therapy—a case report. *J. Perinat. Med.* **16**:45–49.

Rutherford, J. D., and Hands, M. E. (1989). Therapeutics and management during pregnancy. *Cardiovasc. Clin.* **19**:113–125.

Rutherford, S. E., and Phelan, J. P. (1986). Thromboembolic disease in pregnancy. *Clin. Perinatol.* **13**:719–739.

Scharf, S. M., and Cassidy, S. S., eds. (1989). *Heart-Lung Interactions in Health and Disease*. Lung Biology in Health and Disease, Vol. 42. Marcel Dekker, New York.

Schoene, R. B., Robertson, H. T., Pierson, D. J., and Peterson, A. P. (1981). Respiratory drives and exercise in menstrual cycles of athletic and nonathletic women. *J. Appl. Physiol.* **50**:1300–1305.

Schoenfeld, A., Ziv, E., Zeelel, Y., and Ovadia, J. (1986). Catamenial pneumothorax—a literature review and report of an unusual case. *Obstet. Gynecol. Surv.* **41**:20–24.

Shah, A., Sethi, S., and Agarwal, M. K. (1988). Human seminal plasma allergy in India. *J. Asthma* **25**:137–140.

Shahar, J., and Angelillo, V. A. (1986). Catamenial pneumomediastinum. *Chest* **90**:776–777.

Shen, A., Iseman, M. D., Waldron, J. A., and King, T. E. (1987). Exacerbation of pulmonary lymphangioleiomyomatosis by exogenous estrogens. *Chest* **91**:782–785.

Sheth, R. A., Greenberg, S. D., Jenkins, D. E., and Beall, A. C. (1984). Lymphangiomyomatosis with chylous effusions. *South. Med. J.* **77**: 1032–1035.

Sibai, B. M., Taslimi, M. M., El-Nazer, A., Amon, E., Mabie, B. C., and Ryan, G. M. (1986). Maternal-perinatal outcome associated with the syndrome of hemolysis, elevated liver enzymes, and low platelets in severe preeclampsia-eclampsia. *Am. J. Obstet. Gynecol.* **155**:501–509.

Sibai, B. M., Mabie. B. C., Harvey, C. J., and Gonzalez, A. R. (1987). Pulmonary edema in severe preeclampsia-eclampsia: analysis of thirty-seven consecutive cases. *Am. J. Obstet. Gynecol.* **156**:1174–1179.

Smith, J. L., Thomas, F., Orme, J. F., and Clemmer, T. P. (1990). Adult respiratory distress syndrome during pregnancy and immediately postpartum. *West. J. Med.* **153**:508–510.

Snider, D. (1984). Pregnancy and tuberculosis. *Chest* **86**:10S–13S.

Sosin, D., Krasnow, J., Moawad, A., and Hall, J. B. (1986). Successful spontaneous vaginal delivery during mechanical ventilatory support for the adult respiratory distress syndrome. *Obstet. Gynecol.* **68**:19S–23S.

Stark, P., and Pollack, M. S. (1986). Pleural effusions in the postpartum period. *Radiology* **26**:471–73.

Staub, N. C., ed. (1978). *Lung Water and Solute Exchange*. Lung Biology in Health and Disease, Vol. 7. Marcel Dekker, New York.

Sylvester, J. T., Gordon, J. B., Malamet, R. L., and Wetzel, R. C. (1985). Prostaglandins and estradiol-induced attenuation of hypoxic pulmonary vasoconstriction. *Chest* **88**:252S–254S.

Takano, N. (1982) Resting pulmonary ventilation and dead space ventilation during the menstrual cycle. *Jpn. J. Physiol.* **32**:469–473.

Taylor, R. R., Ryi, J., Colby, T. V., and Raffin, T. A. (1990). Lymphangioleiomyomatosis: clinical course in 32 patients. *N. Engl. J. Med.* **323**:1254–1260.

Thaler, I., Bronstein, M., and Rubin, A. E. (1986). the course and outcome of pregnancy associated with bronchiectasis. Case report. *Br. J. Obstet. Gynecol.* **93**:1006–1008.

Turner, E. S., Greenberger, P. A., and Patterson, R. (1980). Management of the pregnant asthmatic patient. *Ann. Intern. Med.* **93**:905–918.

Veille, J-C. (1984). Peripartum cardiomyopathies: a review. *Am. J. Obstet. Gynecol.* **148**:805–818.

Villar, M. A., and Sibai, B. M. (1988). Eclampsia. *Obstet. Gynecol. Clin. North Am.* **15**:355–377.

Wagner, J. M., Morton, M. J., Johnson, K. A., O'Grady J. P., and Speroff, L. (1981). Terbutaline and maternal cardiac function. *JAMA* **246**:2697–2701.

Warrell, D. A. (1987). Pathophysiology of severe falciparum malaria in man. *Parasitology* **94**:S53–S76.

Wasserstrum, N., and Cotton, D. B. (1986). Hemodynamic monitoring in severe pregnancy-induced hypertension. *Clin. Perinatol.* **13**:781–799.

Weinberger, S. E., Weiss, S. T., Cohen, W. R., Weiss, J. W., and Johnson, T. S. (1980). State of the art: pregnancy and the lung. *Am. Rev. Respir. Dis.* **121**:559–581.

Weinmann, G. G., Zacur, H., and Fish, J. E. (1987). Absence of changes in airway responsiveness during the menstrual cycle. *J. Allergy Clin. Immunol.* **79**:634–638.

Weir, E. K., and Reeves, J. T., eds. (1989). *Pulmonary Vascular Physiology and Pathophysiology*. Lung Biology in Health and Disease, Vol. 38. Marcel Dekker, New York.

White, D. P., Douglas, N. J., Pickett, C. K., Weil, J. V., and Zwillich, C. W. (1982). Hypoxic ventilatory response during sleep in normal premenopausal women. *Am. Rev. Respir. Dis.* **126**:530–533.

White, D. P., Douglas, N. J., Pickett, C. K., Weil, J. V., and Zwillich, C. W. (1983). Sexual influence on the control of breathing. *J. Appl. Physiol.* **54**:874–879.

White, D. P., Schneider, B. K., Santen, R. J., McDermott, M., Pickett, C. K., Zwillich, C. W., and Weil, J .V. (1985). Influence of testosterone on ventilation and chemosensitivity in male subjects. *J. Appl. Physiol.* **59**:1452–1457.

Zbella, E. A., Moise, J., and Carson, S. A. (1985). Noncardiogenic pulmonary edema secondary to intrauterine instillation of 32% dextran 70. *Fertil. Steril.* **43**:479–480.

12

Postoperative Complications

JEAN-FRANCOIS PITTET and JEANINE P. WIENER-KRONISH

Cardiovascular Research Institute, University of California, San Francisco
San Francisco, California

I. Introduction

Although the presence of impaired pulmonary function after anesthesia and surgery was reported 80 years ago (Pasteur, 1910), its causes remained unclear until recently. The use of advanced computed tomography (CT) technology during the last 5 years has provided new insights into the pathophysiological mechanisms causing postoperative pulmonary dysfunction. There is now good evidence that the impairment of respiratory muscle function (rib cage and diaphragm) induced by anesthesia and surgery results in the formation of compression atelectasis in dependent lung regions that is associated with the development of shunt and hypoxemia. Therefore, the purpose of this chapter will be to discuss the respective roles of anesthesia and surgery in the formation of postoperative atelectasis in otherwise healthy patients and in high-risk patients and to review the risk factors, pathogenesis, and diagnosis of nosocomial pneumonia and of acute lung injury in postoperative patients.

II. All Patients

A. Postoperative Atelectasis

Postoperative abnormalities in gas exchange present in two temporal patterns (Marshall and Wyche, 1972):

1. A transient postoperative hypoxemia, which is mostly due to a depression of the normal hypoxic and hypercapnic respiratory drive induced by narcotics used for induction and maintenance of anesthesia (particularly in elderly patients); other contributing factors are a residual effect of muscle relaxants used intraoperatively, the loss of pulmonary hypoxic vasoconstrictive reflexes following the administration of inhalational anesthetic agents, and an increased oxygen consumption due to hypertonic muscles and shivering.
2. A prolonged pattern of gas exchange abnormalities that lasts several hours or days, which are due to the effects of anesthesia and surgery on the respiratory system (lungs and chest wall combined); this pattern appears to be an important contributing factor to the postoperative morbidity of anesthesia and surgery.

Effects of Anesthesia on the Respiratory System

Motion and Shape During Anesthesia with Spontaneous Respiration

Induction of general anesthesia in spontaneously breathing subjects reduces the muscle tone of both the intercostals and the diaphragm by two mechanisms: decreasing the drive of respiratory centers that control the diaphragmatic motoneurons and depressing the synaptic transmission of the intercostal motoneurons, which require a summation of both segmental and suprasegmental nonrespiratory inputs of fire (Orem and Dement, 1976). These changes in muscle tone are not affected by anesthetic agents to the same degree. Volatile anesthetics preferentially depress synaptic transmission and, therefore, primarily affect the rib cage muscles (Richard and White, 1975), although they may also produce some inhibition of the respiratory centers and the diaphragm (Dureuil et al., 1987b; Smaje, 1976). Intravenous anesthetics mostly depress the diaphragmatic tonic activity by decreasing the output of the respiratory centers (Morel et al., 1984 and 1986; Germain et al., 1982; Rigg and Rondi, 1981). Therefore, depending on which anesthetic agent is used, the rib cage contribution to the tidal volume, the respiratory drive, or the inspiratory time may be decreased, increased, or unchanged compared to the awake state (Table 1). Despite these differences, induction of general anesthesia by all anesthetic agents but one (ketamine) will produce a cephalad shift of the diaphragm and a decrease in lung volume, primarily in the dependent dorsal regions of the lung. (Froese and Bryan, 1974).

Table 1 Effect of Anesthetic Agents on the Breathing Pattern

	V_T/T_i	Ti/T_{tot}	RC/V_t
Volatile anesthetics	↓	↓	↓
Opiates	↓	→ or ↓	↓
Thiopental	↓ ↓	→	↑
Benzodiazepines	↓	↑	↑
Etomidate	→	→	↑
Droperidol	→	→	→
Ketamine	↑	↑	→ or ↓

V_T/T_i = mean inspiratory flow rate; T_i/T_{tot} = inspiratory time; RC/V_T = percentage of rib cage contribution to tidal volume.

Motion and Shape During Anesthesia with Muscle Paralysis

Although muscle paralysis does not further decrease lung volume, the relative contribution of the diaphragm to the tidal volume and the pattern of diaphragm motion are altered by neuromuscular blockade (Froese and Bryan, 1974; Krayer et al., 1989). (Fig. 1). Interestingly, these changes are dependent on the position of the subjects. In paralyzed subjects lying supine, the motion of the diaphragm is quite small and nearly uniform, and the dependent part of the diaphragm moves less than during spontaneous breathing (Froese and Bryan, 1974; Krayer et al., 1989). In this position, the decrease in thoracic volume is mainly due to a reduction of the cross-sectional area of the chest (Nims et al., 1955). In contrast, in paralyzed subjects lying prone, the diaphragm motion is greater but nonuniform, with most of the motion and cephalad deplacement occurring in the nondependent (dorsal) region (Krayer et al., 1989). This latter observation suggests that after muscle paralysis, the dominant influences on diaphragm motion may be the transdiaphragmatic hydrostatic pressure (Froese and Bryan, 1974) and the anatomical differences between the crural and the costal diaphragmatic regions (Krayer et al., 1989).

Effect on Functional Residual Capacity

The alteration of the shape and motion of the chest wall produced by the induction of general anesthesia causes an increase in lung recoil pressure, a decrease in compliance of the lungs, and a reduction in functional residual capacity (FRC) of approximately 500 ml, or 20% of the awake value for a patient lying supine (Nims et al., 1955; Bergman, 1963; Hedenstierna et al., 1981; Westbrook et al., 1973). The reduction in FRC is observed immediately after induction of anesthesia, whatever anesthetic agent is used (including benzodiazepines) with the

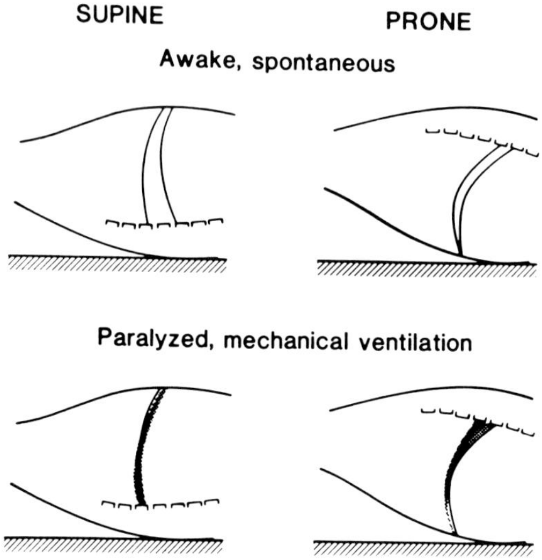

Figure 1 Diaphragm position and displacement for subjects lying supine or prone. Solid lines represent end-expiratory and end-inspiratory diaphragm positions during spontaneous breathing while awake. Stippled areas represent diaphragm excursions during mechanical ventilation while subject was anesthetized and paralyzed.

exception of ketamine (Smaje, 1976; Morel et al., 1986; Froese and Bryan, 1974; Don et al., 1970). The decrease in FRC is not progressive with time.

Many mechanisms have been evoked to explain this reduction in FRC. In 1963, Bendixen and colleagues reported a progressive decrease in the arterial oxygen partial pressure (Pa_{O_2}) during general anesthesia and proposed the concept of absorption atelectasis (Bendixen et al., 1963). However, a similar observation has been not made by other research groups, and the presence of atelectasis was not demonstrated on conventional chest radiographs (Nunn et al., 1965). Others suggested that airway closure may occur during anesthesia and explain this reduction in FRC (Don et al., 1972). Although this observation was confirmed by subsequent studies (Hedenstierna et al., 1976; Gilmour et al., 1976), there were other conflicting results (Juno et al., 1978), and no good correlation between the degree of airway closure and the degree of gas exchange impairment induced by general anesthesia has ever been reported (Hedenstierna et al., 1976; Bergman and Tien, 1983). Moreover, nearly simultaneous measurements of FRC by N_2 clearance and body plethysmography showed similar results, suggesting that very little gas was trapped distal to closed airways (Westbrook et al., 1973). Airway closure is, therefore, no longer considered the major cause of the reduction in FRC or the primary cause of gas exchange impairment during anesthesia, although it may be a contributing factor (Bergman and Tien, 1983).

Using computerized x-ray tomography with transverse exposures of the chest, it has been possible to demonstrate that densities develop in the dependent part of the lung within 5 min. after the induction of anesthesia in 90% of supine subjects without preexisting lung diseases (Brismar et al., 1985; Strandberg et al., 1986a; Tokics et al., 1987a) (Fig. 2). Application of positive end-expiratory pressure (PEEP) of 10 cm H_2O can reduce or eliminate the dense regions, which then reappear within 1 min after the discontinuation of PEEP (Juno et al., 1978) (Fig. 2). These dense areas do not appear to be pleural or interstitial fluid, because they remain in the same anatomical position when the patient is turned from the supine to the lateral position (Brismar et al., 1985). The development of these dense areas is unaffected by changing the inspired oxygen concentration from 40% to 100%, which suggests that these areas are not produced by absorption atelectasis (Brismar et al., 1985). To better characterize these dense areas, this same research group morphologically analyzed these dense regions in anesthetized sheep and found that they corresponded to atelectatic areas of the lung and did not contain interstitial edema (Hedenstierna et al., 1989). Therefore, these dense regions correspond to compression atelectasis produced by the reduction in FRC, probably secondary to the relaxation of the chest wall muscles (rib cage and diaphragm). Interestingly, the formation of compression atelectasis during general anesthesia is not entirely secondary to the decrease in FRC. The application of thoracoabdominal restriction, which reduces the FRC by 20% in awake volunteers, is not accompanied by the development of compression atelectasis, suggesting that the relaxation of the respiratory muscles during general anesthesia is an important factor in the development of this atelectasis (Tokics et al., 1988).

Various anesthetic regimens all cause the development of compression atelectasis. Atelectasis was observed during anesthesia induced by volatile or intravenous anesthetics (with the exception of ketamine), whether or not the trachea was intubated (Strandberg et al., 1986b). The addition of a volatile anesthetic after an anesthesic induction with barbiturates did not increase the area of atelectasis (Strandberg et al., 1986b). After drug-induced muscle paralysis, a small but insignificant increase in the atelectatic areas of the lungs occurred (Strandberg et al., 1986a). Interestingly, there is no compression atelectasis after induction of anesthesia with ketamine, a drug known to maintain the tone of the respiratory muscles (Tokics et al. 1987b). This finding suggests that loss of diaphragmatic and intercostal muscle tone plays a key role in the development of compression atelectasis. This hypothesis has also been supported by the results of studies that show that phrenic nerve stimulation may decrease anesthesia-induced compression atelectasis (Hedenstierna, 1989). The development of compression atelectasis has not been studied using CT scanning during regional

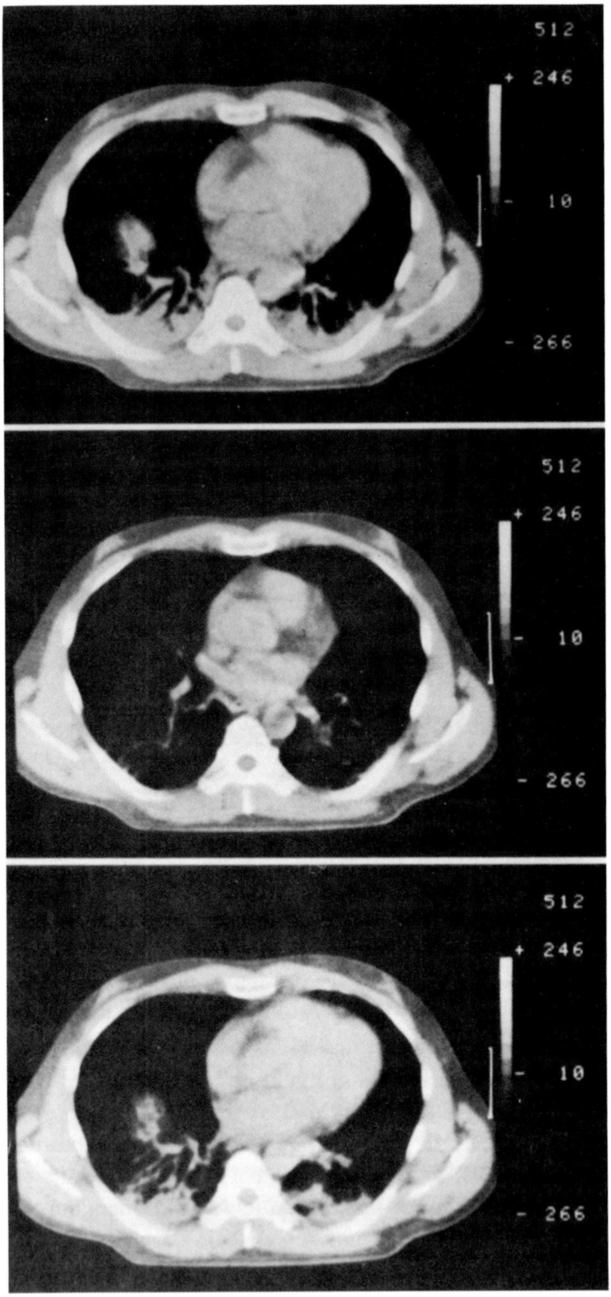

Figure 2 Transverse CT scans of the thorax during anesthesia without and with a positive end-expiratory pressure (PEEP) of 10 cm H_2O (upper and middle panels, respectively) and 10 min after discontinuation of PEEP (lower panel). Note the disappearance of densities in dependent regions during PEEP and their reappearance after discontinuation of PEEP.

anaesthesia procedures, in particular epidural anesthesia for abdominal surgery. The results of some older studies suggest that the function of respiratory muscles may be better preserved during regional anesthesia for abdominal procedures as FRC was not reduced in one study (McCarthy, 1976) and the incidence of airway closure was not increased in another study (Lundh et al., 1983).

No correlation has been found between the age of patients and the formation of compression atelectasis; compression atelectasis has been observed in 1-week-old newborns and in middle-aged or elderly patients (Strandberg et al., 1986a). The size of the atelectasis formed is also variable; 0–10% of the lung, with a mean value of 4–5% of the lung, can be atelectactic (Strandberg et al., 1986a). Although some correlation has been found between the patient's weight and the size of compression atelectasis formed (Strandberg et al., 1987), the cause of the variation in the amount of atelectasis formed remains to be elucidated. Ninety percent of the compression atelectasis that develops during anesthesia is present by 1 hr after the end of surgery, and 50% is still present for 24 hr postoperatively (Strandberg et al., 1986a). This suggests that anesthesia-induced compression atelectasis is an important contributing factor to early postoperative gas exchange impairment.

Atelectasis and Gas Exchange Impairment During Anesthesia

Arterial oxygenation is impaired in most patients during anesthesia whether or not they receive neuromuscular paralytic agents (Marshall and Wyche, 1972). The etiology of this reduced arterial oxygen saturation during anesthesia is dependent on the age of the subjects. In young, healthy patients, hypoxemia appears to be secondary to increased shunt (Rehder et al., 1979; Dueck et al., 1980); in middle-aged patients, there is also an increase in shunt as well as some ventilation-perfusion (V/Q) mismatch (Bindslev et al., 1981). In elderly patients, anesthesia produces both an increase in shunt and an increase in low V/Q regions (Dueck et al., 1980). The relationship between the impairment in V/Q distribution and the development of compression atelectasis has been studied recently, using the multiple inert gas elimination technique and the CT scan (Tokics et al., 1987a). In subjects with healthy lungs, a strong correlation was found during anesthesia between the size of the atelectasis formed and the percentage of shunt (Fig. 2). In patients who did not develop any atelectasis, no increase in shunt and no gas exchange impairment occurred (Tokics et al., 1987a). Interestingly, in patients receiving ketamine intravenously as the anesthetic agent, neither atelectasis nor shunt developed (Tokics et al., 1987b). However, both atelectasis and shunt developed when the patients were paralyzed with muscle relaxant even after ketamine induction (Tokics et al., 1987b). These results confirm the previous reports that shunt is the major cause of gas exchange impairment during anesthesia in subjects with healthy lungs, and that it is due to the perfusion of the atelectatic regions of the dependent regions of the

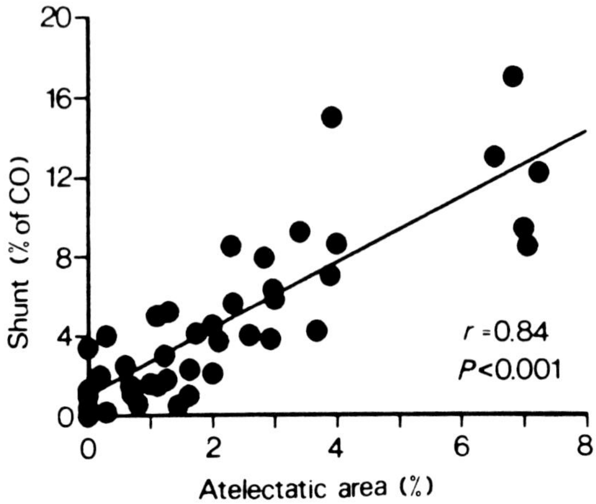

Figure 3 Plot of shunt (Qs) as a percentage of cardiac output versus the atelectatic area as a percentage of the total intrathoracic area, during inhalation anaesthesia with muscle paralysis and mechanical ventilation.

lungs (Fig. 3). The blunting of hypoxic pulmonary vasoconstriction by volatile anesthetics may also increase the alveolar-arterial oxygen difference observed intraoperatively by increasing the perfusion of the atelectatic areas (Sykes et al., 1972). However, this deleterious effect produces minimal gas exchange abnormalities in patients with normal pulmonary function (Marshall, 1990).

In summary, general anesthesia itself produces some decrease in arterial oxygenation by inducing the development of compression atelectasis and decreasing the FRC. These changes in pulmonary function are mainly due to a loss of the tonic activity of the diaphragm and the muscles of the rib cage. Although lasting several hours after the end of anesthesia, the effects of general anesthesia on gas exchange are mild in the absence of preexisting cardiopulmonary diseases.

Effects of Surgery on the Respiratory System

Postoperative lung function abnormalities following cardiothoracic or upper abdominal surgery are characterized by a severe restrictive pattern with a 30–40% reduction of vital capacity and FRC and an increased respiratory frequency. These changes all slowly return toward preoperative values within 2 weeks (Craig, 1981). The primary etiology and time course of this respiratory dysfunction appear to be different from those induced by general anesthesia, although both lead to the formation of atelectasis. In the following section, we will briefly review the effect of both upper abdominal and cardiothoracic surgery on the development of postoperative atelectasis.

Upper Abdominal Surgery

The pulmonary dysfunction induced by upper abdominal surgery (UAS) is characterized by a long-lasting decrease in lung volume leading to the development of atelectasis and hypoxemia (Craig, 1981). Several studies have reported a shift from abdominal to rib cage breathing after UAS, suggesting that diaphragmatic dysfunction may be responsible for the gas exchange impairment induced by this type of surgical procedure (Ford et al., 1988b; Road et al., 1984; Simmoneau et al., 1983). Two main mechanisms have been hypothesized (Ford et al., 1988b): a decrease in the contractility of the diaphragm or a reduction in the activity of the phrenic nerve. The first mechanism is no longer tenable because diaphragmatic contractility was not found to be depressed after UAS in humans, despite a reduction in diaphragmatic function as assessed by the ratio of abdominal to transdiaphragmatic pressure changes during the respiratory cycle (Dureuil et al., 1985). Indeed, the peak transdiaphragmatic pressure generated by bilateral phrenic nerve stimulation was unchanged after UAS compared to preoperative values. Thus, the second proposed mechanism, a decrease in phrenic nerve activity, is now considered to be the main cause of the sustained alteration of diaphragmatic function observed after UAS in humans (Dureuil et al., 1985, 1987a).

The results of animal studies indicate that reflex inhibition of phrenic nerve output occurs during or just after stimulation of visceral or somatic afferents (Ford et al., 1988a; Shannon, 1980; Jammes et al., 1986). After UAS in humans, reflex inhibition of phrenic nerve activity could originate either from an increase in abdominal wall tone or from visceral stimulation. Because diaphragmatic function remains unchanged after lower abdominal surgery (Dureuil et al., 1985), an inhibitory role of parietal receptors in the abdominal wall is probably not contributing to phrenic nerve dysfunction. Nociceptors for pain are also probably not important because the respiratory dysfunction induced by UAS was not modified by selective spinal analgesia with subarachnoid or epidural administration of opiates (Simmoneau et al., 1983; Clergue et al., 1984). However, the administration of local anesthetics in the epidural space has been reported to improve diaphragmatic function after UAS, suggesting that the stimulation of abdominal visceral sympathetic receptors inhibits phrenic activity and in turn, causes the diaphragmatic dysfunction observed after UAS (Albano and Garnier, 1983; Mankikian et al., 1988).

The alleged importance of diaphragmatic dysfunction as the major factor in causing postoperative atelectasis after UAS has recently been challenged (Duggan and Drummond, 1987, 1989). Increased expiratory activity in abdominal and lower intercostal muscles may be responsible for an increase in abdominal pressure and some of the decrease in lung volume that occurs during the first hours after UAS. However, one study of abdominal muscle function found that increased activity during expiration occurred only transiently, for about 24 hr after UAS (Simmoneau et al., 1983; Dureuil et al., 1987a). This suggests that increased expiratory activity of abdominal muscles may explain the early postoperative decrease in lung volume, but that this mechanism did not last long enough to explain the prolonged respiratory effects seen 7–14 days after UAS. Therefore, diaphragm dysfunction and other unknown processes appear to cause the prolonged pulmonary dysfunction that occurs after UAS.

In summary, abnormalities in pulmonary function observed after UAS are believed to be due to decreased diaphragmatic activity produced by stimulation of sympathetic abdominal receptors, and to increased expiratory activity of the abdominal wall muscles. These two mechanisms produce a cephalad deplacement of the diaphragm, which reduces FRC and causes the development of prolonged compression atelectasis postoperatively.

Cardiac and Thoracic Surgery

The postoperative period after cardiothoracic surgery is characterized by a high incidence of respiratory complications (Matthay and Wiener-Kronish, 1988; Slinger 1990). Following cardiac surgery, more than 90% of patients develop significant atelectasis (Markand et al., 1985). Changes in pulmonary function after lung surgery have not been studied extensively. However, the results of some studies suggest that the immediate decrease in lung volume may be less that after UAS (Ali et al., 1974), although the effect of thoracotomy on pulmonary function my persist as long as 6 weeks after surgery (Gorlin et al., 1957).

Postoperative atelectasis is frequently observed after cardiac surgery, although its etiology remains unknown and appears to be multifactorial. Postoperative diaphragmatic dysfunction, as observed after UAS, does not appear to be a major cause of atelectasis after cardiac surgery, because abdominal visceral reflexes are not disturbed. Also, paresis of the phrenic nerve has been found in less than 10% of patients after cardiac surgery (Markand et al., 1985; Wilcox et al., 1988). In one of these studies (Markand et al., 1985), a discriminant analysis of intraoperative variables showed that the incidence of severe atelectasis increased as a larger number of grafts were placed and as a longer operative and bypass time were required. Other factors that increased the incidence of atelectasis included whether the pleural space had been entered and whether an atrial drain or a cardiac insulating pad had not been used.

The most important factor causing atelectasis in these patients appeared to be the effect of cardiopulmonary bypass on respiratory function. It is well established that the duration of cardiopulmonary bypass has some relationship to postoperative pulmonary dysfunction and the development of atelectasis (Edmunds and Alexander, 1980). The mechanism of this dysfunction is not clear.

One possible explanation is that during cardiopulmonary bypass, blood supply to the alveolar epithelium is inadequate, which results in insufficient formation and release of surfactant by type 2 alveolar epithelial cells. There is no direct proof of this explanation, but 90% of patients who have had cardiopulmonary bypass develop atelectasis (Slinger, 1990; Wilcox et al., 1988). Moreover, the results of experimental studies suggest that atelectasis develops when isolated lungs are ventilated without positive end-expiratory pressure, which by increasing end-expiratory lung volume preserves surfactant (Faritty et al., 1966), and that the cold temperature used during bypass may accentuate abnormalities in surfactant production or function (Nagao et al., 1977).

The development of atelectasis is one of the most important causes of postoperative complications in patients undergoing thoracotomy for lung surgery (Kaplan, 1983). The etiology of this atelectasis is not clear and appears to be multifactorial. During the early postoperative period, accumulation of bronchial secretions, increased lung water content, and reduced surfactant activity may lead to the development of atelectasis (Malmkvist, et al., 1989; Karlson, et al., 1965). Diaphragmatic dysfunction does not seem to be an important contributing factor to atelectasis after lung surgery. However, although diaphragmatic contractility is preserved during quiet breathing, the maximal strength of the diaphragm might be reduced in patients who have undergone thoracotomy (Maeda et al., 1988). Nonetheless, phrenic nerve function appears to be normal after thoracotomy (Karlson et al., 1965; De Troyer and Vanderhoest, 1982).

In summary, after cardiac surgery, the most likely explanation for the development of atelectasis is abnormal surfactant release or dysfunction, which may be secondary to pulmonary ischemia or the cold temperature during bypass. After thoracotomies for lung surgery, accumulation of bronchial secretions, increased lung water content, and reduced surfactant activity are also probably important factors that favor the development of atelectasis. In contrast to upper abdominal operations, cardiac and thoracic operations do not appear to produce significant postoperative diaphragmatic dysfunction that contributes to the development of atelectasis.

B. Treatment of Atelectasis

Following cardiothoracic or upper abdominal surgery, patients experience severe immediate postoperative pain and marked respiratory impairment, which is characterized by a restrictive pattern of breathing with significant reductions in forced vital capacity, FRC, tidal volume, and peak expiratory flow rates. The ventilatory changes seen after surgery include monotonous shallow breathing without spontaneous deep breaths, which perpetuates atelectasis, causes increased work of breathing, and perhaps leads to the development of pneumonia. Although there is no therapy that prevents these postoperative alterations in breathing and the development of atelectasis, it has been suggested that effective pain relief and chest physical therapy may normalize the abnormal breathing pattern and minimize the development of significant postoperative complications. The objective of this section is to review the effect of postoperative analgesia and chest physical therapy on postoperative pulmonary function and their role in decreasing postoperative pulmonary complications.

Effect of Analgesia on Postoperative Pulmonary Function

Although any effective analgesic regimen improves the patient's comfort, the route used to administer the agents may influence the effect of analgesia on postoperative pulmonary function. Narcotic drugs given parenterally produce paradoxical breathing and obstructive apnea; these episodes are also associated with decreased lung volumes and with profound oxygen desaturation (Catley et al., 1985). The depressant properties of narcotic analgesia are also enhanced by sleep (Forrest and Bellville, 1964). This fact is particularly important in the postoperative period, as patients spend a large proportion of their time sleeping. These results suggest that narcotic analgesia administered by the conventional parenteral route has serious ventilatory sequelae.

Administration of narcotic analgesia in the epidural space has been shown to provide long-lasting postoperative analgesia (Shulman et al., 1984). Some studies also suggest that epidural narcotic analgesia per se may improve postoperative respiratory mechanics when compared with parenteral narcotic analgesia (Shulman et al., 1984; Miller et al., 1976; Rybro et al., 1982; Welchew and Thornton, 1982). However, these results have not been confirmed by other authors (Bonnet et al., 1984; Rawal et al., 1984; Hjortso et al., 1985; Jayr et al., 1988). The results of studies that have focused on the etiology of the postoperative pulmonary dysfunction have shown that pain is not the key mechanism leading to the development of atelectasis and hypoxemia in the postoperative period. Indeed, diaphragmatic dysfunction, a major cause of respiratory complications after UAS, is not altered by the administration of narcotics in the epidural space, despite the achievement of complete analgesia. Similarly, the shallow and rapid breathing observed after UAS is not abolished by intrathecal injections of morphine even though complete pain relief is obtained (Clergue et al., 1984). Furthermore, the incidence of clinical and radiological postoperative pulmonary complications is not altered by analgesia; Jayr et al. reported a similar incidence of pulmonary complications in a prospective study including 150 patients receiving parental or epidural morphine after abdominal cancer surgery (Jayr et al., 1988).

In contrast, administration of local anesthetics in the epidural space may improve postoperative diaphragm function, probably by interrupting visceral or somatic inhibitory afferents of phrenic activity and increasing abdominal compliance. However, this beneficial effect on the diaphragm function has not always been associated with a decrease in postoperative respiratory complications. Although two reports have shown fewer pulmonary complications with epidural bupivacaine compared to parenteral morphine (Bromage, 1967; Spence and Smith, 1971), other studies did not find any difference in postoperative complications using these two analgesic regimens (Hjortso et al., 1985). This discrepancy may be explained by the fact that some pulmonary complications may not be related to diaphragmatic dysfunction, and that the level of local analgesia was insufficient in some patients to abolish all inhibitory afferents of phrenic activity. Epidural analgesia with local anesthetics is difficult to use in many surgical patients because it is often associated with a bilateral sympathetic blockade resulting in hypotenstion (Logas et al., 1987). This deleterious side effect is also more marked in older patients and in those who have had previous myocardial infarctions (James et al., 1981) or who have had lung resections (Conacher et al., 1983) Intercostal blocks may be an alternative therapy, as they produce similar analgesia (Rawal et al., 1982) and similar improvement in postoperative respiratory function (Faust and Nauss, 1976) as produced by epidural bupivicaine, and intercostal blocks do not produce as severe a decrease in blood pressure (Giesecke et al., 1988). Continuous infusion of small doses of bupivacaine through an indwelling epidural catheter placed extrapleurally is another possible anesthetic technique; this technique obviates the need for repeated intercostal blocks and may also be associated with less hypotension than is seen after ordinary epidural bupivacaine (Sabanathan et al., 1988).

In summary, narcotic analgesia does not appear to improve respiratory function or to decrease the incidence of pulmonary complications after surgery. Regional anesthesia may significantly improve postoperative pulmonary function, but its effect on the incidence of pulmonary complications remains uncertain.

Chest Physical Therapy and Postoperative Pulmonary Function

A decrease in FRC after surgery is due to the persistence of atelectasis and the lack of volitional deep breathing. Periodic maximal inflation restores FRC, normalizes gas exchange, and reduces the incidence of postoperative pulmonary complications (Barlett et al., 1973). Improvement in FRC can be achieved by sitting patients up after surgery (Meyers et al., 1975). Walking is even more effective than sitting, because it further increases FRC and stimulates patients to breathe deeply as a result of movement and exertion (Lewis, 1980). Chest physical therapy, including deep breaths, has been reported to significantly decrease the frequency of postoperative respiratory complications (Morran et al., 1983). The ideal deep breath should be one that is held for 3 sec. A 3-sec deep breath is superior to multiple deep breaths or a single, unsustained deep breath (Ward et al., 1966). A deep breath increases transpulmonary pressure and distends the lungs. However, to be effective, these deep-breath maneuvers must be repeated every 1–2 hr during the waking hours and should be supervised by a nurse or a respiratory therapy practitioner (Ferris and Pollard, 1960). The introduction of aids to deep breathing, including incentive spirometry (IS), intermittent positive pressure breathing (IPPB), or continuous positive airway pressure (CPAP), has added more therapeutic options but may not truly benefit the patient. IS, the most popular lung expansion technique, is prescribed in 95% of hospitals in the United States today. Although IS is superior to no respiratory treatment in preventing postoperative respiratory complications (Celli et al., 1984), there is little evidence from controlled studies that this technique is better than conventional chest physical therapy with deep-breathing exercises in low-risk patients (Celli et al., 1984; Jung et al., 1980; Stock et al., 1985; Schwieger et al., 1986). Interestingly, IS increases the diaphragmetic contribution to the tidal volume preoperatively, but does not do this after surgery; instead, postoperative patients respond to IS by increasing the tidal excursion of their thorax (Chuter et al., 1989). A possible explanation for this is that the patient's attention is focused on the movement of the spirometer ball, which can be moved by increasing chest wall excursion and moving the diaphragm. Not only is IPPB no more effective than other lung expansion techniques, it is very costly and requires specially trained personnel (Celli et al., 1984; Jung et al., 1980; Ali et al., 1984); IPPB also produces abdominal distention in a significant percentage of patients (Celli et al., 1984), all of which make it the least preferred respiratory treatment for the routine management of postoperative surgical patients. Face mask CPAP is an effective treatment for postoperative atelectasis (Stock et al., 1985; Ricksten et al., 1986). The disadvantages of this therapy are its cost, patient discomfort from a tight-fitting mask, and the potential risk of endobronchial aspiration of gastric contents. Nasal CPAP may be an alternative, because it may cause fewer complications (Duncan et al., 1987).

In summary, the present treatment of postoperative atelectasis is only partially successful in patients who have had cardiac, thoracic, or abdominal surgery. The following routine measures should be taken after these operations to help restore pulmonary function and decrease the incidence of pulmonary complications: relieving pain adequately to allow deep breathing, including the use of local analgesia when possible; sitting the patient upright in bed or in a chair as soon as possible after an operation; making the patient take an inspiratory effort of at least 3-sec duration every hour while awake, and finally, using mask or nasal CPAP if other measures have failed.

III. High-Risk Groups

A. Smokers

Postoperative atelectasis is common, particularly after abdominal operations, and does not appear to be associated with any predisposing risk factors (Jayr et al., 1988). In contrast, other postoperative complications, such as fever, productive cough, and pneumonia occur more frequently in certain high-risk groups than in others. Patients who smoke more than 10 cigarettes per day have a sixfold increase in incidence of fever, cough, and pneumonia after surgery (Chalon et al., 1975). Wightman studied patients who had had abdominal operations and found that 14.8% of the patients who smoked had a postoperative complication, whereas only 6.3% of the nonsmoking patients developed pulmonary complications (Wightman, 1968). Lazlo et al. (1973) evaluated all kinds of operations and found that smokers had a 53% incidence of postoperative bronchitis, atelectasis, or pneumonia compared to a 22% incidence in nonsmokers. In a comparison of light smokers (one to nine cigarettes per day) and heavy smokers (>30 cigarettes per day), the incidence of postoperative respiratory complications was found to be 9% and 43%, respectively. Nonsmokers had an incidence of 7.9% of postoperative pulmonary complications (Chalon et al., 1975).

Over 1000 components of cigarette smoke have been identified, and they have wide-ranging effects on the cardiovascular, respiratory, and immune systems, hemostasis, drug metabolism, and patient psychology (Pearce and Jones, 1984). Smoking must be stopped for 4–6 weeks before any beneficial effect can be demonstrated objectively by respiratory function studies (Martin et al., 1975). However, patients will benefit from the elimination of carbon monoxide and the nicotine that occurs after 24 hr of abstinence. After 12–24 hr of smoking cessation, respiratory epithelial cillia beat more effectively, and after several days of not smoking, sputum volume decreases significantly (Pearce and Jones, 1984).

B. Chronic Obstructive Pulmonary Disease

Most investigators have found that patients with abnormal pulmonary function studies are predisposed to an increased incidence of postoperative pulmonary complications, including pneumonia, exacerbation of bronchitis, and fever. Stein and co-workers (1962) were among the first to show that a group of patients with abnormal pulmonary function studies had a 70% risk of developing the pulmonary complications noted above. In a study of 785 patients who underwent elective nonthoracic surgery, 53 of the patients were found to have chronic obstuctive lung disease; of these, 27 (i.e., 50%) developed a pulmonary complication, compared to 44 (or 6%) of the patients without obstructive lung disease. Wightman (1968) also noted that patients who had upper abdominal operations and who also had obstructive lung disease also had a higher incidence of postoperative pulmonary complications than those without airflow obstruction.

Evaluations of more serious postoperative pulmonary complications include Tarhan's study of 63,853 patients who had undergone general anesthesia from 1967 to 1970 (Tarhan et al., 1973); of the 357 patients who had moderate to severe chronic lung disease, 33 (9.2%) died within 9 weeks of their operation secondary to a respiratory complication. Tarhan et al. also found that operations on the thorax and abdomen were associated with a significant increase in mortality (Tarhan et al., 1973). Tarhan's study is not the only study that reported an increased mortality associated with preexisting lung disease. Stein and Cassara (1970) reported that 4 of the 48 (8%) patients who died of postoperative pulmonary complications had abnormal preoperative pulmonary function tests. However, these investigators could not distinguish those patients who died from the other patients with abnormal pulmonary function tests who sustained milder or who had no pulmonary complications postoperatively (Stein and Cassara, 1970). Milledge and Nunn (1975) followed 12 patients with very severe chronic obstructive lung disease (range of FEV_1 1.45–1.04 L) to determine their operative and post operative course. There were no deaths in this group. However, the patients underwent only five abdominal operations and only two had surgery of the upper abdomen; both these patients required prolonged oxygen therapy and one required prolonged ventilatory support. One patient who underwent eye surgery required prolonged postoperative ventilation; this patient had preoperative hypercapnia. Therefore, upper abdominal surgery again appears to be a significant risk factor for mild and severe postoperative pulmonary complications and preoperative hypercapnia appears to be a risk factor for postoperative assisted ventilation.

Other studies have evaluated the need for postoperative ventilation. Cain and associates (1979) evaluated 106 patients who had major thoracic or upper abdominal vascular surgery in an attempt to indentify the preoperative factors that predicted the requirement of prolonged intensive care therapy and found that preoperative pulmonary fuction tests were of no value in predicting the duration of intensive care unit therapy. Jayr and co-workers (1989) evaluated a group of elderly smokers who underwent abdominal vascular surgery to determine the incidence and causes of postoperative respiratory failure. Twelve patients out of 51 required more than 24 hr of mechanical ventilation. Preoperative hypoxemia, an extensive smoking history, and large intraoperative blood loss and fluid administration were associated with the need for postoperative ventilation. These patients did not develop cardiogenic pulmonary edema, but appeared to have increased minute ventilation requirements secondary to severe atelectasis and/or lung injury. Three of these 12 patients died of multisystem organ failure, with respiratory failure contributing to their deaths.

In conclusion, patients who smoke or who have chronic obstructive lung disease appear to be at increased risk for fever, chronic bronchitis, and pneumonia postoperatively. Their risk of developing these complications further increases if they have thoracic or upper abdominal operations, and some reports have shown that patients with chronic obstructive pulmonary disease have an increased mortality from these pulmonary complications. Postoperative ventilation in this group of patients is associated with preoperative hypoxemia and is also found commonly in patients with preoperative hypercapnia. Intraoperative blood loss, possibly a marker of the severity of disease and the difficulty of the surgical repair, also appears to be an important factor in determining postoperative pulmonary ventilation requirements (Jayr et al., 1989).

C. Organ Transplantation

Respiratory infection is a major problem in patients with renal, liver, heart, and lung transplants (Skerrett et al., 1989). Pneumonia often occurs during the early posttransplant period; Kusne and associates (1988) noted that all cases of nosocomial pneumonia in their liver transplant patients occurred within 1 week of surgery, and Dauber and colleagues (1990) reported a 35% incidence of pneumonia in heart-lung and lung transplant patients within the first 2 weeks after transplant. In the first month after renal transplant, enteric gram-negative bacillary pneumonia occurred in the renal transplant patients who remained hospitalized, and *Pseudomonas* pneumonias were found only in patients who were adjacent to other hospitalized patients (Ramsey et al., 1980). Kusnu and colleagues (1988) found that the length of surgery for liver transplant patients also correlated with their risk of infection. However, there have been insufficient studies to allow identification of the factors that distinguish the transplant patients who develop postoperative pneumonia from those who do not. Infections and other pulmonary complications that occur after bone marrow and solid-organ transplantation are discussed in detail in Chapter 2.

IV. Postoperative Pneumonia

A. Factors

The results of several studies have documented an increased risk for the development of postoperative pneumonia after upper abdominal and thoracic surgery (Celis et al., 1988; Scheckler and Peterson, 1986; Hooton et al., 1980; Garibaldi et al., 1981; Salata et al., 1987). However, there have not been any studies that specifically explore the mechanisms that lead to the development of the postoperative pneumonia in these patients. Rather, studies have attempted to find the subpopulations of hospitalized patients who are at risk for the development of nosocomial pneumonia.

Nosocomial infections are those infections that develop in hospitalized patients in whom the infection was not present or not incubating at the time of admission to the hospital (Tobin and Grenvik, 1984). Pneumonia is the third most common nosocomial infection and causes 15% of all deaths in hospitalized patients (Septimus, 1989). Surgery appears to be an independent risk factor for the development of nosocomial pneumonia; in one report, the incidence of nosocomial pneumonia was 22% in a mixed surgical intensive care unit and 12% in a medical intensive care (Tobin and Grenvik, 1984; Septimus, 1989). However, there are several other risk factors for nosocomial pneumonia, and many of these factors occur in postoperative patients. For instance, prolonged intubation and mechanical ventilation have been found to increase the incidence of nosocomial pneumonia in patients (Septimus, 1989; Jimenez et al., 1989; Leu et al., 1989; Celis et al., 1988; Ruiz-Santana et al., 1987; Lowy et al., 1987; Craven and Driks, 1987; Salata et al., 1987; Craven et al., 1986). The chances of developing nosocomial pneumonia increase with an increasing duration of mechanical ventilation. The overall risk of nosocomial pneumonia in a ventilated patient is 9%; however, the risk is 6.5% after 10 days of ventilation, 19% after 20 days of ventilation, and 28% after 30 days of ventilation (Fagon et al., 1989). These data translate into approximately a 1% chance of developing pneumonia per day of mechanical ventilation (Niederman and Fein, 1990). Langer and associates found that 68% of their patients had developed pneumonia after 30 days of mechanical ventilation, but only 10% of the pneumonia appeared after the tenth day of ventilatory support (Langer et al., 1989). Patients who have tracheostomies and require mechanical ventilation have a 66% incidence of nosocomial pneumonia, whereas the patient who has a tracheostomy and does not require mechanical ventilation has a 25% chance of developing a nosocomial pneumonia (Cross and Roup, 1981).

Other important risk factors for the development of nosocomial pneumonia that have been reported reflect the characteristics of the various populations examined. In studies of only ventilated patients, underlying chronic obstructive lung disease has been found to be a risk factor (Jimenez et al., 1989), as was age (Fagon et al., 1989), a depressed level of consciousness, an episode of aspiration (Celis et al., 1988), and the presence of an intracranial pressure monitor, and having the mechanical ventilation circuit changed every 24 hr rather than every 48 hr (Craven et al., 1986). Among an entire group of hospitalized patients, risk factors for the development of nosocomial pneumonia were immunosuppression, leukopenia, nasogastric intubation, and bacteremia (Leu et al., 1989).

B. Pathogenesis

There are four proposed mechanisms for the development of nosocomial pneumonia; inhalation of airborne organisms, aspiration of oropharyngeal contents, direct extension from a contiguous site, and hematogenous spread (Hoyt, 1989). In the 1960s, there were several reported outbreaks of hospital-acquired pneumonia directly related to contaminated respiratory equipment (Ringrose et al., 1968; Reinarz et al., 1965). These findings prompted investigators to evaluate the safe duration for using a ventilator breathing circuit (Craven et al., 1982). Because of these studies, the use of disposable equipment has increased and the risk to the patient of an exogenous source for infection has been significantly reduced (Hoyt, 1989). Therefore, inhalation of airborne organisms does not now appear to be a significant cause of nosocomial pneumonia.

The currently accepted mechanism for the development of nosocomial pneumonia is the aspiration of oropharyngeal contents. Atherton and White (1978) were the first to note that 10 mechanically ventilated patients who had aerobic gram-negative rods in their gastric aspirates were later found to have the same organisms in their tracheal aspirates. Subsequently, it was shown that a majority of critically ill patients become colonized with gram-negative rods in their oropharynx (Tobin and Grenvik, 1984; Johanson et al., 1979; Johanson et al., 1969). The speculation is that oropharyngeal secretions, including the colonized gram-negative bacteria, leak into the trachea, often past an inflated cuff, and lead to lower-airway infection (Dixon, 1983). However, many more patients are colonized with gram-negative bacteria than develop nosocomial pneumonia, which suggests that colonization alone is insufficient for the development of a nosocomial pneumonia and, indeed, may not always be a prerequisite.

An association between colonization of the stomach and tracheal colonization has recently been reported (Garvey et al., 1989). These investigators studied 25 patients whose gastric pH values were alkalinized in an attempt to prevent stress ulcers and found that all 25 had positive bacterial cultures from their stomachs. They also found that, 19% of the time, subsequent cultures from the tracheobronchial tree revealed the same bacteria as in the stomach; however, 22% of the time the bacteria first appeared in the lung and then in the stomach, and 28% of the time the organisms in the stomach never appeared in the tracheobronchial secretions. A more recent study found similar results; 40 neurosurgical patients were randomly assigned to receive or not receive stress ulcer prophylaxis (Reusser et al., 1989). Patients were then followed for the development of stomach colonization, tracheobronchial tree colonization, and pneumonia. The authors found a strong correlation between alkalinization of the stomach and stomach colonization; however, they could only identify one patient from whom the organism was isolated from the stomach first and then the same organism was found in the tracheobronchial tree. Furthermore, there were no significant differences in the rates of pneumonia or septicemia between patients who had and who had not received stress ulcer prophylaxis (Reusser et al., 1989). Therefore, it appears that the stomach may at times be the source of bacteria that subsequently appear in the tracheobronchial secretions and may even be associated with the development of pneumonia. How often this sequence of infection occurs is unclear, and whether one method of gastric alkalinization is more often associated with the development of nosocomial pneumonia than another is not clear from the literature. In conclusion, most authors believe oropharyngeal colonization is a major factor in the development of nosocomial pneumonia; the role of gastric colonization secondary to gastric alkalinization in the development of nosocomial pneumonia is less clear from the current investigations.

C. Diagnosis

The diagnosis of nosocomial pneumonia in a nonintubated patient includes the development of infiltrates on a previously clear chest roentgenogram and the presence of infected sputum; fever and leukocytosis are often present as well. Unfortunately, the diagnosis of nosocomial pneumonia in intubated patients or in patients who have infiltrates already present on their chest radiographs is much more problematic. Experimental studies have shown that sputum samples from infected intubated baboons revealed 78% of the organisms found in their lung autopsy tissue, but the sputum also contained 14 species of bacteria that were not present in the postmortem lung tissue (Johanson et al., 1988). Postmortem needle aspirates of these baboon's lungs contained only 56% of the bacteria found in the autopsied lung tissue, and quantitative bronchoalveolar lavage contained 74% of all the bacteria present in the postmortem lung tissue (Johanson et al., 1988). Therefore, sputum samples contained too many organisms and quantitative bronchoalveolar lavage contained too few bacteria than were found in the lungs at autopsy in this study. Human studies have yielded somewhat different results. Fagon and associates (1989) studied 567 patients who had been mechanically ventilated for more than 3 days. Fiberoptic bronchoscopy for collecting specimens with a protected brush was performed on any patient suspected of having pneumonia; pneumonia, defined by the presence of 10^3 cfu/ml on quantitative culture of the protected brush specimen, was found in only 49% of the patients. The organisms isolated included *Pseudomonas aeruginosa* and *Staphylococcus aureus* in 33% of the pneumonias, and 40% of all the specimens contained more than one organism. Therefore, the majority of patients believed to have pneumonia clinically (because of new infiltrates and infected sputum) did not actually have sufficient bacteria recovered from their protected brush specimens to support the diagnosis.

The use of antibiotics in these intubated patients often changes the bacterial yields of the protected brush procedure, and when and how often the protected brush procedure is performed may also influence the yield of bacteria from this procedure. Nevertheless, these investigators have pursued some of these issues. Fagon and associates (1988) evaluated 147 ventilated patients for suspected pneumonia because of new infiltrates and purulent sputum. Positive cultures ($>10^3$ cfu/ml) from the protected brush were only found in 45 patients. These patients were followed, and in 34/45 of the patients antibiotics had been given and the patients responded to the antibiotics as if they had pneumonia. However, in 4 of the 45 patients, the protected brush specimen proved to be a false positive result. The diagnosis of pneumonia was excluded in 72 of 102 patients by the absence of pneumonia at autopsy or by the patient's recovery without antibiotic therapy. Thus, these results again suggest the appearance of new pulmonary infiltrates and purulent secretions in an intubated patient does *not* necessarily mean that significant numbers of bacteria will be found in the patient's lungs and that pneumonia is present.

Chastre and colleagues (1988) compared bronchoalveolar lavage and the protected brush specimen. Twenty-one ventilated patients who also had new pulmonary infiltrates and purulent tracheal secretions were studied using both the protected brush and bronchoalveolar lavage. The investigators concluded that quantitative culture of the protected brush specimen and microscopic identification of intracellular organisms in cells recovered by bronchoalveolar lavage provided important complementary information, and both procedures should be done to make the diagnosis of nosocomial pneumonia. Another technique, nonbronchoscopic bronchoalveolar lavage, has been recently described to investigate new infiltrates in intubated, ventilated patients (Piperno et al., 1988; Gaussorgues et al., 1989). These investigators performed 435 procedures and made a diagnosis based on the results of 55% of them. In 13 patients who died, an open lung biopsy of the same lobe that was lavaged could be done; all nine patients who had histological evidence of pneumonia also had had positive lavage cultures, whereas one patient without pneumonia on biopsy had a positive culture (75% specificity).

The conclusion from all these studies is that sputum cultures from intubated, mechanically ventilated patients are often inaccurate and do not precisely reveal the organisms found in these patients' lungs. Furthermore, intubated, mechanically ventilated patients can often have new pulmonary infiltrates and purulent sputum and not have significant intrapulmonary bacteria detected by more sensitive tests (i.e., protected brush specimen). A current recommendation for patients who are hemodynamically stable but suspected of having pneumonia is to perform fiberoptic bronchoscopy to obtain a protected brush specimen and perform brochoalveolar lavage (Meduri, 1990). If the patients' preliminary bronchoscopic results are negative, antibiotics should not be initiated and further evaluation should begin (Table 2). However, if the patient has received antibiotics, the results from bronchoscopy can be misleading (Meduri, 1990). Furthermore, if the patient has sepsis syndrome, as manifested by hemodynamic instability or the presence of a metabolic acidosis, empirical antibiotic therapy should be initiated and other sources of infection should also be considered (Table 2). Finally, the impact of these new diagnostic techniques, such as the bronchoscopic protected brush specimen, on a patient's outcome have yet to be established (Meduri, 1990).

Table 2 Evaluation of New Infiltrates and Purulent Sputum in a Ventilated Patient

Rule out extrapulmonary source of sepsis

- Blood culture and sensitivity ×2 from 2 different sites
- Urine for analysis and culture ×2
- Removal of central lines and submit the subcutaneous portion of the catheter for semiquantitative culture
- CT scan of the sinuses to rule out sinusitis
- Echocardiogram to rule out effusion or valvular vegetations

Abdominal x-ray/CT scan of the abdomen

- In patients at High Risk
  - S/P abdominal surgery
  - Pancreatitis
  - GI bleeding or cancer
  - High-dose steroids
- Or with abdominal examination

Rule out atelectasis

- Nebulized beta agonist every 4 hrs
- Chest percussion (over area with new infiltrate) every 2 hrs ×4
- Repeat chest x-ray after 4–8 hrs

Rule out DVT/Pulmonary emboli

- Portable V/Q scan
- Noninvasive evaluation for DVT (IPG or Doppler)

Rule out drug fever

- Discontinue nonessential therapy and observe

Source: Meduri, 1990, with permission.

V. Acute Lung Injury

A. Definition

The pathophysiology and treatment of acute lung injury have recently been reviewed, and therefore only the definition and prognosis of this disorder will be discussed (Wiener-Kronish et al., 1990; Matthay, 1991). Acute lung injury occurs in previously normal patients and can be a fatal postoperative pulmonary complication (Ashbaugh et al., 1967).

The definition of acute lung injury has evolved since the adult respiratory distress syndrome was first described by Ashbaugh and associates (1967). Since then, the heterogeneity of the inciting clinical disorders and the variability of the clinical course have been appreciated, and this information has been incorporated into an expanded definition of the adult respiratory distress syndrome (now referred to as acute lung injury) (Murray et al., 1988). The definition requires describing certain patient information including:

1. The acute lung injury score
2. The clinical risk factors
3. The time course for developing acute lung injury
4. The presence of multiorgan failure or infection

The lung injury score is shown in Table 3. The scoring involves the average of four scores that evaluate the chest radiograph, the arterial blood gas data, the respiratory compliance, and the amount of PEEP a patient is on (Table 3). Acute lung injury is then classified as mild to moderate if the average overall score is 0.1–2.5, and the injury is judged as severe if the averaged score is ≥2.5. Weinberg and colleagues (1984) used this scoring system and found that 25% of septic patients developed severe lung injury and 35% of septic patients developed mild to moderate lung injury. Sepsis is the most common precipitating factor for the development of acute lung injury, but the degree of lung injury produced is variable. The factors that moderate the degree of lung injury produced are still unclear. Investigations of septic patients have generated interest in predicting which septic patient will develop lung injury. Based on the results of experimental studies that have shown that injury to the pulmonary vascular endothelium occurs early in sepsis (Wiener-Kronish et al., 1990), plasma von Willebrand factor (vWF) antigen, a product of both the systemic and pulmonary endothelium, was measured in specific patients; a plasma vWF-antigen concentration >450% of control had a sensitivity of 92% and a specificity of 77% for predicting acute lung injury (Rubin et al., 1990). Moreover, if a patient had nonpulmonary organ failure at entry into the study and also had a plasma vWF antigen >450%, there was an 80% likelihood that the patient would develop lung injury and would die (Rubin et al., 1990).

Other clinical disorders besides sepsis, including gastric aspiration, pulmonary contusion, multiple emergency transfusions, multiple major fractures, pancreatitis, and prolonged hypotension, can lead to the development of acute lung injury. If a postoperative patient has one of these risk factors, his or her chances of developing acute lung injury is about 26%; if the patient has two or more of these risk factors, his chances of developing acute lung injury increase to 37% and 76%, respectively (Pepe et al., 1982). Patients tend to develop acute lung injury rapidly after an inciting event has occurred; for example, 79% of the patients with one of the clinical disorders described developed acute lung injury

Table 3 Components of the Lung Injury Score

1.	Chest radiograph score		
	No alveolar consolidation		0
	Alveolar consolidation in one quadrant		1
	Alveolar consolidation in two quadrants		2
	Alveolar consolidation in three quadrants		3
	Alveolar consolidation in four quadrants		4
2.	Hypoxemia score		
	Pao_2/Flo_2	≥ 300	0
	Pao_2/Flo_2	225–299	1
	Pao_2/Flo_2	175–224	2
	Pao_2/Flo_2	100–174	3
	Pao_2/Flo_2	<100	4
3.	Respiratory system compliance score (when ventilated)		
	Compliance	≥ 80 ml/cm H_2O	0
	Compliance	60–79 ml/cm H_2O	1
	Compliance	40–59 ml/cm H_2O	2
	Compliance	20–39 ml/cm H_2O	3
	Compliance	≤ 19 ml/cm H_2O	4
4.	PEEP score (when ventilated)		
	PEEP	≥ 5 cm H_2O	0
	PEEP	6–8 cm H_2O	1
	PEEP	9–11 cm H_2O	2
	PEEP	12–14 cm H_2O	3
	PEEP	≥ 15 cm H_2O	4

The final value is obtained by dividing the aggregate sum by the number of components that were used:

No lung injury	0
Mild-to-moderate lung injury	0.1–2.5
Severe lung injury (ARDS)	>2.5

Source: Wiener-Kronish et al., 1990, with permission.

within 24 hr after the inciting event and 96% of the patients had developed acute lung injury by 72 hr (Pepe et al., 1982). Therefore, clinical disorders besides sepsis can lead to the development of acute lung injury, and acute lung injury rapidly develops after such an inciting event.

B. Prognosis

Two clinical disorders that occur in postoperative patients appear to lead to an acute lung injury that is associated with a better prognosis for the patients. Patients who develop acute lung injury from fat emboli have a greater than 90% survival (Schonfeld et al., 1983). We have found that patients who develop acute lung injury following cardiopulmonary bypass tend to require less mechanical ventilation and also have a greater survival rate (Matthay and Wiener-Kronish, 1990). The degree of lung injury appears comparable to that observed in patients after other inciting disorders; however, nonpulmonary organ failure may not occur as often in association with these two particular clinical disorders.

The importance of nonpulmonary organ failure in acute lung injury patients is being recognized. Concomitant hepatic failure associated with acute lung injury has nearly a 100% mortality (Schwartz et al., 1989). Patients with acute lung injury who had a pH less than 7.4, a serum bicarbonate concentration of less than 20 mmol/dl (despite mechanical ventilation and other therapies), and a blood urea nitrogen greater than 23 mmol/l (65 mg/dl) had a higher (80%) mortality compared to patients with acute lung injury without these findings. Those patients without these findings had a mortality of 40% (Fowler et al., 1985). Clearly, nonpulmonary factors are also important in affecting a patient's prognosis, and nonpulmonary organ failure is an important factor to consider in categorizing patients with acute lung injury (Table 3).

VI. Summary

In this chapter we have discussed a variety of postoperative pulmonary complications, the mechanisms that may contribute to them, and their diagnosis and treatment. All patients who undergo surgery are vulnerable to the development of postoperative complications, but these are influenced by the type of operation and the presence of certain risk factors. Postoperative atelectasis is extremely common and is difficult to prevent and treat. Pneumonia is also frequent and its prevalence has been linked to several predisposing factors. Acute lung injury, although infrequent in its severe form, is the most devastating because of its high mortality rate.

The radiographic appearance and gas exchange abnormalities of a patient who has acute lung injury are no longer considered adequate in quantifying the extent of the patient's injury. Patients with acute lung injury must now be evaluated in terms of the etiology of their acute lung injury, the duration that their lung injury persists, the severity of their lung injury (based on the lung injury score), and whether other organ failure has occurred. All these factors determine whether the patient will survive and perhaps determine the degree of lung recovery.

References

Albano, J. P., and Garnier, L. (1983). Bulbo-spinal respiratory effects originating from the splanchnic afferents. *Respir. Physiol.* **51**:229–239.

Ali, J., Weisel, R. D., Layug, A. B., Kripke, B. J., and Hechtman, H. B. (1974). Consequences of postoperative alterations in respiratory mechanics. *Am. J. Surg.* **128**:376–382.

Ali, J., Serrette, C., Wood, L. D. H., and Anthonisen, N. R. (1984). Effect of postoperative intermittent positive pressure breathing on lung function. *Chest* **85**:192–196.

Allen, P. D., Walman, T., Concepcion, M., Sheskey, M., Patterson, M. K., Cullen, D., and Covino, B. G. (1986). Epidural morphine provides postoperative pain relief in peripheral vascular and orthopedic surgical patients: a dose-response study. *Anesth. Analg.* **65**:165–170.

Ashbaugh, D. G., Bigelow, D. B., Petty, T. L., and Levine, B. E. (1967). Acute respiratory distress in adults. *Lancet* **2**:319–323.

Atherton, S. T., and White, D. J. (1978). Stomach as a source of bacteria colonizing respiratory tract during artificial ventilation. *Lancet* **2**:968–969.

Barlett, R. H., Brennan, M. L., Gazzangia, A. B., and Hanson, E. L. (1973). Studies on the pathogenesis and prevention of postoperative pulmonary complications. *Surg. Gynecol. Obstet.* **137**:925–933.

Bendixen, H. H., Headley-White, J., and Laver, M. B. (1963). Impaired oxygenation in surgical patients during general anesthesia with controlled ventilation: a concept of atelectasis. *N. Engl. J. Med.* **269**:991–996.

Bergman, N. A. (1963). Distribution of inspired gas during anesthesia and artificial ventilation. *J. Appl. Physiol.* **18**:1085–1089.

Bergman, N. A., and Tien, Y. K. (1983). Contribution of the closure of pulmonary units to impaired oxygenation during anesthesia. *Anesthesiology* **59**:395–401.

Bindslev, L., Hedenstierna, G., Santesson, J., Gotlieb, I., and Carvalhas, A. (1981). Ventilation-perfusion distribution during inhaled anesthesia. Effect of spontaneous breathing, mechanical ventilation and positive end-expiratory pressure. *Acta Anaesth. Scand.* **25**:360–371.

Bonnet, F., Blery, C., Zatan, M., Simonet, O., Brage, D., and Gaudy, J. (1984). Effect of epidural morphine on postoperative pulmonary dysfunction. *Acta Anaesth. Scand.* **28**:147–151.

Brismar, R. B., Hedenstierna, G., Lundquist, H., Strandberg, A., Svensson, L., and Tokics, L. (1985). Pulmonary densities during anesthesia with muscular relaxation-proposal of atelectasis. *Anesthesiology* **62**:422–428.

Bromage, P. R. (1967). Extradural analgesia for pain relief. *Br. J. Anaesth.* **39**:721–729.

Cain, H. D., Stevens, P. M., and Adaniya, R. (1979). Preoperative pulmonary function and complications after cardiovascular surgery. *Chest* **76**:130–135.

Catley, D. M., Thornton, C., Jorddon, C., Lehane, J. R., Royston, D., and Jones, J. G. (1985). Pronounced episodic oxygen desaturation in the postoperative period: its association with ventilatory pattern and analgesic regimen. *Anesthesiology* **63**:20–28.

Celis, R., Torres, A., Gatell, J. M., Almela, M., Rodriguez-Roisin, R., and Agusti-Vidal, A. (1988). Nocosomial pneumonia. A multivariate analysis of risk and prognosis. *Chest* **93**:318–324.

Celli, B. R., Rodriguez, K. S., and Snider, G. L. (1984). A controlled trial of intermittent positive pressure breathing, incentive spirometry and deep breathing exercises in preventing pulmonary complications after abdominal surgery. *Am. Rev. Respir. Dis.* **130**:12–15.

Chalon, J., Tayyab, M. A., and Ramanathan, S. (1975). Cytology of respiratory epithelium as a predictor of respiratory complications after operation. *Chest* **67**:32–35.

Chastre, J., Fagon, J. Y., Soler, P., Bornet, M., Domart, Y., Trouillet, J. L., Gebert, C., and Hance, A. J. (1988). Diagnosis of nosocomial bacterial pneumonia in intubated patients undergoing ventilation: comparison of the usefulness of bronchoalveolar lavage and the protected specimen brush. *Am. J. Med.* **85**:499–506.

Chuter, T. A. M., Weissman, C., Starker, P. M., and Gump, F. E. (1989). Effect of incentive spirometry on diaphragmatic function after surgery. *Surgery* **105**:488–493.

Clergue, F., Montembeault, C., Delpierre, O., Ghesquiere, F., Harari, A., and Viars, P. (1984). Respiratory effects of intrathecal morphine after upper abdominal surgery. *Anesthesiology* **61**:677–685.

Clyburn, P. A., Rosen, M., and Vickers, M. D. (1990). Comparison of respiratory effects of i.v. infusions of morphine and regional analgesia by extradural block. *Br. J. Anaesth.* **64**:446–449.

Conacher, I. D., Paes, M. L., Jacobson, L., Phillips, P. D., and Heariside, D. W. (1983). Epidural analgesia following thoracic surgery: a review of two years experience. *Anesthesiology* **38**:546–551.

Craig, D. B. (1981). Postoperative recovery of pulmonary function. *Anesth. Analg.* **60**:46–52.

Craven, D. E., and Driks, M. R. (1987). Nosocomial pneumonia in the intubated patient. *Semin. Respir. Infect.* **2**:20–33.

Craven, D. E., Connolly, M. G., and Lichtenberg, D. A. (1982). Contamination of mechanical ventilators with tubing changes every 24 or 48 hours. *N. Engl. J. Med.* **306**:1505–1509.

Craven, D. E., Kunches, L. M., Kilinsky, V., Lichtenberg, D. A., Make, B. S., and McCabe, W. R. (1986). Risk factors for pneumonia and fatality in patients receiving continuous mechanical ventilation. *Am. Rev. Respir. Dis.* **133**:792–796.

Craven, D. E., Kunches, L. M., Lichtenberg, D. A., Kollisch, N. R., Barry, A., Heeren, T. C., and McCabe, W. R. (1988). Nosocomial infection and fatality in medical and surgical intensive care unit patients. *Arch. Intern. Med.* **148**:1161–1168.

Cross, A. S., and Roup, B. (1981). Role of respiratory assistance devices in endemic nosocomial pneumonia. *Am. J. Med.* **70**:681–685.

Dauber, J. H., Paradis, I. L., and Dummer, J. S. (1990). Infectious complications in pulmonary allograft recipients. *Clin. Chest Med.* **11**:291–308.

De Troyer, A., and Vanderhoest, P. (1982). Phrenic nerve function after pneumonectomy. *Chest* **81**:212–214.

Dixon, R. E. (1983). Nosocomial respiratory infections. *Infect. Control* **4**: 376–381.

Don, H. F., Wahba, M., Cuadrado, L., and Kelker, K. (1970). The effect of anesthesia and 100% oxygen on the functional residual capacity of the lungs. *Anesthesiology* **32**:521–529.

Don, H. F., Wahba, W. M., and Craig, D. B. (1972). Airway closure, gas trapping, and the functional residual capacity during anesthesia. *Anesthesiology* **36**:533–539.

Dueck, R., Young, I., Clausen, J., and Wagner, P. D. (1980). Altered distribution of pulmonary ventilation and blood flow following induction of inhalational anesthesia. *Anesthesiology* **52**:113–125.

Duggan, J., and Drummond, G. B. (1987). Activity of lower intercostal and abdominal muscle after upper abdominal surgery. *Anesth. Analg.* **66**: 852–855.

Duggan, J. E., and Drummond, G. B. (1989). Abdominal muscle activity and intraabdominal pressure after upper abdominal surgery. *Anesth. Analg.* **69**:598–603.

Dummer, J. S., Montero, C. G., and Griffith, B. P. (1986). Infections in heart-lung transplant recipients. *Transplantation* **41**:725–729.

Duncan, S. R., Negrin, R. S., Mihm, F. G., Guilleminault, C., and Raffin, T. A. (1987). Nasal continuous positive airway pressure in atelectasis. *Chest* **92**:621–624.

Dureuil, B., Vires, N., Cantineau, J. P., Aubier, M., and Desmonts, J. M. (1985). Diaphragmatic contractility after upper abdominal surgery. *J. Appl. Physiol.* **61**:1775–1762.

Dureuil, B., Cantineau, J. P., and Desmonts, J. M. (1987a). Effects of upper or lower abdominal surgery on diaphragmatic function. *Br. J. Anaesth.* **59**:1230–1235.

Dureuil, B., Viires, N., Nivoche, Y., Fiks, M., Pariente, R., Aubier, M., and Desmonts, J. H. (1987b). Different effects of halothane on diaphragm and himblimb muscle in rats. *J. Appl. Physiol.* **63**:1757–1762.

Edmunds, L. H., and Alexander, J. A. (1980). Effect of cardiopulmonary bypass on the lungs. In *Pulmonary Disease and Disorders.* (Edited by A. P. Fishman.) McGraw-Hill, New York, pp. 1728.

Fagon, J. Y., Chastre, J., Hance, A. J., Guiguet, M., Trouillet, J. L., Domart, Y., Pierre, J., and Gebert, C. (1988). Detection of nosocomial lung infection in ventilated patients use of a protected specimen brush and quantitative culture techniques in 147 patients. *Am. Rev. Respir. Dis.* **138**:110–116.

Fagon, J. Y., Chastre, J., Domart, Y., Trouillet, J-L., Pierre, J., Darne, C., and Gibert, C. (1989). Nosocomial pneumonia in patients receiving continuous mechanical ventilation. *Am. Rev. Respir. Dis.* **139**:877–884.

Faritty, E. E., Permutt, S., and Riley, R. L. (1966). Effect of ventilation on surface forces in excised dog lungs. *J. Appl. Physiol.* **21**:1453–1462.

Faust, R. J., and Nauss, L. A. (1976). Postthoracotomy intercostal block: comparison of its effects on pulmonary function with those of intramuscular meperidine. *Anesth. Analg.* **55**:542–546.

Ferris, B., and Pollard, D. S. (1960). Effect of deep and quiet breathing on pulmonary compliance in man. *J. Clin. Invest.* **39**:143–149.

Ford, G. T., Grant, D. A., Rideaout, K. S., Davison, J. S., and Whitelaw, W. A. (1988a). Inhibition of breathing associated with gallbladder stimulation in dogs. *J. Appl. Physiol.* **65**:72–79.

Ford, G. T., Whitelaw, W. A., Rosenal, T. W., Cruse, P. J., and Guenter, C. A. (1988b). Diaphragm function after upper abdominal surgery in humans. *Am. Rev. Respir. Dis.* **127**:431–436.

Forrest, W. H., and Bellville, J. W. (1964). The effect of sleep plus morphine on the respiratory response to carbon dioxide. *Anesthesiology* **25**:137–141.

Fowler, A. A., Hamman, R. F., Zerbe, G. O., Benson, K., and Hyers, T. M. (1985). Adult respiratory distress syndrome; prognosis after onset. *Am. Rev. Respir. Dis.* **132**:472–478.

Froese, A. B., and Bryan, A. C. (1974). Effects of anesthesia and paralysis on diaphragmatic mechanics in man. *Anesthesiology* **41**:242–255.

Garibaldi, R. A., Britt, M. R., Coleman, M. L., Reading, J. C., and Pace, N. L. (1981). Risk factors for postoperative pneumonia. *Am. J. Med.* **70**:677–680.

Garvey, B. M., McCambley, J. A., and Taxen, D. V. (1989). Effects of gastric alkalization on bacterial colonization in critically ill patients. *Crit. Care Med.* **17**:211–216.

Gaussorgues, P., Piperno, D., Bachmann, P., Boyer, F., Jean, G., and Gerard, M. (1989). Comparison of nonbronchoscopic bronchoalveolar lavage to open lung biopsy for bacteriologic diagnosis of pulmonary infections in mechanically ventilated patients. *Intens. Care Med.* **15**:94–98.

Gentry, L. O., and Zeluff, B. (1988). Infection in the cardiac transplant patient. In *Clinical Approach to Infection in the Compromised Host*. (Edited by Y. L. Rubin.) Plenum Press, New York, pp. 623.

Germain, M., Wahba, W. M., and Gillied, D. M. M. (1982). Ventilation following induction of general anesthesia by thiopentone. *Can. Anaesth. Soc. J.* **29**:100–104.

Giesecke, K., Hamberger, B., Jarnberg, P. O., and Klingstedt, C. (1988). Paravertebral block during cholecystectomy: effects on circulation and hormonal responses. *Br. J. Anaesth.* **61**:652–656.

Gilmour, I., Burnham, M., and Craig, D. B. (1976). Closing capacity measurement during general anesthesia. *Anesthesiology* **45**:477–482.

Gorlin, R., Knowles, J. H., Storey, G. H., Fletcher, H. P., and Smith, S. H. (1957). Effects of thoracotomy on pulmonary function. *J. Thorac. Surg.* **34**:242–249.

Gracy, D. R., Divertie, M. B., and Didier, E. P. (1979). Preoperative pulmonary preparation of patients with chronic obstructive pulmonary disease: a prospective study. *Chest* **76**:123–129.

Hedenstierna, G. (1989). New aspects on atelectasis formation and gas exchange impairment during anesthesia. *Clin. Physiol.* **9**:407–417.

Hedenstierna, G., McHarty, G., and Bergstrom, M. (1976). Airway closure during mechanical ventilation. *Anesthesiology* **44**:114–123.

Hedenstierna, G., Lofstrom, B., and Lundh, R. (1981). Thoracic gas volume and chest abdomen dimensions during anesthesia and muscle paralysis. *Anesthesiology* **55**:499–501.

Hedenstierna, G., Tokics, L., Lundh, B., Strandberg, A., Brismar, B., Lindquist, H., and Frostell, C. (1989). Pulmonary densities during anesthesia. An experimental study on lung histology and gas exchange. *Eur. Respir. J.* **2**:528–535.

Hjortso, N. C., Neuman, P., Frosig, F., Andersen, T., Lindhard, A., Rogon, E., and Kehlet, H. (1985). A controlled study on the effect of epidural analgesia with local anesthetics and morphine on morbidity after abdominal surgery. *Acta Anaesth. Scand.* **29**:790–796.

Hooton, T. M., Haley, R. W., Culver, D. H., White, J. W., Morgan, W. M., and Carroll, R. J. (1980). The joint associations of multiple risk factors with the occurrence of nosocomial infection. *Am. J. Med.* **70**:960–970.

Hoyt, J. W. (1989). Nosocomial pneumonia. *Anesth. Clin. North Am.* **7**:869–881.

James, E. C., Kolber, H. L., Iwen, G. W., and Gellatly, T. A. (1981). Epidural anesthesia for post-thoracotomy patients. *J. Thorac. Cardiovasc. Surg.* **82**:898–903.

Jammes, Y., Buchler, B., Delpierre, S., Rasidakis, A., Grimaud, C., and Roussos, C. (1986). Phrenic afferents and their role in inspiratory control. *J. Appl. Physiol.* **60**:854–860.

Jayr, C., Mollie, A., Bourgain, J. L., Alarcon, J., Masselot, J., Lasser, P., Denjean, A., Truffa-Bachi, J., and Henry-Amar, M. (1988). Postoperative pulmonary complications: general anesthesia with postoperative parenteral morphine compared with epidural analgesia. *Surgery* **104**:57–63.

Jayr, C., Matthay, M. A., Lampe, G., Goldstone, J., and Wiener-Kronish, J. P. (1989). Preoperative hypoxemia is a reasonable predictor of severe postoperative pulmonary complications in patients undergoing major abdominal vascular surgery. *Am. Rev. Respir. Dis.* **139**:A151.

Jimenez, P., Torres, A., Rodriguez-Roisin, R., de la Bellasca, J. P., Aznar, R., Gatell, J. M., and Agusti-Vidal, A. (1989). Incidence and etiology of pneumonia acquired during mechanical ventilation. *Crit. Care Med.* **17**:882–885.

Johanson, W. G., Pierce, A. K., and Sanford, J. P. (1969). Changing pharyngeal bacterial flora of hospitalized patients. Emergence of gram-negative bacilli. *N. Engl. J. Med.* **281**:1138–1140.

Johanson, W. G., Woods, E. D., and Chaudhuri, T. (1979). Association of respiratory tract colonization with adherence of gram negative bacilli to epithelial cells. *J. Infect. Dis.* **139**:667–673.

Johanson, W. G., Jr., Seidenfeld, J. J., Gomez, P., de los Santos, R., and Coalson, J. J. (1988). Bacteriologic diagnosis of nosocomial pneumonia following prolonged mechanical ventilation. *Am. Rev. Respir. Dis.* **137**:259–264.

Jung, R., Wight, J., Nusser, R., and Rosoff, L. (1980). Comparison of three methods of respiratory care following upper abdominal surgery. *Chest* **78**:31–35.

Juno, P., Marsh, M., Knopp, T. J., and Rehder, K. (1978). Closing capacity in awake and anesthetized-paralyzed man. *J. Appl. Physiol.* **44**:238–244.

Kaplan, J. A. (1983). *Thoracic Anesthesia*. Churchill-Livingstone, New York.

Karlson, K. E., Seltzer, B., Lee, S., and Gliedman, M. L. (1965). Influence of thoracotomy on pulmonary mechanics: association of increased work of breathing during anesthesia and postoperative pulmonary complications. *Ann. Surg.* **162**:973–980.

Krayer, S., Rehder, K., Vettermann, J., Didier, P., and Ritman, E. L. (1989). Position and motion of the human diaphragm during anesthesia-paralysis. *Anesthesiology* **70**:891–898.

Kusne, S., Dummer, S. J., Singh, N., Iwatsuki, S., Makowka, L., Esquivel, C., Tzakis, A. G., Stanzl, T. E., and Ho, M. (1988). Infections after liver transplant. An analysis of 101 consecutive cases. *Medicine* **67**:132–143.

Langer, M., Mosconi, P., Cigada, M., Mandelli, M., and Intensive Care Unit Group of Infection Control. (1989). Long-term respiratory support and risk of pneumonia in critically ill patients. *Am. Rev. Respir. Dis.* **140**:302–305.

Latimer, R. G., Dickman, M., Day, W. C., Gunn, M. L., and Schmidt, C. D. (1971). Ventilatory patterns and pulmonary complications after upper abdominal surgery determined by preoperative and postoperative computerized spirometry and blood gas analysis. *Am. J. Surg.* **122**:622–632.

Lazlo, G., Archer, G. G., Darrell, J. H., Dawson, J. M., and Fletcher, C. M. (1973). The diagnosis and prophylaxis of pulmonary complications of surgical operation. *Br. J. Surg.* **60**:129–134.

Leu, H. S., Kaiser, D. L., Mori, M., Woolson, R. F., and Wenzel, R. P. (1989). Hospital acquired pneumonia attributable mortality and morbidity. *Am. J. Epidemiol.* **129**:1258–1267.

Lewis, F. R. (1980). Management of atelectasis and pneumonia. *Surg. Clin. North Am.* **60**:1391–1401.

Logas, W. G., El-Blax, N., El-Ganzouri, A., Cullen, M., Staren, E., Faber, P., and Ivankovich, A. D. (1987). Continuous thoracic epidural analgesia for postoperative pain relief following thoracotomy: a randomized, prospective study. *Anesthesiology* **67**:787–791.

Lowy, F. D., Carlisle, P. S., Adams, A., and Feiner, C. (1987). The incidence of nosocomial pneumonia following urgent endotracheal intubation. *Infect. Control* **8**:245–248.

Lundh, R., Hedenstierna, G., and Johansson, H. (1983). Ventilation-perfusion relationships during epidural analgesia. *Acta Anaesth. Scand.* **27**:410–416.

Maeda, H., Nakahara, K., Ohno, K., Kido, T., Ikeda, M., and Kawashima, Y. (1988). Diaphragm function after pulmonary resection. Relationship to postoperative respiratory failure. *Am. Rev. Respir. Dis.* **137**:678–681.

Malmkvist, G., Fletcher, R., Nordstrom, L., and Werner, O. (1989). Effects of lung surgery and one-lung ventilation on pulmonary arterial pressure, venous admixture, and immediate postoperative lung function. *Br. J. Anaesth.* **63**:696–701.

Mankikian, B., Cantineau, J. P., Bertrand, M., Kieffer, E., Sartene, R., and Viars, P. (1988). Improvement of diaphragmatic function by a thoracic extradural block after upper abdominal surgery. *Anesthesiology* **66**:379–386.

Markand, O. N., Moorthy, S. S., Mohomed, Y., King, R. D., and Brown, J. W. (1985). Postoperative phrenic nerve palsy in patients with open-heart surgery. *Ann. Thorac. Surg.* **39**:68–73.

Marshall, B. E., (1990). Hypoxic pulmonary vasoconstriction. *Acta Anaesth. Scand.* **34**(Suppl 94):37–41.

Marshall, B. E., and Wyche, M. Q. (1972). Hypoxemia during and after anesthesia. *Anesthesiology* **37**:178–209.

Martin, R. R., Lindsay, D., Despas, P., Bruce, D., Leroux, M., Anthovisen, N. R., and Macklen, P. T. (1975). The early detection of airway obstruction. *Am. Rev. Respir. Dis.* **111**:119–125.

Matthay, M. A., and Wiener-Kronish, J. P. (1988). Respiratory management after cardiac surgery. *Chest* **95**:424–434.

Matthay, M. A., and Wiener-Kronish, J. P. (1990). Intact epithelial barrier function is critical for the resolution of alveolar edema in humans. *Am. Rev. Respir. Dis.* **142**:1250–1257.

McCarthy, G. S. (1976). The effect of thoracic extradural analgesia on pulmonary gas distribution, functional residual capacity and airway closure. *Br. J. Anaesth.* **48**:243–248.

Meduri, G. (1990). Ventilator-associated pneumonia with respiratory failure. *Chest* **97**:1208–1219.

Meyers, J. R., Lembeck, L., O'Kane, H., and Baue, A. E. (1975). Changes in functional residual capacity of the lung after operation. *Arch. Surg.* **110**:576–583.

Milledge, J. S., and Nunn, J. F. (1975). Criterial of fitness for anesthesia in patients with chronic obstructive lung disease. *Br. Med. J.* **3**:670–673.

Miller, L., Gertel, M., Fox, G. S., and MacLean, L. D. (1976). Comparison of effect of narcotic and epidural analgesia on postoperative respiratory function. *Am. J. Surg.* **131**:291–294.

Morel, D. R., Forster, A., Bachmann, M., and Suter, P. M. (1984). Effect of intravenous midazolam on breathing pattern and chest wall mechanics in humans. *J. Appl. Physiol.* **57**:1104–1110.

Morel, D. R., Forster, A., and Gemperle, M. (1986). Noninvasive evaluation of breathing pattern and thoraco-abdominal motion following the infusion of ketamine or droperidol in humans. *Anesthesiology* **65**:392–398.

Morran, C. G., Finlay, I. G., Mathieson, M., Mckay, A. J., Wilson, N., and McArdle, C. S. (1983). Randomized controlled trial of physiotherapy for postoperative pulmonary complications. *Br. J. Anaesth.* **55**:1113–1117.

Murray, J. F., Matthay, M. A., Luce, J., and Flick, M. R. (1988). An expanded definition of the adult respiratory distress syndrome. *Am. Rev. Respir. Dis.* **138**:720–723.

Nagao, K., Ardila, R., Sugiyama, M., and Hildebrandt, J. (1977). Temperature and hydration: factors affecting increased recoil of excised rabbit lung. *Respir. Physiol.* **29**:11–24.

Niederman, M. S., and Fein, A. M. (1990). Sepsis syndrome, the adult respiratory distress syndrome, and nosocomial pneumonia. *Clin. Chest Med.* **11**:633–656.

Nims, R. G., Conner, E. G., and Comroe, J. H. (1955). The compliance of the human thorax in anesthetized patients. *J. Clin. Invest.* **34**:744–750.

Nunn, J. F., Bergman, N. A., and Coleman, A. J. (1965). Factors influencing the arterial oxygen tension during anesthesia with artificial ventilation. *Br. J. Anaesth.* **37**:898–914.

O'Donohue, W. J. (1985). National survey of the usage of lung expansion modalities for the prevention and treatment of postoperative atelectasis following abdominal and thoracic surgery. *Chest* **87**:76–80.

Orem, J., and Dement, W. C. (1976). Neurophysiological substrates of the changes in respiration during sleep. In *Advances in Sleep Research*. (Edited by E. D. Witzman.) Spectrum, New York, pp. 5–10.

Pasteur, W. (1910). Active lobar collapse of the lung after abdominal operations: a contribution to the study of postoperative lung complications. *Lancet* **2**:1080–1083.

Pearce, A. C., and Jones, R. M. (1984). Smoking and anesthesia: preoperative abstinence and perioperative morbidity. *Anesthesiology* **61**:576–584.

Pepe, P. E., Potkin, R. T., Reus, D. H., Hudson, L. D., and Carrico, C. J. (1982). Clinical predictors of the adult respiratory distress syndrome. *Am. J. Surg.* **144**:124–130.

Pflug, A. E., Murphy, T. M., Butler, S. H., and Tucker, G. T. (1974). The effects of postoperative peridural analgesia on pulmonary therapy and pulmonary complications. *Anesthesiology* **41**:8–17.

Piperno, D., Gaussorgues, P., Bachmann, P., Jaboulay, J. M., and Robert, D. (1988). Diagnostic value of nonbronchoscopic bronchoalveolar lavage during mechanical ventilation. *Chest* **93**:223.

Ramsey, P. G., Rubin, R. H., Tolkoff-Rubin, N. E., Cosimi, A. B., Russell, P. S., and Greene, R. (1980). The renal transplant patient with fever and pulmonary infiltrates: etiology, clinical manifestations and management. *Medicine* **59**:206–222.

Rawal, N., Sjostrand, U. H., Dahlstrom, B., Nydahl, P. A., and Ostelius, J. (1982). Epidural morphine for postoperative pain relief: a comparison with intramuscular narcotic and intercostal nerve block. *Anesth. Analg.* **61**:93–98.

Rawal, N., Sjostrand, U., Christoffersson, E., Dahlstrom, B., Arvill, A., and Rydman, H. (1984). Comparison of intramuscular and epidural morphine for postoperative analgesia in the grossly obese. *Anesth. Analg.* **63**: 583–592.

Rehder, K., Knopp, T. J., Sessler, A. D., and Didier, E. P. (1979). Ventilation-perfusion relationship in young healthy awake and anesthetized-paralyzed men. *J. Appl. Physiol.* **47**:745–753.

Reinarz, J. A., Pierce, A. K., and Maigs, B. B. (1965). The potential role of inhalation therapy equipment in nosocomial pulmonary infection. *J. Clin. Invest.* **44**:831–839.

Reusser, P., Zimmerli, W., Scheidegger, D., Marbet, G. A., Buser, M., and Gyrk. (1989). Role of gastric colonization in nosocomial infections and endotoxemia: a prospective study in neurosurgical patients on mechanical ventilation. *J. Infect. Dis.* **160**:414–421.

Richard, C. D. E., and White, A. E. (1975). The actions of volatile anesthetics on synaptic transmission in the dentate gyrus. *J. Physiol. (Lond.)* **252**:241–257.

Ricksten, S. E., Bengstsson, A., Soderberg, C., Thordon, A., and Kvist, H. (1986). Effects of periodic positive airway pressure by mask on postoperative pulmonary function. *Chest* **89**:774–781.

Rigg, J. R. A., and Rondi, P. (1981). Changes in rib cage and diaphragm contribution to ventilation after morphine. *Anesthesiology* **55**:507–514.

Ringrose, R. E., McKown, B., Felton, F. G., Barclay, B. O., Muchmore, H. G., and Rhoades, E. R. (1968). A hospital outbreak of *Serratia marcescens* associated with ultrasonic nebulizers. *Ann. Intern. Med.* **69**:719–728.

Road, J. D., Burgess, K. R., Whitelaw, W. A., and Ford, G. T. (1984). Diaphragm function and respiratory response after upper abdominal surgery in dogs. *J. Appl. Physiol.* **57**:576–582.

Roukema, J. A., Carol, E. J., and Prins, J. G. (1988). The prevention of pulmonary complications after upper abdominal surgery in patients with noncompromised pulmonary status. *Arch. Surg.* **123**:30–34.

Rubin, D. B., Wiener-Kronish, J. P., Murray, J. F., Green, D. R., Turner, J., Luce, J. M., Montgomery, A. B., Marks, J. B., and Matthay, M. A. (1990). Elevated von Willebrand factor antigen is an early plasma predictor of acute lung injury in nonpulmonary sepsis syndrome. *J. Clin. Invest.* **86**:474–480.

Rubin, R. H. (1988). Infection in the renal and liver transplant patient. In *Clinical Approach to Infection in the Compromised Host*, (2nd ed. Edited by Y. LS.) Plenum Press, New York, pp. 557–621.

Rue, H. S., Kaiser, D. L., Mori, M., Woolson, R. F., and Wenzel, R. P. (1989). Hospital-acquired pneumonia. Attributable mortality and morbidity, *Am. J. Epidemiol.* **129**:1258–1267.

Ruiz-Santana, S., Garcia Jimenez, A., Estaban, A., Guerra, L., Alvarez, B., Corcia, S., Guden, J., Martinez, A., Quintara, E., and Armangol, S. (1987). ICU pneumonias: a multi-institutional study. *Crit. Care Med.* **15**:930–932.

Rybro, L., Schurizek, B. A., Petersen, T. K., and Wernberg, M. (1982). Postoperative analgesia and lung function: a comparison of intramuscular with epidural morphine. *Acta Anaesth. Scand.* **26**:514–518.

Sabanathan, S., Bickford Smith, P. J., Pradhan, G. N., Hashimi, H., Eng, J., and Mearns, A. J. (1988). Continuous intercostal nerve block for pain relief after thoracotomy. *Ann. Thorac. Surg.* **46**:425–426.

Salata, R. A., Lederman, M. M., Shlaes, D. M., Jacobs, M. R., Eckstein, E., Tweardy, D., Toossi, Z., Chmielewski, R., Marino, J., King, C. H., Graham, R. C., and Ellner, J. J. (1987). Diagnosis of nosocomial pneumonia in intubated, intensive care unit patients. *Am. Rev. Respir. Dis.* **135**:426–432.

Scheckler, W. E., and Peterson, P. J. (1986). Nosocomial infections in 15 rural Wisconsin hospitals—results and conclusions from 6 months of comprehensive surveillance. *Infect. Control* **7**:397–402.

Schonfeld, S. A., Ploysongsany, Y., Di Lisio, R., Crissman, J. D., Miller, E., Hammerschmidt, D. E., and Jacob, H. S. (1983). Fat embolism prophylaxis with corticosteroids. *Ann. Intern. Med.* **99**:438–443.

Schwartz, D. A., Bone, R. C., Balk, R. A., and Szidon, J. P. (1989). Hepatic dysfunction in the adult respiratory distress syndrome. *Chest* **95**:871–875.

Schwieger, I., Gamulin, Z., Forster, A., Meyer, P., Gemperle, M., and Suter, P. (1986). Absence of benefit of incentive spirometry in low-risk patients undergoing elective cholecystectomy. A controlled randomized study. *Chest* **89**:652–656.

Septimus, E. J. (1989). Nosocomial bacterial pneumonias. *Semin. Respir. Infect.* **4**:245–252.

Shannon, R. (1980). Intercostal and abdominal muscle afferent influence on medullary dorsal respiratory group neurons. *Respir. Physiol.* **39**:73–94.

Shulman, M., Sandler, A. N., Bradley, J. W., Young, P. S., and Brebner, J. (1984). Postthoracotomy pain and pulmonary function following epidural and systemic morphine. *Anesthesiology* **61**:569–575.

Simmoneau, G., Vivien, A., Sartene, R., Kunstlinger, F., Samii, K., Noviant, Y., and Duroux, P. (1983). Diaphragm dysfunction induced by upper abdominal surgery: role of postoperative pain. *Am. Rev. Respir. Dis.* **128**:899–903.

Skerrett, S. J., Niederman, M. S., and Fein, A. M. (1989). Respiratory infections and acute lung injury in systemic illness. *Clin. Chest Med.* **10**: 469–502.

Slinger, P. D. (1990). Anaesthesia for lung resection. *Can. J. Anaesth.* **37**(4):Sxv–Sxxiv.

Smaje, J. C. (1976). General anaesthetics and the acetylcholine sensitivity of cortical neurones. *Br. J. Pharmacol.* **58**:359–366.

Spence, A. A., and Smith, G. (1971). Postoperative analgesiac and lung function: a comparison of morphine with extradural block. *Br. J. Anaesth.* **43**:144–148.

Stein, M., and Cassara, E. L. (1970). Preoperative pulmonary evaluation and therapy for surgery patients. *JAMA* **211**:787–790.

Stein, M., Koota, G. M., Simon, M., and Frank, H. A. (1962). Pulmonary evaluation of surgical patients. *JAMA* **181**:765–770.

Stinson, E. B., Bieber, C. P., and Griepp, R. B. (1971). Infectious complications after cardiac transplantation in man. *Ann. Intern. Med.* **74**:22–36.

Stock, M. C., Downs, J. B., Gauer, P. K., Alster, J. M., and Imrey, P. B. (1985). Prevention of postoperative pulmonary complications with CPAP, incentive spirometry, and conservative therapy. *Chest* **87**:151–157.

Strandberg, A., Brismar, B., Hedenstierna, G., Lundquist, H., and Tokics, L. (1986a). Atelectasis during anesthesia and in the postoperative period, *Acta Anaesth. Scand.* **30**:154–158.

Strandberg, A., Hedenstierna, G., Tokics, L., Lundquist, H., and Brismar, B. (1986b). Densities in dependent lung regions during anesthesia-atelectasis or fluid accumulation. *Acta Anaesth. Scand.* **30**:256–259.

Strandberg, A., Tokics, B., Brismar, B., Lundquist, H., and Hedenstierna, G. (1987). Constitutional factors promoting development of atelectasis during anaesthesia. *Acta Anaesth. Scand.* **31**:21–24.

Sykes, M. K., Young, W. E., and Robinson, B. E. (1965). Oxygenation during anesthesia with controlled ventilation. *Br. J. Anaesth.* **37**:314–324.

Sykes, M. K., Loh, L., Seed, R. F., Kafer, E. R., and Chakrabarti, N. K. (1972). The effect of inhalational anaesthetics on hypoxic pulmonary vasoconstriction and pulmonary vascular resistance in perfused lungs of the dog and cat. *Br. J. Anaesth.* **44**:776–788.

Tarhan, S., Moffitt, E. A., Sessler, A. D., Douglas, W. W., and Taylor, W. F. (1973). Risk of anesthesia and surgery in patients with chronic bronchitis and chronic obstructive pulmonary disease. *Surgery* **74**:720–726.

Tobin, M. J., and Grenvik, A. (1984). Nosocomial lung infection and its diagnosis. *Crit. Care Med.* **12**:191–199.

Tokics, L., Hedenstierna, G., Strandberg, A., Brismar, B., and Lundquist, H. (1987a). Lung collapse and gas exchange during general anesthesia—effects of spontaneous breathing, muscle paralysis and positive end-expiratory pressure. *Anesthesiology* **66**:157–167.

Tokics, L., Strandberg, A., Brismar, B., Lundquist, H., and Hedenstierna, G. (1987b). Computerized tomography of the chest and gas exchange measurements during ketamine anesthesia. *Acta Anaesth. Scand.* **32**: 684–692.

Tokics, L., Hedenstierna, G., Brismar, B., Strandberg, A., and Lundquist, H. (1988). Thoracoabdominal restriction in supine man: CT and lung function. *J. Appl. Physiol.* **64**:599–604.

Ward, R. J., Danziger, F., and Bonica, J. J. (1966). An evaluation of postoperative respiratory manoeuvre. *Surg. Gynecol. Obstet.* **123**:51–54.

Weinberg, P. F., Matthay, M. A., Webster, R. O., Roskos, K. V., Goldstein, I. M., and Murray, J. F. (1984). Biologically active products of complement and acute lung injury in patients with sepsis syndrome. *Am. Rev. Respir. Dis.* **130**:791–796.

Welchew, E. A., and Thornton, J. A. (1982). Continuous thoracic epidural fentanyl. *Anesthesia* **37**:309–316.

Westbrook, P. R., Stubbs, S. E., Sessler, A. D., Rehder, K., and Hyatt, R. E. (1973). Effects of anesthesia and muscle paralysis on respiratory mechanics in normal man. *J. Appl. Physiol.* **34**:81–86.

Wiener-Kronish, J. P., Gropper, M. A., and Matthay, M. A. (1990). The adult respiratory distress syndrome: definition and prognosis, pathogenesis and treatment. *Br. J. Anaesth.* **65**:107–129.

Wightman, J. A. K. (1968). A prospective survey of the incidence of postoperative pulmonary complications. *Br. J. Surg.* **55**:85–91.

Wilcox, P., Baile, E. M., Hards, J., Muller, N. L., Dunn, L., Pardy, R. L., and Pare, P. D. (1988). Phrenic nerve function and its relationship to atelectasis after coronary artery bypass surgery. *Chest* **93**:693–698.

Wiren, J. E., and Janzon, L. (1983). Respiratory complications following surgery. Improved prediction with preoperative spirometry. *Acta Anaesthesiol. Scand.* **27**:476–479.

AUTHOR INDEX

Italic numbers give the page on which the complete reference is listed.

A

C

E

H

I

J

K

L

Mc

M

O

P

Q

R

S

U

V

W

XYZ

SUBJECT INDEX

A

B

D

L

M

N

O

Q

R

T

U

V

W

Y

PROFESSOR PETER J. BARNES M.A. D.M. FRCP.